Oxford Textbook of
Community Mental Health

Oxford Textbook of
Community Mental Health

Edited by

Graham Thornicroft

Health Service and Population Research Department,
Institute of Psychiatry, King's College London, London, UK

George Szmukler

Health Service and Population Research Department,
Institute of Psychiatry, King's College London, London, UK

Kim T. Mueser

Dartmouth Psychiatry Research Center,
Departments of Psychiatry and of Community and Family Medicine,
Dartmouth Medical School, Lebanon, NH, USA

Robert E. Drake

Dartmouth Psychiatric Research Center, Lebanon, NH, USA

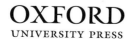

OXFORD
UNIVERSITY PRESS

OXFORD

UNIVERSITY PRESS

Great Clarendon Street, Oxford OX2 6DP

Oxford University Press is a department of the University of Oxford.
It furthers the University's objective of excellence in research, scholarship,
and education by publishing worldwide in

Oxford New York

Auckland Cape Town Dar es Salaam Hong Kong Karachi
Kuala Lumpur Madrid Melbourne Mexico City Nairobi
New Delhi Shanghai Taipei Toronto

With offices in

Argentina Austria Brazil Chile Czech Republic France Greece
Guatemala Hungary Italy Japan Poland Portugal Singapore
South Korea Switzerland Thailand Turkey Ukraine Vietnam

Oxford is a registered trade mark of Oxford University Press
in the UK and in certain other countries

Published in the United States
by Oxford University Press Inc., New York

British Library Cataloguing in Publication Data is available

Library of Congress Cataloging in Publication Data is available

Typeset in Minion
by Glyph International, Bangalore, India
Printed in China
on acid free paper through
Asia Pacific Offset

ISBN 978-0-19-956549-8

10 9 8 7 6 5 4 3 2 1

Contents

List of contributors

Sergio Aguilar-Gaxiola Center for Reduction in Health Disparities,University of California Davis, CA, USA

Ali Obaid AlHamzawi Al-Qadisia University, College of Medicine, Diwania Governorate, Iraq

Jordi Alonso Health Services Research Unit, Institut Municipal d'Investigació Mèdica (IMIM-Hospital del Mar); and CIBER en Epidemiología y Salud Pública (CIBERESP), Barcelona, Spain.

Laura Helena Andrade Section of Psychiatric Epidemiology, Department and Institute of Psychiatry School of Medicine University of São Paulo São Paulo, Brazil

Matthias C. Angermeyer Center for Public Mental Health, Gösing am Wagram, Austria

Paul S. Appelbaum, Division of Psychiatry, Law and Ethics, Department of Psychiatry, Columbia University College of Physicians and Surgeons, NY State Psychiatric Institute, New York, NY, USA

Corrado Barbui Department of Medicine and Public Health, Section of Psychiatry and Clinical Psychology, University of Verona, Verona, Italy

Peter Bartlett Law and Social Sciences, University of Nottingham, Nottingham, UK

Rajaie Batniji Department of Politics and International Relations, University of Oxford, Oxford, UK

Deborah R. Becker Dartmouth Psychiatric Research Center, Lebanon, NH, USA

Thomas Becker Department of Psychiatry and Psychotherapy II, Ulm University, Bezirkskrankenhaus Günzburg, Günzburg, Germany

Gary R. Bond Dartmouth Psychiatric Research Center, Lebanon, NH, USA

Guilherme Borges, Instituto Nacional de Psiquiatria, Universidad Autonoma Metropolitana, Mexico City, Mexico

Evelyn J. Bromet Department of Psychiatry, State University of New York, Stony Brook, NY, USA

Ronny Bruffaerts Department of Neurosciences and Psychiatry, University Hospitals Gasthuisberg, Belgium

Mary F. Brunette Dartmouth Medical School, Lebanon, NH, USA

Brendan Bunting Department of Psychology, University of Ulster, Belfast, Northern Ireland

José Miguel Caldas de Almeida Department of Mental Health, Faculdade de Ciências Médicas, Universidade Nova de Lisboa, Lisbon, Portugal

Mary Cannon Department of Psychiatry, Royal College of Surgeons Ireland, Dublin, Ireland

Amy Cheung Department of Psychiatry, University of Toronto, Toronto, ON, Canada

Dan Chisholm Health Services and Population Research Department, Institute of Psychiatry, King's College London, London, UK; and Department of Health Systems Financing, World Health Organization, Geneva, Switzerland

Delia Cimpean Dartmouth Departments of Medicine and Psychiatry, Lebanon, NH, USA

Andrea Cipriani Department of Medicine and Public Health, Section of Psychiatry and Clinical Psychology, University of Verona, Verona, Italy

Larry Davidson Yale Program for Recovery and Community Health, Yale University School of Medicine, New Haven, CT, USA

Lisa B. Dixon University of Maryland School of Medicine; and VISN 5 Mental Illness Research Education and Clinical Center (MIRECC), VA Maryland Health Care System, Baltimore, MD, USA

Robert E. Drake Dartmouth Psychiatric Research Center, Lebanon, NH, USA

Amy L. Drapalski VISN 5 Mental Illness Research Education and Clinical Center (MIRECC), VA Maryland Health Care System, Baltimore, MD, USA

Martin P. Eccles Institute of Health and Society, Newcastle University

Antonia Errazuriz Department of Psychiatry, University of Cambridge, Herchel Smith Building for Brain & Mind Sciences, Cambridge, UK

Silvia Florescu Scoala Nationala de Sanatate Publica si Perfectionare in Domeniul Sanitar, Bucurest, Romania

Cheryl Forchuk Arthur Labatt School of Nursing, Faculty of Health Sciences, University of Western Ontario; Lawson Health Research Institute, London, ON, Canada

Michelle Funk Department of Mental Health and Substance Abuse, World Health Organization, Geneva, Switzerland

Susan Gingerich Private Practice, Philadelphia, PA, USA

Giovanni de Girolamo IRCCS Centro S. Giovanni di Dio Fatebenefratelli, Brescia, Italy

Ron de Graaf Netherlands Institute of Mental Health and Addiction, Utrecht, The Netherlands

Gyles Glover North East Public Health Observatory, Wolfson Research Institute, Durham University, Stockton on Tees, UK

Jeremy Grimshaw Clinical Epidemiology Program, Ottawa Health Research Institute; Centre for Best Practices, Institute of Population Health, University of Ottawa; Department of Medicine, University of Ottawa, Ottawa, ON, Canada

Gerald N. Grob Institute for Health, Health Care Policy, and Aging Research, Rutgers University, New Brunswick, NJ, USA

Oye Gureje Department of Psychiatry, University College Hospital, Ibadan, Nigeria

Josep Maria Haro Parc Sanitari Sant Joan de Déu, CIBERSAM, Barcelona, Spain

Hristo Ruskov Hinkov Deputy Director of the National Center of Public Health Protection, Sofia, Bulgaria

Lorna Hobbs Sub-department of Clinical Health Psychology, University College London, London, UK

Frank Holloway South London and Maudsley NHS Foundation Trust, Bethlem Royal Hospital, Beckenham, Kent, UK

Chi-yi Hu Shenzhen Institute of Mental Health & Shenzhen Kangning Hospital, Shenzhen, People's Republic of China

Sonia Johnson Department of Mental Health Sciences, University College London, London, UK

Peter B. Jones Department of Psychiatry, University of Cambridge, Herchel Smith Building for Brain & Mind Sciences, Cambridge, UK

Anthony F. Jorm Orygen Youth Health Research Centre, Centre for Youth Mental Health, University of Melbourne, Victoria, Australia

Elie G. Karam St George Hospital University Medical Center, Balamand University, Faculty of Medicine; Institute for Development, Research, Advocacy & Applied Care (IDRAAC); and Medical Institute for Neuropsychological Disorders (MIND), Beirut, Lebanon

Ronald C. Kessler Department of Health Care Policy, Harvard Medical School, Boston, MA, USA

Helen Killaspy Department of Mental Health Sciences, Hampstead Campus, University College London, Royal Free Hospital, London

Kathia Kirschner Harvard Program in Refugee Trauma, Massachusetts General Hospital, Harvard Medical School, MA, USA

Martin Knapp Centre for the Economics of Mental Health, Institute of Psychiatry, King's College London; and Personal Social Services Research Unit, London School of Economics and Political Science London, UK

Markus Koesters Department of Psychiatry and Psychotherapy II, Ulm University, Bezirkskrankenhaus Günzburg,Günzburg, Germany

Viviane Kovess EA 4069 Université Paris Descartes & EHESP School for Public Health Department of Epidemiology, Paris, France

Elizabeth Kuipers King's College London; and Institute of Psychiatry, Department of Psychology, London, UK

Sing Lee The Chinese University of Hong Kong, Hong Kong, People's Republic of China

Daphna Levinson Research & Planning, Ministry of Health, Mental Health Services, Jerusalem, Israel

Glyn H. Lewis Department of Psychological Medicine, University of Wales College of Medicine, Cardiff, UK

Oliver Lewis Mental Disability Advocacy Center (MDAC), Budapest, Hungary

Bruce Link Mailman School of Public Health, New York, NY, USA

Rob Macpherson 2 Gether Partnership NHS Trust, Gloucester, UK

Stephen Marder Ronald Reagan UCLA Medical Center Stewart and Lynda Resnick Neuropsychiatric Hospital at UCLA, Los Angeles, CA, USA

Patrick McGorry Orygen Youth Health, University of Melbourne, Melbourne, Australia

Nisha Mehta King's College Hospital, London, UK

Alexander L. Miller The University of Texas Health Science Center at San Antonio, Department of Psychiatry, San Antonio, TX, USA

Richard F. Mollica Harvard Program in Refugee Trauma, Massachusetts General Hospital, Harvard Medical School, MA, USA

Troy A. Moore The University of Texas Health Science Center at San Antonio, Department of Psychiatry, San Antonio, TX, USA

Craig Morgan Health Service and Population Research Department, Institute of Psychiatry, King's College London, London, UK

Jodi Morris Department of Mental Health and Substance Abuse, World Health Organization, Geneva, Switzerland

Kim Mueser Dartmouth Psychiatric Research Center, Departments of Psychiatry and of Community and Family Medicine, Dartmouth Medical School, Lebanon, NH, USA

Quyen Ngo-Metzger Bureau of Primary Health Care Health Resources and Services Administration, Washington, D.C, USA

Mark van Ommeren Department of Mental Health and Substance Abuse, World Health Organization, Geneva, Switzerland

Yutaka Ono Health Center, Keio University, Tokyo, Japan

Maria Petukhova Department of Health Care Policy, Harvard Medical School, Boston, MA, USA

Jo Phelan Department of Sociomedical Sciences, Columbia University, New York, NY, USA

José Posada-Villa Colegio Mayor de Cundinamarca University, Bogota, Colombia

Paddy Power LEO Services, South London & Maudsley NHS Foundation Trust, London, UK

Martin Prince Health Service and Population Research Department, Institute of Psychiatry, London, UK

Nikolas Rose Martin White Professor of Sociology, London School of Economics and Political Science, London, UK

Alan Rosen Department of Psychiatry, Royal North Shore Hospital, New South Wales, Australia

Abraham Rudnick Departments of Psychiatry and Philosophy, Division of Social and Rural Psychiatry, University of Western Ontario;, Psychosis Program, Regional Mental Health Care, London, ON, Canada

Rajesh Sagar Department of Psychiatry, All India Institute of Medical Sciences, New Delhi, India

Benedetto Saraceno Department of Mental Health and Substance Abuse, World Health Organization, Geneva, Switzerland

Shekhar Saxena Department of Mental Health and Substance Abuse, World Health Organization, Geneva, Switzerland

Aart H. Schene Department of Psychiatry, Academic Medical Center, University of Amsterdam, Amsterdam, The Netherlands

Lloyd I. Sederer New York State Office of Mental Health; and Columbia School of Public Health, New York, NY, USA

Soraya Seedat MRC Research Unit on Anxiety and Stress Disorders, Cape Town, South Africa

Jonathan Shaywitz Anxiety Disorders Program, Cedars–Sinai Hospital, Los Angeles, CA, USA

Geoff Shepherd Health Service and Population Research Department, Institute of Psychiatry, University of London, London, UK

Mike Slade Health Service and Population Research Department, Institute of Psychiatry, King's College London, London, UK

R. Srinivasa Murthy Association for the Mentally Challenged, Dharmaram College, Bangalore, India

Margaret (Peggy) Swarbrick Collaborative Support Programs of New Jersey, Freehold, NJ; and University of Medicine and Dentistry of New Jersey, School of Health Related Professionals, Department of Psychiatric Rehabilitation and Counseling, Newark, NJ, USA

George Szmukler Health Service and Population Research Department, Institute of Psychiatry, King's College London, London, UK

Michele Tansella University of Verona, Faculty of Medicine and Medicine and Surgery, Verona, Italy

Hollie V. Thomas Department of Psychological Medicine,University of Wales College of Medicine, Cardiff, UK

Graham Thornicroft Health Service and Population Research Department, Institute of Psychiatry, King's College London, London, UK

William C. Torrey Dartmouth Medical School, Lebanon, NH, USA

Jonathan Totman Department of Mental Health Sciences University College London, London, UK

Peter Tyrer Centre for Mental Health, Imperial College, London, UK

Philip S. Wang Division of Services and Intervention Research, National Institute of Mental Health, Bethesda, MD, USA

J. Elisabeth Wells Department of Public Health and General Practice, Christchurch School of Medicine, Christchurch, New Zealand

Harvey Whiteford University of Queensland, Brisbane, Australia

Rob Whitley Department of Psychiatry, Dartmouth Medical School, Dartmouth Psychiatric Research Center, Lebanon, NH, USA

Paula Whitty Institute of Health and Society, Newcastle University, Newcastle, UKContents

SECTION 1

Introduction

CHAPTER 1

Introduction to community mental health care

Robert E. Drake, George Szmukler,
Kim T. Mueser, and Graham Thornicroft

Community mental health care has evolved as a discipline for over 50 years now. In describing this evolution as well as current approaches, this book combines traditional concepts, such as community-based interventions and an epidemiological perspective, with newer concepts, such as recovery philosophy, evidence-based practices, and implementation fidelity, which have shaped the field over the past decade. Like community mental health care itself, the book is multidisciplinary and pluralistic. It addresses controversies and also emphasizes areas of convergence, where social values, medical science, and policy forces agree on specific directions.

Defining community mental health

Our definition of community mental health, shown in Box 1.1, highlights several fundamental issues. First, community mental health assumes a public health perspective (Levine and Petrilla, 1996). As summarized by Thornicroft and Tansella (2009), this encompasses: 1) a population view, 2) patients in a socioeconomic context, 3) generating information on primary prevention, 4) individual as well as population-based prevention, 5) a systemic view of service provision, 6) open access to services, 7) team-based services, 8) a long-term, longitudinal, life-course perspective, and 9) cost-effectiveness in population terms. This perspective also includes a commitment to social justice by addressing the needs of traditionally underserved populations, such as ethic minorities, homeless persons, and immigrants, and to provision of services where those in need are located and in a fashion that is acceptable as well as accessible (Thornicroft et al., 2010).

Second, community mental health care focuses primarily on the people who experience mental illnesses. It emphasizes not just their deficits, needs, and disabilities (an illness perspective), but also their strengths, capacities, and aspirations (a recovery perspective). Services and supports thus aim to enhance a person's ability to develop a positive identity, to frame the illness experience, to self-manage the illness, and to pursue personally valued social roles (Slade, 2009).

Third, community mental health care includes the community in a broadly defined sense. As a corollary of the second point, it emphasizes not just the reduction or management of environmental adversity, but also the strengths of the families, social networks, communities, and organizations that surround people who experience mental illnesses (Rapp and Goscha, 2006; Warner, 2000). Mental illnesses are embedded in and partially determined by social and environmental contexts. Services must therefore comprise a wide network of interlocking components, including physical health care, housing, social services, religious organizations, peer supports, self-help organizations, and informal support systems. Because social and environmental forces impinge strongly on people who experience mental illnesses, community mental health must attend to these larger social forces in ways that are both ethical and pragmatic.

Fourth, community mental health melds medical science and recovery philosophy. A scientific approach to services prioritizes using the best available data on the effectiveness of interventions. At the same time, people who experience mental illnesses have the right to understand their illnesses (to the extent that professionals understand them), to consider the available options for interventions and whatever information is available on their effectiveness and side effects, and to have their preferences included in a process of shared decision-making (Drake et al., 2009a). In recent years, traditional definitions of recovery that focus on the complete remission of symptoms and illness-related deficits have been replaced by definitions that view recovery as a personally meaningful process that involves growth and adaptation in the community, irrespective of symptoms and impairments (Davidson et al., 2009; Slade, 2009). A commitment to recovery emphasizes helping people to overcome their illnesses and achieve their goals to the greatest extent possible and values their full participation in the service system and in their communities.

Community mental health care is shaped by a variety of values and forces that often conflict. Some values derive from the larger society—especially those expressed through a government's social policy on the one hand, and through medical science on

---

Box 1.1 Definition of community mental health care

Community mental health care comprises the principles and practices needed to promote mental health for a local population by: 1) addressing population-based needs in ways that are accessible and acceptable; 2) building on the goals and strengths of people who experience mental illnesses; 3) promoting a wide network of supports, services, and resources of adequate capacity; and 4) emphasizing services that are both evidence-based and recovery-oriented.

---

the other; while others derive from the smaller groups of participants directly engaged in mental health issues—those of service users, carers, and health professionals (Banton, 1985; Perkins and Repper, 1998). An analysis of community mental health thus requires an examination from multiple perspectives. It also requires the application of the methods of a variety of academic disciplines, including the behavioural and social sciences, history, politics, and, since questions of value are so central, moral philosophy and ethics.

The evolution of community mental health care

In the initial phases of deinstitutionalization, attempts to recreate the hospital service environment in the community had the unintended effect of perpetuating segregation, paternalism, passivity, dependency, low expectations, stagnation, stigma, and hopelessness (Nelson et al., 2001). At that time, community-based alternatives, such as nursing homes, group homes, day hospitals, day treatment programmes, and sheltered workshops, commonly replicated the stultifying environments of long-term hospitals. The typical 'deinstitutionalized' mental health client trudged from a supervised group home to a supervised group day programme and then perhaps to a supervised group outing. Segregation, dependence, and stigma were blatant aspects of such care. Mental health clients in these settings were often treated as though they were incompetent children who could not make decisions, manage their own illnesses, live on their own, integrate into their communities, work competitively, or pursue friendships and leisure activities. In retrospect, community mental health care of this era can be seen as inadvertently perpetuating stigma and as continuing to socialize people into disability. Many people with mental illnesses rejected this approach.

The search to improve community mental health care has steadily evolved. Over the past five decades, numerous ideas and voices have shaped this evolution. People who experience mental illnesses, their families, mental health professionals, policy makers, administrators, insurers, theorists, advocates, judges, guild organizations, for-profit industries, media, public safety officials, and researchers are among those who have expressed views. The voices have often been conflicting and discordant rather than unified and clear (Banton et al., 1985; Levine, 1981). Consensus has rarely been achieved. And when consensus has developed, the instantiation of new models of care has often been characterized by rhetoric, inadequate funding, and failure, rather than by genuine commitment, faithful implementation, and success (Drake and Essock, 2009; Geddes and Harrison, 1997).

Some ideas have been validated by scientific evidence; many remain largely untested. Nonetheless, ideas have strongly influenced

the mental health service system and the field of community mental health. Several of these notions are discussed in detail throughout this text. Among the most prominent are the following:

From ethical and legal perspectives, people who experience mental illnesses have the same rights as others in society—the same rights to pursue their own health care preferences, functional goals, and happiness as others (Davidson et al., 2009). Legal rights include not only freedom from abusive treatments but also freedom to live and receive services in the 'least restricted environment'. They also include the right to be considered competent to make decisions about one's life. These rights can be abridged only if the individual meets specific legal standards. Thus, communities, clinicians, and families can no longer decide that an individual is incompetent on the basis of ad hoc criteria.

From a philosophical perspective, people with an illness are considered 'people first'. Neither illness nor disability determines personhood; humanity defines a person. Because an individual who experiences a mental illness should not defined by the illness, current usage prefers language such as 'a person who has experienced mental illness' or 'a person with schizophrenia' rather than 'a schizophrenic'.

From a clinical perspective, community mental health now assumes that people with even the most severe mental illnesses have a significant capacity to manage their own illnesses and to pursue personally meaningful goals, often in spite of ongoing symptoms (Mueser et al., 2002). Current mental health philosophies and interventions thus emphasize strengths, resilience, self-management, self-agency, and capacity for functional recovery.

From a socioenvironmental perspective, the strengths of the individual's social network and community are also more salient (Warner, 2000). The professional view of families has transitioned from causing illness (schizophrenogenic mothers) to exacerbating illness (high expressed emotion), to ameliorating illness (families with a member who experiences mental illness). Many families can provide considerable supports to their relatives who are experiencing mental illnesses, especially when the families themselves are helped to acquire appropriate education, skills, and supports. Similarly, the community environment is now viewed as a potential salutary force. Like the rest of us, people with mental illnesses grow and mature through participating in regular jobs, educational experiences, integrated social settings, normal housing arrangements, and routine community activities (Becker and Drake, 2003). In addition, we recognize that the public's misperceptions about mental illness can be extremely damaging and can be overcome by direct contacts and community integration (Thornicroft, 2010).

From a psychological perspective, as Alcoholics Anonymous and religious communities have long recognized, helping others promotes and enhances the process of recovery from a major illness. Peer supports and clients as mental health employees have become prominent features of the mental health system in many areas (Solomon, 2004). Although lacking controlled research, these movements continue to grow steadily and to be supported by numerous personal testimonies.

From a research perspective, community mental health continues to move steadily toward becoming a scientific practice. Beliefs in the mysteries of psychotherapy, untested theories and interventions, and the authority of senior clinicians and professional societies have gradually been replaced by scientific methods. While many interventions have been proven ineffective or harmful, an increasing number of interventions have been shown to be efficacious and many have also been shown to be effective in real-world settings (New Freedom Commission on Mental Health, 2003; U.S. Department of Health and Human Services, 1999). Research standards, transparency, and unbiased review processes have enabled progress. Evidence-based medicine and evidence-based practices have largely replaced the acceptance of outpatient mental health as a cottage industry with few standards. Debates continue regarding what outcomes to study, appropriate research methods, and the emerging efforts to study service systems.

From a systems perspective, research on unmet needs has also expanded considerably (Thornicroft, 2000). Despite increased knowledge of effective clinical interventions for most mental disorders, the gap between science and service remains large. Most of the people who experience mental disorders are unable to access effective treatments, even in the wealthiest countries (Mojtabai et al., 2009). When access is not a problem, acceptability often is—many people reject the services that are offered (Kreyenbuhl et al., 2009). Further, most mental health practitioners and systems do not use the most effective practices (Drake et al., 2009b). Continuing education programmes typically do not result in learning and using new skills. Information systems do not deliver useful point-of-contact information that would enhance collaborative decision-making. Finally, mental health treatment systems typically do not track quality of care and outcomes. Information systems for mental health often record amounts of services delivered rather than the quality or outcomes related to those services.

From an international perspective, as globalization, migration, and cultural pluralism transform the world, community mental health systems have not responded adequately to the challenges afforded by these trends. People from minority cultures and those who speak other languages have difficulty accessing services that they find welcoming and acceptable. Disparities in mental health services affect virtually every country (Desjarlais et al., 1995; Thornicroft et al., 2010).

The structure of this book

We have organized this book to reflect the large diversity of perspectives on community mental health but also to attempt a synthesis of perspectives and our convergence of views. Across two countries (the United Kingdom and the United States) and over several decades of working in, studying, and thinking about community mental health, we share a remarkable convergence of ideas.

Community mental health should respond to the needs, goals, and preferences of people who experience mental illnesses. Following a brief introduction (Chapter 1) and historical review (Chapters 2 and 3), the book provides overviews of recovery as a central organizing vision in community mental health (Chapter 4) and of the needs for a community mental health system (Chapters 5–10). We begin with the epidemiological data that underlie a public health approach to community mental health. People are not merely numbers, of course, and Chapter 8 includes the perspectives of those who experience mental illnesses themselves. Because we are concerned with social justice, we emphasize the needs of specific groups, such as ethno-cultural minorities and immigrants,

which are often overlooked in establishing mental health services (Chapters 10 and 11).

Specific components of community mental health and how they are organized constitute the heart of community mental health. They are discussed in Chapters 12 to 24.

Ethical and legal perspectives, including the difficult issue of coercive interventions, are discussed in Chapters 25 to 27.

Countervailing the recovery vision are public attitudes that can be characterized as stigma and discrimination. These issues and efforts to overcome them are discussed in Chapters 28 to 30.

Mental health policies and financing mechanisms determine the structure of potentially available services. Chapters 31 to 33 cover these issues.

Within the parameters of governmental policies and funding, professionals are responsible for implementing a service system that is as effective as possible. Chapters 34 to 38 discuss the mechanisms used to ensure effective care, in low- and middle-income countries as well as wealthy ones.

Intervention science—how we know what interventions and services are effective—is another critical building block for a community mental health system.

Finally, we consider the future of community mental health, again across the broad spectrum of countries, in Chapter 43.

References

Banton R., Clifford P., Frosch S., Lousada J., and Rosenthall J. (1985). *The Politics of Mental Health*. London: Macmillan.

Becker, D.R. and Drake, R.E. (2003). *A Working Life for People with Mental Illness*. New York: Oxford Press.

Davidson, L., Tondora, J., Lawless, M.S., O'Connell, M.J., and Rowe, M. (2009). *A Practical Guide to Recovery-Oriented Practice: Tools for Transforming Mental Health Care*. New York: Oxford University Press.

Desjarlais R., Eisenberg L., Good B., and Kleinman A. (1995). *World Mental Health. Problems and Priorities in Low-Income Countries*. Oxford: Oxford University Press.

Drake, R.E. and Essock, S.M. (2009). The science to service gap in real world schizophrenia treatment. *Schizophrenia Bulletin*, **35**, 677–8.

Drake, R.E., Cimpean, D., and Torrey, W.C. (2009a). Shared decision making in mental health: Prospects for personalized medicine. *Dialogues in Clinical Neuroscience*, **11**, 319–32.

Drake, R.E., Essock, S.M., and Bond, G.R. (2009b). Implementing evidence-based practices for the treatment of schizophrenia patients. *Schizophrenia Bulletin*, **35**, 704–13.

Geddes, L. and Harrison, P. (1997). Closing the gap between research and practice. *British Journal of Psychiatry*, **171**, 220–5.

Kreyenbuhl J., Buchanan R.W., Dickerson F.B., and Dixon, L.B. (2009). The schizophrenia patient outcomes research team (PORT): updated treatment recommendations. *Schizophrenia Bulletin*, **36**, 94–103.

Levin, B. and Petrila, J. (1996) *Mental Health Services. A Public Health Perspective*. Oxford: Oxford University Press.

Levine, M. (1981). *The History and Politics of Community Mental Health*. New York: Oxford University Press.

Mojtabai R., Fochtmann L., Chang S., Kotov R., Craig T.J., and Bromet, E. (2009). Unmet need for mental health care in schizophrenia: an overview of literature and new data from a first-admission study. *Schizophrenia Bulletin*, **35**, 679–95.

Mueser, K.T., Corrigan, P.W., Hilton, D.W., Tanzman, B., Schaub, A., Gingerich, S., *et al.* (2002). Illness management and recovery: A review of the research. *Psychiatric Services*, **53**, 1272–84.

Nelson, G., Lord, J., and Ochocka, J. (2001). *Shifting the Paradigm in Community Mental Health: Towards Empowerment and Community*. Toronto: University of Toronto Press.

New Freedom Commission on Mental Health. (2003). *Achieving the Promise: Transforming Mental Health Care in America. Final Report.* Publication SMA-03-3832. Rockville, MD: US Department of Health and Human Services.

Perkins R. and Repper J. (1998). *Dilemmas in Community Mental Health Practice.* London: Radcliffe Medical Press.

Rapp, C. and Goscha, R. (2006). *The Strengths Model: Case Management with People with Psychiatric Disabilities.* New York: Oxford University Press.

Slade, M. (2009). *Personal Recovery and Mental Illness: A Guide for Mental Health Professionals.* New York: Cambridge University Press.

Solomon P. (2004). Peer support/peer provided services underlying processes, benefits, and critical ingredients. *Psychiatric Rehabilitation Journal,* **27**, 392–401.

Thornicroft G. (ed) (2000). *Measuring Mental Health Needs,* 2nd edn. London: Royal College of Psychiatrists (Gaskell).

Thornicroft, G. (2010). Discrimination against people with mental illness: what can psychiatrists do? *Advances in Psychiatric Treatment,* **16**, 53–9.

Thornicroft, G. and Tansella, M. (2009). *Better Mental Health Care.* Cambridge: Cambridge University Press.

Thornicroft, G., Alem, A., Dos Santos, R.A., Barley, E., Drake, R.E., Gregorio, G., *et al.* (2010). Lessons learned in the implementation of community mental health care. *World Psychiatry,* **9**, 67–77.

U.S. Department of Health and Human Services. (1999). *Mental Health: A Report of the Surgeon General.* Rockville, MD: U.S. Department of Health and Human Services, Substance Abuse and Mental Health Services Administration, Center for Mental Health Services, National Institutes of Health, National Institute of Mental Health.

Warner, R. (2000). *The Environment of Schizophrenia: Innovations in Practice, Policy, and Communications.* London: Brunner-Routledge.

SECTION 2

Origins of 'community psychiatry'

CHAPTER 2

Historical changes in mental health practice

Nikolas Rose

Introduction

However we define 'community psychiatry', it is clear that, in contemporary societies, practices addressed to the mental troubles of individuals have proliferated across everyday life.[1] Psychiatric interventions occur in mental hospitals, psychiatric wards in general hospitals, special hospitals, medium secure units, day hospitals, outpatient clinics, child guidance clinics, prisons, children's homes, sheltered housing, drop-in centres, community mental health centres, domiciliary care by community psychiatric nurses, multiple forms of psychological therapies, and, of course, in the general practitioner's surgery, not least through the increasing prescription of psychiatric drugs. No phase of life is unknown to these practices: infertility, pregnancy, birth and the postpartum period; infancy; childhood at home and at school; sexual normality, perversion, impotence, and pleasure; family life, marriage and divorce, employment and unemployment, mid-life crises, and failures to achieve; old age, terminal illness, and bereavement.

Wherever problems arise—in our homes, on the streets, in factories, schools, hospitals, the army, courtroom, or prison—experts with specialist knowledge of the nature, causes, and remedies for mental distress are on hand to provide its diagnoses and propose remedial action. And, of course, there is a wider penetration of psychiatry, broadly defined, into popular culture, as psychiatrists, mental hospitals, those with mentally illness, and the problems of mental health feature daily in political and social debates, in our newspapers, in television documentaries, exposés, talk shows, and soap operas. The languages that have been disseminated have

given us new vocabularies in which to think and talk about our problems—stress, trauma, depression, neuroses, compulsions, phobias. They have also provided us with new ways of explaining, judging, and accounting for our personal miseries, of distinguishing the normal and the abnormal, identifying what is illness, when to seek assistance and from whom. It would not, therefore, be too much of an exaggeration to say that we lived in a 'psychiatric society'.

'Community psychiatry', then, is one dimension of the 'psychiatric societies' that have taken shape over the course of the 20th century. There have been many international variations in the historical paths followed in different national contexts, but the rationalities and practices that have taken shape are remarkably similar across the Western world. In this chapter, focusing upon the United Kingdom, I want to sketch out some of the key moments in this history.[2]

The territory of psychiatry

The early decades of the 20th century are usually understood as a period when 'organicism' in psychiatry was in its heyday, when therapeutic pessimism dominated, and when psychiatry and its practitioners, like their patients, were entrapped within the enclosed institutional spaces that were the legacy of the asylum movement of the previous hundred years: asylums that had now become little more than vast warehouses for containment of those thought to be of unsound mind. At the outbreak of the First World War, there were nearly 140,000 patients in mental hospitals and other institutions in England and Wales, and the average county asylum housed over 1000 inmates. These figures were to increase over the subsequent four decades, reaching a peak of over 150,000 inmates by 1954 (Jones, 1972: appendix 1). Conventional psychopathology by and large saw mental pathology in terms of a relation between an inherited constitution and the life stresses to which it was subject. The inherited nervous

---

1 This is a revised and updated version of a chapter entitled 'Psychiatry: The Discipline of Mental Health, which appeared in *The Power of Psychiatry* edited by Peter Miller and Nikolas Rose (1986), Cambridge: Polity Press. More detailed references to original texts can be found there, and in Rose (1985). Thanks to Diana Rose for her advice in preparing this version. Note that at each point in the history that I describe, I have adopted the vocabulary that was used—the absence of repeated 'scare quotes' should not be taken for agreement.

2 Except where specifically stated, reference is to developments in England and Wales.

system might be insufficiently equipped with nerve cells, association fibres, or be otherwise organically flawed. After conception, including during the *in utero* period, the nervous system might be damaged by stress. The brain might be injured, or harmed by toxins such as alcohol or by lack of nutrition or defects in the blood supply. In addition to such direct stress, the nervous system was also subject to the effects of indirect stress. Anxiety, inappropriate or over-demanding education, worries about employment or finance, intemperance or sexual excess, even religious fanaticism could adversely affect the nervous system (Rose, 1985: pp.177–9; Rosen, 1959).

But this organicism still allowed psychiatry to play a role outside the asylum. Epilepsy, alcoholism, mental defect, mania, melancholia, and other personal and social ills were regarded as expressions of an inherited neuropathic constitution which might lead to antisocial and immoral conduct. Such undesirable behaviour might also provoke the onset of explicit pathology in those with such a predisposition, and thus could be criticized on medical as well as moral grounds. Careful management of infants was essential. For those children whose families had shown pathology, this would strengthen the constitution and build up habits which would minimize the risk of onset. It was also vital in other families, for not even the strongest constitution was immune to damage. And, of course, the profligate breeding of those with severely tainted constitutions could lead to a swamping of the nation with neuropaths and a decline in national efficiency and the quality of the race. Hence the involvement of many key figures from the field of mental medicine in eugenic campaigns for the medical inspection, sterilization, or permanent segregation of mental defectives and others of the social problem group, and for their sterilization or permanent segregation (Farrall, 1985; Searle, 1976).

The wider sociopolitical role for psychiatry at this time was thus largely reactive and defensive: to help minimize and control the threat posed by insanity. But in the period following the First World War, a number of psychiatrists developed a more positive strategy. This modelled itself on the arguments of the new public health that claimed to be able to address large-scale problems concerning the size and quality of the population and its consequences (Armstrong, 1983). In this preventive medicine, the political fortunes of the nation came to be seen as dependent upon the physical health of each individual; simultaneously individuals were thought to play a significant part in the spread of ill health through their personal conduct. Hence reform of this conduct could promote social well-being. A complex apparatus of medical inspection, education in domestic hygiene, registration of births, infant welfare clinics, health visitors, school milk and meals, health clinics, and so forth was established to investigate these habits and to educate citizens to conduct their personal lives in a hygienic manner; and, indeed, to encourage them to want to be healthy. The new social psychiatry adopted many of these principles, and actively tried to promote mental welfare and mental hygiene. The first focus of this strategy was 'the neuroses'. This term was applied to conditions that were considered to be mild mental disturbances: they did not disable the individual completely, but were sufficient to cause social inefficiency and personal unhappiness. If left untreated, these minor troubles were thought likely to develop into more serious mental problems. And it was argued that many of those in workhouses and prisons—vagrants, criminals, delinquents, and others who were socially or industrially inefficient—suffered from mental pathology which had probably begun in a small way in treatable neurosis.

Hence the neuroses of childhood were of particular concern. They provided a fortunate early warning of troubles to come, and, given the malleability of the child, it was thought that, in the majority of cases, they could be successfully treated.

The neuroses came to light in all those sites where individuals could now be judged to fail in relation to institutional norms and expectations—in the production-line routines of factory labour, in the new expectations of universal schooling, in the newly established juvenile courts, and, especially, in the unprecedented demands upon the military in the First World War. Shell shock accounted for 10% of officer casualties in the 1914–1918 war, and for 4% of casualties from other ranks. More than 80,000 such cases were estimated to have occurred over the course of the war, and some 65,000 ex-servicemen were still receiving disability pensions in 1921 because of shell shock. While senior military officers frequently regarded shell shock as merely a disguise for cowardice, organicist physicians considered the condition to be a genuine one resulting from minute cerebral haemorrhages caused by the blast (Hearnshaw, 1964: pp.245–6; Rose, 1985: pp.182–3). But doctors working in the shell-shock clinics and specialized hospitals that were set up to deal with these cases were unconvinced by such organic explanations, especially given the lack of independent evidence of the postulated lesions. Versions of the therapeutic methods invented by Janet in Paris and Freud in Vienna were tried out on the shell-shocked with some success. Shell shock appeared to respond to a variety of approaches ranging from occupational training, through persuasion and a form of rational re-education, the use of suggestion, to a type of psychotherapy using hypnosis or free association. Experience with this treatment converted many to a kind of dynamic theory of the will, using concepts such as instinct and repression, and attentive to the intermixing of physical and mental symptoms. These beliefs played a key role in the mental hygiene movement: for the first time, psychiatrists would collaborate with other professionals in a strategy for the prevention, the early detection, and the voluntary treatment of mental ill-health.

The rationale of mental hygiene, with its belief in a continuity between minor and major mental disorders and in the importance of early intervention for individual adjustment and social efficiency, underpinned the argument made in a series of official reports from the 1920s to the outbreak of the Second World War (discussed in detail in Rose, 1985: pp.197–209). Poor mental hygiene was thought to be the cause of all sorts of social ills, preventable by education in proper techniques for mental welfare and mental hygiene, and by early detection of the signs of trouble followed by prompt and efficient treatment. It was believed that this was hampered by the stigma which surrounded lunacy, by the isolation of the asylum from other medical facilities, and by the legal procedures of 1890 which allowed asylums only to take patients certified through a cumbersome legal process. This discouraged individuals with mild problems from seeking help, and discouraged doctors from utilizing asylums, turning them into institutions for the incarceration of those considered beyond hope. Not only was this a counterproductive method of organizing services, it was also conceptually unwarranted. As the Royal Commission on Lunacy and Mental Disorder put it in 1926: 'insanity is, after all, only a disease like other diseases…a mind deranged can be ministered to no less effectively than a body deranged… The problem of insanity is essentially a public health problem to be dealt with on modern public health lines.' (1926: pp.16–22.)

Treatment should not require certification, compulsion, or incarceration. Facilities should be available in hospitals for outpatient and voluntary treatment to encourage easy access to help at an early stage of the disease (Rees, 1945: p.29). This was the rationale that had led to the establishment of the Maudsley Hospital, which was completed in 1915 and the Cassel Hospital, which opened in 1919 (Barnes, 1968: pp.10–15; Jones, 1972: pp.235–6). It was for similar reasons that the Mental Treatment Act 1930 renamed asylums 'mental hospitals' and stipulated that, in the majority of cases, lunatics should be termed simply 'persons of unsound mind'. Patients could now be received for inpatient treatment on voluntary application, and local authorities were to make provision for the establishment of psychiatric outpatient clinics at general and mental hospitals.[3]

Disturbed individuals could come to the clinics themselves, once they or others were educated in the signs of mental disturbance, and now free of the fears of stigma or incurability. Others were to be referred to them from school, court, and elsewhere by statutory and voluntary agencies. In the clinics, assessment and treatment would be carried out, reports would be supplied to courts or schools, individuals would be referred to other institutions. But the clinics would also provide the base for a system of mental hygiene which could act more widely on the lives of patients, ex-patients, and potential patients. Social workers, psychiatric social workers, probation officers, school attendance officers, and others would operate between the clinic and home, school, or courtroom, conveying information, advice, and education. The new mental hygiene was to provide the basis of a project of general public education as to the habits likely to promote mental welfare. Mental health was to be a personal responsibility and a national objective.

Community as therapy

Despite these developments, in practice the pre-Second World War psychiatric population was split between the 'neurotics'—maladjusted and delinquent children, inefficient workers, and shell-shocked soldiers and the like—and the 'psychotics'. These latter were those certified under mental health legislation, segregated from the sufferers of physical illness, and confined in the large, isolated, custodial mental hospitals. The provision of outpatient clinics was confined to a few geographical areas; only a small number of the more recently built asylums had established separate facilities for new acute patients; very few beds for inpatient treatment were provided in wards of general hospitals; some, but not all, municipal hospitals had set up 'observation wards' where mental patients could be confined under short sections for limited periods for assessment and diagnosis before being discharged or committed to a mental hospital.

In the 1930s, mental hospitals in England and Wales had an average population of around 1200, but some contained up to 3000 patients. The majority were there for long periods—if not permanently—and active therapeutic intervention was spasmodic. It was accepted that the majority of patients were suffering from psychoses which were often hereditary in origin and mostly incurable. The old ideals of moral treatment had largely been discarded, though, for the most fortunate patients, asylums did operate as communities where they 'lived a life of contented servitude, working as orderlies, storemen, or domestic servants in a cosier world than that outside' (Clark, 1964). With the melancholic, paraphrenic or deluded, certain attachments formed between staff and patients; for others, the regimen varied from neglect, through surveillance and containment, to degradation and brutality.

However questionable their claims to efficacy, the new physical treatments developed in the 1930s did disrupt this stasis. They offered asylum doctors an image of themselves as healers of the sick and not merely superintendents of the institution. Waves of enthusiasm for these treatments swept through the hospitals. Physical treatments— from removal of tonsils to varieties of convulsion therapy—were selected according to the latest reports in the medical literature or the predilections of the medics. As with the claims for bleedings and purgings of the 18th century and for the use of sedatives such as chloral hydrate and bromides in the 19th century, such hopes were usually short-lived. But despite limited experimentation in asylums, or in units attached to them, the principal task of asylum doctors remained the containment of chronic patients, it often required the use of coercion, and offered few prospects for innovation other than more efficient administration.

Within mental medicine, hostility was growing between the long-established sector of asylum superintendents who dominated the Board of Control, defenders of the need for separate and distinct institutions for the treatment of the mentally ill, and physicians who sought the integration of the practice, training, and facilities of psychiatry with those of the general hospital. The future of psychiatry was being shaped outside the asylum mainstream, in specialist units in general hospitals, in outpatient clinics, in private practice, in psychotherapy and psychoanalysis. The Second World War was decisively to shift the balance between these two wings of psychiatry (cf. Baruch and Treacher, 1978).

John Rawlings Rees, Director of the Tavistock Clinic, was appointed consulting psychiatrist to the Army, perhaps because the problems at issue in wartime were precisely those of functional nerve disorder over which the Tavistock had established its jurisdiction. In any event, the consequence was that the new tasks of psychiatry were to be thought from within the rationale of mental hygiene. Psychiatrists tried to develop methods of selection, both for the weeding out of potential problem cases and in the selection of those suitable for promotion. They tried to adjust military training techniques in order to enhance the fit between the mental and the organizational, and sought to maximize morale by methods of man-management which would promote solidarity through acting on the psychiatrically important aspects of group life. Whilst each of these developments would have significance for the expanded role of the 'psy' professions in the post-war period, most important for psychiatry itself was the issue of treatment.[4] Psychiatrists were involved in the treatment of casualties: in the army alone they saw almost a quarter of a million cases during the Second World War, even discounting those referred from army intakes, those seen in selection testing and patients seen in

---

3 The responsibilities of local authorities for lunacy and mental deficiency services and aftercare had already been widened by provisions of the Local Government Act of 1929 which followed the recommendations of the Royal Commission on Lunacy and Mental Disorder. cf. Rose (1985): pp.158–163.

4 On the concept of the psy professions (psychiatrists, psychologists, psychiatric social workers, and many more) see Rose (1996).

psychiatric hospitals (Rees, 1945: p.46). Whilst only about 8000 of these were diagnosed as psychotics, about 130,000 were considered to be neurotics. The invaliding rate for psychiatric disabilities was over 30% of all discharges for medical causes. Whilst military neurosis centres did manage to return about 80% of their cases to duty, the results of treatment overall were poor. This emphasized the need for new treatment techniques. More fundamentally, it confirmed that psychiatry should not focus upon the confinement of the small number of psychotically deranged persons. To fulfil the task that society required, it needed to shift its attention to the detection and treatment of those large numbers of the population who were now known to be liable to neurotic breakdown, maladjustment, inefficiency, and unemployability on the grounds of poor mental health (cf. Jones, 1972: pp.262–82).

Perhaps the most significant invention in treatment concerned the institution itself. At the start of the Second World War, whilst confinement might have been a condition for certain types of treatment, it was not in itself considered to be therapeutic. But in the course of the war, for the first time since the heyday of moral treatment, some at least began to argue that the institution itself could be a therapeutic technology. Maxwell Jones credits Wilfred Bion with the first recognition of the principle underlying the social therapies that 'social environmental influences are themselves capable of effectively changing individual and group patterns of behaviour' (M. Jones, 1952: p.519 c.f. Kraüpl Taylor, 1958; Manning, 1976). In 1943, Bion undertook an experiment in which he treated the unruly conduct of the inmates of the Training Wing of Northfield Military Hospital through manipulating authority relations, believing that if the men themselves had to take responsibility for organizing tasks, and for defining and disciplining miscreants, they would learn that the disruption was not grounded **in** authority but in their psychological relations **to** authority.

Although the authorities terminated this experiment after 6 weeks, it was followed by a second 'Northfield experiment' in which Thomas Main sought to produce what he referred to as a 'therapeutic community' in which the hospital was to be used 'not as an organization run by doctors in the interests of their own greater technical efficiency, but as a community with the immediate aim of full participation of all its members in its daily life and the eventual aim of the resocialization of the neurotic individual for life in ordinary society… a spontaneous and emotionally structured (rather than medically dictated) organization in which all staff and patients engage' (Main, 1946: p.67). At the same time, Maxwell Jones became joint director of the Mill Hill Neurosis Unit, set up by the Ministry of Health for the treatment of 'effort syndrome' and concluded that the patient's reactions to the hospital community mirrored his reactions to the community outside, and hence that the hospital itself might be an instrument to be used to explore and improve the patients condition.

At the end of the war, Jones was put in charge of one of the units for labour resettlement set up by the Ministry of Labour with the aim of rehabilitating ex-prisoners of war for civilian life. The techniques deployed in these 'transitional communities' for 'social reconnection' were those which had been developed in the community treatment of neurotic soldiers, with the addition of attempts to connect up the 'transitional community' with the local community which surrounded it (Curle, 1947; Wilson et al., 1947, c.f. Kraüpl Taylor, 1958). Where rehabilitation had previously been a mere adjunct to therapy conducted by other

means—mediating between life under the dominance of medicine and life as a private matter—it was now seen as the essence of the therapeutic intervention itself. The patient was one who had lost his or her capacity to function as an adjusted social individual; treatment was to reinvest them with the rights, privileges, capacities, moralities, and responsibilities of personhood. This way of thinking, in which mental ill-health is identified in terms of a failure to cope, and treatment becomes a matter of the restoration of coping capacities, would spread widely through psychiatric practice in the post-war period, and indeed would become the practical rationale of much of community psychiatry in the 1970s and beyond.

In the immediate post-war period, Jones argued that the techniques he had developed could be applied to any other socially maladjusted individuals—in particular, to 'psychopaths' (Jones, 1952: introduction). In 1947 he moved to the Industrial Neurosis Unit at Belmont Hospital and applied these methods to the 'chronic unemployed neurotics' it received from all over England included inadequate and aggressive psychopaths, schizoid personalities, early schizophrenics, various drug addictions, sexual perversions, and chronic psychoneurotics. Through a variety of discussion groups, intense small groups, and psychodrama, sexual, criminal, industrial or social deviants, whose behaviour was now construed as a manifestation of an underlying personality disorder, were to be managed back to a state of adjustment in which they could function smoothly within the institutional regimes which they had previously disrupted.

It required but a simple shift of perspective to see that the traditional mental hospital violated all these therapeutic maxims. Hence in the 1950s, a two-pronged attack on such institutions was mounted under the banner of the 'therapeutic community'. On the one hand, a series of research studies of psychiatric institutions confirmed the pathogenic features of their organization and management (e.g. Caudill, 1958; Stanton and Schwartz, 1954). On the other, a series of 'adventures in psychiatry' were undertaken, notably at the Cassel, Claybury, and Fulbourn, which sought to reorganize the mental hospital more or less according to the new rationale and to incorporate some or all of the new techniques of administrative therapy into their institutions, sometimes in combination with chemotherapy or psycho-analytically inspired individual therapy (Barnes, 1968: pp.4–15; Clark, 1964; Martin, 1962). These developments were isolated and short-lived. Many psychiatrists were scandalized by the reported 'goings on' in such hospitals. They criticized the therapeutic efficacy of these attempts to use the institution as a positive element in the production of the cure, and they used arguments about the negative effects of mental hospital life in order to support their case. But, in fact, this new 'social' vision of the psychiatric institution reverberated through the system, leading to the widespread unlocking of wards throughout the 1950s, coupled with reductions in the regimentation of the lives of confined patients, and a policy of accelerated discharge.[5]

---

5 T.P. Rees at Warlingham Park Hospital opened the doors of 21 out of his 23 wards in the early fifties; by 1956 22 out of 37 wards at Netherne Hospital were opened and 60% of patients were allowed out on parole within the boundaries of the estate; MacMillan opened the doors at Mapperly Hospital Nottingham in 1954, Stern did likewise at the Central Hospital Warwick in 1957 as did Mandelbrote at Coney Hill, Gloucester. Details are in Kraüpl Taylor 1958: pp.155–6.

This attention to the organizational and interpersonal features of the psychiatric setting offered new opportunities for psychiatric nurses. The new therapeutic vision of the interpersonal relations of the hospital enabled them to stake a claim for a more autonomous type of expertise. Doctors could not claim special skills in the manipulation of the dynamic relations between members of the institutional community, yet these were now to be systematically utilized in the construction of a normal identity for the patient. At its high point, which was probably in the 1970s, this underpinned a new 'psychotherapeutic' vision of psychiatric nursing as an activity which could itself be curative through working upon the patient's relationships with the situations he or she encountered in the everyday life of the ward.

In the psychiatric wards of old mental hospitals and new psychiatric units, and in the day hospitals and half-way houses that began to proliferate, new techniques of nursing were developed and deployed. Nurses, in psychiatric and in general nursing, gradually altered their view of the patient: no longer merely a series of tasks, the patient was a sick person who needed to be actively engaged in the process of getting better.[6] These developments in nursing were accompanied by the growth of other forms of institutional therapy that owed something to the therapeutic community idea. Occupational and industrial therapies sought not only to increase muscular coordination, and hence self-confidence, but also to encourage the habits of labour. As mental disorder began to be seen, at least in part, as an inability to cope with the demands of employment, work itself began to be seen as a vital element in the treatment of mental disorder (Miller, 1986). The developing programme of hospital closure allowed these practices to develop in new psychiatric spaces—in day hospitals run by the hospital service, day centres run by local authorities, half-way houses, hostels, group homes, and a variety of other residential and non-residential institutions. In the 1970s and 1980s, these professionals and their techniques would find their homes in the new institutions of the psychiatric community.

A place would also be found for the authentic therapeutic communities. There were not only Belmont, now known as Henderson Hospital, and the Cassel, but also 'mini'-therapeutic communities (Clark, 1970; Manning and Hinshelwood, 1979). These were characterized by such techniques as large and small group meetings, projective and expressive therapies involving art and drama, occupational therapies, and individual therapies—developed in psychiatric units in general hospitals, in rehabilitative institutions in the prison system, in institutions for maladjusted, delinquent, and criminal youths, in houses for drug users and alcoholics often run by ex-patients, in the work of Richmond Fellowship, and in many other residential establishments in the public, grant-aided, charitable, and private sectors. These institutions provide a therapeutic rationale for the confinement of young neurotics and the personality disordered, the persistently self-damaging, the repetitively suicidal, the ostentatiously antisocial, those who continually act out, and those who are continually manipulated by others: those whose illness appears to consists only in a disruptive failure

of social adjustment and whose treatment can thus be seen as co-extensive with, and exhausted by, a systematic programme of resocialization.

Accounting for community psychiatry

Conventional accounts of the move of psychiatry 'into the community' in the second half of the 20th century in the United Kingdom, the United States, and much of Europe stress two factors: the discovery of genuinely effective psychotropic drugs and the recognition that confinement could be damaging. On the one hand, drugs offered the possibility of amelioration of symptoms if not cure, and did away with the necessity for long periods of institutional confinement—whilst also validating the medical mandate over problems of mental health. On the other, the discovery of the poor conditions within mental institutions and the pathogenic effects of confinement itself, led to a view that long periods of confinement were damaging and antitherapeutic. In the United States, Albert Deutsch documented the shameful conditions in the asylums that were reminiscent of those in the concentration camps, and Erving Goffman published his sociological account of the effects of the 'total institution' in stripping away the personality and identity of the inmate (Deutsch, 1948; Goffman, 1962). In Britain, Russell Barton diagnosed a condition he christened 'institutional neurosis'—a form of illness produced by the institution itself and John Wing demonstrated that institutionalism—apathy, resignation, dependence, depersonalization, and reliance on fantasy—was common to long-stay inmates of even well-run mental hospitals, and that reforms centring upon enriching the institutional environment were difficult to maintain in the face of institutional exigencies (Barton, 1959; Wing, 1962; see also Lomax, 1921). It appeared that the pathogenic effects of the mental hospital were intractable; the solution was not to reform the institution but to do away with it. Such accounts suggest that these developments led to changes in policy, based on the view that mental hospitals did little good but much harm, and consumed scarce resources which were better directed to more effective forms of provision. Wherever possible hospitalization should be avoided, where necessary it should be in the ordinary medical system, the length of stay should be minimized, and individuals should be maintained 'in their communities' where, rather than suffering the pathogenic consequences of institutionalization, they would be subject to the benign influences of normality.

Critics of this account of psychiatric progress point out that critiques of 'museums of madness' were nothing new, and so other factors must account for their effects at this particular moment in psychiatric history (e.g. Baruch and Treacher, 1978; Scull, 1985; Treacher and Baruch, 1981). They also dispute the significance accorded to the new discoveries in psychopharmacology, pointing to the repetitious history of enthusiastic claims for the efficacy of physical treatments of mental disorder followed by disillusionment occasioned by relapse, side effects, or other disappointments. And it is true that there is little correlation between patterns of hospital bed use and discharge rates and the use of such drugs in different areas and countries; the role of phenothiazine drugs in the 1950s was more for control within the hospital than to facilitate discharge. Thus sociologists and historians have suggested that the determinants of the move away from custodial responses to mental disorder must be found elsewhere. They suggest

---

6 Developments in nursing can be traced through the articles and letters in *Nursing Mirror* and *Nursing Times* over this period. See also Meacher (1979) and Barnes (1968). These developments in nursing are consonant with the shift in medical perception noted in Armstrong (1984).

that what was at stake was not a desegregation of the mentally ill, but a desegregation of psychiatry—a desire of psychiatrists to end their isolation and gain access to the power, careers, and status of other medical specialisms. They regard the 'drug revolution' not as the origin of the move away from the mental hospital but as a pseudoscientific legitimation for it (Treacher and Baruch, 1981). And they argue that the political rationale for a shift away from the custodial institution lay in a 'fiscal crisis of the state': the cost of incarceration, of maintaining the buildings, and paying the increased wages won by the unions were harder and harder to justify, in a situation where the state was finding it increasingly difficult to fund its welfare activities through the taxation system without unacceptable demands upon private profit (Scull, 1985).

The truth probably lies somewhere between these two narratives. Whilst the cost of maintaining mental hospitals, which were largely built in the 19th century, was a significant factor, as we have seen, the events that led to unlocking the wards and the run-down of the mental hospital system began much earlier, predating any 'fiscal crisis'. Indeed, cross-national comparisons show no correlation between moves away from incarceration and economic prosperity or crisis. However, the development of post-war welfare states did provide crucial conditions for this shift in policy. Whilst in the 19th century, institutional confinement was seen as the condition for social support, in the era of the welfare state and social insurance this was no longer the case. Social insurance made it possible for individuals without wage labour to be maintained without incarceration. Public housing facilities provided the conditions for such persons to be physically sheltered outside institutions, as did the development of private and charitable housing schemes. The foundation of a comprehensive system of primary medical care enabled general practitioners to play a key role in dispensing pharmaceutical treatments without the need for hospital admission. The consolidation of medical and psychiatric social work within the local authorities and the hospitals enabled supervision of the patients outside hospitals.

However, it would be wrong to see the changes in psychiatry as merely a fortunate beneficiary of the new rationale of welfare. The post-war modernization of psychiatry was neither a mere rationalization for financial savings nor a consequence of psychopharmacology: it was the generalization of a sociopolitical strategy whose rudiments had been put in place over a 50-year period.

Blurring the boundaries of the institution

Official discussions of psychiatry in the post-Second World War period appear merely to reiterate and extend the themes concerning the need for early and voluntary treatment and the organizational and clinical similarities and interdependencies between mental and physical ills. The Royal Commission on Mental Illness and Mental Deficiency, which was set up in 1954 and reported in 1957, posed the issues in a similar way, as did the Mental Health Act 1959 which followed on from its recommendations. As the Minister put it, what was involved was a 're-orientation of mental health services away from institutional care towards care in the community'. Hence the Act extended the open-door policy, established informal admissions as the norm, extended local authority powers, encouraged liaison between health and social services, and so forth (see, for the above, Jones, 1972: p.307). This strategy linked up with developments in the post-war apparatus of the welfare state. Psychiatric social work had extended from the child guidance clinics and mental hospitals into the heart of social casework (Younghusband, 1978). Psychiatric social workers were employed not only in the prison and borstal services, in care committees, and so forth, but also in the extensive work of rehabilitation of ex-service men and women, working in the mental health advisory services set up for this purpose under the National Health Service Act of 1946. And, further, psychiatrically trained social workers were now operating as Children's Officers under the Children Act of 1948: all social work now attended, to a greater or lesser extent, to the psychological investments and conflicts which underpinned even those presenting problems which were apparently entirely practical.

While the Mental Health Act of 1959 allocated considerable discretionary powers to doctors in respect of involuntary admission to mental hospital and the administration of treatment without the patient's consent, this was neither an extension of the coercive powers of the authorities nor a triumph of organicist medicine over other theories of the origin of mental disorder or other professional claims for a role in a mental health system. On the contrary, the strategy sought to minimize the role of incarceration in the social responses to mental distress, to establish links and alliances between medicine and other social agencies, to facilitate the movement of individuals amongst and between the different branches of the mental health system, and to encourage each of us to take responsibility for the preservation and promotion of mental health.

But despite these conceptual continuities, the transformations of the psychiatric system in the 1950s and 1960s do mark a significant shift in the spatial dispensation of psychiatry. Whilst neither criticisms of the asylum nor claims for the efficacy of physical treatments were new, in the context of the new rationale for psychiatry as a part of public health, they enabled an extension of psychiatric modernization to those sectors of the psychiatric system which had previously been most difficult to access. On the one hand, it was now argued that the closed asylums with their populations of chronic and psychotic patients were not only sucking in social resources which were more usefully deployed in the other sectors of the system, but were also actively damaging in their effects. On the other, whatever their real efficacy, the new pharmacological technologies of treatment, made it possible to imagine that people with severe psychiatric problems could be managed outside the hospital. The medical complex of general practitioners, outpatient departments, and ordinary general hospitals could administer the drug-based therapeutics without the segregative institution. Social insurance and social workers could service the ill person without confinement. And madness—understood now merely as illness, unhappiness, and inefficiency—no longer constituted a fundamental threat to reason and order which required incarceration. The asylum had become unnecessary.

The policy landmarks of the new configuration are clear enough (Jones, 1972: pp.321–34). Enoch Powell, Minister of Health, in his 1961 speech to the National Association of Mental Health, announced the objective of halving the number of places in hospitals for mental illness over the next 15 years, and the closure of the majority of the existing mental hospitals. The Ministry circular following this speech confirmed the decline in bed spaces, urged planning for closure of 'large, isolated and unsatisfactory buildings', and laid out the four kinds of accommodation to be provided in the new system: acute units for short-stay patients, usually in general hospitals; medium-stay units for medium-stay patients; units for long-stay patients, often in hostels or annexes of general hospitals; and secure units provided on a regional basis. In 1962 the Hospital Plan for the next 15 years envisaged the phasing out of all specialist hospitals, such as those for the mentally ill and the chronically sick, and their incorporation into District General Hospitals. In 1963, *Health and Welfare: the Development of Community Care* urged the desirability of 'community care', but did not specify what this entailed. By 1971, *Hospital Services for the Mentally Ill* proposed the complete abolition of the mental hospital system, with all inpatient, day-patient, and outpatient services provided by departments of District General Hospitals, linked in to services provided by the local authority social services, general practitioners, and in consultation with the Department of Employment.

This policy was continued throughout the 1970s, irrespective of the political complexion of the government of the day. The lines of argument were similar in *Better Services for the Mentally Ill*, produced by Barbara Castle's Labour ministry in 1975, and in *Care in Action* and *Care in the Community* produced in 1981 under the aegis of the monetarist conservatism represented by Patrick Jenkin. The strategy was now more clearly developed: articulated in terms of the creation of a comprehensive psychiatric service, a continuum of care, and a community psychiatric system; prevention through education and the encouragement of practices to promote mental health; early treatment entailing the removal of stigma, ease of access, minimization of legal formalism, and the education of professionals so that they may pick up the early signs of mental disorder; outpatient treatment in clinics, sheltered housing, through domiciliary services, and with social work support; inpatient treatment to be minimized, for as short a period as possible and within the district general hospital; aftercare on discharge provided by the outpatient services. Despite the controversies over the passage of the 1983 Mental Health (Amendment) Act, its emphases on care in the community, on the minimization of hospitalization and compulsory detention, and so forth, were entirely consonant with the direction of psychiatric modernization.

The psychiatric system which had taken shape in England, Europe, and the United States by the 1980s was not primarily an apparatus of coercion and segregation, delineated by the mental hospital and monopolized by the medical profession. At the programmatic level, it aspired towards a 'continuum of care' which would run from custodial measures for those with major mental derangements, through voluntary treatment for minor mental troubles, to prophylactic work by propaganda, advice, and the reform of personal life in the interests of mental health. The psychiatric population was highly differentiated and distributed across a range of specialized sites: secure units, local authority group homes, specialized units for children, alcoholics, anorexics, drug users, and so forth. And relations had been established between such institutions and other sites where psychiatric expertise was deployed: the child guidance clinic, the courtroom, the counselling centre, the prison, and the classroom. In this 'advanced' psychiatric system (Castel, 1982), key roles were played by non-medical professions—nursing, social work, probation, psychology, education, occupational therapy—and increasingly by quasi-professional 'voluntary' or self-help organizations.

Nor was this psychiatric complex dominated by a socially blind organicism at the level of theory or treatment. Most psychiatric professionals allowed a key role for 'social factors' in the precipitation and prevention of mental distress, sought to inject psychiatric considerations into debates over social policies, and established collaborative relations between medical treatment in hospital and the aid of other social agencies. A practical eclecticism enabled the coexistence of therapeutic ideologies and techniques which appear fundamentally opposed: from individual psychotherapy to co-counselling, from dynamic group therapy to behaviour modification, from drug treatment to family therapy. Hospitals using psychotropic medications, therapeutic communities, feminist self-help groups, social work group homes, community nurses, and many other strange bedfellows combined to chart the domain of mental health and develop technologies for its management. The move away from the asylum extended the range of social ills seen to be flowing from psychiatric disturbance and simultaneously psychiatrized new populations. Children, delinquents, criminals, vagrants and the work shy, the aged, unhappy marital and sexual partners all became possible objects for explanation and treatment in terms of mental disturbance. And, in the majority of cases, such treatment was not imposed coercively upon unwilling subjects but sought out by those who had come to identify their own distress in psychiatric terms, believed that psychiatric expertise would help them, and were thankful for the attention they received.

Community and control

The shifts in psychiatric policy over the closing two decades of the 20th century entailed a critique of many of these assumptions, and a reshaping of the practices to which they were linked. Many approaches that had been developed over the previous 50 years fell into disrepute, as expensive, lengthy, and unproven: the demand for 'evidence-based treatments' was a key factor in displacing psychodynamically-inspired therapies with interventions that sought rapid and measurable transformations in specific pathologies of thought or conduct. In this and other ways, the conceptual and practical boundaries between minor and severe mental illness were reconfigured. Many psychiatrists questioned the conception of a continuum of mental distress and argued for the need to concentrate on the severe conditions—which were increasingly thought to have an organic basis—which should be principal target of treatment and the principal concern of publicly funded psychiatric services. 'Care in the community' was criticized from all sides.[7] Critics drew attention to the neglect, homelessness, and degradation that had been produced in the name of an unrealistic policy of reduction of hospitalization, which was, in any event, hampered by inadequate funding, incompetent management, and service rivalry. Newspaper headlines focused upon the despairing plight of former mental patients isolated in bedsits, vagrancy, homelessness, despair, and suicide and claimed that this was a policy which, under the guise of reform, amounted to abandonment. Many psychiatrists began to argue that the key factor for a successful life in the community for those with mental health problems was the maintenance of psychotropic medication: community psychiatry required not so much 'a continuum of care' but effective measures to ensure drug-compliance outside the hospital.

---

7 In this section I am drawing on my 1998 paper 'Governing risky individuals: the role of psychiatry in new regimes of control', in *Psychiatry, Psychology and Law*, **5**, 177–95.

By the close of the 20th century, assertions that care in the community had 'failed' no longer focused on the neglect of the vulnerable in the community but on the supposed threat to 'the community' by the mentally ill in their midst. A concerted campaign of 'scare in the community' had generated a new popular conception of 'mental illness' in terms of the propensity to violence (Philo, 1996; D. Rose, 1998). Hence a new sociopolitical demand was placed on psychiatry: it should take as its principal objective the surveillance and control of the mentally ill in the name of the protection and security of 'the community' (cf. Crichton, 1995). The little phrase 'care in the community patient' came to identify certain persons who, because illness had stripped them of their normal moral safeguards, posed a threat to the tranquillity, order, and safety of 'the public'. The issue of homicides by those suffering from mental illness, previously a matter for a small number of forensic psychiatrists concerned with a small minority of 'dangerous individuals' who were 'mentally abnormal offenders', came to shape arguments about the sociopolitical obligations of psychiatrists and other mental health professions to secure the security of 'the public'. One word characterizes the new demands placed on psychiatry: risk (Rose, 1998, c.f. Castel, 1991; Duggan, 1997; Steadman et al., 1993). Mechanisms for the control of risk became central to the operation of all psychiatry—identification of risk factors, risk assessment, risk schedules, risk registers, risk management (Royal College of Psychiatrists, 1996).

The role of mental health professionals was less that of cure or care than of the administration of dangerous, damaged, or desperate individuals across a complex institutional field comprising institutions of various levels of security, half-way houses of various types, day centres, drop-in centres, hospital hostels, clinics, sheltered housing, assertive outreach teams, and much more. The failures of psychiatry were now posed in terms of the failure of prediction and control of risky individuals, and hence the placing of 'the community' at risk. And there was a growing demand for the extension of coercive powers of mental health law—measures to secure drug compliance, provisions for preventive detention…—in the belief that this was the only way to mitigate the dangers posed by the severely mentally ill to themselves, their families, psychiatric professionals and 'the public' (c.f. Pratt, 1995; Simon, 1997).

As concerns about risk came to the fore, so did new divisions among those who it treated: low risk, medium risk, and high risk. In the zone of low risk, quasi-therapeutic techniques of control proliferated across everyday life, regulating and reshaping of individual conduct according to norms of autonomy, responsibility, competence, and self-fulfilment. Here one found counselling, mediation, conciliation, cognitive therapies, behavioural techniques, and the like within the school, the factory, the training programme for the unemployed, and in hospital clinics, tutors' studies, the work of health visitors and social workers, and, of course, the prescription of psychiatric medication from the surgeries of general practitioners. These practices for the management of the self operated in a much broader therapeutic habitat: a culture in which radio, television, and cinema offer us psychologized images of ourselves, and a whole range of practices of life are shaped and organized in therapeutic terms.

The zone of medium risk was marked out by psychiatric wards on general hospitals, the practices of social workers, together with quasi public provision provided under contract by 'voluntary agencies'. Alongside this public provision, a private market opened up for the management of acute mental health problems which do not appear immediately linked to danger to others. The new private arrangements were supported by the growth of private health insurance and by the emergence of market-style arrangements for the purchase of care by publicly funded health services. In this zone of medium risk, mental health was increasingly governed through the family, by means of strategies that sought to enhance, intensify, and instrumentalize the apparently 'natural' bonds of obligation between members of domestic units: the self-governing family was urged, educated, and obliged to take on itself the sociopolitical responsibility of managing its own mental health problems and its own problematic members.

The work of public agencies and state institutions increasingly came to focus on the issue of 'high risk'. Mental health professionals were given a key role within an extending apparatus charged with the obligation of the continuous and unending management of permanently problematic persons in the name of community safety. Different tactics were involved: 24-hour nursed care, community treatment orders, assertive outreach, crisis intervention and the like. Within this way of thinking about 'the community at risk', the different types of psychiatric institutions are virtually defined in terms of the need for security rather than those of therapy or care (Grounds, 1995). A new archipelago of islands of confinement were created: special hospitals, medium secure units, re-locked wards in psychiatric hospitals, units for those deemed to have 'dangerous and severe personality disorders'. At the same time, new proposals were formulated for the confinement of certain 'monstrous individuals': those who, although they may have served a sentence for their crimes, and have not been diagnosed with a treatable mental illness, were considered too risky to the general public to be allowed to go free. As the 20th century closed, across the English-speaking world, strategies were developed for the preventive detention of sexual predators, paedophiles, the incorrigibly antisocial—of those thought to pose a risk to the community on the basis not so much of what they have done, but of what they are and what they might do (e.g. Greig, 1997 for Australia; Pratt, 2000; for New Zealand; Scheingold et al., 1994 for the United States).

The assessment and management of risk has become part of the political obligation of psychiatry and the professional obligation of all those working with issues of mental health (Alberg et al., 1996; Snowden, 1997). Psychiatry and law are intrinsically bound together within these new strategies of regulation and the mechanisms of law play a key role in shaping the conduct of psychiatric professionals. The shadow of the law—the real or imagined fear of prosecution or of censure by quasi-judicial public inquiries—shapes professional conduct, and provides the legitimization for the relentless task of documentation intrinsic to these new risk-based psychiatric technologies. Psychiatric judgement has become enwrapped in a grid of legal and quasi-legal obligations (such as codes of practice, notes of guidance, and so forth) within a new regime of blame, in which mental health professionals operate under the threat of being held accountable for any harm to 'the community' which might result from the actions of those with whom they have been involved.

'Madness' has come to be emblematic of all the threats that are ascribed by those who think of themselves as 'normal' to those who they marginalize or exclude. Within this perception, difference is recoded as danger, and a constant labour is required to mark out and police those differences that are no longer demarcated by the walls of an asylum or the closed doors of the hospital ward.

In this new problems space, not merely those with mental health problems, not only psychiatric professionals, but everyday life itself is 'governed through madness'—that is to say, regulated and shaped in terms of the fear of those with mental health problems and the need to reduce risks. At a time when the 'users', 'consumers', and 'survivors' of psychiatry are, at last, demanding their own say in the practices of mental health, one principal challenge for psychiatrists 'in the community' over the next decades lies in their capacity to manage these new tensions between their obligations to their patients and these sociopolitical demand for control.

Coda

As we reach the end of the first decade of the 21st century, the dilemmas of risk management in the community have become intertwined with another set of dilemmas concerning the proper scope of psychiatry (Rose, 2006b). Epidemiological data appears to show nothing less than an epidemic of mental health problems—with over one-quarter of the general population deemed to be suffering from a DSM (*Diagnostic and Statistical Manual of Mental Disorders*) diagnosable mental disorder in any one year, and around one-half across a lifetime (Kessler et al., 2005; Wittchen and Jacobi, 2005). The use of psychiatric medication continues to increase worldwide (Olfson and Marcus, 2009; Rose, 2006a,b). Controversies flare over the increasing diagnosis of children with such conditions as autism spectrum disorder, attention deficit hyperactivity disorder, and even bipolar disorder. The profession struggles with the attempts to align definitions and classifications of disorder based on symptomatology with the belief that all psychiatric disorders are disorders of the brain, or at the very least have neural underpinnings and neural correlates (Hyman, 2007; Regier et al., 2009). The logic of prevention leads some to argue for screening of asymptomatic intervention using biomarkers with the aim of early intervention to forestall the later development of psychiatric illness or antisocial conduct (Singh and Rose, 2009). Thus the questions are posed: Is there really so much undiagnosed and untreated psychiatric illness, requiring greater disease awareness among professionals and public, more effective diagnosis, ready provision of psychiatric drugs, and an expanding community mental health which will reduce stigma? Or are doctors and psychiatrists too ready to diagnose disorder for variations in mood or behaviour once considered normal ups and downs of life? Are actual and potential consumers of psychiatry too ready to understand what ails them in psychiatric terms? What are the roles of the pharmaceutical companies, patients' pressure groups, and psychiatrists themselves in this expansion of the territory of psychiatry? What is the proper scope of psychiatry in relation to community mental health? Perhaps we should reflect on some words of Aubrey Lewis, almost half a century ago, which have lost none of their relevance (Lewis, 1967: pp.277–8):

> We can… agree that the practice of psychiatry should be limited to illness and its prevention, and that illness occurs broadly where there is disabling of distressing interference with normal function But in the last thirty years the impatience and perhaps the credulity of public opinion has pressed upon the psychiatrist requests that he treat people who are not ill and advise on problems that are not medical. It needs no logician to detect the fallacy in the syllogism which runs: psychiatrists are experts in mental disorder; mental disorder is a form of abnormal behaviour; therefore psychiatrists are experts in abnormal behaviour of every sort. Yet in matters touching upon misbehaviour in children,

vocational selection, troubles in marriage, crime, and many other tribulations, the psychiatrist has sometimes assumed responsibility, or had responsibility thrust upon him, beyond the range of his medical functions…. There is no other branch of medicine which finds it so difficult to say 'no'; and is so often blamed when it says 'yes'.

References

Alberg, C., Hatfied, B., and Huxley, P. (1996). *Learning Materials on Mental Health: Risk Assessment.* Manchester: University of Manchester.

Armstrong, D. (1983). *Political Anatomy of the Body: medical knowledge in Britain in the twentieth century*, Cambridge: Cambridge University Press.

Armstrong, D. (1984). The patient's view. *Social Science and Medicine*, **18**, 737–44.

Barnes, E. (ed.) (1968). *Psychosocial nursing: studies from the Cassel Hospital.* London: Tavistock.

Barton, R. (1959). *Institutional Neurosis.* Bristol: Wright.

Baruch, G. and Treacher, A. (1978). *Psychiatry Observed.* London: Routledge and Kegan Paul.

Castel, R. (1991). From Dangerousness to Risk. In: Burchell, G., Gordon, C., and Miller, P. (eds.) *The Foucault Effect: Studies in Governmentality*, pp. 281–98. Hemel Hempstead, Harvester Wheatsheaf.

Castel, R., Castel, F., and Lovell, A. (1982). *The Psychiatric Society*, Goldhammer, A. (trans.). New York. Columbia University Press.

Caudill, W. (1958). *The Psychiatric Hospital as a Small Society.* Cambridge, MA: Harvard University Press.

Clark, D.H. (1970). The therapeutic community: concept, practice, future. *British Journal of Psychiatry*, **117**, 375–88.

Clark, D.H. (1964). *Administrative Psychiatry.* London: Tavistock.

Crichton, J. (ed.) (1995). *Psychiatric Patient Violence: Risk and Response.* London: Duckworth.

Curle, A. (1947). Transitional communities and social reconnection. A follow-up study of the civil resettlement of British prisoners of war. *Human Relations*, **1**, 42–68.

Deutsch, A. (1948). *The Shame of the States.* Reprinted in 1973. New York: Arno.

Duggan, C. (ed.) (1997). Assessing risk in the mentally disordered, Supplement 32 to the *British Journal of Psychiatry.* London: Royal College of Psychiatrists.

Farrall, L.A. (1985). *The origins and growth of the English eugenics movement, 1865-1925.* New York: Garland.

Goffman, E. (1962). *Asylums.* New York: Doubleday.

Greig, D. (1997). Shifting the boundary between psychiatry and law. *Liberty: Journal of the Victorian Council of Civil Liberties*, February.

Grounds, A. (1995). Risk assessment and management in a clinical context. In: Crichton, J. (ed.) *Psychiatric Patient Violence: Risk and Response*, pp. 43–59. London: Duckworth.

Hearnshaw, L.S. (1964). *A Short History of British Psychology, 1840-1940.* London: Methuen.

Hyman, S.E. (2007). Can neuroscience be integrated into the DSM-V? *Nature Reviews Neuroscience*, **8**, 725–32.

Jones, K. (1972). *A History of the Mental Health Services*, London: Routledge and Kegan Paul.

Jones, M. (1952). *Social Psychiatry.* London: Tavistock.

Kessler, R.C., Demler, O., Frank, R.G., Olfson, M., Pincus, H.A., Walters, E.E., *et al.* (2005). Prevalence and treatment of mental disorders, 1990 to 2003. *New England Journal of Medicine* **352**, 2515–23.

Kräupl Taylor, F. (1958). A history of group and administrative therapy in Great Britain. *British Journal of Medical Psychology*, **31**, 153–73.

Lewis, A.J.S. (1967). *Medicine and the affections of the mind. In: The State of Psychiatry. Essays and addresses*, pp. 273–97. London: Routledge & Kegan Paul.

Lomax, M. (1921). *Experiences of an Asylum Doctor.* London: Allen and Unwin.

Main, T. (1946). The hospital as a therapeutic institution. *Bulletin of the Menninger Clinic*, **10**, 66–70.

Manning, N. and Hinshelwood, R. (eds.) (1979). *The Therapeutic Community: Reflections and Progress*. London: Routledge and Kegan Paul.

Manning, N.P. (1976). Innovation in social policy – the case of the therapeutic community. *Journal of Social Policy*, **5**, 265–79.

Martin, D. (1962). *Adventure in Psychiatry*. Oxford: Cassirer.

Meacher, M. (ed.) (1979). *New Methods of Mental Health Care*. Oxford: Pergamon.

Miller, P. (1986). The psychotherapy of employment and unemployment. In: Miller P. and Rose, N. (eds.) *The Power of Psychiatry*, pp. 143–76. Cambridge: Polity.

Philo, G. (1996). *Media and Mental Distress*. London: Longmans.

Pratt, J. (2000). Sex crimes and the new punitiveness. *Behavioral Sciences & The Law*, **18**, 135–51.

Olfson, M., and Marcus, S. C. (2009). National patterns in antidepressant medication treatment. *Archives of General Psychiatry*, **66**, 848–56.

Pratt, J. (1995). Dangerousness, risk and technologies of power. *Australia and New Zealand Journal of Criminology*, **28**, 3–31.

Rees, J.R. (1945). *The Shaping of Psychiatry by War*. London: Chapman and Hall.

Regier, D.A., Narrow, W.E., Kuhl, E.A., and Kupfer, D.J. (2009). The conceptual development of DSM-V. *American Journal of Psychiatry* **166**, 645–50.

Rose, D. (1998). Television, madness and community care. *Journal of Community and Applied Social Psychology*, **8**, 213–28.

Rose, N. (1985). *The Psychological Complex: Psychology, politics and society in England, 1869-1939*. London: Routledge and Kegan Paul.

Rose, N. (1996). *Inventing Ourselves: Psychology, Power and Personhood*. Cambridge, MA: Cambridge University Press.

Rose, N. (1998). Governing risky individuals: the role of psychiatry in new regimes of control, *Psychiatry, Psychology and Law*, 1998, **5**, 177–95.

Rose, N. (2006a). Psychopharmaceuticals in Europe. In: Knapp, M., McDaid, D., Mossialos, E., and Thornicroft, G. (eds.) *Mental Health Policy and Practice Across Europe*, pp. 146–87. Milton Keynes: Open University Press.

Rose, N. (2006b). Disorders without borders? The expanding scope of psychiatric practice. *BioSocieties*, **1**, 465–84.

Rosen, G. (1959). Social stress and mental disease from the 18th century to the present: some origins of social psychiatry. *Millbank Memorial Fund Quarterly*, **37**, 5–32.

Royal College of Psychiatrists (1996). *Assessment and Clinical Management of Risk of Harm to Other People*. London: Royal College of Psychiatrists.

Royal Commission on Lunacy and Mental Disorder (1926). *Report*, Cmd. 2700. London: HMSO.

Scheingold, S., Pershing, J., and Olson, T. (1994). Sexual violence, victim advocacy and Republican criminology. *Law and Society Review*, **28**, 729–63.

Scull, A. (1985). *Decarceration*, 2nd edn. Cambridge: Polity.

Searle, G.R. (1976). *Eugenics and politics in Britain, 1900-1914*. Leyden: Noordhoff.

Simon, J. (1997). Governing through crime. In: Friedman L. and Fisher, G. (eds.) *The Crime Conundrum: Essays on Criminal Justice*, pp. 171–80. Boulder, CO: Westview Press.

Singh, I. and Rose, N. (2009). Biomarkers in psychiatry. *Nature*, **460**, 202–7.

Snowden, P. (1997). Practical aspects of clinical risk assessment and management. In: Duggan, C. (ed.) *Assessing risk in the mentally disordered, Supplement 32 to the British Journal of Psychiatry*, pp. 32–34. London: Royal College of Psychiatrists.

Stanton, A.H. and Schwartz, M.S. (1954). *The Mental Hospital*. London: Tavistock.

Steadman, H.J., Monahan, J., Clark Robbins, P., Appelbaum, P. Grisso, T., Klassen, D., *et al.* (1993). *From dangerousness to risk assessment: implications for appropriate research strategies*. In: Hodgins, S. (ed.) *Mental Disorder and Crime*, pp. 297–318. Newbury Park, CA: Sage.

Treacher, A. and Baruch, G. (1981). Towards a critical history of the psychiatric profession. In: Ingleby, D. (ed.) *Critical Psychiatry*, pp. 120–59. Harmondsworth: Penguin.

Wilson, A.T.M., Doyle, M., and Kelnar, J. (1947). Group techniques in a transitional community. *Lancet*, **1**, 735–8.

Wing, J. (1962). Institutionalism in mental hospitals. *British Journal of Social and Clinical Psychology*, **1**, 38.

Wittchen, H.U., and Jacobi, F. (2005). Size and burden of mental disorders in Europe – a critical review and appraisal of 27 studies. *European Neuropsychopharmacology*, **15**, 357–76.

Younghusband, E. (1978). *Social Work in Britain: 1950-1975*. London: George Allen and Unwin.

CHAPTER 3

Mental health policy in modern America

Gerald N. Grob[1]

In the United States a variety of factors have shaped and continuously modified mental health policy: the changing composition of the population with severe mental disorders; concepts of the aetiology and nature of mental illnesses; shifting diagnostic systems; the organization and ideology of psychiatry; funding mechanisms; and existing popular, political, social, and professional attitudes and values. Equally significant has been the structure of the American political system, which divides authority between local, state, and national government.

Few policies are formulated *de novo*, and this is particularly true of mental health. The changes that occurred during the last half of the 20th century require an understanding of earlier developments. Before 1900, responsibility for social welfare (with the exception of a federal programme providing disability and old-age pensions for Civil War veterans and their dependents) lay largely with state governments. Beginning in the early 19th century, states created a vast public hospital system to care for persons with severe mental disorders. Mental health, as a matter of fact, remained the single largest item in their budgets. Many states also required local governments to contribute funds to care for their residents in state hospitals. This created an incentive to retain residents with mental disorders in almshouses where the cost of care was lower.

Toward the end of the 19th century, states began to assume total responsibility for funding its mental hospitals. A curious and unforeseen development followed. Local communities saw an entrepreneurial opportunity to reduce their own expenditures. In brief, they began to redefine senility in psychiatric terms, and thus to transfer aged persons from local almshouses (which in the 19th century served in part as old age homes) to state mental hospitals. The structural context of policymaking thus altered coverage patterns, which in turn transformed in part the mission of state hospitals by converting them into institutions that provided custodial care for large numbers of elderly disabled persons. As late as 1958, nearly one-third of all patients in state hospitals were over the age of sixty-five (American Psychiatric Association 1960; Grob 1991).

At the end of World War II the nation's public hospitals faced a crisis of unprecedented proportions. Between 1930 and 1945 state governments were preoccupied with the problems growing out of the Great Depression and World War II, and paid little attention to the deteriorating conditions within their public hospital system. Despite problems caused by declining appropriations, an aging physical plant, and staff shortages, the daily census of hospitals rose steadily. In 1945 their average daily resident population was about 430,000; approximately 85,000 were first-time admissions. A decade later the number had risen to 558,000. That elderly persons constituted a large proportion of the patient population only reinforced perceptions that such institutions were preoccupied with custodial rather than therapeutic functions (Grob 1991).

Few public policies, however long established or stable, remain immune from broader social, economic, intellectual, and scientific currents. Beginning with World War II, the faith that institutionalization was the appropriate policy choice slowly began to erode. Within two decades the very legitimacy of mental hospitals had been undermined by individuals and groups committed to a new policy paradigm, namely, that the care and treatment of persons with severe mental disorders should take place in the community. By 2005 the number of institutionalized patients had fallen to slightly less than 50,000; the overwhelming majority of persons with severe disorders were now treated in general hospitals or other outpatient facilities (Atay et al., 2007).

What accounts for such a dramatic policy shift? The answer to this question is by no means simple. The changes in post-war mental health priorities had diverse roots. The military experiences of World War II allegedly demonstrated that community and outpatient treatment of persons with mental disorders was superior and more efficient. A simultaneous shift in psychiatric thinking fostered receptivity toward a psychodynamic and psychoanalytic model that emphasized life experiences, the importance of socioenvironmental factors, and psychotherapy of one form or another. The belief that early identification of individuals at risk and intervention in

[1] Author's or Editor's contribution to the Work was done as part of the Author's or Editor's official duties as a NIH employee and is a Work of the United States Government. Therefore, copyright may not be established in the United States.

the community would be effective in preventing subsequent hospitalization became popular. This belief was especially encouraged by psychiatrists and other mental health professionals holding a public health orientation. They also shared a faith that psychiatry, in collaboration with other social and behavioural sciences, could ameliorate those social and environmental conditions that in their eyes played an important role in the aetiology of mental disorders. The introduction of new psychosocial and biological therapies—including but not limited to psychotropic drugs—held out the promise of a better and more productive life for persons who in the past were institutionalized. At the same time psychiatrists began to abandon mental hospital employment for private and community practice. Finally, a series of journalistic and media exposés seemed to confirm the belief that mental hospitals were simply incarcerating persons and providing little in the way of therapy (Grob 1991).

All of these developments, by themselves or in conjunction with each other, would surely have promoted change. Nevertheless, the entry of the federal government into the mental health policy arena proved crucial, for it altered the very ways in which policy was conceptualized and implemented. After 1945 new structural relations were forged among federal agencies; federal funding for biomedical research increased precipitously; and the role of the Public Health Service expanded dramatically. The passage of the Hill–Burton Act in 1946 provided generous subsidies for hospital construction, and third-party medical insurance programmes expanded rapidly. The emergence of a health lobby that included members of Congress and influential laypersons hastened the expansion of federal health activities.

The growing role of the federal government in health affairs did not necessarily imply that it would seek to pre-empt the traditional role of states in providing care and treatment for persons with severe mental disorders. The passage of the National Mental Health Act of 1946 and subsequent creation of the National Institute of Mental Health (NIMH), however, proved critical in hastening change (Public Law Chap. 538, 1946). The act was conceived and orchestrated through Congress by Dr Robert H. Felix, the first director of the NIMH from 1949 to 1964. One of the shrewdest and most effective federal bureaucrats of his generation, Felix worked to end institutional care and employ federal prestige and resources to create a new community-oriented policy. His underlying belief was that mental disorders represented 'a true public health problem', the resolution of which required knowledge about the aetiology and nature of mental illnesses, more effective means of prevention and treatment, and better trained personnel. Public health, according to Felix, was concerned with the 'collective health' of the community. The NIMH mental health programme was designed 'to help the individual by helping the community, to make mental health a part of the community's total health program, to the end that all individuals will have greater assurance of an emotionally and physically healthy and satisfying life for themselves and their families.' Felix was able to frame a national agenda that assumed that community care and treatment would replace archaic and obsolete mental hospitals (Felix 1945, 1949; Felix and Bowers 1948).

During the 1950s, interest in community alternatives to mental hospitalization mounted. The development of psychosocial and milieu therapies, as well as the introduction of psychotropic drugs, gave impetus to the belief that early identification and treatment would obviate the need for hospitalization. Support for a community mental health programme came from a variety of constituencies. The Council of State Governments and Governors Conferences in the 1950s endorsed this approach as a means of arresting the seemingly inevitable growth of the institutionalized population. Private foundations such as the Milbank Memorial Fund as well as leading university departments of psychiatry added their voices to the chorus promoting change. The growing faith in community mental health services led New York State in 1954 and California in 1957 to enact legislation encouraging communities to expand their mental health services (Grob 1991).

Nevertheless, activists faced a daunting problem, namely, that responsibility for policy still resided with 48 state governments. In the hope of altering intergovernmental relations and forging a national policy, they created the Joint Commission on Mental Illness and Health. A private undertaking, the commission received congressional endorsement with the passage of the Mental Health Study Act of 1955, which authorized the Public Health Service to provide federal grants. After nearly 6 years of work and the publication of nine monographs, the commission issued its final report, *Action for Mental Health*, which presented a large number of general recommendations and a plea for a dramatic increase in federal funding (Grob 1991; Joint Commission on Mental Illness and Health 1961).

Although President John F. Kennedy was sympathetic to *Action for Mental Health*, he faced conflicting pressures. On the one side were those pushing for legislation dealing with mental retardation; on the other side were key congressional figures determined to secure legislation dealing with mental health. Faced with a split, Kennedy sidestepped the issue by appointing an interagency task force on mental health. Because its members were not especially knowledgeable about the subject, they relied on Felix and the NIMH to guide their deliberations. Felix adroitly used his position to further his agenda. He and his staff had little use for the recommendations of the Joint Commission. Whereas the commission had emphasized the care and treatment of persons with severe disorders, the NIMH favoured a more comprehensive policy focusing on 'the improvement of the mental health of the people of the country through a continuum of services, not just upon the treatment and rehabilitative aspects of these programs'. Radical rather than incremental change was required. Felix and his staff therefore recommended the adoption of a comprehensive community programme that would make it possible 'for the mental hospital as it is now known to disappear from the scene within the next twenty-five years'. Its place would be taken by a new institution—a community mental health centre (CMHC)—that would offer comprehensive services to all Americans (National Institute of Mental Health, 1961, 1962a,b).

Felix's views prevailed, and in 1963 Congress enacted the Community Mental Health Centers Act, which provided a 3-year authorization of $150 million dollars for construction. Two years later it enacted legislation that offered financial support for staffing (Public Law 88-164, 1963; Public Law 89-105, 1965). The passage of this legislation, however, represented the victory of ideology over reality. The functions of a CMHC remained vague and undefined. A community programme, moreover, was based on certain assumptions: that patients had a home in the community; that a sympathetic family would assume responsibility for the care of the released patient; that the organization of the household would not impede rehabilitation; and that the patient's presence would not cause undue hardships for other family members. In 1960, however, 48% of the hospitalized population was unmarried, 12% widowed, and 13% either divorced or separated. The assumption that patients would be able to reside in the community with their families while undergoing rehabilitation was hardly supported by such data, especially since the legislation said little or nothing about income support, occupation, or housing (Kramer, 1956, 1967; Kramer et al., 1968; Pollack et al., 1959).

Nor was there evidence that CMHCs could provide care and treatment for a severely disabled population in the community. Indeed, the legislation and the subsequent regulations governing CMHCs provided no links with state hospitals. State authorities, which had administrative responsibilities for overseeing policy implementation, were also bypassed in favour of a federal–local partnership. The result was that CMHCs had considerable autonomy and freedom from state regulations. This permitted centres to focus on a new set of clients who better fitted the orientations of mental health managers and professionals trained in psychodynamic and preventive orientations. The treatment of choice at most centres was individual psychotherapy, an intervention especially adapted to a middle-class, educated clientele without severe disorders and one that was congenial to the professional staffs composed largely of social workers and clinical psychologists. In effect, CMHCs broadened the clientele of the mental health system, but did not provide services for persons with severe mental disorders. Centres, according to Donald G. Langsley (president of the American Psychiatric Association) in 1980, had 'drifted away from their original purpose' and featured 'counseling and crisis intervention for predictable problems of living'. The changing nature of staffing at CMHCs reflected its new functions; an absolute decline in the number of psychiatrists was matched by an increase in psychologists and social workers (Grob, 1991; Langsley, 1980; Musto, 1975).

In the 1960s, faith in the efficacy of prevention and community mental health reinforced the belief that institutionalization could eventually become a relic of the past. To be sure, mental hospital populations, which peaked at 558,000 in 1955, thereafter began an uneven decline. Between 1955 and 1965 state hospital populations fell by only 15%. During the following decade, the decline was 60%, although rates varied sharply from state to state. The belief that CMHCs played a role in what subsequently became known as deinstitutionalization was widespread (Mechanic and Rochefort, 1992).

In some respects even the term 'deinstitutionalization' is somewhat of a misnomer. Indeed, the first wave of deinstitutionalization actually involved a lateral transfer of patients from state hospitals to long-term nursing facilities because states were motivated to benefit from a windfall of new federal dollars. Between 1900 and 1960, state hospitals were serving in part as old age homes. The enactment of Medicaid in 1965 encouraged the construction of nursing home beds because it provided a payment source for patients transferred from state mental hospitals or admitted to nursing homes and general hospitals. Although states were responsible for the full costs of patients in their public mental hospitals, they could transfer patients to other facilities and have the federal government assume from half to three-quarters of the cost, depending on the state's economic status. This incentive encouraged a mass transinstitutionalization of long-term patients with dementia who had been previously housed in public mental hospitals for lack of other institutional alternatives. In 1963, nursing homes cared for nearly 220,000 individuals with mental disorders, of whom 188,000 were 65 or older. Six years later the comparable numbers were 427,000 and 368,000 (Goldman et al., 1983; Gronfein, 1985; Kramer, 1977; National Institute of Mental Health, 1974). Within a short time, according to a 1977 study by the General Accounting Office, Medicaid had become 'one of the largest single purchasers of mental health care and the principal federal program funding the long-term care of the mentally disabled'. It was also the most significant 'federally sponsored program affecting deinstitutionalization' (General Accounting Office, 1977). The shift from mental hospital to nursing facility care was a development driven by a desire to promote the use of federal resources rather than by a desire to improve the lot of elderly persons and others with a severe and persistent mental disorder.

A second wave of deinstitutionalization began in the early 1970s that included new cohorts of persons with mental disorders coming to public notice for the first time. Between 1946 and 1960 more than 59 million births were recorded. The disproportionately large size of this age cohort meant that the number of persons (most of whom were young) at risk from developing a severe mental illness was very high. They were also highly mobile and often had a dual diagnosis of a mental disorder and substance abuse. The availability of a series of federal entitlement programmes—including Social Security Disability Insurance (SSDI), Supplementary Security Income for the Aged, the Disabled, and the Blind (SSI), Medicare, and food stamps—encouraged states to make admission to mental hospitals more difficult, if only because resources for persons with severe mental disorders in the community were available.

Treatment in the community for clients with multiple needs, as compared with mental hospital care, posed severe challenges. In the community (and particularly in large urban areas) clients were widely dispersed and their successful management depended on bringing together needed services administered by a variety of bureaucracies, each with its own culture, priorities, and preferred client populations. Although there were sporadic and occasionally successful efforts to integrate these services (psychiatric care and treatment, social services, housing, social support) in meaningful ways, the results in most areas were dismal. These new patients were typically treated during short inpatient stays in general hospitals and in other outpatient settings; they had to make do with whatever services they could garner.

The decentralization of services and lack of integration made it extraordinarily difficult to deal with persons with severe disorders in the community, and many became part of the street culture where the use of alcohol and drugs was common. Individuals with a dual diagnosis of a serious mental disorder and substance abuse presented such serious problems that many mental health professionals refused to deal with them despite their growing numbers. Moreover, the decline in institutional care created a situation where the 'criminalization' of persons with serious mental illnesses became more common. If such individuals were on the streets, they were more likely to engage in acts that attracted the attention of authorities and that ended in arrest and detention. Many persons with serious mental illnesses had encounters with the police, and a significant number were caught up in the criminal justice rather than the mental health system and incarcerated in prisons. To be sure, collaboration between the two systems was possible, but often different perspectives, values, and cultures placed formidable barriers in the way of cooperation.

In the last third of the 20th century, states pursued a policy of reducing their mental hospital populations by placing barriers in the way of new admissions and only as a last resort. This policy, in conjunction with the vast expansion in the clientele and diagnoses (as exemplified in the third and subsequent editions of the American Psychiatric Association's *Diagnostic and Statistical Manual of Mental Disorders* since 1980), shifts in public attitudes and perceptions, changing treatment strategies, and social and economic factors, led to the emergence of a confusing array of organized and unorganized settings for the treatment of persons with mental illnesses. State mental health agencies, which in theory were responsible for administering the mental health system, found themselves faced with declining resources and an increasing inability to influence policy. Multiple sources of funding from a variety of federal programmes administered by independent agencies made it difficult to develop and implement comprehensive, integrated, and effective community-based services. Many of the components of community mental health care—income support, housing, social support networks—were designed for other populations and often did not fit the needs of persons with severe and cyclic persistent mental illnesses.

When the General Accounting Office prepared a comprehensive report to Congress in 1977, it laid bare the problems of a disorganized and uncoordinated mental health system. Although endorsing deinstitutionalization, the report was extraordinarily critical of the manner in which it was implemented. Responsibility for the care, support, and treatment of persons with serious disorders was 'frequently diffused among several agencies and levels of government'. The dramatic growth of federal involvement in mental health had not produced the anticipated benefits, if only because there was little or no coordination between the 135 federal programmes administered by eleven major agencies and departments (General Accounting Office, 1977).

By the 1970s most knowledgeable observers recognized that the mental health system was in disarray. Upon taking office in early 1977, Jimmy Carter created a presidential commission to investigate the mental health system and present its recommendations to the president. After public hearings and months of deliberations, the commission presented its final report in the spring of 1978. It included more than 100 recommendations that affected not only relations among federal, state, and local governments but also public and private agencies and such federal programmes as Medicare and Medicaid. In many ways the heterogeneous character of the commission's work was influenced by a political climate in which debates were shaped by the demands of groups that defined themselves in terms of class, ethnicity, gender, and race. By that time neither state hospitals nor persons with serious and persistent mental disorders were at the centre of policy debates. The commission's final report was neither a blueprint for legislative action nor the expression of a particular group. The diversity of its recommendations could not easily be translated into legislation (Grob and Goldman, 2006; Report to the President, 1978).

For more than 2 years the administration and Congress struggled in an effort to draft appropriate legislation. The problem was the absence of any consensus on mental health policy. Deinstitutionalization—whatever its meaning—was coming under widespread criticism by a variety of interest groups, each with its own agenda. In October 1980, Congress finally enacted and Carter signed into law the Mental Health Systems Act. While in theory assigning the highest priority to individuals with long-term mental disorders, the legislation also recognized the claims of various other groups whose needs were quite different, including children and adolescents, the elderly, rural residents, and victims of rape. The absence of new resources and vague generalizations about the kinds of services required, however, raised doubts about the legislation's effectiveness. Indeed, in order to make it through Congress, the legislation offered something to everyone, and as a result lacked any focus. Moreover, some provisions—especially those dealing with the prevention of mental illnesses and the promotion of mental health—reflected ideology and were little more than attractive slogans that had no basis in empirical data. Nor did the legislation offer any guidelines to assist persons with severe mental disorders to negotiate a myriad of programmes administered by independent agencies (Foley and Sharfstein, 1983; Grob and Goldman, 2006; Mechanic, 1999; Public Law 96-398, 1980).

No sooner had the Mental Health Systems Act become law when its provisions were rendered moot. The inauguration of Ronald Reagan in January 1981 led to an immediate reversal of policy. In the summer of 1981 the Omnibus Budget Reconciliation Act became law. Under its provisions the federal government provided block grants to states for mental health and substance abuse services. States were given considerable leeway in spending their allocations. With but a few exceptions, the Mental Health System and CMHC Acts were repealed, thus—at least in theory—diminishing the direct role of the federal government in mental health (Public Law 97-35, 1981).

In the short run, the work of Carter's President's Commission on Mental Health appeared to have had relatively little influence on the evolution of mental health policy. Yet serendipity is often an unrecognized force in human affairs. This was particularly true of the section in the final report calling for the establishment of a national priority and a national plan to meet the needs of individuals with long-term mental illnesses. As a result of this recommendation, a Department of Health, Education and Welfare task force proposed that the secretary of the agency appoint a group to develop a 'national plan for the chronically mentally ill' (Report of the HEW Task Force 1979; Report to the President 1978). Completed in December 1980, the plan laid out a blueprint for future action (Koyanagi and Goldman, 1991a,b; U.S. Department of Health and Human Services, 1980).

In the 1980s the Reagan administration was committed to policies that were designed to limit if not reduce the social welfare functions of the federal government. The means chosen involved sharp reductions in taxation and the transfer of many social welfare functions downward to state and local governments. Although successful to some degree, the impact of these policies was mitigated by administrative actions taken by individuals within the federal bureaucracy under pressure from advocates and members of Congress. Concerned that preoccupation with tax reductions and the shrinkage or elimination of social programmes might have devastating consequences for persons with severe and persistent mental illnesses, Congress enacted legislation that ensured that this group would retain access to resources necessary to survive in the community. Thus the abortive effort to enact a programme of broad comprehensive reform during the Carter administration was replaced instead by an emphasis on sequential incremental change that over time at least mitigated some of the difficult conditions faced by persons whose severe and persistent mental disorders created a state of dependency.

The National Plan embodied a strategy that went beyond simple incremental change. It provided a blueprint of specific recommendations suggesting a clear direction and a sequence of steps to achieve desired changes. Specifically, it offered recommendations to change both statutes and regulations governing important mainstream health and social welfare programmes, including Medicare, Medicaid, and the disability programmes of the Social Security Administration (e.g. SSDI, SSI), which affected people with severe and persistent mental disorders. During the 1980s, many of the recommendations of the National Plan were implemented both by statutory enactments and administrative actions within the federal bureaucracy. By the 1990s, Medicaid and Medicare eclipsed state categorical dollars as a source of mental health funding. While the new federalism restored some of the lost state authority in mental health services policy, the federal government actually picked up more of the bill (Grob and Goldman, 2006).

For all of the successes of mental health policy in the 1980s, policies and programmes remained fragmented (President's New Freedom Commission on Mental Health, 2003). Federal agencies in charge of entitlement programmes were separated by bureaucratic walls from the Department of Health and Human Services and other departments with some influence on the lives of individuals experiencing a mental disorder, including the Department of Housing and Urban Development and the Departments of Labor and Education. A range of new social problems involving people with mental illnesses (homelessness, substance abuse, HIV/AIDS) created new pressures. Medicaid and Medicare may have improved mental health benefits, but these benefits had more limitations than those of general health benefits. The system remained fragmented; no single agency accepted responsibility.

In the 1990s, the gap between research and practice led to the publication of the Surgeon General's *Mental Health*. Its policy recommendations were general in scope: the necessity of building the science base; the need to overcome stigma; the importance of improving public awareness of effective treatments; the need for an adequate supply of mental health services and providers; the importance of delivering state-of-the-art treatments; the need to tailor treatment to age, gender, race, and culture; and the importance of facilitating entry into treatment as well as reducing barriers to treatment (U.S. Department of Heath and Human Services, 1999).

In 2002, George W. Bush created a President's New Freedom Commission on Mental Health. The executive order establishing the commission had limited boundaries but also reflected a wish for 'transformation'. During its deliberations the commission struggled with the tensions of encouraging change while coping with a mandate for limited resources. As Michael F. Hogan, the commission's chair observed, the nation's mental health system remained 'fragmented, disconnected and often inadequate, frustrating the opportunity for recovery. Today's mental health care system is a patchwork relic—the result of disjointed reforms and policies. Instead of ready access to quality of care, the system presents barriers that all too often add to the burdens of mental illnesses for individuals, their families, and our communities.' The commission argued that mental health care had to be consumer and family driven. It made the concept of recovery a basic theme and outlined a number of goals for a transformed mental health system, Its recommendations, however, were not specific, nor could they be linked to federal, state, or local mental health policy. The report also came at a time when health policy occupied a very low priority for the administration, which by then was deeply involved in foreign wars (President's New Freedom Commission on Mental Health, 2003).

Both the Surgeon General and New Freedom Commission reports made the concept of 'recovery' the central theme in guiding mental health policy and practice. Nevertheless, the concept was unclear, confusing, and even contradictory. Much of its appeal was due to optimistic rhetoric rather than substance. Persons with a serious mental illness are not a homogeneous population. Some have only one episode and then return to their previous functioning. Others recover only after years of being disabled by their illness. Focusing solely on cure or recovery runs the risk of abandoning people whose serious mental illnesses leads to prolonged disability. Even when their disorder is in complete remission, such individuals do not always achieve functional recovery. Indeed, Robert P. Liberman and Alex Kopelowicz have suggested that the concept of recovery from schizophrenia is a 'concept in search of research'. A more realistic and modest definition is that recovery incorporates the important idea that careful attention to and prevention of secondary disabilities can limit some of the adverse effects of serious mental disorders and thus make it possible for persons with such disorders to realize some of their goals and have reasonable lives in the community (Liberman and Kopelowicz, 2005).

Similarly, rhetorical claims about the effectiveness of clinical interventions have often concealed underlying problems and contradictions. For more than half a century antipsychotic drugs had been the mainstay of psychiatric practice. Though indispensable for the treatment of severe and persistent mental illnesses—especially schizophrenia—they neither cured the illness nor were their side effects negligible. Marketing and advertising by pharmaceutical companies of allegedly new and more effective drugs only exacerbated a difficult situation. Indeed, recent studies of new antipsychotic drugs failed to show any advantage over their older first-generation counterparts, to say nothing about their metabolic side effects. These new drugs, Jeffrey A. Lieberman recently observed, 'represent an incremental advance at best. This underscores the urgent need for greater progress in developing novel therapeutics for schizophrenia and related disorders' (Freedman 2006; Lieberman 2006; Lieberman et al., 2005).

Are there 'lessons' that can be drawn from knowledge of the past? At the very least, history suggests that there is a price to be paid for implementing ideology ungrounded in empirical reality and for making exaggerated rhetorical claims. The sustained attack on a century-old institutional policy, for example, was based on a superficial if not misreading history of mental health policy in the United States and was advanced as part of a campaign to justify the new community-oriented policy that became known as deinstitutionalization. The ideology of community mental health and the facile assumption that residence in the community would promote adjustment and integration was illusory and did not take into account the extent of social isolation, exposure to victimization, inducement to substance abuse, homelessness, and criminalization of persons with mental disorders. The assumption that CMHCs would assume responsibility for aftercare and rehabilitation of persons discharged from mental hospitals proved erroneous. The absence of mechanisms of control and accountability permitted CMHCs to focus on new populations of more amenable and attractive clients with far less severe disorders. Nor does the recent move to enrol persons with serious mental disorders in managed care offer assurances that the varied needs of this group will finally be met. Preliminary evidence suggests that a 'democratization' of services reduces the intensity of services for patients with more profound disabilities and needs (Mechanic and McAlpine, 1999).

Equally notable are the roles played by rhetoric and ideology in the development of mental health policy during past decades and a view of past policy that bore little relationship to reality. To dismiss rhetoric and ideology as simply forms of public posturing is to ignore their consequences. Rhetoric and ideology shape agendas and debates; they create expectations that in turn mould policies, and they inform the socialization, training, and education of those in professional occupations. The concept of community care and treatment and the corresponding attack on institutional care—all of which played significant policy roles during the last half century—were not inherently defective. But states, communities, and policy advocates lacked the foresight or commitment to ensure adequate financing and to provide needed services. In addition, optimistic claims about the prevention of mental disorders had little or no basis in empirical evidence; they represented the height of rhetorical fancy.

The history of mental health policy in the United States also provides a fascinating if largely ignored case study of the interaction of political structure and ideology. In the 19th century a faith in the efficacy of institutionalization led to the creation of a vast system of public hospitals that at their peak contained more than half a million patients. Yet an incremental policymaking process and intergovernmental rivalries led to a series of unanticipated consequences. By the early 20th century mental hospitals were providing care for a large number of elderly persons at a time when other alternatives for this group were non-existent. A half century later, dissatisfaction with the existing state of affairs led to demands that an obsolete and archaic institutional system be replaced by a new community-oriented policy. Each of these stages was shaped by intergovernmental rivalries that maximized efforts to shift costs to different levels and ideological claims that bore little relationship to reality. Moreover, the growth of a system of public welfare that included a myriad of entitlement programmes to deal with sickness and dependency had the inadvertent effect of diminishing the central policy focus on persons with severe and persistent mental illnesses. As long-term institutionalization diminished and was replaced by a variety of public programmes that focused on different populations, the latter group was faced by a fragmented system of services ill-suited to their complex needs. Americans at the beginning of the 21st century still faced the problem of shaping a policy that meets the needs of a people whose severe mental disorders creates dependency.

References

American Psychiatric Association (1960). *Report on Patients Over 65 in Public Hospitals*. Washington, DC: American Psychiatric Association.

Atay, J.E. and Foley, D. (2007). *Background Report, Admissions and Resident Patients, State and County Mental Hospitals, United States, 2005*. Rockville, MD: Center for Mental Health Services.

Felix, R.H. (1945). Mental Public Health: A Blueprint. Presentation at St. Elizabeths Hospital, 21 April 1945. *Robert H. Felix Papers*. Bethesda, MD: National Library of Medicine.

Felix, R.H. (1949). Mental disorders as a public health problem. *American Journal of Psychiatry*, **106**, 401–6.

Felix, R.H. and Bowers, R.V. (1948). Mental hygiene and socio-environmental factors. *Milbank Memorial Fund Quarterly*, **26**, 125–47.

Foley, H.A. and Sharfstein, S.S. (1983). *Madness and Government: Who Cares for the Mentally Ill?* Washington, DC: American Psychiatric Press.

Freedman, R. (2006). The choice of antipsychotic drugs for schizophrenia. *New England Journal of Medicine, 353*, 1286–88.

General Accounting Office (1977). *Returning the Mentally Disabled to the Community: Government Needs to do More* (HRD-76-152). Washington, DC: General Accounting Office.

Goldman, H.H., Adams, N.H., and Taube, C.A. (1983). Deinstitutionalization: The data demythologized. *Hospital & Community Psychiatry*, **34**, 129–34.

Grob, G.N. (1983). *Mental Illness and American Society, 1875-1940*. Princeton, NJ: Princeton University Press.

Grob, G.N. (1991). *From Asylum to Community: Mental Health Policy in Modern America*. Princeton, NJ: Princeton University Press.

Grob, G.N. and Goldman, H.H. (2006). *The Dilemma of Federal Mental Health Policy: Radical Reform or Incremental Change?* New Brunswick, NJ: Rutgers University Press.

Gronfein, W. (1985). Incentives and intentions in mental health policy: A comparison of the Medicaid and Community Mental Health Programs. *Journal of Health and Social Behavior*, **26**, 192–206.

Joint Commission on Mental Illness and Health (1961). *Action for Mental Health: Final Report of the Joint Commission on Mental Illness and Health*. New York: Basic Books.

Koyanagi, C. and Goldman, H.H. (1991a). *Inching Forward: A Report on Progress Made in Federal Mental Health Policy in the 1980s*. Alexandria, VA: National Mental Health Association.

Koyanagi, C. and Goldman, H.H. (1991b). The quiet success of the National Plan for the chronically mentally ill. *Hospital & Community Psychiatry*, **42**, 899–905.

Kramer, M. (1956). *Facts Needed to Assess Public Health and Social Problems in the Widespread Use of the Tranquilizing Drugs*. Washington, DC: U.S. Public Health Service, Publication No. 486.

Kramer, M. (1967). *Some Implication of Trends in the Usage of Psychiatric Facilities for Community Mental Health Programs and Related Research*. Washington, DC: U.S. Public Health Service, Publication No. 1434.

Kramer, M. (1977). *Psychiatric Services and the Changing Institutional Scene, 1950-1985*. DHEW Publication No. [ADM] 77–433. Washington DC: Government Printing Office.

Kramer, M., Taube, C., and Starr, S. (1968). Patterns of use in psychiatric facilities by the aged: current status, trends, and implications. American Psychiatric Association, *Psychiatric Research Reports*, **23**, 89–150.

Langsley, D.G. (1980). The community mental health center: Does it treat patients? *Hospital & Community Psychiatry*, **21**, 815–19.

Liberman, R.P. and Kopelowicz, A. (2005). Recovery from schizophrenia: A concept in search of research. *Psychiatric Services*, **56**, 735–42.

Lieberman, J.A. (2006). Comparative effectiveness of antipsychotic drugs. *Archives of General Psychiatry*, **63**, 1069–72.

Lieberman, J.A., Stroup, T.S., McEvoy, J.P., Swartz, M.S., Rosenheck, R.A., Perkins, D.O., *et al*. (2005). Effectiveness of antipsychotic drugs in patients with chronic schizophrenia. *New England Journal of Medicine*, **353**, 1209–23.

Mechanic, D. (1999). *Mental Health and Social Policy: The Emergence of Managed Care*, 4th edn. Boston, MA: Allyn and Bacon.

Mechanic, D. and McAlpine, D.D. (1999). Mission unfulfilled: Potholes on the road to mental health parity. *Health Affairs*, **18**, 7–21.

Mechanic, D. and Rochefort, D.A. (1992). A policy of inclusion for the mentally ill. *Health Affairs*, **11**, 128–50.

Musto, D.F. (1975). Whatever happened to community mental health? *Public Interest*, **39**, 53–79.

National Institute of Mental Health (1961). National Institute of Mental Health Position Paper on the Report of the Joint Commission on Mental Illness and Health. *National Institute of Mental Health Records 1965-1967, Box 1, Record Group 511.2*. Washington, DC: National Archives.

National Institute of Mental Health (1962a). Preliminary Draft Report of NIMH Task Force on Implementation of Recommendations of the Report of the Joint Commission on Mental Illness and Health. *National Institute of Mental Health, Miscellaneous Records, 1956-1967, Box 1, Record Group 511.2*. Washington, DC: National Archives.

National Institute of Mental Health (1962b). A Proposal for a Comprehensive Mental Health Program to Implement the Findings of the report of the Joint Commission on Mental Illness and Health. *National Institute of Mental Health Miscellaneous Records, 1956-1967, Box 1, Record Group 511.2*. Washington, DC: National Archives.

National Institute of Mental Health (1974). *Statistical Note No. 107*. Rockville, MD: National Institute of Mental Health.

Pollack, E.S. Person, P. H., Kramer, M., and Goldstein, H. (1959). *Patterns of Retention, Release, and Death of First Admissions to State Mental Hospitals*. Washington, DC: U.S. Public Health Service, Publication No. 672.

President's New Freedom Commission on Mental Health (2003). *Achieving the Promise: Transforming Mental Health Care in America: Final Report*. DHHS Pub. No. SMA-03-3832. Washington, DC: U.S. Department of Health and Human Services.

Public Law Chap. 538 (1946). *U.S. Statutes at Large*, **60**, 421–6.

Public Law 88-164 (1963). *U.S. Statutes at Large*, **77**, 282–99.

Public Law 89-105 (1965). *U.S. Statutes at Large*, **79**, 427–30.

Public Law 96-398 (1980). *U.S. Statutes at Large*, **94**, 1564–613.

Public Law 97-35 (1981). *U.S. Statutes at Large*, **95**, 535–98.

Report of the HEW Task Force of the Report to the President from the President's Commission on Mental Health, December 15, 1978 (1979) Washington, DC: U.S. Government printing office.

Report to the President from the President's Commission on Mental Health (1978). 4 vols. Washington, DC: Government Printing Office.

U.S. Department of Health and Human Services (1980). *Steering Committee on the Chronically Mentally Ill: Toward a National Plan for the Chronically Mentally Ill*. Washington, DC: U.S. Public Health Service.

U.S. Department of Health and Human Services (1999). *Mental Health: A Report of the Surgeon General*. Rockville, MD: U.S. Public Health Service.

CHAPTER 4

Recovery as an integrative paradigm in mental health

Mike Slade and Larry Davidson

What is recovery?

The term 'recovery' is at the heart of a debate about the core purpose of mental health services. It is a contested term, with at least two meanings. We call these two meanings recovery from mental illness, or 'clinical recovery', on the one hand, and being in recovery with a mental illness, or 'personal recovery', on the other (Davidson and Roe, 2007). Each meaning is underpinned by a set of values, and creates role expectations for mental health professionals. We begin by differentiating these two meanings.

Meaning 1: clinical recovery or recovery 'from' mental illness

The first meaning of recovery has emerged from professional-led research and practice. Clinical recovery has four key features:

1 It is an outcome or a state, generally dichotomous

2 It is observable—in clinical parlance, it is objective, not subjective

3 It is rated by the expert clinician, not the patient

4 The definition of recovery is invariant across individuals

Various definitions of recovery have been proposed by mental health professionals. A widely-used definition is that recovery comprises full symptom remission, full- or part-time work or education, independent living without supervision by informal carers, and having friends with whom activities can be shared, all sustained for a period of 2 years (Libermann and Kopelowicz, 2002). Defining recovery has allowed epidemiological research to establish recovery rates. In Table 4.1 we show all 20-year or longer follow-up studies published until 2008.

These empirical data challenge the applicability of a chronic disease model to mental illness, with its embedded assumption that conditions like schizophrenia are necessarily lifelong and have a deteriorating course.

However, deep assumptions about normality are embedded in clinical recovery. As Ruth Ralph and Patrick Corrigan comment in relation to clinical recovery:

This kind of definition begs several questions that need to be addressed to come up with an understanding of recovery as outcome: How many goals must be achieved to be considered recovered? For that matter, how much life success is considered 'normal'? (Ralph and Corrigan, 2005: p.5.)

Table 4.1 Recovery rates in long-term follow-up studies of psychosis

Study authors	Location	Year	n	Mean length of follow-up (years)	% recovered or significantly improved
Huber et al.	Bonn	1975	502	22	57
Ciompi and Muller	Lausanne	1976	289	37	53
Bleuler	Zurich	1978	208	23	53–68
Tsuang et al.	Iowa	1979	186	35	46
Harding et al.	Vermont	1987	269	32	62–68
Ogawa et al.	Japan	1987	140	23	57
Marneros et al.	Cologne	1989	249	25	58
DeSisto et al.	Maine	1995	269	35	49
Harrison et al.	18-site	2001	776	25	56

As a result, and as a product of the user/survivor movement spanning the last 40 years, people who use mental health services have called for a new approach. As Ridgway (2001) argues:

> The field of psychiatric disabilities requires an enriched knowledge base and literature to guide innovation in policy and practice under a recovery paradigm. We must reach beyond our storehouse of writings that describe psychiatric disorder as a catastrophic life event.

The second meaning of 'recovery' provides the rubric under which such an enriched knowledge base has been accruing.

Meaning 2: personal recovery or being 'in' recovery

People personally affected by mental illness have become increasingly vocal in communicating both what their life is like with the mental illness and what helps in moving beyond the role of a patient with mental illness. Early accounts were written by individual pioneers (Coleman, 1999; Davidson and Strauss, 1992; Deegan, 1988; Fisher, 1994; O'Hagan, 1996; Ridgway, 2001). These brave, and sometimes oppositional and challenging, voices provide ecologically valid pointers to what recovery looks and feels like from the inside.

Once individual stories were more visible, compilations and syntheses of these accounts began to emerge from around the (especially Anglophone) world, e.g. from Australia (Andresen et al., 2003), New Zealand (Barnett and Lapsley, 2006; Goldsack et al., 2005; Lapsley et al., 2002; Mental health Commission, 2000), Scotland (Scottish Recovery Network, 2006, 2007), the United States (Davidson et al., 2005; Ridgway, 2001; Spaniol and Koehler, 1994), and England (Barker et al., 1999; McIntosh, 2005). The understanding of recovery which has emerged from these accounts has a different focus from clinical recovery, for example in emphasizing the centrality of hope, identity, meaning, and personal responsibility (Andresen et al., 2003; Ralph, 2000; Spaniol et al., 2002).

We will refer to this consumer-based understanding of recovery as **personal recovery**, to reflect its individually defined and experienced nature. To note, other distinguishing terms have also been used, including clinical recovery versus social recovery (Secker et al., 2002), scientific versus consumer models of recovery (Bellack, 2006), and service-based recovery versus user-based recovery (Schrank and Slade, 2007).

Many definitions of recovery have been proposed by those who are experiencing it:

> Recovery refers to the lived or real life experience of people as they accept and overcome the challenge of the disability…they experience themselves as recovering a new sense of self and of purpose within and beyond the limits of disability. (Deegan, 1988.)
>
> For me, recovery means that I'm not in hospital and I'm not sitting in supported accommodation somewhere with someone looking after me. Since I've recovered, I've found that in spite of my illness I can still contribute and have an input into what goes on in my life, input that is not necessarily tied up with medication, my mental illness or other illnesses. (Scottish Recovery Network, 2006.)

The most widely-cited definition, which underpins most recovery policy internationally, is by Bill Anthony (1993):

> Recovery is a deeply personal, unique process of changing one's attitudes, values, feelings, goals, skills, and/or roles. It is a way of living a satisfying, hopeful, and contributing life even within the limitations caused by illness. Recovery involves the development of new meaning

and purpose in one's life as one grows beyond the catastrophic effects of mental illness.

It is consistent with the less widely-cited but more succinct definition proposed by Retta Andresen and colleagues, that recovery involves:

> The establishment of a fulfilling, meaningful life and a positive sense of identity founded on hopefulness and self determination. (Andresen et al., 2003.)

For those who value succinctness, the definition we use in our (MS) local service is:

> Recovery involves living as well as possible. (South London and Maudsley NHS Foundation Trust, 2007.)

Recovery as an integrative paradigm

The recovery approach is based on personal recovery. Personal recovery represents a paradigm shift, in which the intellectual challenge emerges from outside the dominant scientific paradigm (the understanding of recovery emerges from people who have experienced mental illness, not from mental health professionals). Previous preoccupations (e.g. risk, symptoms, hospitalizations) become seen as a subset or special case of the new paradigm. By contrast, what was previously of peripheral interest (i.e. the patient's perspective) becomes central. This involves a reversal of some traditional clinical assumptions. Mental illness is a part of the person, rather than the person being a mental patient. Having valued social roles improves symptoms and reduces hospitalization, rather than treatment being needed before the person is ready to take on responsibilities and life roles. The recovery goals come from the patient and the support to meet these goals comes from the clinician among others, rather than treatment goals being developed which require compliance from the patient. Assessment focuses more on the strengths, preferences, and skills of the person than on what they cannot do. The normal human needs of work, love and play **do** apply—they are the ends to which treatment may or may not contribute. People with mental illness are fundamentally normal, i.e. like everyone else in their aspirations and needs. They will, over time, make good decisions about their lives if they have the opportunity, support, and encouragement, rather than being people who will in general make bad decisions so professionals need to take responsibility for them.

Recovery is also an **integrative** paradigm, at both the personal and the system level. For the individual, it integrates the experience of mental illness with the person, by giving primacy to personhood over illness. For example, person-first language—talking about the person experiencing psychosis or the person with schizophrenia (or, even better, the person with a diagnosis of schizophrenia) rather than the schizophrenic or the schizophrenic patient—serves to remind that diagnoses classify illnesses, not people (Davidson and Flanagan, 2007). Recovery also integrates levels of experience, such as political, cultural, life events (trauma, loss, etc.), and personal values, rather than segmenting into professionally-defined components of identity (Barrett, 1996). It addresses the call for culturally competent or responsive services, by highlighting the fact that a person's cultural background, affiliations, and affinities are all crucial aspects of who he or she is, and thereby influence help-seeking, treatment response, and ways of managing the illness.

For the mental health system, the recovery paradigm similarly involves integration of the function of traditionally separate professional disciplines in the service of action planning oriented around the individual's goals. This contrasts with care planning oriented around each discipline's specialist skills. Likewise, recovery can be used as a bridge to integrate treatment for co-occurring psychiatric and substance use disorders, or mental health and physical illnesses, rather than leaving the individual to navigate complex health and social care systems to get his or her needs met through fragmented or uncoordinated care (Davidson and White, 2007). Overall, a recovery-oriented system is an integrated system which wraps around the individual to meet his or her needs.

We now describe a theoretical framework intended to guide mental health professionals in their efforts to support recovery.

The personal recovery framework

Supporting recovery will involve giving primacy to identity over illness. What is identity? Three perspectives have evolved in the humanities. Psychologists focus on personal identity—the things that make a person unique. This individuality is the reason why there cannot be one model of recovery, why professionals should be cautious about saying (or thinking) 'we do recovery', and why the individual's views on what matters to them has to be given primacy. Sociologists more commonly refer to social identity—the collection of group memberships that define the individual. Social identity is damaged when the person experiences entrapment in a low-value and stigmatized social role, such as a mental health service user. Philosophers relate identity to the existence of a persisting entity particular to a given person. Ongoing growth and transformation are central to human development, which is why the goal of returning to a premorbid state is neither attainable nor desirable. Combining these perspectives, **identity comprises those persistent characteristics which make us unique and by which we are connected to the rest of the world.** This definition underpins the Personal Recovery Framework (Slade, 2009a) shown in Fig. 4.1, which illustrates the identity challenges which occur for people experiencing mental illness.

The social environment comprises the world and others in it. Identity enhancing relationships can be with the self, the mental illness, or with the social environment. Figuratively, the process of recovery involves reclaiming a positive identity in two ways (shown as arrows in Fig. 4.1): by identity-enhancing relationships and promotion of well-being which push the mental illness into being a smaller component of identity, and by framing and self-managing which pull the mental illness part. These processes take place in a social context which provides scaffolding for the development of an identity as a person in recovery.

In the Personal Recovery Framework, the individual experiences recovery through undertaking four inter-related and overlapping recovery tasks. First, **developing a positive identity** outside of being a person with a mental illness. This process involves establishing the conditions in which it is possible to experience life as a person not an illness. Second, **developing a personally satisfactory meaning** to frame the experience which professionals would understand as mental illness. This involves making sense of the experience so that it can be put in a box: framed as a part of the person but not as the whole person. This meaning might be expressed as a diagnosis or a

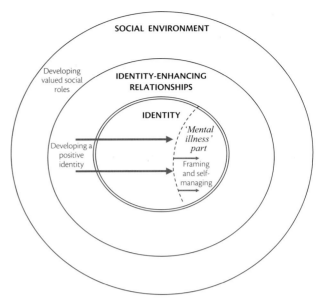

Fig. 4.1 The Personal Recovery Framework.

formulation, or it may have nothing to do with clinical models—a spiritual or cultural or existential crisis. The actual meaning matters less than the degree to which it provides both a constraining frame for the experience and an impetus to move from being clinically managed to the third task of **taking personal responsibility** through self-management: being responsible for your own well-being, including seeking help and support from others when necessary. The final recovery task involves the acquisition of previous, modified, or new **valued social roles**. These normally have nothing to do with mental illness.

The job of mental health professionals

The Personal Recovery Framework points to four ways in which clinicians can support an individual's recovery: fostering relationships, promoting well-being, offering treatments, and improving social inclusion (Slade, 2009b). Mental health services need to be oriented around these four recovery support tasks if they are to maximally support recovery.

Fostering relationships includes those with a higher being, with family and informal carers, with other people with lived experience of mental illness, and with mental health professionals. For example, exposure to people who are further along their recovery journey is profoundly hope-creating, and this is one reason to employ people with experience of mental illness in the mental health workforce. For the same reason, involvement in mutual self-help groups and intentional recovery communities (Whitley et al., 2008) can provide a safe space in which to create a positive personal narrative and challenge the constraints of an illness-defined identity. For professionals, the ability to connect with people during a chaotic period of their life is a recovery support when used as a springboard towards a partnership relationship, in which coaching and mentoring skills are employed by the professional to promote self-management (Borg and Kristiansen, 2004).

Promoting well-being involves the use of expertise on mental well-being, drawing from the science of positive psychology.

For example, the Authentic Happiness theory identifies different types of good life: pleasant, engaged, meaningful, and achieving (Seligman, 2002). The pleasant life (i.e. filled with positive emotions, symptom-free) is not the only type of good life, so supporting recovery also involves putting resources into, for example, spiritual development (for a meaningful life) or promoting activism (for an engaged life). The New Economics Foundation (http://www.neweconomics.org) identifies five-a-day for well-being: Connect, Be active, Take notice, Keep learning, and Give. Mental health services which are promoting well-being will focus efforts in these areas.

Offering treatments involves the use of evidence-based interventions, but oriented around recovery goals rather than treatment goals. Treatment goals are set by the clinician, and will normally relate to avoiding bad things happening, such as relapse, hospitalization, harmful risk, etc. Recovery goals are the person's dreams and aspirations. They are unique, often idiosyncratic. They are forward-looking, although they may of course involve the past. They focus on what the person actively wants, rather than what the person wants to avoid. Recovery goals are strengths-based and orientated towards reinforcing a positive identity and developing valued social roles. They can be challenging to mental health professionals, either because they seem unrealistic or inappropriate, or because supporting them seems to lie outside the professional role. They sometimes involve effort by the professional, or they may have nothing to do with mental health services. They always require the service user to take personal responsibility and put in effort. Recovery goals are set by the service user. Treatment supports recovery when it is offered to the person in support of his or her recovery goals.

Finally, improving social inclusion is central, because hope without opportunity dies. Amartya Sen (awarded the Nobel Prize for Economics in 1998) identified the notion of substantial freedom, meaning that even where legally codified, freedom is effectively restrained when a lack of psychological, social, and financial resources make it impossible to achieve goals and live a meaningful life. The experience (and anticipation) of discrimination blights the lives of many people with mental illness. To support recovery, the focus of a clinician's role needs to enlarge beyond the level of treatment. Helping local employers to make accommodations for employees experiencing mental illness, or working with user activists to challenge discrimination, are just as much a part of the job as treating illness. Free guides for mental health professionals wishing to take up these tasks are becoming increasingly available (Shepherd et al., 2008; Slade, 2009c).

Change in values and behaviour is difficult. For people using services, this is why recovery can take a long time. For people working in services, it is just as difficult, but also just as necessary if recovery is to become a reality. We illustrate some of the implications of recovery for two concrete areas of clinical activity: person-centred care planning and prescribing of medication.

Person-centred care planning and recovery

One way of understanding the application of person-centred care planning in mental health is to place it within the context of evidence-based medicine. Evidence-based medicine is based on the confluence of four factors: 1) the empirical evidence that exists related to the effectiveness of various interventions; 2) the individual practitioner's clinical experience, expertise, and judgement; 3) the resources available to the person; and 4) patient choice (Davidson et al., 2009a; Guyatt and Rennie, 2002; Sackett et al., 1996). An underlying assumption of evidence-based medicine is that all individuals have the right to make their own health care decisions. Since the person is free to ultimately make his or her own decisions, it becomes incumbent upon practitioners to understand this fact and to communicate with the person and his or her family in as accurate, informative, culturally, and personally responsive, and perhaps even persuasive, a way as possible so as to maximize outcomes. In order to do so, the practitioner needs to attend to the person's role as decision-maker, including his or her needs, values, and preferences, within the context of a collaborative relationship.

Person-centred care planning results from accepting and emphasizing the person's role as decision-maker and the importance of his or her needs, values, and preferences in the care planning process. What is unique about the application of person-centred care planning in mental health is that is makes explicit the underlying assumption that people with mental illnesses are first and foremost people, and therefore more specifically, citizens of their respective societies. They were born with the same rights to citizenship as anyone else, and any limitations placed upon those rights will have to be justified and sanctioned by law. Beginning with this assumption means that we need not argue for or justify offering person-centred care to persons with mental illnesses as a separate population. Persons with mental illnesses are 'entitled' to person-centred care to the same degree and for the same reasons as are any other citizens: because it is in accord with the emphasis democratic societies place on autonomy and personal sovereignty. These values apply in health care as well as in other spheres of society, and they apply equally as well to persons with mental illnesses as they do to any other persons... until, unless, and then only for as long as limitations placed on these values are justified and sanctioned by law.

That is, person-centred care, like evidence-based medicine more broadly, is considered the default condition; it should be provided unless there are clear and persuasive, and legally valid, reasons for not doing so. The onus is on those who wish to limit the applicability of this approach to any given population, whether that be persons with mental illnesses, those with developmental disabilities, those with Alzheimer's, those knocked unconscious by a car accident, or those with any other special considerations (e.g. forensic populations).

Understanding person-centred care planning as the default condition has both advantages and disadvantages. The advantage is that this simple understanding of person-centred care is consistent with the focus on rights and personal sovereignty emphasized above and therefore is hard to challenge based purely on principle. Few can argue that people do not want to make their own decisions or that people do not want care that is consistent with their personal values, needs, and preferences. The apparent simplicity of this explanation makes it hard to discount. Unfortunately, the disadvantage of framing this issue in this way stems precisely from this same advantage. Because it is hard to discount, person-centred care comes to be equated with 'motherhood and apple pie' (an American phrase for things that are undeniably good), and, as a result, everyone claims to be doing it already. At this vague level, it is easy for people to dismiss the challenges inherent in having to change their practice by insisting that they already practise in a person-centred way. In addition, the range of accommodations required to offer this approach to persons with mental illnesses are overlooked or under-appreciated. We address a few of these below, framing questions that can be used to determine the degree to which mental health care is being provided in a person-centred fashion (Davidson et al., 2009b).

Is the care centered on an individual person?

Person-centred care can only be carried out at the level of each individual, unique person within the context of his or her family and life. Each person-centred care plan should look different from any others, and be based squarely on this particular person's goals, needs, values, and preferences. This does not mean that person-centred plans cannot include traditional treatments, such as taking prescribed medication or participating in cognitive behavioural psychotherapy. It does mean, however, that these interventions—and such traditional clinical goals as symptom reduction and abstinence from drugs and alcohol—are only included to the degree that the person decides to use or pursue them, which will be based on whether or not the person sees these interventions or goals as contributing to his or her achievement of other personally relevant recovery goals, such as attaining decent housing, getting a job, or returning to school. Relevant questions would thus include: Does the plan provide a roadmap for where the person is headed and what he or she is trying to do in his or her life, or does it merely stipulate what treatment he or she needs? Can you tell from the plan what the care team is trying to accomplish, not just what they are trying to avoid? Does the plan address a life outside of or beyond formal mental health services, or does it remain within the boundaries of the mental health system? If medication is part of the plan, can you tell what the medication is to be used for? Is adherence an end in itself, or is it viewed as a route to some other, personally desirable end? Will the services being offered limit the person to the passive role of mental patient, or will they lead to some worthwhile and wished for changes in the person's life? As mentioned above, the process begins with these goals and works backwards to what is needed for the person to advance toward his or her goals, rather than insisting that the person be adherent to treatment goals first in order to then decide on and pursue his or her own personal aspirations.

Is the care based on the person's strengths?

Is it clear how the plan will utilize identified strengths, both within the person and within his or her social milieu? Can you tell from the plan what the person's specific interests are, and how these interests have contributed to the formulation of goals and objectives? Does the plan help to move the person towards what interests him or her, or does it simply move him or her away from problematic behaviours or activities? If substance abuse is identified as a problem to be addressed, for example, does the plan also address what kind of sober activities the person may want to participate in instead? Are community activities and resources identified in the plan that would support the person in pursing his or her interests? Are there people identified in the plan with whom the person can share these interests?

Does the plan clearly delineate the tasks and roles to be performed and the parties responsible for each? Of particular importance is, does the plan clearly identify the person's own sphere of responsibility and the tasks that he or she agrees to take on?

These questions address one of the more important reasons to adopt person-centred care planning in mental health; i.e. recognizing and incorporating the person's own role in his or her recovery. What does the person need to do to promote or progress in his or her own recovery? What kind of support will the person need in order to carry out these responsibilities successfully? These two questions provide the key focus of recovery-oriented care for people with mental illnesses, and require in-depth knowledge of the person, his or her capacities and needs, and the resources available in his or her social milieu. Based on this knowledge, the care team is able to identify what might be the next one or two steps in the person's recovery and to sketch out what will be involved in the person taking these next few steps. This is how the plan becomes more than a piece of paper that satisfies regulatory, accrediting, and/or reimbursing bodies and to be more of an organic and useful work in progress.

Does the plan and the care provided change over time with the person's evolving goals and needs?

Person-centred care plans do not accept maintenance as a valid goal, as people do not want merely to be 'maintained'. It is quite possible for people to want to maintain a level of clinical stability, though, or to want to remain at a plateau of functioning for an extended period of time. Few people like change for the sake of change, and many people with mental illnesses are afraid of taking risks or trying new things out a very legitimate fear that they might suffer a setback (a fear often reinforced by caring practitioners who do not want to see people relapse). But life also does not stand still. Therefore, while containing the illness may be a very real concern and goal for some people at some times, it is not possible to do so simply by maintaining one's life; i.e. by trying to stand still. Care plans therefore anticipate that change is inevitable and that people will need to continue to adapt to new situations and new challenges, whether they like to or not. One important contribution care plans, and person-centred care more broadly, can make in such situations is to help the person identify those things that he or she wants to keep the same while other things are changing around them.

Are the plan, and the services offered, understandable to the person?

Just as the plan needs to identify the person's own role in promoting or pursuing recovery, the plan and the care offered need to be accessible to and understandable by the person. This is one area in which psychiatric person-centred care may need to incorporate the use of tools and aids to help the person compensate for cognitive impairments or a history of educational deprivation. Does the plan address those aspects of the person's experiences that are of concern to him or her, and in a language that he or she will be able to understand (e.g. voices as opposed to auditory hallucinations, feelings of being unsafe, vulnerable, or unprotected as opposed to paranoia, etc.)? Does the person know what he or she has agreed to receive or participate in? Has his or her consent been truly informed, or will things be done to him or her to which he or she has not agreed? Even in the case of people receiving treatment involuntarily, or individuals who have legal conservators or guardians, have concerted efforts been made to inform the person of the available options and to explain what he or she can expect to happen, including what needs to happen for him or her to no longer be receiving care involuntarily or no longer need a guardian?

Finally, does the plan encourage and support the person in assuming increasing control over his or her life, including the power to make his or her own decisions?

Here, too, psychiatric person-centred care plans may need to focus specifically on these issues of control, empowerment, and decision-making more than care plans in other specialty areas of medicine. This is not only because of the impact of mental illness on the person's life, but also because of the history of mental health care and its tendency to socialize people into a passive and helpless patient role. People may need to be encouraged to take back control of certain parts of their life, the responsibility for which may have been assumed by others. They may also need to be encouraged to view themselves as capable, and as having intact domains of functioning beyond the reach of the illness. They may need to be reminded of, or introduced to, their strengths and gifts, they may need a series of small successes, easy wins, in order to rebuild their self-confidence and sense of personal efficacy. And they may need encouragement and support in taking risks and trying new things—perhaps even some gentle prodding to get unstuck, to be liberated from the inertia of chronic illness. We turn now to our second example: the contribution of medication to personal recovery.

Medication and recovery

In a recovery-focused mental health service, a full range of psychotropic medication is available. However, the job of the service is not to get medication taken, whatever the cost. The job is to support personal recovery. This may or may not involve use of medication for an individual at a particular point in their life journey. So medication is one potential recovery support, among many. The job of the clinician is to give genuine choice and control about medication to the service user. This means that the person may decide to use medication as the prescriber recommends, or may modify the recommendations of the prescriber, or may decide not to take medication. Genuine choice is available only where any of these choices is allowable, which is why prescribing levels are a litmus test for a recovery focus (Slade et al., 2008). The content of the individual's decision about medication is in this sense irrelevant—what matters is the extent to which the person is taking personal responsibility for their well-being.

So what does a recovery-focused approach to medication look like? Of course, many clinicians will place great importance on medication. Their psychopharmacological expertise may be well developed. This is an important resource to bring to the decision-making process. The change in a recovery-focused service is that this expertise is meshed with the consumer's expertise about their own values, beliefs, goals, and preferred approaches to meeting challenges. The job of the clinician is to help people come to the

best choice **for them**. Medication may or may not be necessary for recovery—the journey of recovery involves finding out whether it has a part to play. Since medication will be a tool for many people, at points in their life, it is often important to discuss. The discussion needs to focus on what will be helpful for the individual, and in order to have that discussion the first thing that needs clarifying are the person's recovery goals. Once it is clear what the person is trying to achieve in life, then the role of medication can be discussed in a more focused way. Some people will want to be prescribed medication, and it should be fully available. Some people will experience decisional uncertainty, and the clinical task is then to support decision-making through crystallizing questions, providing unbiased information, and supporting the person to plan and undertake experiments. This will involve truly shared decision-making—two experts in the room, jointly undertaking information exchange and (always) clarification of values. Decisions about medication, just like any other form of treatment, are personal not medical decisions.

How is this done? This is an area where mental health services can learn from innovative approaches to supporting the decision-making process in general medicine (e.g. www.dhmc.org/shared_decision_making.cfm, http://decisionaid.ohri.ca/odsf.html). Some of these decision-support approaches are now being evaluated in mental health services, e.g. CommonGround (Deegan et al., 2008). One such approach is to reframe medicine—in the sense of things that help you to feel better—as much more than solely pharmacological. Pat Deegan's notion of personal medicine (Deegan, 2005) includes all the things that people do to feel better: laughter, love, hope, caffeine, exercise, chocolate, etc. In other words, medicine is what you do, not just what you take. Pill medicine (i.e. psychotropic prescribed medication) is then a subset of personal medicine. This approach is of course already used, such as when prescribing exercise (Meyer and Broocks, 2000), nutrition therapy (Lakhan and Vieira, 2008), or bibliotherapy (Gregory et al., 2004). This has two implications.

First, the prescriber is not the arbiter of the best medicine—only the consumer can judge what medicines are helpful. This is facilitated by the development of what Deegan calls power statements which reflect the person's goals for using psychiatric medication:

For example, a husband developed the following power statement to share with his psychiatrist:

'My marriage is powerful personal medicine, and is the most important thing in my life. I don't want paranoia or sexual side effects from medication to stress my marriage. You and I have to find a medication that supports me in my marriage so that my marriage can support my recovery.'

Notice how the power statement contextualizes the use of medication within the overarching goal for recovery. Also, notice how the power statement acts as an invitation to collaboration and shared decision-making between the prescriber and the client. (Deegan, 2007.)

Second, it highlights that finding the balance between pill medicine and other forms of personal medicine is central. If the most important medicine **to the individual** is pill medicine, then a focus on medication is appropriate. If, by contrast, the most important medicine (i.e. what gets and keeps the person well) is some other form of personal medicine, then an exclusive focus on psychopharmacology will hinder recovery.

A recovery-promoting approach is thus to view medication as an '**exchangeable protection against relapse**' (Libermann, 2002), in which pharmacological and psychosocial approaches both buffer the individual against relapse. For example, framing medication as a potential tool for sustaining well-being creates a very different dialogue (Copeland, 1999). The advantage of this view is that it creates a focus on promoting resilience (which definitely matters) rather than on medication (which may or may not matter). Resilience can be supported by working with the consumer to identify answers to the statements 'I have…' (external supports of people and resources), 'I am…' (inner personal strengths) and 'I can…' (social and interpersonal skills) Mental Health Commission (2001). Medication is thus one potential external support, alongside a whole range of other types of resilience-promoting supports, skills, and strengths. Finding a balance between personal medicine and pill medicine is an essential ingredient of recovery. Both prescribers and consumers will benefit from exposure to the resources which are becoming available to support people who want to come off their psychiatric medication, including websites (e.g. http://www.comingoff.com), booklets published by voluntary sector groups (Darton, 2005; Icarus Project and Freedom Center, 2007), and books (Breggin and Cohen, 2007; Lehman, 2004; Watkins, 2007).

Conclusion

Recovery-oriented care addresses all of these things and more, helping the person to gradually piece back together a meaningful and self-determined life out of the ravages wrought by mental illness. While much work remains to be done in developing the technologies and tools that will be needed for the design and implementation of such services and supports, the fruits of these labours will more than justify the efforts involved.

Further reading

Amering, M. and Schmolke, M. (2009). *Recovery in mental health. Reshaping scientific and clinical responsibilities.* Chichester: Wiley.

Davidson, L., Tondora, J., Lawless, M.S., O'Connell, M., and Rowe, M. (2009). *A Practical Guide to Recovery-Oriented Practice Tools for Transforming Mental Health Care.* Oxford: Oxford University Press.

Hopper, K., Harrison, G., Janca, A., and Sartorius, N. (2007). *Recovery From Schizophrenia: An International Perspective. A Report From the WHO Collaborative Project, the International Study of Schizophrenia.* Oxford: Oxford University Press.

Perkins, R. and Repper, J. (2003). *Social Inclusion and Recovery.* London: Baillière Tindall.

Ralph, R.O. and Corrigan, P.W. (eds). (2005). *Recovery in mental illness. Broadening our Understanding of Wellness.* Washington, DC: American Psychological Association.

Slade, M. (2009). *Personal recovery and mental illness. A guide for mental health professionals.* Cambridge: Cambridge University Press.

References

Andresen, R., Oades, L., and Caputi, P. (2003). The experience of recovery from schizophrenia: towards an empirically-validated stage model. *Australian and New Zealand Journal of Psychiatry*, 37, 586–94.

Anthony, W.A. (1993). Recovery from mental illness: the guiding vision of the mental health system in the 1990s. *Innovations and Research*, 2, 17–24.

Barker, P.J., Davidson, B., and Campbell, P. (eds.) (1999). *From the Ashes of Experience.* London: Whurr Publications.

Barnett, H. and Lapsley, H. (2006). *Journeys of Despair, Journeys of Hope. Young Adults Talk About Severe Mental Distress, Mental Health Services and Recovery.* Wellington: Mental Health Commission.

Barrett, R.J. (1996). *The psychiatric team and the social definition of schizophrenia: An anthropological study of person and illness.* London: Cambridge University Press.

Bellack, A. (2006). Scientific and consumer models of recovery in schizophrenia: concordance, contrasts, and implications. *Schizophrenia Bulletin*, 32, 432–42.

Bleuler, M. (1978). *The schizophrenic disorders.* New Haven, CT: Yale University Press.

Borg, M. and Kristiansen, K. (2004). Recovery-oriented professionals: Helping relationships in mental health services. *Journal of Mental Health*, 13, 493–505.

Breggin, P. and Cohen, D. (2007). *Your Drug May Be Your Problem: How and Why to Stop Taking Psychiatric Medications.* Reading, MA: Perseus Books.

Ciompi, L. and Muller, C. (1976). *The life-course and aging of schizophrenics: a long-term follow-up study into old age.* Berlin: Springer.

Coleman, R. (1999). *Recovery – an Alien Concept.* Gloucester: Hansell.

Copeland, M.E. (1999). *Wellness Recovery Action Plan.* Brattleboro: VT: Peach Press.

Darton, K. (2005). *Making sense of coming off psychiatric drugs.* London: Mind.

Davidson, L. and Flanagan, E.H. (2007). 'Schizophrenics,' 'borderlines,' and the lingering legacy of misplaced concreteness: An examination of the persistent misconception that the DSM classifies people instead of disorders. *Psychiatry*, 70, 100–112.

Davidson, L. and Roe, D. (2007). Recovery from versus recovery in serious mental illness: One strategy for lessening confusion plaguing recovery. *Journal of Mental Health*, 16, 459–70.

Davidson, L. and White, W. (2007). The concept of recovery as an organizing principle for integrating mental health and addiction services. *Journal of Behavioral Health Services & Research*, 34, 109–20.

Davidson, L. and Strauss, J. (1992). Sense of self in recovery from severe mental illness. *British Journal of Medical Psychology*, 65, 131–45.

Davidson, L., Sells, D., Sangster, S., and O'Connell, M. (2005). Qualitative studies of recovery: what can we learn from the person? In: Ralph, R.O. and Corrigan, P.W. (eds.) *Recovery in Mental Illness. Broadening our Understanding of Wellness*, pp. 147–70. Washington, DC: American Psychological Association.

Davidson, L., Drake, R.E., Schmutte, T., Dinzeo, T., and Andres-Hyman, R. (2009a). Oil and water or oil and vinegar? Evidence-based medicine meets recovery. *Community Mental Health Journal*, 45, 323–32.

Davidson, L., O'Connell, M., and Tondora, J. (2009b). Conclusion: Making sure the person is involved in person-centred care. In: Rudnick, A. and Roe, D. (eds.), *Serious mental illness (SMI): person-centered approaches.* London Routledge, in press.

Deegan, P. (1988). Recovery: the lived experience of rehabilitation. *Psychosocial Rehabilitation Journal*, 11, 11–19.

Deegan, P. (2005). The importance of personal medicine. *Scandinavian Journal of Public Health*, 33, 29–35.

Deegan, P. (2007). The lived experience of using psychiatric medication in the recovery process and a shared decision-making program to support it. *Psychiatric Rehabilitation Journal*, 31, 62–9.

Deegan, P., Rapp, C., Holter, M., and Riefer, M. (2008). A program to support shared decision making in an outpatient psychiatric medication clinic. *Psychiatric Services*, 59, 603–5.

DeSisto, M.J., Harding, C.M., McCormick, R.V., Ashikage, T., and Brooks, G. (1995). The Maine and Vermont three-decades studies of serious mental illness: II. *Longitudinal course. British Journal of Psychiatry*, 167, 338–42.

Fisher, D.V. (1994). Health care reform based on an empowerment model of recovery by people with psychiatric disabilities. *Hospital and Community Psychiatry*, 45, 913–15.

Goldsack, S., Reet, M., Lapsley, H., and Gingell, M. (2005). *Experiencing a Recovery-Oriented Acute Mental Health Service: Home Based Treatment from the Perspectives of Services Users, their Families and Mental Health Professionals.* Wellington: Mental Health Commission.

Gregory, R.J., Canning, S.S., Lee, T.W., and Wise, J.C. (2004). Cognitive bibliotherapy for depression: A meta-analysis. *Professional Psychology: Research and Practice*, **35**, 275–80.

Guyatt, G. and Rennie, D. (eds.) (2002). *Users' guide to the medical literature: A manual for evidence-based clinical practice*. Chicago, IL: American Medical Association Press.

Harding, C.M., Brooks, G., Ashikage, T., Strauss, J.S., and Brier, A. (1987). The Vermont longitudinal study of persons with severe mental illness II: long-term outcome of subjects who retrospectively met DSM-III criteria for schizophrenia. *American Journal of Psychiatry*, **144**, 727–35.

Harrison, G., Hopper, K., Craig, T., Laska, E., Siegel, C., Wanderling, J., *et al.* (2001). Recovery from psychotic illness: a 15- and 25-year international follow-up study. *British Journal of Psychiatry*, **178**, 506–17.

Huber, G., Gross, G., and Schuttler, R. (1975). A long-term follow-up study of schizophrenia: Psychiatric course and prognosis. *Acta Psychiatrica Scandinavica*, **52**, 49–57.

Icarus Project and Freedom Center (2007). *Harm Reduction Guide to Coming Off Psychiatric Drugs*. http://theicarusproject net/ HarmReductionGuideComingOffPsychDrugs.

Lakhan, S.E. and Vieira, K.F. (2008). Nutritional therapies for mental disorders. *Nutrition Journal* **7**, 2.

Lapsley, H., Nikora, L.W., and Black, R. (2002). *Kia Mauri Tau! Narratives of Recovery from Disabling Mental Health Problems*. Wellington: Mental Health Commission.

Lehmann, P. (ed.) (2004). *Coming off Psychiatric Drugs: Successful Withdrawal from Neuroleptics, Antidepressants, Lithium, Carbamazepine and Tranquilizers*. Shrewsbury: Peter Lehmann Publishing.

Libermann, R.P. (2002). Future directions for research studies and clinical work on recovery from schizophrenia: Questions with some answers. *International Review of Psychiatry*, **14**, 337–42.

Libermann, R.P. and Kopelowicz, A. (2002). Recovery from schizophrenia: a challenge for the 21st century. *International Review of Psychiatry*, **14**, 242–55.

Marneros, A., Deister, A., Rohde, A., Steinmeyer, E.M., and Junemann, H. (1989). Long-term outcome of schizoaffective and schizophrenic disorders, a comparative study, I: Definitions, methods, psychopathological and social outcome. *European Archives of Psychiatry and Clinical Neuroscience*, **238**, 118–25.

McIntosh, Z. (2005). *From Goldfish Bowl to Ocean: personal accounts of mental illness and beyond*. London: Chipmunkapublishing.

Mental Health Commission (2000). *Three forensic service users and their families talk about recovery*. Wellington: Mental Health Commission.

Mental Health Commission (2001). *Recovery Competencies. Teaching Resource Kit*. Wellington: Mental Health Commission.

Meyer, T. and Broocks, A. (2000). Therapeutic impact of exercise on psychiatric diseases: guidelines for exercise testing and prescription. *Sports Medicine*, **30**, 269–79.

Ogawa, K., Miya, M., Watarai, A., Nakazawa, M., Yuasa, S., and Utena, H. (1987). A long-term follow-up study of schizophrenia in Japan, with special reference to the course of social adjustment. *British Journal of Psychiatry*, **151**, 758–65.

O'Hagan, M. (1996). Two accounts of mental distress. In: Read, J. and Reynolds, J. (eds.) *Speaking our Minds*, pp. 44–50. London: Macmillan.

Ralph, R.O. (2000). Recovery. *Psychiatric Rehabilitation Skills*, **4**, 480–517.

Ralph, R.O. and Corrigan, P.W. (eds.) (2005). *Recovery in mental illness. Broadening our Understanding of Wellness*. Washington, DC: American Psychological Association.

Ridgway P. (2001). Restorying psychiatric disability: Learning from first person narratives. *Psychiatric Rehabilitation Journal*, **24**, 335–43.

Sackett, D., Rosenberg, W.M.C., Gray, J.A.M., Haynes, R.B., and Richardson, W.S. (1996). Evidence based medicine: what it is and what it isn't: It's about integrating individual clinical expertise and the best external evidence. *British Medical Journal*, **312**, 71–2.

Schrank, B. and Slade, M. (2007). Recovery in psychiatry. *Psychiatric Bulletin*, **31**, 321–5.

Scottish Recovery Network (2006). *Journeys of Recovery. Stories of hope and recovery from long term mental health problems*. Glasgow: Scottish Recovery Network.

Scottish Recovery Network (2007). *Routes to recovery. Collected wisdom from the SRN Narrative Research Project*. Glasgow: Scottish Recovery Network.

Secker, J., Membrey, H., Grove, B., and Seebohm, P. (2002). Recovering from illness or recovering your life? Implications of clinical versus social models of recovery from mental health problems for employment support services. *Disability & Society*, **17**, 403–18.

Seligman, M. (2002). *Authentic happiness: Using the new positive psychology to realize your potential for lasting fulfillment*. New York: Free Press.

Shepherd, G., Boardman, J., and Slade, M. (2008). *Making recovery a reality*. Briefing Paper. London: Sainsbury Centre for Mental Health.

Slade, M. (2009a). *Personal recovery and mental illness. A guide for mental health professionals*. Cambridge: Cambridge University Press.

Slade, M. (2009b). The contribution of mental health services to recovery. *Journal of Mental Health*, 18, 367–71.

Slade, M. (2009c). *100 ways to support recovery*. London: Rethink.

Slade, M., Amering, M., and Oades, L. (2008). Recovery: an international perspective. *Epidemiologia e Psichiatria Sociale*, **17**, 128–37.

South London and Maudsley NHS Foundation Trust (2007). *Social Inclusion, Rehabilitation and Recovery Strategy 2007–2010*. London: South London and Maudsley NHS Foundation Trust.

Spaniol, L. and Koehler, M. (eds) (1994). *The experience of recovery*. Boston, MA: Center for Psychiatric Rehabilitation.

Spaniol, L., Wewiorski, N., Gagne, C., and Anthony, W. (2002). The process of recovery from schizophrenia. *International Review of Psychiatry*, **14**, 327–36.

Tsuang, M.T., Woolson, R.F., and Fleming, J. (1979). Long-term outcome of major psychosis. *Archives of General Psychiatry*, **36**, 1295–301.

Watkins, J. (2007). *Healing Schizophrenia: Using Medication Wisely*. Victoria: Michelle Anderson.

Whitley, R., Harris, M., Fallot, R.D., and Berley, R.W. (2008). The active ingredients of intentional recovery communities: Focus group evaluation. *Journal of Mental Health*, **17**, 173–82.

SECTION 3

Needs: perspectives and assessment

CHAPTER 5

The application of epidemiology to mental disorders

Glyn H. Lewis, Antonia Errazuriz, Hollie V. Thomas, Mary Cannon, and Peter B. Jones

Introduction

In this chapter we shall present the main tools used by epidemiologists to measure the occurence and aetiology of disease in populations, and we shall summarize the results of epidemiological studies when applied to mental disorders.

Epidemiology of neurosis

Diagnostic boundaries

There is a long-running controversy over the nature and relevance of diagnoses in studies of common mental disorders involving mood disturbance, particularly depression, and anxiety. Studies have tended either to concentrate on depression or treated psychiatric disorder in the community as a single category. Much of the literature has concentrated on investigating depression despite the evidence that depression and anxiety disorders have different risk factors being relatively sparse (Eaton and Ritter, 1988). There is also evidence that depression and generalized anxiety disorder have the same genetic vulnerability (Kendler et al., 1993) The main difference between the mental health of individuals can be explained in terms of a single dimension, but there are also likely to be factors that increase the risk of, e.g. depression, over and above the risk of common mental disorder. We acknowledge, too, that the term neurosis is, itself, controversial, but consider it to retain enough useful meaning in the current context.

Descriptive epidemiology

In community surveys the majority of the population have at least one neurotic symptom at any one time. For example, in the British Health and Lifestyle survey (Cox et al., 1987), 70% of the population reported at least one of the symptoms on the General Health Questionnaire (GHQ) (Goldberg and Williams, 1988). In that sense, the abnormal individuals are those without a neurotic symptom. Fatigue and sleep problems were the most common symptoms in two, consecutive major surveys of psychiatric morbidity in Great Britain in 1993 and 2000, being present in 27% and

29% of the population, respectively (Jenkins et al., 1997; Singleton et al., 2001). Irritability and worry are also more common than depression and anxiety.

In the first of these, the Office of Population Censuses and Surveys (OPCS) National Survey of Psychiatric Morbidity (Jenkins et al., 1997), about 15% of the population had a neurotic psychiatric disorder in the week before interview. The threshold in this study indicates a degree of symptomatology that would concern a primary care physician. Twenty-one per cent of those studied in the multinational World Health Organization (WHO) study of common mental disorders in primary care fulfilled one or more diagnoses from the 10th revision of the International Classification of Disease (ICD-10), mostly neurotic conditions (Ormel et al., 1994). Table 5.1 shows the prevalence of the main neurotic disorders from four population-based studies and the WHO study of primary care. There are quite marked differences in prevalence between the surveys. These result from using different diagnostic criteria, different assessments for psychiatric disorders, and geographical and temporal variation.

Gender

Women generally have more neurotic disorders, of whatever type, than men in community surveys. It is usually stated that there are two exceptions, social phobias and obsessive–compulsive disorder, but this was not the case in the three United Kingdom surveys of 1993, 2000, and 2007 where obsessive–compulsive disorder was consistently more prevalent in women (Jenkins et al., 1997; McManus et al., 2009; Singleton et al., 2001). There are also some studies where the gender difference is less marked than those done in the United Kingdom and United States (Jenkins, 1985).

There are a number of possible explanations for neurosis being more common in women than in men. Many of the studies are cross-sectional and so the excess prevalence may result from either a higher incidence in women or a longer duration of illness though longitudinal studies have usually confirmed a higher incidence. The difference between the sexes may result because women are more likely to divulge details of their emotional life or be more aware of them. One other possibility is some underlying inherited

Table 5.1 Prevalence (%) of neurotic disorders from four population surveys, and from an international primary care study

	ECA, US[1]	OPCS, UK[2]	ONS, UK[3]	NCS, US[4]	WHO, PHC[5]
Period prevalence	1 month	1 week	1 week	12 months	12 months
Depression	2.4	2.2	2.6	10.3	10.5
Phobias total	6.7[a]	2.2	2.6		
Agoraphobia	7.6[a]			2.8	1.5
Social phobia	3.2[a]			7.9	
Specific phobia	15.1[a]			8.8	
Panic disorder	0.5	1.0	1.2	2.3	1.1
Obsessive–compulsive disorder	1.3	1.4	1.3		
Generalized anxiety disorder	1.3	4.4	4.7	3.1	7.9
Any common mental disorder or 'neurosis'		15.5	17.6		
Diagnostic criteria	DSM-III	ICD-10	ICD-10	DSM-III-R	ICD-10

[1] ECA 5 US sites (Robins and Regier, 1991).
[2] 1993 OPCS National Survey of Psychiatric Morbidity. Results taken from Table 2.4 (McManus et al., 2009).
[3] Adult psychiatric morbidity in England, 2007: Results of a household survey (McManus et al., 2009).
[4] US National Comorbidity Survey (Kessler et al., 1994).
[5] WHO Primary Care study (Ormel et al., 1994).
[a] Lifetime prevalence.

or acquired characteristic, e.g. related to endocrine differences or differences in upbringing. Alternatively, differences between the sexes may result from differences in environmental factors in development, e.g. sexual abuse is more common in girls than in boys.

One of the most likely explanations for the gender difference concerns the different social roles occupied by men and women. Women are more likely to be in low status jobs and are also more likely to have many competing roles, e.g. most women continue to provide childcare and home keeping while out at work. Studies that investigate relatively homogenous groups of men and women, e.g. civil servants of the same grade, find that there is no gender difference in psychiatric disorder (Jenkins, 1985).

Socioeconomic status

There are some contradictory results concerning whether neurotic disorders are commoner in those with lower socioeconomic status. It is likely that these can be accounted for by the varying way of measuring or conceptualizing socioeconomic status. There are three aspects of socioeconomic status that are commonly measured: occupational status, such as Registrar General Social Class as used in the United Kingdom, educational attainment, and standard of living. In a recent study it has been argued that a poor standard of living does show a consistent independent relationship with an increased prevalence of common mental disorder (Lewis et al., 1998). It is likely that this is mediated by delaying recovery from

episodes of depression. This is also probably true of the association between unemployment and psychiatric disorder (Weich and Lewis, 1998).

Geographical variation

Geographical variation in the rates of disease can help provide clues to aetiology and are also useful in planning services. There have been many reports that neurotic psychiatric disorders are commoner in urban areas, at least in Western societies (Blazer et al., 1985; Lewis and Booth, 1994). The reasons for this are not understood, though Brown and colleagues found that stressful life events were commoner in South London than North Uist in the Outer Hebrides, Scotland (Brown et al., 1977).

Disability

Major depression and other neurotic disorders are associated with profound morbidity and social impairment, equal to or in excess of that seen in many chronic physical illnesses (Wells et al., 1989). There is considerable impact on industry of neurotic disorder as well as direct costs on the health service (Croft-Jeffreys and Wilkinson, 1989; Smith et al., 1995). This can be forgotten by the psychiatrist or other mental health professional in secondary care where psychotic disorders are abound and are more disabling for the individual. For the community as a whole, though, depression and anxiety disorders are sufficiently common that they lead to a considerable aggregate burden that falls, mainly, on primary care. If one takes account of morbidity as well as mortality, then by the year 2020 unipolar depression will account for over 5% of the disability-adjusted life years lost to ill-health (Murray and Lopez, 1997), second only to ischaemic heart disease.

Epidemiology of needs assessment

It is important to remember that the epidemiological assessment of neurotic symptoms is different from an assessment of needs. It is relatively difficult to make assessments of need in this area as more knowledge is needed about the relationship between the epidemiological criteria for defining a case and the criteria for defining who would benefit from particular interventions. One study has attempted to relate the criteria used in admission to antidepressant trials to the assessment used in the OPCS National Survey in the UK. They concluded that up to 6% of the population might have a neurotic disorder that is severe enough to benefit from antidepressant medication. However, such figures have a number of limitations and need to be interpreted with caution.

Aetiology of common mental disorder

In the long term, preventive strategies for neurotic disorder will need to be based upon sound epidemiological findings concerning the environmental causes of the conditions. At the moment a public health approach towards preventing these conditions is premature but an important priority for research must be to understand more about the aetiology of these conditions and translate the findings into practical preventive strategies.

The literature on the aetiology of common mental disorder is voluminous and the suggestions of important aetiological factors correspondingly large. Three main areas have been studied: childhood experience, adult experience, and current stressors and personality. A genetic contribution has also been established but its nature is as yet unknown.

Childhood experience

Parental loss and separation

The seminal studies of Brown and Harris (1978) suggested that loss of the mother before 11 years increased the risk of adult depression. Subsequent studies have produced contradictory findings (Parker et al., 1992). Separation or loss of a parent rarely occurs in isolation and any association with neurotic disorder may be confounded by other variables. For example, childhood parental loss is often followed by socioeconomic disadvantage and inconsistent or inadequate parenting by alternative care-givers. Parker's work from Australia has also linked style of parenting during childhood to later depression, but also, albeit to a lesser extent, anxiety (Parker et al., 1979).

Other early experiences

There is considerable interest in the possibility that childhood sexual abuse increases the risk of neurotic disorder in adulthood. Community-based studies find that adults with a variety of neurotic diagnoses report increased rates of early traumatic sexual encounters (Angst and Vollrath, 1991; Brown et al., 1993). Disentangling the links between abuse and adult disorder is not easy, since child sexual abuse does not happen randomly, and is associated with other adversity, including poverty, parental discord, inadequate parenting, and physical abuse. However, child sexual abuse was independently associated with the prevalence of adult psychiatric disorder in a community survey from New Zealand (Mullen et al., 1993).

Although childhood experiences are important in the aetiology of adult neurosis, there is no simple relationship between childhood and adult neurotic disorder. Most emotionally disordered children do not become neurotic adults, and most neurotic disorders develop in adult life (Rutter, 1985). However, there is a striking continuity between depression as a child and depression as an adult (Harrington et al., 1990).

Adolescent experiences

In general, the literature on the social aetiology of neurosis concentrates on childhood predictors of adult disorder, and adult experiences. Mental health in childhood is also frequently addressed but the change from childhood to adulthood has received less attention. Specific issues such as unemployment (Banks and Jackson, 1982) and acute life events have been addressed (Goodyer et al., 1987). A recent community-based study showed that 17% of girls living at home showed evidence of psychiatric disorder—independent risk factors were maternal distress and the quality of the parental marriage (Monck et al., 1994).

Adult experiences and current stressors

Life events

The relationship between life events and neurotic disorder has been extensively reviewed elsewhere. This body of work has provided some of the most convincing evidence for establishing psychosocial environmental stresses as an important cause of depression. In particular, George Brown's work has been influential in arguing that the social context of life events and the meaning attached to them by the individual is also an important determinant of the likelihood of developing depression.

One of the limitations of the life-event approach is that it seems to have a limited relevance to public health. Life events, such as bereavement, are an inevitable part of the human condition.

Though other life events such as redundancy could, in principle, be influenced by economic policy, it is more likely that the context of the life event is more amenable to policy changes than the occurrence of life events themselves. Future research should include the role of the context of life events, e.g. poor housing, financial problems, or inadequate child care, in the hope of drawing conclusions that could potentially influence government policy or give more insight into the social and psychological mechanisms leading to depression.

Social support and social networks

One consistent finding is an association between poor social support and neurotic disorder. Brown and Harris (1978) found that women who lacked an intimate or confiding relationship had an increased risk of depression (in the presence of a life event). Scott Henderson and colleagues (1981) in Australia went on to find a more general association between neurotic disorder and lack of satisfaction with the social network. In the Epidemiologic Catchment Area (ECA) study, all anxiety disorders were commoner among the separated or divorced, whilst in New Zealand, females who were widowed, separated, or divorced were more likely to have neurotic disorder than those currently married (Romans et al., 1993).

There are two areas of controversy in this area. The first is the rather technical point of whether social support interacts with life events in increasing the risk of depression. In other words, is there a stronger association between life events and depression in the presence of poor social support? This issue depends upon the nature of the statistical model that is being used by the researchers (Alloway and Bebbington, 1987). Of more importance, however, is the question whether the association between poor social support and disorder is causal, or whether the association results from either a personality attribute or measurement bias resulting from depression. Henderson has argued for the latter while Brown maintains the former position.

Unemployment

Unemployment is associated with higher rates of neurosis (Jenkins et al., 1997). Warr has conducted some elegant studies showing that men made unemployed are at increased risk of developing neurotic disorder and their mental health improves when they return to work (Warr, 1987). The situation for women is more complicated because of the expectation of work within the home.

Physical illness

Physical and psychiatric illnesses are associated more than by chance alone. In general, there is a threefold increase in psychological disorder in people with medical illness. The relationship between physical and psychological illness is complex. Psychological disorder may result from illness or chronic disability. Sometimes physical and psychological illness may have a common aetiology, e.g. diseases of the central nervous system are more likely to have a coexistent psychiatric disorder. There may also be a Berksonian, or referral bias that leads to the association seen in health care settings. However, the commonest reason for the association between physical and psychological illness is somatization, illness behaviour, and its effect on symptom reporting.

Personality

It is widely assumed that personality characteristics are an important risk factor for developing neurotic disorder. Eysenck's neuroticism scale is claimed to be such a dimension, those scoring high on neuroticism having an increased risk of developing neurotic illness (Eysenck and Eysenck, 1964). However, there is a considerable overlap between the questions asked by neuroticism scales and the actual symptoms of neurotic disorder. A number of studies (Coppen and Metcalfe, 1965; Hirschfeld et al., 1983; Kendell and DiScipio, 1968) have found that neuroticism scale scores are closely correlated with measures of neurotic disorder and change with recovery from depression. Duncan-Jones et al. (1990) have also argued, with evidence from statistical models, that the neuroticism scale is effectively measuring the same thing as the average level of neurotic psychiatric disorder measured by the GHQ. Nevertheless the idea of a general liability to develop neurotic symptoms, with a genetic contribution, is probably an important part of the aetiology of neurotic disorder.

An alternative and perhaps complementary approach is based upon theories of personality developed by social learning theorists. For example, Warr's studies on unemployment have found that 'commitment to work' is related to poor mental health during unemployment and good mental health in employment (Warr, 1987). Work commitment was assessed by a short and simple scale incorporating attitudinal questions such as 'If you had won a million pounds would you still want to work?'. This series of studies provides a model for studying personal attributes and their relationship with mental illness and show an interaction between personality and the impact of a life event. They also illustrate the link between an individual's attitudes and societal norms, in this instance, the social and economic importance of the 'work ethic'.

The role of genetic factors

We have already noted that genetic factors, known to be important in a wide range of mental disorders, are most likely shared between different diagnoses or manifestations of illness (Kendler et al., 1993). Recent studies involving scans of the entire genome looking for particularly relevant genes (genome-wide association studics (GWAS); Donnelly, 2008) indicate that many, rather than few genes appear to contribute to an individual's risk and that even with this formulation the size of genetic effects in terms of single genes or systems are likely to be very small in comparison with the environmental and interpersonal events discussed in the preceding paragraphs (Bosker et al., 2010). The conceptual problem is that these events and the likely combinations of risk genes are so common. One intriguing possibility is that it is the interactions between genetic diathesis, or risk, and life events that determine vulnerability, perhaps interacting with other factors such as stage of the life course at which adversity is encountered. Thus, having particular sets of genes, and particular adversities during a certain window of vulnerability and on top of specific personality characteristics, might be each be considered to have a probability akin to throwing a six with a die, but throwing four sixes with four dice at the same time is a rarer event; in fact, neurotic disorder is more common than this.

Evidence for such interactions has been sought in appropriate samples over the recent decade. An initial finding in the Dunedin birth cohort of moderation by a polymorphism in the serotonin transporter gene (a biologically plausible candidate) of the effect of early childhood life stress on risk of depression in adult life stimulated enormous interest in this formulation of the illness (Caspi et al., 2003). Many replications followed though have tailed-off such that a recent meta-analysis indicated no such interactional effect (Risch et al., 2009), a controversial finding that is likely to trigger rather than prevent further work in this area for depression as well as other disorders such as the psychoses, considered below.

Epidemiology of psychosis

Diagnostic preamble

As for neurosis, the question as to what is a case is fundamental to counting, treating, or establishing cause. The debate surrounding the definition of diagnostic categories within psychosis has been fierce (Clare, 1980) and continues to this day as numerous committees meet to debate how the *Diagnostic and Statistical Manual of Mental Disorders* (DSM) and ICD classifications (see below) are to be recast such that their members can agree. As now, over the century since our modern concepts of schizophrenia and bipolar affective disorder were first described, opinion has varied considerably as to how best to define them and, indeed, whether they existed at all. This is esoteric stuff for the clinician and service planner faced with the imperative of people with delusions, hallucinations, thought disorder, negative features, severe depression, or mania.

The disturbance and disability involving individuals, carers, and community seem a long way from academic arguments about operational criteria. Current research is focusing once more on diagnostic boundaries, but is more inclusive within the psychoses. Ultimately, a classification based upon causes or mechanisms may be a goal. For the moment, many services are making routine diagnoses and management returns using standard operational criteria such as those defined in the ICD-10 (World Health Organization, 1994). This is favoured by European psychiatrists and is similar to its American step-sister, DSM-IV (American Psychiatric Association, 1994). Both these systems have undergone a 'narrowing' in their definitions of schizophrenia and other psychotic syndromes from previous to present versions. Together with a more general recent history of the schizophrenia concept, these are considered by Cannon and Jones (1996).

From the point of view of a community psychiatric service, the majority of people with psychosis will have syndromes adequately described by schizophrenia or non-affective psychosis. These will outnumber those with affective psychoses, such as bipolar disorder and psychotic depression, by about fivefold, although the needs of this group may be high (see below). There will be smaller group with other psychotic syndromes, including those related to drugs.

In some quarters the pendulum has swung towards talk of 'severe mental illness' (SMI), a catch-all term, too loose for epidemiology. The term is of some use to service planning where many requirements are common across diagnoses, and where there is heterogeneity of needs within any one diagnosis. Post hoc attempts to define this term have invoked composite notions of diagnosis, severity, disability and duration. As mentioned above, the majority of this 'SMI' comprises schizophrenia.

The advantage of the term is that it puts the concept of needs to the fore. The danger is that aspects of care specific to individual diagnoses may be forgotten. This is particularly the case for those people with neurotic syndromes that may be severe, disabling, and long-lasting. A person with severe OCD may benefit from common aspects of a service designed for the majority of people with SMI who have schizophrenia. However, they also need distinct therapy that will be left untried if diagnostic accuracy and precision are neglected. Similarly, 'blue skies' research concerning causes and mechanisms, referred to earlier in this chapter may be impossible if there are no boundaries, although some research is relevant to a wider group. Just the same problems apply to another catch-all term, first episode psychosis, or the so-called, at-risk mental states. These have become popular over the past decade with the establishment of specialist services to target those in the early stages of disorder when intervention may be more effective. In this chapter we have been using recent operational definitions when we refer to schizophrenia but stick to that term because the majority of epidemiological evidence refers to that concept.

Descriptive epidemiology

The low incidence (10–40 cases per 100,000 per year) and assumptions about relatively low lifetime prevalence (0.5–1%) of schizophrenia in the population has led to a reliance on case–control study designs in research. Chronic patients recruited from hospital wards are compared with volunteer controls from the community and consequent problems of bias and confounding have led to many contradictory findings that are not replicated. For a time, it looked as though schizophrenia would prove to be the undoing of epidemiologists (Cannon and Jones, 1996) just as it had once been the 'graveyard of neuropathologists' (Plum, 1972). Over the past two decades, however, the application of advances in cohort and case–control methodology to psychiatric epidemiology, have led increasingly to more robust results (Lewis and Pelosi, 1990).

Incidence and time trends

Examination of incidence rates may be potentially more informative than prevalence of schizophrenia. The latter can be influenced by many factors such as changes in treatment and changes in mortality rate; both are affected by changes in the age and sex structure of the population (see below). Ideally, incidence studies should be based on community incidence samples but, as this is difficult to achieve, case registers and hospital admission data are commonly used. A recent systematic review of the international literature on the incidence of schizophrenia using the best quality evidence available reported a median incidence per person (10–90% quartile) of 15.2 (7.7–43.0) per 100,000 (McGrath et al., 2004). The broad precision estimate shows that the estimates from different samples must vary as well as being a comment on the rarity of the condition.

Whether or not the occurrence of schizophrenia is changing is an even more difficult question to answer than is merely trying to estimate incidence at any one time. Eagles and Whalley first reported a decline in the diagnosis of schizophrenia among first admissions in Scotland between 1969 and 1978 (Eagles and Whalley, 1985). There have since been 22 further papers examining this issue in England (Bamrah et al., 1991; Boydell et al., 2003; Castle et al., 1991; Crow et al., 1990; Der et al., 1990; Harrison et al., 1991; Kirkbride et al., 2009; Nixon and Doody, 2005), Scotland (Allardyce et al., 2000; Eagles et al., 1988; Geddes et al., 1993; Kendell et al., 1993), Denmark (Munk-Jørgensen, 1986; Munk-Jorgensen and Mortensen, 1992; Tsuchiya and Munk-Jørgensen, 2002), Sweden (Ösby et al., 2001), Finland (Suvisaari et al., 1999), New Zealand (Joyce, 1987), Canada (Nicole et al., 1992), Ireland (Waddington and Youssef, 1994), the United States (Stoll et al., 1993), and the Netherlands (Oldehinkel and Giel, 1995). Those based on national statistics have found a large (40–50%) decline in first admission rates for schizophrenia

during the 1970s and the 1980s (Bamrah et al., 1991; Castle et al., 1991; Joyce, 1987; Munk-Jorgensen and Mortensen, 1992). Findings based on case-register data have had less consistent findings and indeed, three such studies from Camberwell (Boydell et al., 2003; Castle et al., 1991) and Salford (Bamrah et al., 1991) in the United Kingdom actually found an increase in the incidence of schizophrenia during the same period. Others have reported no change in the incidence of schizophrenia over time (Kirkbride et al., 2009; Nixon and Doody, 2005) or a decrease in first-admission rates only among women (Kendell et al., 1993; Oldehinkel and Giel, 1995; Waddington and Youssef, 1994).

The major question is whether the decrease noted in first admission rates corresponds to an actual decrease in the incidence of the condition. Many factors influence this apparent 'administrative decline' in schizophrenia. The introduction of more restrictive diagnostic criteria for schizophrenia may cause a shift to diagnoses such as 'borderline states' (Munk-Jørgensen, 1986) or affective psychosis (Oldehinkel and Giel, 1995; Stoll et al., 1993). The move to community care over the past two decades could have affected hospital admission rates (Nicole et al., 1992). Clinicians' attitudes have changed and they are now more reluctant to make a diagnosis of schizophrenia on the first hospital admission (Munk-Jørgensen, 1986), and this could lead to a spurious fall in incidence rates over the last few years of the period under observation. Private health insurance companies' policies regarding schizophrenia may be partly responsible for this effect (Stoll et al., 1993). Changes in the age, sex, and ethnic structure of the population over the period under study have not been taken into account in most studies. The two areas of the United Kingdom that have shown an increased incidence of schizophrenia—Camberwell and Salford—are both areas with a high proportion of immigrants (Bamrah et al., 1991; Boydell et al., 2003; Castle et al., 1991). Unfortunately, schizophrenia has such a low incidence that it may be impossible to disentangle all these effects and reach any firm conclusions regarding changes in incidence in the developed world in recent decades (Jablensky, 1995).

Geographical variation

In 1978 a large multicentre study of schizophrenia was initiated by WHO, the Ten-Country Study, to provide information about the incidence, course, and outcome of schizophrenia in different cultures (Jablensky et al., 1992). Two case-definitions of schizophrenia were used: a broad, clinical definition comprising ICD-9 schizophrenia and paranoid psychoses, and a narrow, restrictive definition including only cases classified as 'nuclear' schizophrenia using the CATEGO computer program (Wing et al., 1974). For narrowly defined schizophrenia rates ranged only between 7 and 14 per 100,000 per year. The parsimonious conclusion is that rates for narrowly-defined schizophrenia are the same in all centres. However, confidence intervals for these estimates were wide and there may not have been sufficient statistical power to detect differences.

The incidence rates for broadly-defined schizophrenia do seem to vary between countries, (range 16–42 per 100,000), and the rates for centres in the developing world were about twice as high as those in the developed world. However, the variation in incidence rates for schizophrenia worldwide is very small compared with illnesses such as ischaemic heart disease or cancer which are known to have major environmental risk factors.

Prevalence

The lifetime prevalence of schizophrenia in the Western world seems to lie somewhere between 0.4% and 1.4%, and may have decreased over the past decade with a major systematic review conducted in 2005 estimating it to be at the lower end of this estimate (0.4%, 0.02–1.21) (Saha et al., 2005). However, a more recent study from Finland indicates that the lifetime prevalence for any psychotic disorder is between 2.7% and 3.5% (Perala et al., 2007). This disparity reinforces the point that narrow definitions of disorders can lead to considerable underestimates of morbidity in the population.

Two major prevalence studies of psychiatric illness have been carried out in the United States and indicate a decrease in prevalence of schizophrenia over one decade. The ECA programme (Keith et al., 1991) surveyed 17,803 persons between 1980 and 1984 and found a lifetime prevalence of schizophrenia of 1.4%. The National Co-morbidity Survey (NCS) (Kessler et al., 1994) interviewed 8098 people between 1990 and 1992 and found that lifetime prevalence for the summary category of non-affective psychosis was 0.7%. This discrepancy may be related to issues of sampling, interview methodology, or actual change over time and remain to be clarified by future reports.

The 1993 OPCS Psychiatric Morbidity Survey (Jenkins et al., 1997; Mason and Wilkinson, 1996; Meltzer et al., 1996) indicated that 4 per 1000 people of working age living in private households had experienced psychosis in the previous 12 months. This has been remarkably consistent over the two subsequent household surveys by the Office of National Statistics (ONS) in 2000 and 2007 with the authors commenting in 2009 that there had been no change in the occurrence of probably psychosis between the two later surveys in which 0.5% of 16- to 74-year-olds screened positively in both studies (McManus et al., 2009). These British prevalence estimates are lower than those found in the NCS although 37% of those who screened positive for psychosis in the British studies refused a second diagnostic interview, so the true prevalence may be been somewhat higher. Furthermore, some people with psychosis will have been in residential care so outside the scope of these household surveys.

A number of other studies have been undertaken in the United Kingdom and Ireland to define the prevalence of a more tightly defined schizophrenia syndrome. Some of these have been summarized by Jeffreys et al. (1997) and are shown in Table 5.2, adapted and updated, together with rates from more recent studies. The results show a fairly tight range, with studies yielding prevalence estimates of between 1.7 to 7.8 cases per 1000 after correction for the age of the population. Such age correction is useful given the fact that schizophrenia is a disorder of adult life, rather than of the extremes of age. This range is consistent with a point prevalence rate of 4.6 per 1000 persons (1.9–10.0) estimated in a recent systematic review of international studies on schizophrenia (Saha et al., 2005).

The more recent studies indicate that the prevalence may be higher in urban than in rural populations. This has already been alluded to in terms of incidence, but a similar finding is of key importance for service planning, and for understanding the factors associated with causation and determinants of outcome.

Age and sex distribution

Total lifetime risk for schizophrenia appears to be just about equal in both sexes (Jablensky et al., 1992; Keith et al., 1991) but the details of the relationship with the life course differ for men and women.

Table 5.2 Prevalence studies of schizophrenia in the United Kingdom and Ireland

Study (type of study)	Place	Schizophrenia prevalence rate per 1000 total population
Wing (1976)[1] (CR, U:point)	Camberwell	2.0
Wing (1976)[1] (CR, U:point)	Salford	2.8
Freeman and Alpert (1986)[2] (CR, U: 1 year)	Salford Nithsdale	6.8* a 2.4
McCreadie (1982)[2] (K, R: point)	Dublin, Ireland	1.7
Walsh (1986)[1] (CR, U:point)	Three Counties, Ireland	2.5*
Walsh (1986)[1] (CR, R:point)	Co. Cavan, Ireland	4.9
Youssef et al. (1991)[2] (K, R: 1 year)	S. Camden[3] N. Camden[3]	7.1* [3.3]
Harvey et al. (1996) (K, U:point)	Hampstead South London	[4.6]* 7.3
Jeffreys et al. (1997) (K, U:point)	England, Scotland and Wales	[4.9] 4.7
Thornicroft et al. (1998)[2] (K, U, 1 year; all psychosis)		[2.2] 5.1
Leask et al. (2000) (CR, lifetime up to age 28)		[3.0] 5.9* [3.5]* 7.7 a [6.7] 4
Leask et al. (2000) (CR, lifetime up to age 43)	England, Scotland, and Wales	(2.3) 4
Ruggeri et al. (2000) (HSS, U:1 year)	South London	[[7.8]] *** a
Macpherson et al. (2003) (HSS, U: 2 month)	Gloucester	3.3 ** a
McCullagh et al. (2003) (HSS, point)	Eastern England	1.8 **** b

CR, case register; K, key informant: HSS, Health Service Survey; U, urban; R, rural
* Age correction (15 plus). ** Age correction (18–65). *** Age correction (19 plus). **** Age correction (18–64).
a All psychosis.b Non-affective psychosis
[1] Data available in Torrey (1987).
[2] Data available in Jeffreys et al. (1997).
[3] Camden data based on population estimates near census (Harvey, 1996; Harvey et al., 1996).
[4] Details available from authors.
Figures in [] refers to patients with DSM-III-R diagnosis of schizophrenia.
Figures in () refers to patients with CATEGO narrow diagnosis of schizophrenia (S+)
Figures in [[]] refers to diagnosis of with Severe Mental Illness (broad psychosis) using OPCRIT

Schizophrenia can occur at any age (Asarnow and Asarnow, 1994; Castle et al., 1991; Van Os et al., 1995); but onset is commonly in early adulthood. The mean age of onset for males is 3 to 4 years earlier than for females, irrespective of whether 'onset' of schizophrenia is defined as first sign of mental disorder, first psychotic symptom, or first hospital admission (Häfner et al., 1993). The peak age of onset for males is between 15 and 30 years while females have a slower and more even rate of onset with a peak between the ages of 20 and 35 years and a second smaller peak after the age of 45 years. No satisfactory explanation yet exists for this sex difference.

Social class

An association between schizophrenia and low social class was confirmed by the ECA prevalence study which showed that schizophrenic patients in the United States were 10 times more likely to be in the lowest socioeconomic group than the highest. Evidence from birth cohorts in Britain, (Done et al., 1994; Jones et al., 1994) and Finland (Aro et al., 1995) show that this relationship is not causal, as schizophrenic patients at birth have the same socioeconomic distribution as the general population. What is remarkable is the steep decline in social status that accompanies the illness and is evident even before the clinical onset (Jones et al., 1993). This decline is far greater than that experienced by patients with severe affective disorder. Recent evidence (Croudace et al., 2000) suggests a non-linear gradient between summary scores of deprivation and occurrence of psychosis in the United Kingdom This study demonstrated a disproportionate amount of incidence and administrative prevalence (admissions) in the most deprived areas (Dauncey et al., 1993). These findings have been taken further by recent studies investigating the quality of the social and interpersonal environment at the neighbourhood level. Compared with neighbourhoods with medial levels of social cohesion and trust, incidence rates of schizophrenia have been found to be significantly higher in neighbourhoods with low (incidence rate ratio (IRR) 2.0) and high (IRR 2.5) levels of these characteristics (Kirkbride et al., 2008).

Marital status

People with schizophrenia are unlikely to be married though, if they are, they have a better clinical and social outcome than single patients (Jablensky et al., 1992). Marriage may, of course, merely reflect better premorbid social adjustment and later age at onset, both independent predictors of good outcome. However the prevalence of schizophrenia among separated or divorced people in the United States (2.9%) is similar to that among single people (2.1%), suggesting that marriage may confer an independent protective effect (Keith et al., 1991). An interaction between marital status and gender was found in the 1-year follow-up of the ECA study (Tien and Eaton, 1992). Single women were 14 times more likely to develop schizophrenia than married women, but single men were almost 50 times more likely to develop schizophrenia than their married counterparts. The role of marital status as a risk indicator or modifier for schizophrenia requires further study. However, it is clear that the basic characteristics of a population will predict some of the requirements of a community psychiatric service, in terms of its provision for those with psychosis.

Ethnicity and migrant status

Gender, age, and social characteristics of a community all, therefore, have a bearing on service requirements. However, migration and ethnic group are the two least understood and emotive factors that have a massive effect on the services that must be provided and that may hold keys to understanding the genesis of psychosis.

To date no single indigenous ethnic group appears to have a significantly higher occurrence of schizophrenia than any other, although some 'pockets' of high prevalence may exist in isolated areas such as North Sweden (Böök et al., 1978). The west of Ireland (Torrey, 1980, 1987) and the Istrian peninsula in Croatia (Crocetti et al., 1971) had previously been identified as 'high-risk' cultures but the higher incidence and prevalence rates originally found among these peoples are now thought to be due to bias (Eaton, 1991), The ECA study (Keith et al., 1991) found a higher prevalence for schizophrenia among black people than among white people in the United States (2.1% vs. 1.4%). However, controlled for age, gender, marital status, and, most importantly, socioeconomic group, the difference disappeared. The ÆSOP study conducted in the United Kingdom has reported remarkably high IRRs for both schizophrenia and manic psychosis in both African-Caribbeans (schizophrenia 9.1, manic psychosis 8.0) and black Africans (schizophrenia 5.8, manic psychosis 6.2) in both men and women (Fearon et al., 2006).

Schizophrenia in immigrants

The report of a 10-fold increase in the incidence of schizophrenia among the African-Caribbean population in Nottingham (Harrison et al., 1988) is yet to be explained. It has been convincingly replicated in other centres in the United Kingdom (King et al., 1994; Thomas et al., 1993; Van Os et al., 1994; Wessely et al., 1991), again in Nottingham (Harrison et al., 1997), and in the Netherlands (Selten and Sijben, 1994). In these replications the incidence ratio has been rather lower (3–4) when the denominator has been adjusted for possible under-reporting in census data (King et al., 1994; Van Os et al., 1995, 1996), An increased incidence ratio for schizophrenia has also been found among African and Asian (King et al., 1994) immigrants in the United Kingdom, indicating that the effect is not confined solely to a single ethnic minority, a conclusion supported by the ÆSOP study mentioned previously (Fearon et al., 2006). Whether some migrant groups escape the increased risk is a matter of current research.

The hospital admission rate for schizophrenia among migrants is higher in their host country than in their country of origin, (Burke, 1974; Hickling, 1991; Odegaard, 1932) implicating factors occurring principally after migration. The risk of schizophrenia is greater for second-generation migrants than first-generation migrants (Coid et al., 2008; McGovern and Cope, 1987) arguing against selective migration of pre-schizophrenic individuals. Both first- and second-generation migrants are exposed to psychosocial stresses, but these may have differential effects on generations exposed to different socioeconomic climates or other epigenetic events (Sugarman and Craufurd, 1994). The fact that immigrants from poor countries tend to show higher rates of schizophrenia than immigrants from affluent countries, implicates factors associated with improved living conditions, industrialization, or urbanization. There is as yet little evidence to support more 'biological' explanations (Eagles, 1991; Warner, 1995) and the emphasis for research is on the effect of stress associated with being a visible minority in a host country, an effect that trickles down generations and is probably amplified by more general socioeconomic disadvantage.

Thus, the evidence for a unique epidemic of schizophrenia among certain immigrant groups is not conclusive, but is intriguing. Possible confounders such as low socioeconomic and marital status may reduce the incidence ratio even further. Ethnicity probably represents a 'proxy' variable for a variety of social and perhaps biological factors. Once these are controlled, there may be little or no residual effect of ethnicity but we would gain information about other, perhaps preventable, risk factors. The most parsimonious conclusion would be that schizophrenia in immigrants is caused by the same factors that cause schizophrenia in other groups but that these factors are more common, (and therefore more conspicuous), following migration; there is some evidence in favour of this in terms of parental separation during childhood that is much more common in African-Caribbean children, though the strength of the association of this factor with schizophrenia does not differ between ethnic groups (Fisher et al., 2010).

Course and outcome

The definition of schizophrenia or other psychoses is of importance here, as some have an element of chronicity built in to them. Outcome studies are usually based on hospital treatment samples and so may not be representative (Ram et al., 1992); indeed, the true natural course of schizophrenia is nowadays always masked by treatment. The results of outcome studies are difficult to summarize because the definitions of outcome and methods of assessment used are so varied. However, all show marked heterogeneity in course and outcome (Ram et al., 1992). At the extremes of outcome, about a fifth of patients seem to recover after a single episode of psychosis (Geddes et al., 1994; Leff et al., 1992; Tohen et al., 1992) while about the same proportion, perhaps a little less, develop a chronic unremitting psychosis and never fully recover (Jablensky et al., 1992; Leff et al., 1992; Shepherd et al., 1989). Clinical outcome at 5 years can be summarized by the rule of thirds with approximately 35% of patients in the poor outcome category (Leff et al., 1992; Shepherd et al., 1989); 36% in the good outcome category (Bleuler, 1978; Hegarty et al., 1994) and the remainder with intermediate outcome. Prognosis does not appear to worsen after 5 years (Bleuler, 1978; Hegarty et al., 1994; Jablensky et al., 1992; Mason and Wilkinson, 1996).

Predictors of course and outcome
Mutable factors
Mutable factors represent important targets for psychiatric services. High levels of 'expressed emotion' among close relatives, i.e. criticism, hostility, and over-involvement (Brown et al., 1972; Leff et al., 1983), predict early relapse. Substance abuse (Jablensky et al., 1992; Linszen et al., 1994) also predicts poor prognosis. Delay in receiving treatment results in poorer outcome (Johnstone et al., 1986; Loebel et al., 1992; Wyatt, 1991). This intriguing finding might be due to reverse causality, with poorer prognosis itself resulting in delayed treatment. However, it is possible that a more biological process is involved where untreated positive symptoms alter the 'hard-wiring' in the brain. Alternatively, or in addition, secondary disabilities and the ongoing psychological impact of psychosis are both likely to affect outcome.

Immutable factors
Patients from developing countries have a better outcome than patients from developed countries (Jablensky et al., 1992). It is not yet known which aspects of non-Western 'culture' are responsible for this effect. Possible social factors include lower levels of 'expressed emotion' (Leff et al., 1990), stronger social support networks, or lack of 'stigma'. Ethnicity does not appear to be strongly associated with outcome (Harrison et al., 1999). Other favourable prognostic factors are good premorbid social adjustment, female sex, being married, and later age at onset (Jablensky et al., 1992) but these factors are unlikely to act independently (Eaton, 1991). Acute onset of illness and the experience of negative life events prior to illness are also related to better outcome (Leff et al., 1992; Van Os et al., 1994).

Aetiology

Genetic and epigenetic events are involved in causation, and it appears that events over the life course may interact to form complete causal constellations. The aetiology of the psychoses is complex and not yet understood. Table 5.3, adapted and updated from Cannon and Jones (1996) and Jones and Cannon (1998), summarizes some of the factors that have been implicated. The examination of relative risks can give clues to causation.

Table 5.3 shows that only genetic risk factors come anywhere near the effect size expected for a strong causal agent. However, we cannot ignore the existence of so many pre- and postnatal risk factors with small effect sizes. These environmental risk factors of small effect could be 'proxy' measures for an unrecognized major environmental causal agent, or may act additively with each other, or with chance events. They could also indicate the existence of gene–environment interactions. This last possibility is currently considered highly likely, in which case all the average effect sizes in Table 5.3 will be uninterpretable; some people at genetic risk will be far more likely to develop psychosis in the presence of the factors, others will be resilient or at low risk despite their presence. Thus, we suggest caution in interpreting these effects, with some such as city birth being common and, in itself, unavoidable for most. Nevertheless, we point out two things. First, these effects are larger than any potential genetic effect at the molecular level as demonstrated in the GWAS studies referred to earlier with respect to depression and anxiety. The other is that the field is at an early stage in terms of gene–environment studies; again, the model of neurotic disorders probably pertains to psychosis.

One key point is the emergence of the whole life course as a period during which genetic or epigenetic events may increase the risk for psychosis (Jones, 1999), the effects not being specific for schizophrenia (Jones and Tarrant, 1999). Moreover, the effects of early events may be apparent, albeit in subtle ways, many years before psychosis emerges. This developmental reformulation has had a considerable effect on biological views of the causes and mechanisms of schizophrenia, although most would now concede that psychosocial stress and other precipitants ought to be included in any complete causal model. Biological or organic factors (including genetics) may account for the majority in liability for predisposition (vulnerability or diathesis), with psychosocial factors being important for precipitation or triggering in what is essentially a 'stress-diathesis' model (Zubin and Spring, 1977). This dichotomy in timing of effects whereby biological effects (including genetics) act early and psychosocial effects are triggers is unlikely to be valid. Certainly, only complex models drawing from genetic and epigenetic factors, and across the life course, are likely to explain the main epidemiological variations for psychosis such as sex differences in incidence, and migrant group effects.

Are prediction and primary prevention feasible?
Another important issue for community psychiatry that arises from new, developmental views of the aetiology of psychosis is the prospect of prediction and primary prevention (Jones, 1999). Theoretical attempts are being made (Davidson et al., 1999). However, useful prediction is not yet feasible because the predictive power of any models in current cohort studies is so low, and there is no science of prepsychotic interventions. The problem with low power of models is due to the combination of modest relative risks, involving fairly

Table 5.3 'Best-estimate' effect sizes of various genetic and environmental risk factors for schizophrenia (expressed as odds ratios or relative risks)

Category of risk factor	Specific risk factors	'Best-estimate' of effect size[a]
Genetic[b]	Monozygotic twin of schizophrenic patient	46
	Child of 2 schizophrenic parents	40
	Dizygotic twin of schizophrenic patient	14
	Child or sibling of schizophrenic patient	10
	Parent of schizophrenic patient	5
Developmental[c]	Childhood central nervous system infection	5
	Delayed milestones	3
	Speech problems	3
	Cerebral ventricular enlargement	2
Postnatal environment[c]	Pre-eclampsia	9
	Perinatal brain damage	7
	Rhesus incompatibility	3
	Immigrant/ethnic minority status	3
	Unwanted pregnancy	2
	Solitariness as child	2
Pre- and perinatal environment[c]	Birth complications	2
	Severe undernutrition (1st trimester)	2
	Maternal influenza (2nd trimester)	2
	Born in city	1.4
	Born in winter/early spring	1.2
Adolescent and early adult life[c, d]	Cannabis use[6]	2

[a] Rounded to nearest whole number >1.
[b] Relative risk.
[c] Odds ratio.
[d] Effect from a systematic review; estimate may vary according to dose and strength of cannabis, and be subject to gene–environment interaction such that the effect is much greater for some individuals.
Adapted from Cannon and Jones (1996) and Jones and Cannon (1998).
[6] Data available in (Moore et al., 2007).

common characteristics and, thankfully, a relatively rare outcome. With lifetime odds in the general population of 99% for not getting schizophrenia, it is a much safer proposition to identify who will not get the disorder, than it is those who will. Improving prediction by adding more variables to a model may not be helpful in a real-life setting; data on cognition and family history are candidates but would have to be available on a routine basis.

Current evidence does allow some comments to be made. Prediction in high-risk samples, where the likelihood of disorder is an order of magnitude higher than in the general population, is much more feasible. Those known to be at genetic high risk, or in clinics taking referrals for possible psychosis are examples (McGorry and Jackson, 1999). If there were a feasible intervention, the number needed to treat in order to prevent one case of schizophrenia may be in the realm of acceptability once side effects (including stigma and fear) are taken into account (Jones and Croudace, 2001). Such an equation, though, is radically different for different interventions; drugs psychotherapy, for instance.

Dose–response relationships between possible causes and risk of schizophrenia give rise to some exciting possibilities. Those being described for psychosis are similar in nature to those between smoking and lung cancer, blood pressure and cerebrovascular disease. The majority of cases arise from the majority of the population at medium risk. High-risk individuals are rare and account for only a small proportion of disorder. Rose pointed out that, in these situations, the most efficient interventions are not those aimed at the few cases arising from the high-risk population (Rose, 1989). Rather, they are aimed at the majority at medium risk from which most cases would arise. Thus, the exciting public health implications of the new epidemiology of psychosis (Jones and Cannon, 1998) are very similar to those for common mental disorder, though the true impact of the latter is likely to be greater.

But there is a problem for all outcomes. Most people in this majority will not become ill; certainly they will not get schizophrenia. Most people have to suffer an intervention unnecessarily. Rose called this the prevention paradox. However, there is another paradox; this is where the lack of specificity between developmental deviance and later schizophrenia may even turn out to be an advantage. Other outcomes after developmental problems encompass a church broader than just affective disorder. They include conduct disorder and sociopathic personality disorder, criminality, poor educational achievement, and a penumbra of other outcomes. If widespread interventions aimed at children and adolescents were relatively inefficient at preventing schizophrenia but also impinged upon the incidence of more common, deleterious outcomes then the population may benefit. If such interventions were generally beneficial with no 'side effects' (better education, for instance) then the prevention paradox is low. The data suggest that this kind of situation would be a stark contrast to a hypothetical programme using current antipsychotic drugs in children at high risk for schizophrenia but not yet psychotic. Thus, in terms of prediction and prevention of schizophrenia, the scope for community psychiatry may lie way beyond secondary and tertiary prevention, or the 'firefighting' that drives it today.

Conclusions

The epidemiological approach is an essential element when applied to planning services, evaluating interventions, investigating aetiology, and devising and evaluating preventive strategies.

Acknowledgement

PBJ acknowledges support from the National Institute of Health Research and its Collaboration for Leadership in Applied Health

Research and Care for Cambridgeshire and Peterborough, and the Wellcome Trust.

References

Allardyce, J., Morrison, G., McCreadie, R.G., Van Os, J., Kelly, J., and Murray, R.M. (2000). Schizophrenia is not disappearing in south-west Scotland. *British Journal of Psychiatry*, **177**, 38–41.

Alloway, R. and Bebbington, P. (1987). The buffer theory of social support? a review of the literature. *Psychological Medicine*, **17**, 91–108.

American Psychiatric Association (1994). *Diagnostic and Statistical Manual*, 4th edn. Washington, DC: American Psychiatric Association.

Angst, J. and Vollrath, M. (1991). The natural history of anxiety disorders. *Acta Psychiatrica Scandinavica*, **84**, 446–52.

Aro, S., Aro, H., and Keskimaki, I. (1995). Socio-economic mobility among patients with schizophrenia or major affective disorder. *A 17-year retrospective follow-up. British Journal of Psychiatry*, **166**, 759–67.

Asarnow, R.F. and Asarnow, J.R. (1994). Childhood-onset schizophrenia: Editors' introduction. *Schizophrenia Bulletin*, **20**, 591–7.

Bamrah, J.S., Freeman, H.L., and Goldberg, D.P. (1991). Epidemiology of schizophrenia in Salford, 1974–84. *Changes in an urban community over ten years. British Journal of Psychiatry*, **159**, 802–10.

Banks, M.H. and Jackson, P.R. (1982). Unemployment and risk of minor psychiatric disorder in young people: cross-sectional and longitudinal evidence. *Psychological Medicine*, **12**(, 789–98.

Blazer, D., George, L.K., Landerman, R., Pennybacker, M., Melville, M.L., Woodbury, M., *et al.* (1985). Psychiatric disorders: A rural/urban comparison. *Archives of General Psychiatry*, **42**, 651–6.

Bleuler, M. (1978). *The Schizophrenic Disorders: Long-term Patient and Family studies*. New Haven, CT: Yale University Press.

Böök, J.A., Wetterberg, L., and Modrzewska, K. (1978). Schizophrenia in a North Swedish geographical isolate, 1900–1977. Epidemiology, genetics and biochemistry. *Clinical Genetics*, **14**, 373–94.

Bosker, F.J., Hartman, C.A., Nolte, I.M., Prins, B.P., Terpstra, P., Posthuma, D., *et al.* (2010). Poor replication of candidate genes for major depressive disorder using genome-wide association data. *Molecular Psychiatry* (advance online publication, March 30).

Boydell, J., Van Os, J., Lambri, M., Castle, D., Allardyce, J., McCreadie, R.G., *et al.* (2003). Incidence of schizophrenia in south-east London between 1965 and 1997. *British Journal of Psychiatry*, **182**, 45–9.

Brown, G.W., Birley, J.L.T., and Wing, J.K. (1972). Influence of family life on the course of schizophrenic disorders: A replication. *British Journal of Psychiatry*, **121**, 241–58.

Brown, G.W. and Harris, T. (1978). *Social Origins of Depression*. London: Tavistock.

Brown, G.W., Davidson, S., Harris, T., Maclean, U., Pollock, S., and Prudo, R. (1977). Psychiatric disorder in London and North Uist. *Social Science and Medicine (1967)*, **11**, 367–77.

Brown, G.W., Harris, T.O., and Eales, M.J. (1993). Aetiology of anxiety and depressive disorders in an inner-city population. *2. Comorbidity and adversity. Psychological Medicine*, **23**, 155–65.

Burke, A.W. (1974). First admissions and planning in Jamaica. *Social Psychiatry and Psychiatric Epidemiology*, **9**, 39–45.

Cannon, M. and Jones, P. (1996). Schizophrenia. *Journal of Neurology, Neurosurgery and Psychiatry*, **60**, 604–13.

Caspi, A., Sugden, K., Moffitt, T.E., Taylor, A., Craig, I.W., Harrington, H., *et al.* (2003). Influence of life stress on depression: moderation by a polymorphism in the 5-HTT gene. *Science*, **301**, 386–9.

Castle, D., Wessely, S., Der, G., and Murray, R.M. (1991). The incidence of operationally defined schizophrenia in Camberwell, 1965–84. *British Journal of Psychiatry*, **159**, 790–4.

Clare, A. (1980). *Psychiatry in Dissent. Controversial Issues in Thought and Practice*, 2nd edn. London: Tavistock.

Coid, J.W., Kirkbride, J.B., Barker, D., Cowden, F., Stamps, R., Yang, M., *et al.* (2008). Raised incidence rates of all psychoses among migrant groups: Findings from the East London First Episode Psychosis Study. *Archives of General Psychiatry*, **65**, 1250–8.

Coppen, A. and Metcalfe, M. (1965). Effect of a depressive illness on M.P.I. scores. *British Journal of Psychiatry*, **111**, 236–9.

Cox, B.D., Blaxter, M., Buckle, A.L.J., Fenner, N.P., Golding, J.F., Gore, M., *et al.* (1987). *The Health and Lifestyle Survey*. Cambridge: Health Promotion Research Trust.

Crocetti, G., Lemkau, P.V., Kulcar, Z., and Kesic, B. (1971). Selected aspects of the epidemiology of psychoses in Croatia, Yugoslavia. *III. The cluster sample and the results of the pilot survey. American Journal of Epidemiology*, **94**, 126–34.

Croft-Jeffreys, C. and Wilkinson, G. (1989). Estimated costs of neurotic disorder in UK general practice 1985. *Psychological Medicine*, **19**, 549–58.

Croudace, T.J., Kayne, R., Jones, P.B., and Harrison, G.L. (2000). Non-linear relationship between an index of social deprivation, psychiatric admission prevalence and the incidence of psychosis. *Psychological Medicine*, **30**, 177–85.

Crow, T.J., Prince, M., Phelan, M., Graham, P., De Alarcon, J., Seagroatt, V., *et al.* (1990). Trends in schizophrenia. *Lancet*, **335**, 851–3.

Dauncey, K., Giggs, J., Baker, K., and Harrison, G. (1993). Schizophrenia in Nottingham: lifelong residential mobility of a cohort. *British Journal of Psychiatry*, **163**, 613–19.

Davidson, M., Reichenberg, A., Rabinowitz, J., Weiser, M., Kaplan, Z., and Mark, M. (1999). Behavioral and intellectual markers for schizophrenia in apparently healthy male adolescents. *American Journal of Psychiatry*, **156**, 1328–35.

Der, G., Gupta, S., and Murray, R. M. (1990). Is schizophrenia disappearing? *Lancet*, **335**, 513–16.

Done, D.J., Crow, T.J., Johnstone, E.C., and Sacker, A. (1994). Childhood antecedents of schizophrenia and affective illness: social adjustment at ages 7 and 11. *British Medical Journal*, **309**, 699–703.

Donnelly, P. (2008). Progress and challenges in genome-wide association studies in humans. *Nature*, **456**, 728–31.

Duncan-Jones, P., Fergusson, D.M., Ormel, J., and Horwood, L.J. (1990). A model of stability and change in minor psychiatric symptoms: results from three longitudinal studies. *Psychological Medicine Monograph Supplement*, **18**, 1–28.

Eagles, J.M. (1991). The relationship between schizophrenia and immigration. *Are there alternatives to psychosocial hypotheses? British Journal of Psychiatry*, **159**, 783–9.

Eagles, J.M. and Whalley, L.J. (1985). Decline in the diagnosis of schizophrenia among first admissions to Scottish mental hospitals from 1969-78. *British Journal of Psychiatry*, **146**, 151–54.

Eagles, J.M., Hunter, D., and McCance, C. (1988). Decline in the diagnosis of schizophrenia among first contacts with psychiatric services in north-east Scotland, 1969-1984. *British Journal of Psychiatry*, **152**, 793–8.

Eaton, W.W. (1991). Update on the Epidemiology of Schizophrenia. *Epidemiologic Reviews*, **13**, 320–28.

Eaton, W.W. and Ritter, C. (1988). Distinguishing anxiety and depression with field survey data. *Psychological Medicine*, **18**, 155–66.

Eysenck, H.J. and Eysenck, S.B.G. (1964). *Manual of the Eysenck personality inventory*. London: University of London Press.

Fearon, P., Kirkbride, J.B., Morgan, C., Dazzan, P., Morgan, K., Lloyd, T., *et al.* (2006). Incidence of schizophrenia and other psychoses in ethnic minority groups: results from the MRC AESOP Study. *Psychological Medicine*, **36**, 1541–50.

Fisher, H.L., Jones, P.B., Fearon, P., Craig, T.K., Dazzan, P., Morgan, K., *et al.* (2010). The varying impact of type, timing and frequency of exposure to childhood adversity on its association with adult psychotic disorder. *Psychological Medicine*, **40**, 1967–78.

Geddes, J., Mercer, G., Frith, C.D., MacMillan, F., Owens, D.G., and Johnstone, E.C. (1994). Prediction of outcome following a first episode of schizophrenia. A follow-up study of Northwick Park first episode study subjects. *British Journal of Psychiatry*, **165**, 664–8.

Geddes, J.R., Black, R.J., Whalley, L.J., and Eagles, J.M. (1993). Persistence of the decline in the diagnosis of schizophrenia among first admissions to Scottish hospitals from 1969 to 1988. *British Journal of Psychiatry*, **163**, 620–6.

Goldberg, D. P. and Williams, P. (1988). *The User's Guide to the General Health Questionnaire*. Windsor: NFER-Nelson.

Goodyer, I.M., Kolvin, I., and Gatzanis, S. (1987). The impact of recent undesirable life events on psychiatric disorders in childhood and adolescence. *British Journal of Psychiatry*, **151**, 179–84.

Häfner, H., Maurer, K., Loffler, W., and Riecher-Rossler, A. (1993). The influence of age and sex on the onset and early course of schizophrenia. *British Journal of Psychiatry*, **162**, 80–6.

Harrington, R., Fudge, H., Rutter, M., Pickles, A., and Hill, J. (1990). Adult outcomes of childhood and adolescent depression: I. Psychiatric status. *Archives of General Psychiatry*, **47**, 465–73.

Harrison, G., Owens, D., Holton, A., Neilson, D., and Boot, D. (1988). A prospective study of severe mental disorder in Afro-Caribbean patients. *Psychological Medicine*, **18**, 643–57.

Harrison, G., Cooper, J.E., and Gancarczyk, R. (1991). Changes in the administrative incidence of schizophrenia. *British Journal of Psychiatry*, **159**, 811–16.

Harrison, G., Glazebrook, C., Brewin, J., Cantwell, R., Dalkin, T., Fox, R., *et al.* (1997). Increased incidence of psychotic disorders in migrants from the Caribbean to the United Kingdom. *Psychological Medicine*, **27**, 799–806.

Harrison, G., Amin, S., Singh, S.P., Croudace, T., and Jones, P. (1999). Outcome of psychosis in people of African-Caribbean family origin. Population-based first-episode study. *British Journal of Psychiatry*, **175**, 43–9.

Harvey, C.A. (1996). The Camden schizophrenia surveys. I. The psychiatric, behavioural and social characteristics of the severely mentally ill in an inner London health district. *British Journal of Psychiatry*, **168**, 410–17.

Harvey, C.A., Pantelis, C., Taylor, J., McCabe, P.J., Lefevre, K., Campbell, P.G., *et al.* (1996). The Camden schizophrenia surveys. *II. High prevalence of schizophrenia in an inner London borough and its relationship to socio-demographic factors. British Journal of Psychiatry*, **168**, 418–26.

Hegarty, J.D., Baldessarini, R.J., Tohen, M., Waternaux, C., and Oepen, G. (1994). One hundred years of schizophrenia: a meta-analysis of the outcome literature. *American Journal of Psychiatry*, **151**, 1409–16.

Henderson, A.S., Byrne, D.G., and Duncan-Jones, P. (1981). *Neurosis and the Social Environment*. Sydney: Academic Press.

Hickling, F.W. (1991). Psychiatric hospital admission rates in Jamaica, 1971 and 1988. *British Journal of Psychiatry*, **159**, 817–21.

Hirschfeld, R.M., Klerman, G.L., Clayton, P.J., Keller, M.B., McDonald-Scott, P., and Larkin, B. H. (1983). Assessing personality: effects of the depressive state on trait measurement. *American Journal of Psychiatry*, **140**, 695–9.

Jablensky, A. (1995). Schizophrenia: recent epidemiologic issues. *Epidemiologic Reviews*, **17**, 10–20.

Jablensky, A., Sartorius, N., Ernberg, G., Anker, M., Korten, A., Cooper, J. E., *et al.* (1992). Schizophrenia: manifestations, incidence and course in different cultures A World Health Organization Ten-Country Study. *Psychological Medicine Monograph Supplement*, **1**, 1–97.

Jeffreys, S.E., Harvey, C.A., McNaught, A.S., Quayle, A.S., King, M.B., and Bird, A.S. (1997). The Hampstead Schizophrenia Survey 1991. I: Prevalence and service use comparisons in an inner London health authority, 1986-1991. *British Journal of Psychiatry*, **170**, 301–6.

Jenkins, R. (1985). Sex differences in minor psychiatric morbidity. *Psychological Medicine Monograph Supplement*, **7**, 1–53.

Jenkins, R., Lewis, G., Bebbington, P., Brugha, T., Farrell, M., Gill, B., *et al.* (1997). The National Psychiatric Morbidity Surveys of Great Britain: initial findings from the Household Survey. *Psychological Medicine*, **27**, 775–89.

Johnstone, E.C., Crow, T.J., Johnson, A.L., and MacMillan, J.F. (1986). The Northwick Park Study of first episodes of schizophrenia. *I. Presentation of the illness and problems relating to admission. British Journal of Psychiatry*, **148**, 115–20.

Jones, P., Murray, R., Rodgers, B., and Marmot, M. (1994). Child developmental risk factors for adult schizophrenia in the British 1946 birth cohort. *Lancet*, **344**, 1398–402.

Jones, P.B. (1999). Longitudinal approaches to the search for the causes of schizophrenia: Past, present and future. In Gattaz, W.F. and Hafner, H. (eds.) *Search for the Causes of Schizophrenia Vol. IV Balance of the Century*, pp. 91–119. Berlin: Darmstadt: Steinkopff (Springer).

Jones, P.B. and Cannon, M. (1998). The new epidemiology of schizophrenia: Common methods for genetics and the environment. *Psychiatric Clinics of North America*, **21**, 1–26

Jones, P.B. and Croudace, T. (2001). Predicting schizophrenia from teachers' reports of behaviour. Results from a general population birth cohort. In Miller, T., Mednick, S.A., McGlashan, T.H., Libiger, J. and Johannessen, J.O. (eds.) *Early Intervention in Psychotic Disorders*, Vol. **91**, pp. 1–29. Dordrecht: Kluwer Academic Publishers.

Jones, P.B. and Tarrant, C.J. (1999). Specificity of developmental precursors to schizophrenia and affective disorders. *Schizophrenia Research*, **39**, 121–5.

Jones, P.B., Bebbington, P., Foerster, A., Lewis, S.W., Murray, R.M., Russell, A., *et al.* (1993). Premorbid social underachievement in schizophrenia. Results from the Camberwell Collaborative Psychosis Study. *British Journal of Psychiatry*, **162**, 65–71.

Joyce, P.R. (1987). Changing trends in first admissions and readmissions for mania and schizophrenia in New Zealand, 1974 to 1984. *Australian and New Zealand Journal of Psychiatry*, **21**(1), 82–6.

Keith, S.J., Regier, D.A., and Rae, D.S. (1991). Schizophrenic disorders. In Robins, L.N. and Regier, D.A. (eds.) *Psychiatric disorders in America: the epidemiologic catchment area study*, pp. 33–52. New York: The Free Press.

Kendell, R.E. and DiScipio, W.J. (1968). Eysenck Personality Inventory Scores of patients with depressive illnesses. *British Journal of Psychiatry*, **114**, 767–70.

Kendell, R.E., Malcolm, D.E., and Adams, W. (1993). The problem of detecting changes in the incidence of schizophrenia. *British Journal of Psychiatry*, **162**, 212–18.

Kendler, K.S., Kessler, R.C., Neale, M.C., Heath, A.C., and Eaves, L.J. (1993). The prediction of major depression in women: toward an integrated etiologic model. *American Journal of Psychiatry*, **150**, 1139–48.

Kessler, R.C., McGonagle, K.A., Zhao, S., Nelson, C.B., Hughes, M., Eshleman, S., *et al.* (1994). Lifetime and 12-month prevalence of DSM-III-R psychiatric disorders in the United States. Results from the National Comorbidity Survey. *Archives of General Psychiatry*, **52**, 8–19.

King, M., Coker, E., Leavey, G., Hoare, A., and Johnson-Sabine, E. (1994). Incidence of psychotic illness in London: comparison of ethnic groups. *British Medical Journal*, **309**, 1115–19.

Kirkbride, J.B., Boydell, J., Ploubidis, G.B., Morgan, C., Dazzan, P., McKenzie, K., *et al.* (2008). Testing the association between the incidence of schizophrenia and social capital in an urban area. *Psychological Medicine*, **38**, 1083–94.

Kirkbride, J.B., Croudace, T., Brewin, J., Donoghue, K., Mason, P., Glazebrook, C., *et al.* (2009). Is the incidence of psychotic disorder in decline? Epidemiological evidence from two decades of research. *International Journal of Epidemiology*, **38**, 1255–64.

Leask, S.J., Jones, P.B., Done, D.J., Crow, T.J., and Richards, M. (2000). No association between breast-feeding and adult psychosis in two national birth cohorts. *British Journal of Psychiatry*, **177**, 218–21.

Leff, J., Kuipers, L., Berkowitz, R., Vaughn, C., and Sturgeon, D. (1983). Life events, relatives' expressed emotion and maintenance neuroleptics in schizophrenic relapse. *Psychological Medicine*, **13**, 799–806.

Leff, J., Wig, N.N., Bedi, H., Menon, D.K., Kuipers, L., Korten, A., *et al.* (1990). Relatives' expressed emotion and the course of schizophrenia in Chandigarh. A two-year follow-up of a first-contact sample. *British Journal of Psychiatry*, **156**, 351–6.

Leff, J., Sartorius, N., Jablensky, A., Korten, A., and Ernberg, G. (1992). The International Pilot Study of Schizophrenia: five-year follow-up findings. *Psychological Medicine*, **22**, 131–45.

Lewis, G., and Booth, M. (1994). Are cities bad for your mental health? *Psychological Medicine*, **24**, 913–15.

Lewis, G. and Pelosi, A.J. (1990). The case-control study in psychiatry. *British Journal of Psychiatry*, **157**, 197–207.

Lewis, G., Bebbington, P., Brugha, T., Farrell, M., Gill, B., Jenkins, R., *et al.* (1998). Socioeconomic status, standard of living, and neurotic disorder. *Lancet*, **352**, 605–9.

Linszen, D.H., Dingemans, P.M., and Lenior, M.E. (1994). Cannabis abuse and the course of recent-onset schizophrenic disorders. *Archives of General Psychiatry*, **51**, 273–9.

Loebel, A.D., Lieberman, J.A., Alvir, J.M., Mayerhoff, D.I., Geisler, S.H., and Szymanski, S.R. (1992). Duration of psychosis and outcome in first-episode schizophrenia. *American Journal of Psychiatry*, **149**, 1183–8.

Macpherson, R., Haynes, R., Summerfield, L., Foy, C., and Slade, M. (2003). From research to practice. *Social Psychiatry and Psychiatric Epidemiology*, **38**, 276–81.

Mason, O. and Wilkinson, G. (1996). The prevalence of psychiatric morbidity. OPCS survey of psychiatric morbidity in Great Britain. *British Journal of Psychiatry*, **168**, 1–3.

McCullagh, M., Morley, S., and Dodwell, D. (2003). A systematic, confidential approach to improving community care for patients with non-affective psychosis. *Primary Care Psychiatry*, **8**, 127–30.

McGorry, P.D. and Jackson, H.J. (1999). *The recognition and management of early psychosis. A preventive approach*. Cambridge: Cambridge University Press.

McGovern, D. and Cope, R.V. (1987). First psychiatric admission rates of first and second generation Afro Caribbeans. *Social Psychiatry and Psychiatric Epidemiology*, **22**, 139–49.

McGrath, J., Saha, S., Welham, J., El Saadi, O., MacCauley, C., and Chant, D. (2004). A systematic review of the incidence of schizophrenia: the distribution of rates and the influence of sex, urbanicity, migrant status and methodology. *BMC Medicine*, **2**, 13.

McManus, S., Meltzer, H., Brugha, T., Bebbington, P., and Jenkins, R. (2009). *Adult psychiatric morbidity in England, 2007: results of a household survey, NHS Information Centre for health and social care*. Leeds: NHS Information Centre for Health and Social Care.

Meltzer, H., Gill, B., Petticrew, M., and Hinds, K. (1996). *Economic activity and social functioning of adults with psychiatric disorders*. London: HMSO.

Monck, E., Graham, P., Richman, N., and Dobbs, R. (1994). Adolescent girls. II. *Background factors in anxiety and depressive states. British Journal of Psychiatry*, **165**, 770–80.

Moore, T.H.M., Zammit, S., Lingford-Hughes, A., Barnes, T.R.E., Jones, P.B., Burke, M., *et al.* (2007). Cannabis use and risk of psychotic or affective mental health outcomes: a systematic review. *Lancet*, **370**, 319–28.

Mullen, P.E., Martin, J.L., Anderson, J.C., Romans, S.E., and Herbison, G.P. (1993). Childhood sexual abuse and mental health in adult life. *British Journal of Psychiatry*, **163**, 721–32.

Munk-J rgensen, P. (1986). Decreasing first-admission rates of schizophrenia among males in Denmark from 1970 to 1984. *Acta Psychiatrica Scandinavica*, **73**, 645–50.

Munk-Jorgensen, P. and Mortensen, P.B. (1992). Incidence and other aspects of the epidemiology of schizophrenia in Denmark, 1971-87. *British Journal of Psychiatry*, **161**, 489–95.

Murray, C.J.L., and Lopez, A.D. (1997). Alternative projections of mortality and disability by cause 1990-2020: Global Burden of Disease Study. *Lancet*, **349**, 1498–504.

Nicole, L., Lesage, A., and Lalonde, P. (1992). Lower incidence and increased male:female ratio in schizophrenia. *British Journal of Psychiatry*, **161**, 556–7.

Nixon, N.L. and Doody, G.A.(2005)Official psychiatric morbidity and the incidence of schizophrenia 1881–1994. *Psychological Medicine*, **35**, 1145–53.

Odegaard, O. (1932). Emigration and insanity: a study of mental disease among Norwegian-born population in Minnesota. *Acta Psychiatrica et Neurologica Scandinavica*, **7**, 1–206.

Oldehinkel, A.J. and Giel, R. (1995). Time trends in the care-based incidence of schizophrenia. *British Journal of Psychiatry*, **167**, 777–82.

Ormel, J., VonKorff, M., Ustun, T.B., Pini, S., Korten, A., and Oldehinkel, T. (1994). Common mental disorders and disability across cultures: Results From the WHO Collaborative Study on Psychological Problems in General Health Care. *Journal of the American Medical Association*, **272**, 1741–8.

Ösby, U., Hammar, N., Brandt, L., Wicks, S., Thinsz, Z., Ekbom, A., *et al.* (2001). Time trends in first admissions for schizophrenia and paranoid psychosis in Stockholm County, Sweden. *Schizophrenia Research*, **47**, 247–54.

Parker, G., Tupling, H., and Brown, L. (1979). A parental bonding instrument. *British Journal of Medical Psychology*, **52**, 877–85.

Parker, G.B., Barrett, E.A., and Hickie, I.B. (1992). From nurture to network: examining links between perceptions of parenting received in childhood and social bonds in adulthood. *American Journal of Psychiatry*, **149**, 877–85.

Perala, J., Suvisaari, J., Saarni, S.I., Kuoppasalmi, K., Isometsa, E., Pirkola, S., *et al.* (2007). Lifetime prevalence of psychotic and bipolar I disorders in a general population. *Archives of General Psychiatry*, **64**, 19–28.

Plum, F. (1972). Prospects for research on schizophrenia. 3. Neurophysiology. Neuropathological findings. *Neurosciences Research Program Bulletin*, **10**, 384–8.

Ram, R., Bromet, E.J., Eaton, W.W., Pato, C., and Schwartz, J.E. (1992). The natural course of schizophrenia: A review of first-admission studies. *Schizophrenia Bulletin*, **18**, 185–207.

Risch, N., Herrell, R., Lehner, T., Liang, K.-Y., Eaves, L., Hoh, J., *et al.* (2009). Interaction between the serotonin transporter gene (5-HTTLPR), stressful life events, and risk of depression: A meta-analysis. *Journal of the American Medical Association*, **301**, 2462–71.

Robins, L. and Regier, D. (1991). *Psychiatric disorders in America: the epidemiological catchment area study*. New York: The Free Press.

Romans, S.E., Walton, V.A., McNoe, B., Herbison, G.P., and Mullen, P.E. (1993). Otago Women's Health Survey 30-month follow-up. I: Onset patterns of non-psychotic psychiatric disorder. *British Journal of Psychiatry*, **163**, 733–8.

Rose, G. (1989). The mental health of populations. In Williams, G. and Wilkinson, P. (eds.) *The Scope of Epidemiological Psychiatry*, pp. 75–85. London: Routledge.

Ruggeri, M., Leese, M., Thornicroft, G., Bisoffi, G., and Tansella, M. (2000). Definition and prevalence of severe and persistent mental illness. *British Journal of Psychiatry*, **177**, 149–55.

Rutter, M. (1985). Resilience in the face of adversity. Protective factors and resistance to psychiatric disorder *British Journal of Psychiatry*, **147**, 598–611.

Saha, S., Chant, D., Welham, J., and McGrath, J. (2005). A systematic review of the prevalence of schizophrenia. *PLoS Med*, **2**, e141.

Selten, J. P. and Sijben, N. (1994). First admission rates for schizophrenia in immigrants to the Netherlands. *Social Psychiatry and Psychiatric Epidemiology*, **29**, 71–7.

Shepherd, M., Watt, D., Falloon, I., and Smeeton, N. (1989). The natural history of schizophrenia: a five-year follow-up study of outcome and prediction in a representative sample of schizophrenics. *Psychological Medicine Monograph Supplement*, **15**, 1–46.

Singleton, N., Bumpstead, R., O'Brien, M., Lee, A., and Meltzer, H. (2001). *Psychiatric morbidity among adults living in private households*: London: The Stationery Office.

Smith, K., Shah, A., Wright, K., and Lewis, G. (1995). The prevalence and costs of psychiatric disorders and learning disabilities. *British Journal of Psychiatry*, **166**, 9–18.

Stoll, A.L., Tohen, M., Baldessarini, R.J., Goodwin, D.C., Stein, S., Katz, S., *et al.* (1993). Shifts in diagnostic frequencies of schizophrenia and major affective disorders at six North American psychiatric hospitals, 1972–1988. *American Journal of Psychiatry*, **150**, 1668–73.

Sugarman, P. A. and Craufurd, D. (1994). Schizophrenia in the Afro-Caribbean community. *British Journal of Psychiatry*, **164**, 474–80.

Suvisaari, J.M., Haukka, J.K., Tanskanen, A.J., and Lonnqvist, J.K. (1999). Decline in the incidence of schizophrenia in Finnish cohorts born from 1954 to 1965. *Archives of General Psychiatry*, **56**, 733–40.

Thomas, C.S., Stone, K., Osborn, M., Thomas, P.F., and Fisher, M. (1993). Psychiatric morbidity and compulsory admission among UK-born Europeans, Afro-Caribbeans and Asians in central Manchester. *British Journal of Psychiatry*, **163**, 91–9.

Tien, A.Y. and Eaton, W.W. (1992). Psychopathologic precursors and sociodemographic risk factors for the schizophrenia syndrome. *Archives of General Psychiatry*, **49**, 37–46.

Tohen, M., Stoll, A.L., Strakowski, S.M., Faedda, G.L., Mayer, P.V., Goodwin, D.C., *et al.* (1992). The McLean First-episode Psychosis Project: Six-month recovery and recurrence outcome. *Schizophrenia Bulletin*, **18**, 273–82.

Torrey, E.F. (1980). *Schizophrenia and Civilization*. New York: Jason Aronson.

Torrey, E.F. (1987). Prevalence studies in schizophrenia. *British Journal of Psychiatry*, **150**(5), 598–608.

Tsuchiya, K.J. and Munk-J rgensen, P. (2002). First-admission rates of schizophrenia in Denmark, 1980-1997: have they been increasing? *Schizophrenia Research*, **54**, 187–91.

Van Os, J., Fahy, T.A., Bebbington, P., Jones, P., Wilkins, S., Sham, P., *et al.* (1994). The influence of life events on the subsequent course of psychotic illness: A prospective follow-up of the Camberwell Collaborative Psychosis Study. *Psychological Medicine*, **24**, 503–13.

Van Os, J., Howard, R., Takei, N., and Murray, R. (1995). Increasing age is a risk factor for psychosis in the elderly. *Social Psychiatry and Psychiatric Epidemiology*, **3**, 161–4.

Van Os, J., Castle, D.J., Takei, N., Der, G., and Murray, R.M. (1996). Psychotic illness in ethnic minorities: clarification from the 1991 census. *Psychological Medicine*, **26**, 203–8.

Waddington, J.L. and Youssef, H.A. (1994). Evidence for a gender-specific decline in the rate of schizophrenia in rural Ireland over a 50-year period. *British Journal of Psychiatry*, **164**, 171–6.

Warner, R. (1995). Time trends in schizophrenia: changes in obstetric risk factors with industrialization. *Schizophrenia Bulletin*, **21**, 483–500.

Warr, P. (1987). *Work, Unemployment and Mental Health*. Oxford: Oxford Science Publications.

Weich, S. and Lewis, G. (1998). Poverty, unemployment, and common mental disorders: population based cohort study. *British Medical Journal*, **317**, 115–19.

Wells, K.B., Stewart, A., Hays, R.D., Burnam, M.A., Rogers, W., Daniels, M., *et al.* (1989). The functioning and well-being of depressed patients: Results from the Medical Outcomes Study. *Journal of the American Medical Association*, **262**, 914–19.

Wessely, S., Castle, D., Der, G., and Murray, R. (1991). Schizophrenia and Afro-Caribbeans. *A case-control study. British Journal of Psychiatry*, **159**, 795–801.

Wing, J.K., Cooper, J.E., and Sartorius, N. (1974). *The Measurement and Classification of Psychiatric Symptoms*. Cambridge: Cambridge University Press.

World Health Organization (1994). *The ICD-10 Classification of Mental and Behavioural Disorders: Diagnostic Criteria for Research*. Geneva: World Health Organization.

Wyatt, R.J. (1991). Neuroleptics and the natural course of schizophrenia. *Schizophrenia Bulletin*, **17**, 325–51.

Zubin, J. and Spring, B. (1977). Vulnerability: A new view of schizophrenia. *Journal of Abnormal Psychology*, **86**, 103–26.

CHAPTER 6

Treated and untreated prevalence of mental disorders: results from the World Health Organization World Mental Health (WMH) surveys[1]

Philip S. Wang,[2] Sergio Aguilar-Gaxiola, Ali Obaid AlHamzawi, Jordi Alonso, Laura Helena Andrade, Matthias C. Angermeyer, Guilherme Borges, Evelyn J. Bromet, Ronny Bruffaerts, Brendan Bunting, José Miguel Caldas de Almeida, Silvia Florescu, Giovanni de Girolamo, Ron de Graaf, Oye Gureje, Josep Maria Haro, Hristo Ruskov Hinkov, Chi-yi Hu, Elie G. Karam, Viviane Kovess, Sing Lee, Daphna Levinson, Yutaka Ono, Maria Petukhova, José Posada-Villa, Rajesh Sagar, Soraya Seedat, J. Elisabeth Wells, and Ronald C. Kessler

Overview

Twelve-month prevalence and treatment of common mental disorders were assessed in 24 countries in the World Health Organization (WHO) World Mental Health (WMH) surveys. Assessments were based on the WMH Composite International Diagnostic Interview. 16.7% of respondents (interquartile range (IQR): 10.0–20.7% across surveys) met criteria for any 12-month disorder, 24.5% of which (IQR: 18.6–25.8%) were classified serious (serious mental illness; SMI). The proportion of respondents who received treatment for these disorders was much lower in low/lower-middle- (3.4%) than upper-middle- (8.7%) and high-income (12.0%) countries. Although proportional treatment was much higher among respondents with SMI (44.4%) than less severe disorders, only a minority of people with even serious disorders received treatment judged to be at least minimally adequate (40.4% overall, 43.7%/38.4/22.2% in high-, upper-middle-, and low/lower-middle-income countries). These results show that

1 Portions of this chapter appeared previously in Wang, P.S., Aguilar-Gaxiola, S., Alonso, J., Angermeyer, M.C., Borges, G., Bromet, E.J., *et al.* (2007). Use of mental health services for anxiety, mood, and substance disorders in 17 countries in the WHO World Mental Health Surveys. *Lancet*, **370**, 841–50. © Elsevier Ltd. Used with permission.

2 Author's or Editor's contribution to the Work was done as part of the Author's or Editor's official duties as a NIH employee and is a Work of the United States Government. Therefore, copyright may not be established in the United States.

unmet need for mental health treatment is pervasive and especially dire in less developed countries. Alleviating these unmet needs will require expansion and optimal allocation of treatment resources.

Introduction

Neuropsychiatric disorders are leading causes of disability worldwide, accounting for 37% of all healthy life years lost from disease (Lopez et al., 2006). They are among the most disabling conditions even in low-income countries, where detection of emotional problems and access to treatment are lowest. Although efficacious and tolerable treatments for these disorders are increasingly available, even economically-advantaged societies experience competing priorities and budgetary constraints (Tasman et al., 2003). Knowing how to provide effective treatment is consequently a worldwide imperative (Hu, 2003). Unfortunately, most countries suffer from a lack of data to guide decisions, absent or competing visions for resources, and near constant pressures to cut insurance and entitlements (Mechanic, 1994).

How can countries redesign their mental health care systems and optimally allocate resources? A first step is to document the services currently being used as well as the extent and nature of unmet needs for treatment. A second step may be to conduct cross-national comparisons of service use and unmet needs in countries with different mental health care systems. Such comparisons have the potential to help uncover optimal financing, national policies, and delivery systems for the care of mental disorders. Unfortunately, few cross-national studies of such differences are available (Bijl et al., 2003; Kessler et al., 1997).

For these reasons, WHO established the WMH Survey Initiative in 1998 (Demyttenaere et al., 2004). Coordinated surveys of the prevalence of mental disorders, their severity, impairments, and treatments have been implemented and analysed in 24 developing and developed countries. The current report describes the levels, types, and adequacy of mental health service use in these countries. We also examine unmet needs for treatment among strata defined by the seriousness of mental disorders. Finally, we identify sociodemographic correlates of unmet needs for treatment to guide the design and targeting of future resources, policies, and interventions.

Survey samples

In terms of the methods used, the WMH surveys were carried out in 24 countries in the following regions: Africa (Nigeria, South Africa), the Americas (Brazil, Colombia, Mexico, United States), Asia and the Pacific (India, Japan, New Zealand, Beijing-Shanghai and Shenzhen in the People's Republic of China), Europe (Belgium, Bulgaria, France, Germany, Italy, Netherlands, Northern Ireland, Portugal, Romania, Spain, Ukraine), and the Middle East (Iraq, Israel, Lebanon). Using World Bank criteria (World Bank, 2003), countries were classified as low/lower-middle income (Colombia, India, Iraq, Nigeria, People's Republic of China, Ukraine), higher-middle income (Brazil, Bulgaria, Lebanon, Mexico, Romania, South Africa), and high income (all others). Surveys were conducted face-to-face by trained lay interviewers with respondents selected using probability procedures from multistage clustered area probability household samples (Table 6.1). The total sample

size of respondents aged 18 and older was 121,902 with individual country samples ranging from a low of 2357 in Romania to a high of 12,790 in New Zealand. The weighted average response rate across all countries was 72.0%, with individual country response rates ranging from a low of 45.9% in France to a high of 98.8% in Pondicherry, India.

The interview was divided into two parts. All respondents completed Part I, which contained core diagnostic assessments and basic information about sociodemographics. All Part I respondents who met criteria for any lifetime core disorder plus a probability subsample of approximately 25% of all other Part I respondents were administered Part II, which assessed disorders of secondary interest along with predictors and consequences of disorders and service use. The Part I data were weighted to adjust for differential probabilities of selection within and between households, for non-response bias, and for residual discrepancies between the sample and census population distributions of a profile of sociodemographic and geographic variables. The Part II data were additionally weighted to adjust for the differential sampling of Part I respondents into Part II as a function of the presence of Part I core disorders. WMH weighting procedures are discussed in more detail elsewhere (Heeringa et al., 2008).

Standardized procedures were used consistently across all WMH sites for interviewer training, WHO translation and back-translation and harmonization of all study materials, and quality control of interviewer work. These procedures are described in detail elsewhere (Harkness et al., 2008; Pennell et al., 2008). Informed consent was obtained before beginning interviews in each country. Procedures for obtaining informed consent and protecting human subjects were approved and monitored by the Institutional Review Boards of the organizations coordinating the survey in each country.

Twelve-month mental disorders

Mental disorders present at any time in the 12 months before interview were assessed in the WMH surveys with Version 3.0 of the WHO Composite international Diagnostic Interview (CIDI) (Kessler and Üstün, 2004), a fully-structured diagnostic interview designed to be administered by trained lay interviewers. Disorders were defined according to the definitions and criteria of the American Psychiatric Association's *Diagnostic and Statistical Manual of Mental Disorders*, Fourth Edition (DSM-IV). The disorders considered in the current report include anxiety disorders (agoraphobia with or without panic disorder, generalized anxiety disorder, panic disorder with or without agoraphobia, post-traumatic stress disorder, obsessive–compulsive disorder, social phobia, and specific phobia), mood disorders (bipolar disorder including bipolar I and II, dysthymic disorder, and major depressive disorder), impulse-control disorders (intermittent-explosive disorder, attention deficit hyperactivity disorder, oppositional defiant disorder, and conduct disorder), and substance disorders (alcohol and drug abuse with or without dependence). All diagnoses were made with CIDI organic exclusion rules. Clinical reappraisal studies of CIDI diagnoses in a number of WMH countries (Haro et al., 2006) documented generally good concordance between diagnoses based on the CIDI and diagnoses based on independent clinical interviews with the Structured Clinical Interview for DSM-IV (SCID) (First et al., 2002).

Table 6.1 WMH Sample Characteristics by World Bank income categories[1]

	Survey[2]	Sample characteristics[3]	Field dates	Age range	Sample size		Response rate[4]
					Part I	Part II	
I. Low/lower-middle-income countries							
Colombia	NSMH	Stratified multistage clustered area probability sample of household residents in all urban areas of the country (approximately 73% of the total national population)	2003	18–65	4426	2381	87.7
India	WMHI	Stratified multistage clustered area probability sample of household residents in Pondicherry region. NR	2003–5	18+	2992	1373	98.8
Iraq	IMHS	Stratified multistage clustered area probability sample of household residents. NR	2006–7	18+	4332	4332	95.2
Nigeria	NSMHW	Stratified multistage clustered area probability sample of households in 21 of the 36 states in the country, representing 57% of the national population. The surveys were conducted in Yoruba, Igbo, Hausa and Efik languages	2002–3	18+	6752	2143	79.3
PRC	B-WMH S-WMH	Stratified multistage clustered area probability sample of household residents in the Beijing and Shanghai metropolitan areas	2002–3	18+	5201	1628	74.7
PRC	Shenzhen	Stratified multistage clustered area probability sample of household residents and temporary residents in the Shenzhen area	2006–7	18+	7134	2476	80.0
Ukraine	CMDPSD	Stratified multistage clustered area probability sample of household residents. NR	2002	18+	4725	1720	78.3
Total					35562	16053	82.6
II. Upper-middle-income countries							
Brazil	São Paulo Megacity	Stratified multistage clustered area probability sample of household residents in the São Paulo metropolitan area.	2005–7	18+	5037	2942	81.3
Bulgaria	NSHS	Stratified multistage clustered area probability sample of household residents. NR	2003–7	18+	5318	2233	72.0
Lebanon	LEBANON	Stratified multistage clustered area probability sample of household residents. NR	2002–3	18+	2857	1031	70.0
Mexico	M-NCS	Stratified multistage clustered area probability sample of household residents in all urban areas of the country (approximately 75% of the total national population).	2001–2	18–65	5782	2362	76.6
Romania	RMHS	Stratified multistage clustered area probability sample of household residents. NR	2005–6	18+	2357	2357	70.9
South Africa	SASH	Stratified multistage clustered area probability sample of household residents. NR	2003–4	18+	4315	4315	87.1
Total					25,666	15,240	76.6
III. High-income countries							
Belgium	ESEMeD	Stratified multistage clustered probability sample of individuals residing in households from the national register of Belgium residents. NR	2001–2	18+	2419	1043	50.6
France	ESEMeD	Stratified multistage clustered sample of working telephone numbers merged with a reverse directory (for listed numbers). Initial recruitment was by telephone, with supplemental in-person recruitment in households with listed numbers. NR	2001–2	18+	2894	1436	45.9
Germany	ESEMeD	Stratified multistage clustered probability sample of individuals from community resident registries. NR	2002–3	18+	3555	1323	57.8
Israel	NHS	Stratified multistage clustered area probability sample of individuals from a national resident register. NR	2002–4	21+	4859	4859	72.6
Italy	ESEMeD	Stratified multistage clustered probability sample of individuals from municipality resident registries. NR	2001–2	18+	4712	1779	71.3
Japan	WMHJ2002–2006	Un-clustered two-stage probability sample of individuals residing in households in 11 metropolitan areas	2002–6	20+	4129	1682	55.1

(Continued)

Table 6.1 (*Contd.*) WMH Sample Characteristics by World Bank income categories

	Survey[2]	Sample characteristics[3]	Field dates	Age range	Sample size		Response rate[4]
					Part I	Part II	
Netherlands	ESEMeD	Stratified multistage clustered probability sample of individuals residing in households that are listed in municipal postal registries. NR	2002–3	18+	2372	1094	56.4
New Zealand[5]	NZMHS	Stratified multistage clustered area probability sample of household residents. NR	2003–4	18+	12790	7312	73.3
N Ireland	NISHS	Stratified multistage clustered area probability sample of household residents. NR	2004–7	18+	4340	1986	68.4
Portugal	NMHS	Stratified multistage clustered area probability sample of household residents. NR	2008–9	18+	3849	2060	57.3
Spain	ESEMeD	Stratified multistage clustered area probability sample of household residents. NR	2001–2	18+	5473	2121	78.6
United States	NCS-R	Stratified multistage clustered area probability sample of household residents. NR	2002–3	18+	9282	5692	70.9
Total					60,674	32,387	65.4
IV. Total					121,902	63,680	72.0

[1] The World Bank (2008). *Data and Statistics*. Accessed 12 May 2009 at: http://go.worldbank.org/D7SN0B8YU0

[2] NSMH (The Colombian National Study of Mental Health); WMHI (World Mental Health India); IMHS (Iraq Mental Health Survey); NSMHW (The Nigerian Survey of Mental Health and Wellbeing); B-WMH (The Beijing World Mental Health Survey); S-WMH (The Shanghai World Mental Health Survey); CMDPSD (Comorbid Mental Disorders during Periods of Social Disruption); NSHS (Bulgaria National Survey of Health and Stress); LEBANON (Lebanese Evaluation of the Burden of Ailments and Needs of the Nation); M-NCS (The Mexico National Comorbidity Survey); RMHS (Romania Mental Health Survey); SASH (South Africa Health Survey); ESEMeD (The European Study Of The Epidemiology Of Mental Disorders); NHS (Israel National Health Survey); WMHJ2002–2006 (World Mental Health Japan Survey); NZMHS (New Zealand Mental Health Survey); NISHS (Northern Ireland Study of Health and Stress); NMHS (Portugal National Mental Health Survey); NCS-R (The US National Comorbidity Survey Replication).

[3] Most WMH surveys are based on stratified multistage clustered area probability household samples in which samples of areas equivalent to counties or municipalities in the US were selected in the first stage followed by one or more subsequent stages of geographic sampling (e.g. towns within counties, blocks within towns, households within blocks) to arrive at a sample of households, in each of which a listing of household members was created and one or two people were selected from this listing to be interviewed. No substitution was allowed when the originally sampled household resident could not be interviewed. These household samples were selected from Census area data in all countries other than France (where telephone directories were used to select households) and the Netherlands (where postal registries were used to select households). Several WMH surveys (Belgium, Germany, Italy) used municipal resident registries to select respondents without listing households. The Japanese sample is the only totally un-clustered sample, with households randomly selected in each of the four sample areas and one random respondent selected in each sample household. 18 of the 24 surveys are based on nationally representative (NR) household samples.

[4] The response rate is calculated as the ratio of the number of households in which an interview was completed to the number of households originally sampled, excluding from the denominator households known not to be eligible either because of being vacant at the time of initial contact or because the residents were unable to speak the designated languages of the survey.

[5] New Zealand interviewed respondents 16+ but for the purposes of cross-national comparisons we limit the sample to those 18+

Severity of mental disorders

Disorder severity was defined using the criteria of the US Substance Abuse and Mental Health Services Administration (SAMHSA), which defines a **serious mental illness** (SMI) as 'a diagnosable mental, behavioral, or emotional disorder of sufficient duration to meet diagnostic criteria specified within DSM-III-R, and that resulted in functional impairment which substantially interferes with or limits role functioning in family, work, or community activities' (Substance Abuse and Mental Health Services Administration, 1993). This was operationalized in the WMH surveys by requiring either bipolar I disorder or substance dependence with a physiological dependence syndrome, a suicide attempt in conjunction with any 12-month DSM-IV disorder, severe role impairment due to a mental disorder in at least two areas of functioning measured by the disorder-specific Sheehan Disability Scales (SDS) (Leon et al., 1997), or overall functional impairment from any disorder consistent with a Global Assessment of Functioning (GAF) (Endicott et al., 1976) score of 50 or less. Disorders not classified as meeting criteria for SMI were classified as **moderate** in

severity if the respondent had either substance dependence without a physiological dependence syndrome or at least moderate interference in any SDS domain. All other disorders were classified as **mild** in severity. Some evidence for the validity of these ratings comes from statistically significant monotonic associations in the vast majority of surveys between severity and days in the prior year that respondents were totally unable to carry out normal daily activities because of these mental disorders (Kessler et al., 2008).

Twelve-month mental health service use

Services received for the treatment of mental disorders in the 12 months prior to the WMH interview were assessed by asking respondents if they ever during that time period saw any of a number of different types of professionals, either as an outpatient or inpatient, for problems with emotions, nerves, mental health, or use of alcohol or drugs. Included were mental health professionals (e.g. psychiatrist, psychologist), general medical professionals (e.g. general practitioner, specialist, nurse, occupational therapist), religious counsellors (e.g. minister, sheikh), and traditional healers (e.g. herbalist, spiritualist). Examples of these types of providers were presented in a Respondent Booklet as a visual recall aid and varied somewhat across countries depending on local circumstances. Follow-up questions were asked about number and duration of visits in the past 12 months.

Reports of 12-month service use were classified into the following sectors: mental health specialty (MHS; including psychiatrist, psychologist, other mental health professional in any setting, social worker or counsellor in a mental health specialty setting, use of a mental health hotline), general medical (GM; including primary care doctor, other general medical doctor, nurse, any other health professional not previously mentioned), human services (HS; including religious or spiritual advisor, and social worker or counsellor in any setting other than a specialty mental health setting), and complementary alternative medicine (CAM, including any other type of healer such as a chiropractor or faith healer as well as participation in a support group or self-help group).

Continuity and adequacy of treatment

We also studied intensity of treatment, but found that only a very small proportion of patients in most countries had a large enough number of visits for treatment to meet even the most minimal standards of being considered to have adequate care. In order to make at least some distinction regarding intensity, then, we classified patients as receiving follow-up care if they returned for a second visit in any service sector (one visit for presumptive evaluation/diagnosis and one or more visits for treatment or monitoring). Because respondents who began treatments shortly before interview may not have had time to fulfil these requirements, anyone reporting being in ongoing treatment at interview was considered to have met this definition.

Patients were classified as potentially having received at least **minimally adequate treatment** according to available evidence-based guidelines (Agency for Health Care Policy and Research, 1993; American Psychiatric Association, 2006; Lehman and Steinwachs, 1998) if they received either at least a minimum intensity of pharmacotherapy (at least 1 month of a medication plus four or more visits to any type of medical doctor) or psychotherapy (eight or more visits with any professional). The decision to require at least four physician visits for pharmacotherapy was based on the fact that four or more visits for medication evaluation, initiation, and monitoring are generally recommended during the acute and continuation phases of treatment (Agency for Health Care Policy and Research, 1993; American Psychiatric Association, 2006; Lehman and Steinwachs, 1998). At least eight sessions were required for psychotherapy based on the fact that clinical trials demonstrating effectiveness have generally included eight or more visits (Agency for Health Care Policy and Research, 1993; American Psychiatric Association, 2006; Lehman and Steinwachs, 1998).

Sociodemographic predictor variables

We examined a small number of sociodemographic correlates of treatment, including gender and family income. Family income was defined in each country in relation to within-country medians, where **low** income was defined as less than half the country median, **low average** as between low and the within-country median, **high-average** as between low-average and three times the within-country median, and **high** as more than three times the within-country average median.

Analysis procedures

Data analysis began by computing the proportions of respondents with 12-month disorders and the proportions of the latter who received any treatment in any or specific sectors within 12 months of the survey. We then examined the proportions of those in treatment who received follow-up care and minimally adequate care. We then examined how these basic patterns of service use differed across strata defined by the severity of disorders. Logistic regression analysis was then used to study sociodemographic predictors of receiving any 12-month treatment. Because the WMH data were weighted and clustered, standard errors of parameter estimates were obtained using the Taylor series method as implemented in the SUDAAN software system (Research Triangle Institute, 2002). Two-sided 0.05-level significance tests were used to judge the statistical significance of logistic regression coefficients. Wald χ^2 tests based on Taylor series coefficient variance–covariance matrices were used to evaluate the significance of sets of coefficients.

Twelve-month prevalence of DSM-IV/CIDI mental disorders

The proportion of respondents estimated to have any DSM-IV/CIDI disorder in the 12 months before interview averaged (mean) 16.7% across surveys, with a median of 13.6% (Table 6.2). The highest prevalence was 29.6% in São Paulo and the lowest 6.0% in Nigeria. The interquartile range (IQR: 25th–75th percentiles) of prevalence estimates across surveys was 10.0-20.7%. Relative prevalence estimates were quite consistent across surveys, with anxiety disorders the most common disorders in 22 of 24 countries (Table 6.2). The two exceptions are Israel and Ukraine, where mood disorders were estimated to be the most common disorders. Mood disorders were the next most common class of disorders in all but two other countries. The exceptions were South Africa, where substance use disorders were more common than mood disorders, and Beijing-Shanghai and the United States where behaviour disorders were more common than mood disorders.

Roughly one-fourth (24.5%) of all disorders were classified serious (SMI) using the definition of that term described above in the section on measurement (Table 6.3). The median proportion of cases with SMI across surveys was 22.3%. The range was 6.2–36.9% and the IQR was 18.6–25.8%. A higher proportion of all disorders was classified moderate (mean 37.8%, median 38.7%). The range was 12.5–50.6% and the IQR was 32.7–42.9%. A roughly similar proportion of all disorders was classified mild (mean and median both 37.7%). The range was 28.3-74.8% and the IQR was 34.9–42.1%.

The 12-month prevalence of having any disorder varied significantly across countries (χ^2_{24}= 1401.2, p <0.001). The severity distribution among cases also varied significantly across countries (χ^2_{48} = 352.9, p <0.001). Prevalence and severity (the proportion of respondents with a disorder who qualify for a diagnosis of SMI) among cases both varied significantly by country income level (χ^2_2 = 34.5, p = <0.001 for prevalence; χ^2_2 = 54.1, p = <0.001 for severity), although these associations were modest in substantive terms, with a Pearson contingency coefficient of 0.02 for the association between country income level and prevalence and of 0.06 for the association between income level and disorder severity. There were much more substantial positive associations (Pearson correlations) of overall disorder prevalence with both the proportion of cases

Table 6.2 Twelve-month prevalence of DSM-IV/CIDI disorders[1] in the WMH surveys[1]

	Any disorder[2]		Anxiety disorders[2]		Mood disorders[2]		Impulse-control disorders[2,3]		Substance disorders[2]	
	%	(se)	%	(se)	%	(se)	%	(se)	%	(se)
I. Low/lower-middle-income countries										
Colombia	21.0	(1.0)	14.4	(1.0)	6.9	(0.4)	4.4	(0.4)	2.8	(0.4)
India: Pondicherry	20.0	(1.1)	10.5	(0.8)	5.5	(0.5)	4.3	(0.7)	5.3	(0.6)
Iraq	13.6	(0.8)	10.4	(0.7)	4.1	(0.4)	1.7	(0.3)	0.3	(0.1)
Nigeria	6.0	(0.6)	4.2	(0.5)	1.2	(0.2)	0.1	(0.0)	0.9	(0.2)
PRC: Beijing, Shanghai	7.1	(0.9)	3.0	(0.5)	2.2	(0.4)	2.7	(0.6)	1.6	(0.4)
PRC: Shenzhen	16.0	(0.9)	11.4	(0.9)	4.8	(0.4)	2.9	(0.3)	0.0	(0.0)
Ukraine	21.4	(1.3)	6.8	(0.7)	10.0	(0.8)	5.1	(0.8)	6.4	(0.8)
Total	14.8	(0.4)	9.2	0.3	4.8	(0.2)	2.7	(0.2)	1.9	(0.1)
II. Upper-middle-income countries										
Brazil: São Paulo	29.6	(1.0)	19.9	(0.8)	11.8	(0.7)	5.3	(0.7)	3.8	(0.4)
Bulgaria	11.2	(0.8)	7.6	(0.7)	3.2	(0.3)	0.8	(0.3)	1.2	(0.3)
Lebanon	17.9	(1.6)	12.1	(1.2)	7.0	(0.8)	2.6	(0.7)	1.3	(0.8)
Mexico	13.4	(0.9)	8.4	(0.6)	5.0	(0.4)	1.6	(0.3)	2.5	(0.4)
Romania	8.2	(0.7)	4.9	(0.5)	2.5	(0.3)	1.9	(0.7)	1.0	(0.2)
South Africa	16.9	(0.9)	8.4	(0.6)	4.9	(0.4)	1.9	(0.3)	5.7	(0.6)
Total	16.7	(0.4)	10.2	(0.3)	5.8	(0.2)	2.5	(0.2)	3.2	(0.2)
III. High-income countries										
Belgium	13.2	(1.5)	8.4	(1.4)	6.1	(0.8)	1.7	(1.0)	1.3	(0.4)
France	18.9	(1.4)	13.7	(1.1)	6.8	(0.7)	2.4	(0.6)	0.8	(0.3)
Germany	11.0	(1.3)	8.3	(1.1)	3.4	(0.3)	0.6	(0.3)	1.2	(0.4)
Israel	10.0	(0.5)	3.6	(0.3)	6.4	(0.4)	0.0	(0.0)	1.3	(0.2)
Italy	8.8	(0.7)	6.5	(0.6)	3.6	(0.3)	0.4	(0.2)	0.1	(0.1)
Japan	8.0	(0.7)	4.8	(0.6)	2.8	(0.4)	0.2	(0.1)	1.0	(0.3)
Netherlands	13.6	(1.0)	8.9	(1.0)	5.5	(0.7)	1.9	(0.7)	1.7	(0.5)
New Zealand	20.7	(0.6)	15.0	(0.5)	8.0	(0.4)	0.0	(0.0)	3.4	(0.3)
Northern Ireland	23.1	(1.4)	14.6	(1.0)	10.6	(0.9)	4.5	(1.0)	3.5	(0.5)
Portugal	22.9	(1.0)	16.5	(1.0)	8.3	(0.6)	3.5	(0.4)	1.6	(0.3)
Spain	9.7	(0.8)	6.6	(0.9)	4.4	(0.4)	0.5	(0.2)	0.3	(0.2)
United States	27.0	(0.9)	19.0	(0.7)	9.8	(0.4)	10.5	(0.7)	3.8	(0.4)
Total	17.7	(0.3)	11.9	(0.2)	7.2	(0.2)	2.7	(0.2)	2.2	(0.1)
IV. Total	16.7	(0.2)	10.8	(0.2)	6.2	(0.1)	2.6	(0.1)	2.4	(0.1)

[1] See the section on measurement of disorders in the text for a list of the disorders assessed

[2] Between-country differences in prevalence are significant both for any disorder ($\chi^2_{24} = 1401.2$, p <0.001) and for each class of disorder ($\chi^2_{24} = 715.4-1099.9$, p <0.001).

[3] Prevalence of impulse-control disorders was estimated in the subsample of respondents who were 44 years of age or younger at the time of the interview.

classified as serious (0.30) and the proportion of cases classified as either serious or moderate (0.40).

The finding of a positive association between estimated prevalence and severity across countries is potentially important because it speaks to an issue that has been raised in the methodological literature regarding the possibility of biased prevalence estimates. Two separate research groups found an opposite sort of pattern than the one found in the WMH surveys. The first was a study comparing results from the Korean Epidemiologic Catchment

Area (KECA) Study (Chang et al., 2008) with results from parallel surveys in other countries. The authors argued that the lower estimated prevalence of major depression in the KECA than the other surveys was due, at least in part, to a higher threshold for reporting depression among people in the Korean population than in population studies in the other surveys. In support of this assertion, the investigators showed that Koreans diagnosed as depressed with an earlier version of the CIDI, which was the diagnostic instrument used in the KECA survey, had considerably higher levels of role

Table 6.3 Twelve-month prevalence of DSM-IV/CIDI disorders by severity in the WMH surveys[1]

	Unconditional prevalence[2]						Conditional prevalence[2]					
	Disorders						Disorders					
	Serious		Moderate		Mild		Serious		Moderate		Mild	
	%	(se)	%	(se)	%	(se)	%	(se)	%	(se)	%	(se)
I. Low/lower-middle-income countries												
Colombia	4.9	(0.5)	8.6	(0.7)	7.5	(0.5)	23.3	(2.1)	41.2	(2.6)	35.5	(2.1)
India: Pondicherry	4.3	(0.3)	7.8	(0.7)	7.9	(0.8)	21.7	(1.6)	39.0	(3.1)	39.3	(2.8)
Iraq	3.0	(0.4)	4.9	(0.4)	5.7	(0.6)	21.9	(2.3)	36.0	(2.6)	42.1	(2.9)
Nigeria	0.8	(0.3)	0.8	(0.2)	4.5	(0.5)	12.8	(3.8)	12.5	(2.6)	74.8	(4.2)
PRC: Beijing, Shanghai	1.0	(0.3)	2.3	(0.5)	3.8	(0.6)	13.8	(3.7)	32.2	(4.9)	54.0	(4.6)
PRC: Shenzhen	1.0	(0.3)	5.2	(0.5)	9.8	(0.8)	6.2	(1.6)	32.7	(2.9)	61.2	(3.6)
Ukraine	4.9	(0.4)	8.4	(0.8)	8.1	(1.0)	22.9	(1.8)	39.4	(2.9)	37.7	(3.5)
Total	2.8	(0.2)	5.3	(0.2)	6.7	(0.3)	18.8	(0.9)	35.9	(1.2)	45.3	(1.3)
II. Upper-middle-income countries												
Brazil: São Paulo	10.0	(0.6)	9.8	(0.5)	9.8	(0.6)	33.9	(1.4)	33.0	(1.8)	33.2	(1.4)
Bulgaria	2.3	(0.3)	3.6	(0.5)	5.4	(0.5)	20.3	(2.8)	32.1	(3.6)	47.7	(2.7)
Lebanon	4.0	(0.7)	7.7	(1.0)	6.2	(1.2)	22.3	(3.1)	42.9	(4.9)	34.9	(5.6)
Mexico	3.5	(0.4)	4.7	(0.4)	5.2	(0.5)	26.3	(2.4)	34.8	(2.2)	38.9	(2.5)
Romania	2.3	(0.4)	2.4	(0.3)	3.5	(0.5)	27.9	(3.4)	29.3	(3.7)	42.8	(3.5)
South Africa	4.3	(0.4)	5.3	(0.5)	7.2	(0.6)	25.7	(1.8)	31.4	(2.1)	43.0	(2.1)
Total	4.7	(0.2)	5.5	(0.2)	6.5	(0.3)	28.0	(0.9)	33.1	(1.1)	39.0	(1.0)
III. High-income countries												
Belgium	4.3	(0.8)	5.1	(0.8)	3.8	(0.6)	32.6	(4.2)	38.7	(3.4)	28.8	(4.8)
France	3.5	(0.5)	8.1	(0.8)	7.2	(0.9)	18.6	(2.5)	43.1	(3.0)	38.3	(3.6)
Germany	2.4	(0.4)	4.8	(0.8)	3.9	(0.7)	21.6	(2.5)	43.2	(4.5)	35.2	(4.1)
Israel	3.7	(0.3)	3.5	(0.3)	2.8	(0.2)	36.9	(2.4)	34.8	(2.3)	28.3	(2.1)
Italy	1.4	(0.2)	4.2	(0.5)	3.2	(0.5)	15.9	(2.7)	47.8	(3.9)	36.3	(3.9)
Japan	1.3	(0.4)	3.8	(0.5)	2.9	(0.4)	16.1	(4.5)	47.2	(4.8)	36.7	(3.7)
Netherlands	4.2	(0.6)	4.2	(0.5)	5.2	(0.8)	31.1	(3.5)	31.1	(3.6)	37.8	(4.7)
New Zealand	5.3	(0.3)	8.6	(0.4)	6.7	(0.3)	25.8	(1.0)	41.7	(1.4)	32.5	(1.2)
Northern Ireland	6.7	(0.7)	7.7	(0.7)	8.7	(1.1)	28.8	(3.0)	33.4	(2.6)	37.8	(3.3)
Portugal	4.0	(0.4)	11.6	(0.6)	7.3	(0.5)	17.5	(1.5)	50.6	(2.0)	31.9	(1.9)
Spain	1.9	(0.2)	4.2	(0.5)	3.6	(0.6)	19.9	(2.4)	43.5	(4.1)	36.6	(4.8)
United States	6.9	(0.4)	10.7	(0.5)	9.4	(0.6)	25.5	(1.4)	39.7	(1.2)	34.8	(1.4)
Total	4.5	(0.1)	7.2	(0.2)	6.0	(0.2)	25.4	(0.6)	40.7	(0.7)	33.9	(0.7)
IV. Total	4.1	(0.1)	6.3	(0.1)	6.3	(0.1)	24.5	(0.5)	37.8	(0.5)	37.7	(0.6)

[1] See the section on measurement of disorders in the text for a list of the disorders assessed and a description of how severity was operationalized.

[2] Unconditional prevalence is prevalence in the total sample. Conditional prevalence is prevalence among cases. For example, the 4.9% of respondents in the Colombia survey with a 12-month serious disorder represent 23.3% of the 21.0% of respondents in the Colombia who had any 12-month DSM-IV/CIDI disorder. (The 21.0% total prevalence is reported in Table 6.2.)

[3] Between-country differences in prevalence are significant both for unconditional prevalence for each class of disorders (χ^2_{24} = 377.9–741.6, p <0.001) and for conditional prevalence for each class of disorders (χ^2_{24} = 146.8–187.2, p <0.001).

impairment than respondents diagnosed as depressed using the same instrument in the US.

The second relevant previous study was carried out as part of the WHO Collaborative Study on Psychological Problems in General Health Care (PPG) (Üstün and Sartorius, 1995). In that study, nearly 26,000 primary care patients in 14 countries were assessed using an earlier version of the CIDI that included an evaluation of current symptoms of depression. As in the WMH surveys, substantial cross-national variation was found in the prevalence of major depression. However, the investigators found that the average amount of impairment associated with depression across countries was inversely proportional to the estimated prevalence of depression in those countries (Chang et al., 2008; Simon et al., 2002).

This result is consistent with the possibility that the substantial cross-national variation in estimated prevalence of depression in the PPG study might be due, at least in part, to cross-national differences in diagnostic thresholds. However, we do not find results consistent with these in the WMH surveys, where the countries with the lowest prevalence estimates of the DSM-IV/CIDI disorders assessed in the surveys also had the lowest reported levels of impairment associated with those disorders.

Twelve-month use of mental health services

The proportion of respondents using any mental health services in the 12 months prior to the WMH surveys averaged (mean) 9.0% across surveys, with a median of 6.8% and an IQR of 4.3–10.9 (Table 6.4). This proportion varied significantly across countries, from a low of 1.6% in Nigeria to a high of 18.0% in the US ($\chi^2_{24} = 1324.1$, p <0.0001), with much lower proportions in low/lower-middle-income countries (3.4%) than in upper-middle- (8.7%) or high-income countries (12.0%). The largest proportions of patients were seen in the general medical (GM) sector in all but six surveys (the exceptions being Colombia, Israel, Japan, Mexico, São Paulo, and Shenzhen, where specialty mental health treatment was somewhat more common than GM treatment). The proportion of patients seen in the GM sector averaged (mean) 58.7% with a median of 64.9% with an IQR of 42.5% to 68.5%. This proportion varied significantly by country income level ($\chi^2_2 = 24.7$, p <0.001) and was higher in high- (61.1%) and upper-middle- (56.7%) than low/lower-middle-income (45.9%) countries. The next highest proportion of patients was seen in the mental health specialty (MHS) sector, with a mean 40.4%, median 44.3%, and IQR of 24.3% to 50.5%. As with GM treatment, the proportion of patients seen in the MHS sector varied significantly by country income level ($\chi^2_2 = 54.6$, p <0.001) and was higher in high- (44.2%) and upper-middle- (33.1%) than low/lower-middle-income (31.2%) countries. Much lower proportions of patients were seen in the human services (HS) sector (mean 13.8%, median 9.2%, IQR 5.4–18.0%) and CAM sector (mean 14.0%, median 7.4%, IQR 3.5–15.5%). As with GM and MH treatment, the proportions of patients seen in the HS and CAM sectors varied significantly by country income level ($\chi^2_2 = 11.7$–15.6, p <0.001). Unlike GM and MH treatment, though, the proportions of patients seen in the HS and CAM sectors were higher in low/lower-middle-income countries (18.3% and 15.1% in HS and CAM, respectively) than in upper-middle- (16.9% and 17.0%) or high-income (12.1% and 12.8%) countries.

Service use by severity of disorders

Significant monotonic relationships were found between disorder severity and probability of service use in 21 of the 25 WMH surveys ($\chi^2_2 = 34.9$–672.1, p <0.001) (Table 6.5). The exceptions were the two surveys in the People's Republic of China and the surveys in Pondicherry, India and South Africa. Even in the latter four surveys, though, the association between severity and probability of treatment was significant ($\chi^2_2 = 12.8$–41.5, p = 0.005–<0.001) and generally monotonic in that the lowest rates in treatment were among those with no disorders or, in the case of Beijing-Shanghai, mild disorders and treatment rates were higher among those with moderate-serious disorders than none-mild disorders in all but one comparison (higher treatment among those with mild than moderate disorders in Pondicherry). However, there were also inversions in three of these four surveys (the exception being Pondicherry) due to higher treatment rates among respondents with moderate than serious disorders.

The association of disorder severity with MH specialty treatment among patients

Not only was disorder severity associated with probability of receiving any treatment, but severity was also related significantly to treatment being received in the specialty mental health sector ($\chi^2_2 = 109.3$, p <0.001) (Table 6.6). As noted above, 40.4% of patients across surveys were seen in the MHS sector. This proportion was significantly higher among patients with serious (55.8%) than moderate-mild (39.7–34.7%) or no (35.7%) disorders. The same generally monotonic association between severity and proportional MH treatment among patients was found in high- ($\chi^2_2 = 72.5$, p <0.001) and upper-middle-income ($\chi^2_2 = 62.3$, p <0.001) countries, but not in low/lower-middle-income countries ($\chi^2_2 = 6.4$, p = 0.09).

Continuity and adequacy of treatments

Although the vast majority of people who received treatment (84.9%) had follow-up care, this varied significantly across surveys ($\chi^2_{24} = 83.1$, p <0.001) and as a function of country income level ($\chi^2_2 = 31.6$, p <0.001), with considerably higher proportions receiving follow-up care in high (86.2%) and upper-middle-income (85.3%) countries than in low/lower-middle-income countries (74.9%) (Table 6.7). A much stronger association was found, furthermore, between disorder severity and probability of receiving follow-up care among patients in high-income countries ($\chi^2_3 = 46.4$, p <0.001) than in either upper-middle-income countries ($\chi^2_3 = 8.4$, p = 0.039) or low/lower-middle-income countries ($\chi^2_3 = 6.1$, p = 0.11).

Treatment adequacy could be defined in only 19 of the 25 surveys due to information needed to define adequacy not being collected in all WMH surveys. Only a minority of patients (29.0%) in these 19 surveys received minimally adequate treatment (Table 6.8). This percentage varied significantly across surveys ($\chi^2_{18} = 88.8$, p <0.001) and as a function of country income level ($\chi^2_2 = 19.9$, p <0.001), with considerably higher proportions receiving adequate treatment in high- (30.9%) and upper-middle-income (28.8%) countries than in low/lower-middle-income countries (15.2%). A much stronger association was found, furthermore, between disorder severity and probability of receiving minimally adequate treatment among patients in high-income countries

Table 6.4 Treatment of 12-month DSM-IV/CIDI disorders overall and by service sector in the WMH surveys

| | Unconditional[1] | | | | | | | | | | Conditional[1] | | | | | | | |
| | Any[2] | | Specialty[2] | | General medical[2] | | Human service[2] | | CAM[2] | | Specialty[2] | | General medical[2] | | Human Service[2] | | CAM[2] | |
	%	(se)	%	(se)	%	(se)	%	(se)	%	(se)	%	(se)	%	(se)	%	(se)	%	(se)
I. Low/lower-middle-income countries																		
Colombia	5.5	(0.6)	3.0	(0.4)	2.3	(0.4)	0.5	(0.2)	0.2	(0.1)	53.4	(4.8)	41.7	(5.1)	9.2	(2.8)	3.7	(1.4)
India: Pondicherry	1.9	(0.3)	0.3	(0.2)	0.8	(0.1)	0.7	(0.3)	0.1	(0.1)	18.1	(8.3)	42.5	(7.0)	37.1	(11.0)	4.7	(3.2)
Iraq	2.2	(0.4)	0.7	(0.2)	0.9	(0.3)	0.7	(0.2)	0.1	(0.0)	33.4	(7.4)	41.3	(8.3)	32.2	(7.4)	2.9	(1.9)
Nigeria	1.6	(0.3)	0.1	(0.1)	1.1	(0.2)	0.5	(0.2)	0.0	(0.0)	8.3	(3.6)	66.6	(10.0)	30.9	(10.1)	1.1	(1.1)
PRC: Beijing, Shanghai	3.4	(0.6)	0.6	(0.2)	2.3	(0.5)	0.3	(0.1)	0.7	(0.3)	18.0	(5.9)	68.5	(7.1)	7.4	(3.7)	21.2	(7.2)
PRC: Shenzhen	3.3	(0.7)	1.2	(0.4)	0.7	(0.2)	0.1	(0.1)	1.8	(0.5)	37.1	(9.9)	20.9	(5.7)	4.2	(1.8)	54.2	(7.6)
Ukraine	7.2	(0.8)	1.2	(0.3)	4.0	(0.7)	1.7	(0.4)	1.0	(0.3)	17.2	(3.8)	55.4	(7.1)	24.1	(5.1)	14.4	(4.0)
Total	3.4	(0.2)	1.1	(0.1)	1.6	(0.1)	0.6	(0.1)	0.5	(0.1)	31.2	(2.7)	45.9	(3.1)	18.3	(2.3)	15.1	(2.1)
II. Upper-middle-income countries																		
Brazil: São Paulo	10.1	(0.6)	6.3	(0.4)	3.3	(0.3)	1.5	(0.3)	1.4	(0.2)	62.4	(2.2)	32.7	(2.6)	14.6	(2.4)	13.7	(2.2)
Bulgaria	5.6	(0.6)	1.4	(0.2)	4.5	(0.5)	0.2	(0.1)	0.1	(0.0)	24.3	(2.6)	81.2	(2.5)	3.4	(1.8)	1.2	(0.8)
Lebanon	4.4	(0.6)	1.0	(0.3)	2.9	(0.5)	0.8	(0.3)	0.0	(0.0)	22.3	(5.7)	66.6	(7.4)	17.5	(6.1)	0.0	(0.0)
Mexico	5.1	(0.5)	2.8	(0.3)	1.7	(0.3)	0.3	(0.1)	1.0	(0.2)	53.6	(4.2)	33.1	(4.0)	6.2	(2.0)	20.0	(3.4)
Romania	3.4	(0.4)	1.7	(0.3)	2.0	(0.4)	0.1	(0.1)	0.1	(0.1)	51.5	(7.6)	57.8	(7.9)	3.4	(1.5)	1.9	(1.9)
South Africa	15.4	(1.0)	2.5	(0.4)	10.2	(0.8)	3.7	(0.4)	3.7	(0.3)	16.3	(2.2)	66.4	(2.5)	24.0	(1.9)	23.8	(2.1)
Total	8.7	(0.4)	2.9	(0.2)	5.0	(0.3)	1.5	(0.1)	1.5	(0.1)	33.1	(1.4)	56.7	(1.6)	16.9	(1.3)	17.0	(1.1)
III. High-income countries																		
Belgium	10.9	(1.4)	5.2	(0.7)	8.2	(1.3)	0.4	(0.2)	0.7	(0.3)	47.9	(4.4)	75.5	(3.8)	3.7	(1.8)	6.5	(2.9)
France	11.3	(1.0)	4.4	(0.5)	8.8	(0.9)	0.4	(0.2)	0.5	(0.3)	39.4	(3.6)	78.4	(3.3)	3.4	(1.2)	4.3	(2.1)
Germany	8.1	(0.8)	3.9	(0.6)	4.2	(0.6)	1.0	(0.4)	0.6	(0.2)	48.5	(4.8)	51.7	(5.1)	12.2	(4.5)	7.4	(2.5)
Israel	8.8	(0.4)	4.4	(0.3)	3.6	(0.3)	1.6	(0.2)	0.8	(0.1)	50.5	(2.6)	40.4	(2.6)	18.0	(2.0)	9.6	(1.5)
Italy	4.3	(0.4)	2.0	(0.3)	3.0	(0.3)	0.4	(0.1)	0.1	(0.0)	47.1	(5.1)	70.9	(4.8)	9.1	(2.4)	1.5	(0.7)
Japan	5.3	(0.6)	2.7	(0.3)	2.4	(0.3)	0.6	(0.3)	0.9	(0.2)	50.1	(4.2)	45.5	(5.5)	11.3	(4.6)	16.6	(3.9)
Netherlands	10.9	(1.2)	5.5	(1.0)	7.7	(1.1)	0.6	(0.2)	1.5	(0.4)	51.0	(6.0)	71.2	(6.1)	5.4	(1.6)	13.5	(3.8)
New Zealand	13.8	(0.5)	5.2	(0.3)	9.2	(0.4)	1.6	(0.2)	2.6	(0.3)	37.6	(1.8)	66.5	(1.8)	11.5	(1.1)	19.0	(1.7)
Northern Ireland	14.2	(0.9)	4.7	(0.5)	12.3	(0.8)	0.8	(0.2)	1.5	(0.3)	33.0	(2.7)	86.1	(2.7)	5.7	(1.3)	10.7	(2.2)
Portugal	15.0	(0.8)	6.6	(0.6)	9.8	(0.7)	0.9	(0.2)	0.7	(0.2)	44.3	(3.1)	65.2	(3.0)	5.8	(1.3)	5.0	(1.0)
Spain	6.8	(0.5)	3.6	(0.4)	4.4	(0.4)	0.1	(0.1)	0.2	(0.1)	52.2	(3.6)	64.9	(3.4)	2.1	(0.8)	3.5	(1.0)
United States	18.0	(0.7)	8.8	(0.5)	9.3	(0.4)	3.4	(0.3)	2.8	(0.2)	48.9	(1.7)	51.6	(1.3)	18.9	(1.2)	15.5	(1.0)
Total	12.0	(0.2)	5.3	(0.1)	7.3	(0.2)	1.5	(0.1)	1.5	(0.1)	44.2	(0.8)	61.1	(0.8)	12.1	(0.6)	12.8	(0.6)
IV. Total	9.0	(0.2)	3.7	(0.1)	5.3	(0.1)	1.2	(0.1)	1.3	(0.1)	40.4	(0.8)	58.7	(0.8)	13.8	(0.6)	14.0	(0.5)

[1] The entries in the unconditional treatment columns represent treatment in the total sample. The entries in the conditional treatment columns represent the proportion of patients who received treatment in specific sectors. For example, the 3.0% of respondents in the Colombia sample who received treatment in the Mental Health Specialty sector represent 53.4% of the 5.5% of respondents who received any type of treatment.

[2] See the section on measurement of 12-month service use in the text for a description of how treatment within sectors was operationalized. Treatment rates differ significantly across countries for each column in the table, with χ^2_{24} values in the range 261.1–1324.1, p <0.001.

Table 6.5 Treatment of 12-month DSM-IV/CIDI disorders by severity of disorder in the WMH surveys

	Serious disorders		Moderate disorders		Mild disorders		No disorder	
	%	(se)	%	(se)	%	(se)	%	(se)
I. Low/lower-middle-income countries								
Colombia	27.7	(4.8)	10.3	(2.0)	7.8	(1.6)	3.4	(0.6)
India: Pondicherry	9.7	(2.8)	6.6	(1.2)	8.1	(3.2)	0.4	(0.2)
Iraq	23.7	(6.2)	9.2	(3.2)	5.3	(2.5)	0.9	(0.2)
Nigeria	21.3	(10.2)	13.8	(7.1)	10.0	(2.7)	1.0	(0.3)
PRC: Beijing, Shanghai	11.0	(5.9)	23.5	(10.6)	1.7	(1.1)	2.9	(0.6)
PRC: Shenzhen	4.3	(1.8)	10.0	(3.4)	3.9	(1.0)	2.8	(0.7)
Ukraine	25.7	(3.2)	21.2	(3.6)	7.6	(2.6)	4.4	(0.8)
Total	21.7	(2.5)	12.0	(1.4)	6.2	(0.9)	2.1	(0.2)
II. Upper-middle-income countries								
Brazil: São Paulo	34.5	(2.1)	21.3	(2.8)	12.7	(1.5)	4.7	(0.5)
Bulgaria	31.0	(4.6)	21.4	(3.6)	16.5	(4.7)	3.6	(0.5)
Lebanon	20.1	(5.2)	11.4	(3.1)	4.0	(1.6)	3.0	(0.7)
Mexico	25.8	(4.3)	17.9	(2.9)	11.9	(2.4)	3.2	(0.4)
Romania	36.4	(7.3)	17.4	(6.2)	14.4	(4.4)	1.8	(0.4)
South Africa	26.2	(3.6)	26.6	(3.9)	23.4	(3.2)	13.3	(0.9)
Total	30.4	(1.5)	21.1	(1.5)	16.0	(1.4)	6.1	(0.3)
III. High-income countries								
Belgium	60.9	(9.1)	36.5	(8.6)	13.9	(4.3)	6.7	(1.1)
France	48.0	(6.4)	28.8	(3.9)	21.1	(3.5)	7.0	(1.1)
Germany	40.0	(8.5)	23.9	(4.6)	20.3	(5.1)	5.9	(0.9)
Israel	52.5	(3.9)	32.3	(3.7)	13.9	(3.1)	5.9	(0.4)
Italy	51.0	(6.4)	25.5	(4.1)	17.3	(4.3)	2.1	(0.4)
Japan	44.1	(11.8)	19.7	(3.8)	15.9	(4.6)	3.9	(0.6)
Netherlands	50.4	(6.8)	30.5	(7.1)	15.8	(5.9)	7.7	(1.3)
New Zealand	56.6	(2.2)	39.9	(1.9)	22.2	(1.9)	7.3	(0.5)
Northern Ireland	72.8	(4.7)	34.5	(4.1)	17.4	(4.2)	6.7	(0.8)
Portugal	66.4	(4.6)	35.0	(2.5)	18.2	(3.0)	9.0	(0.8)
Spain	58.7	(4.9)	36.9	(4.8)	17.0	(3.9)	3.9	(0.5)
United States	59.7	(2.4)	40.0	(1.3)	26.4	(1.7)	9.7	(0.6)
Total	58.4	(1.2)	36.2	(0.9)	21.2	(1.0)	6.7	(0.2)
IV. Total	44.4	(0.9)	27.8	(0.7)	16.0	(0.7)	5.3	(0.1)

[1] See the section on measurement of 12-month disorders in the text for a description of how severity was operationalized. Treatment rates differ significantly by severity within each of the surveys, with χ^2_3 values in the range 12.0–672.1, p = 0.050–<0.001. Treatment rates also differ significantly across countries within each disorder severity subsample (χ^2_{16} = 107.8–354.9, p <0.001, with only 17 countries with combined number of serious and moderate cases greater than 60 used in the tests).

(χ^2_3 = 59.8, p <0.001) than in either upper-middle-income countries (χ^2_3 = 9.3, p = 0.025) or low/lower-middle-income countries (χ^2_2 = 7.5, p = 0.059). Yet even serious cases in high-income countries had less than a 50:50 chance (43.7%) of receiving minimally adequate treatment.

Predictors of any 12-month service use

Women were more likely than men with the same disorder severity to receive treatment in 24 of the 25 surveys (the exception being Shenzhen in the People's Republic of China, where there was no significant gender difference), with female:male odds ratios (ORs) in the range 1.1 to 2.5. These ORs were statistically significant in 14 of the 24 surveys (χ^2_1 = 5.3–66.3, p = 0.021–<0.001). The association between income and treatment among people with the same disorder severity, in comparison, was surprisingly inconsistent, as this association was statistically significant in only eight of the 25 surveys (χ^2_3 = 8.9–25.2, p = 0.030–<0.001), in seven of which the association was positive. Three of these seven

Table 6.6 Proportional treatment of 12-month DSM-IV/CIDI disorders in the mental health specialty section by severity of disorder[1]

	Serious disorders		Moderate disorders		Mild disorders		No disorder	
	%	(se)	%	(se)	%	(se)	%	(se)
I. Low/lower-middle-income countries								
Colombia	62.9	(8.3)	47.1	(8.0)	62.2	(10.3)	48.8	(8.3)
India: Pondicherry[2]	–	(–)	–	(–)	–	(–)	–	(–)
Iraq[2]	23.4	(10.1)	23.4	(10.1)	44.4	(10.4)	44.4	(10.4)
Nigeria[2]	–	(–)	–	(–)	9.5	(4.4)	9.5	(4.4)
PRC: Beijing, Shanghai[2]	–	(–)	–	(–)	16.7	(6.8)	16.7	(6.8)
PRC: Shenzhen[2]	24.3	(10.9)	24.3	(10.9)	39.7	(11.0)	39.7	(11.0)
Ukraine	34.8	(6.8)	16.2	(8.2)	–	(–)	12.5	(5.3)
Total	41.9	(6.1)	22.0	(4.3)	34.3	(6.4)	30.2	(4.4)
II. Upper-middle-income countries								
Brazil: São Paulo	70.8	(4.8)	60.7	(7.5)	53.0	(6.9)	58.5	(5.5)
Bulgaria	39.7	(8.6)	36.1	(13.6)	–	(–)	17.8	(5.0)
Lebanon[2]	35.6	(9.2)	35.6	(9.2)	14.0	(7.3)	14.0	(7.3)
Mexico	60.3	(8.0)	59.1	(6.8)	51.0	(11.2)	50.4	(7.0)
Romania[2]	44.4	(9.3)	44.4	(9.3)	55.6	(8.0)	55.6	(8.0)
South Africa	35.9	(7.6)	19.7	(5.9)	14.9	(5.5)	14.1	(2.0)
Total	57.0	(3.3)	40.5	(3.5)	31.1	(3.8)	25.2	(1.9)
III. High-income countries								
Belgium	58.6	(9.8)	48.6	(10.9)	–	(–)	44.0	(7.4)
France	49.7	(8.6)	33.6	(8.3)	34.1	(7.0)	40.3	(6.9)
Germany	46.4	(12.1)	69.3	(8.8)	–	(–)	47.2	(6.2)
Israel	47.2	(5.6)	53.2	(7.0)	–	(–)	50.7	(3.2)
Italy	–	(–)	31.7	(10.1)	–	(–)	65.8	(7.4)
Japan[2]	70.7	(9.4)	70.7	(9.4)	44.0	(5.2)	44.0	(5.2)
Netherlands	64.9	(7.1)	45.2	(15.5)	–	(–)	48.2	(9.2)
New Zealand	57.4	(2.9)	34.9	(3.4)	26.3	(4.3)	31.8	(2.9)
Northern Ireland	48.3	(5.9)	23.5	(5.8)	21.2	(8.2)	27.3	(6.3)
Portugal	58.6	(6.2)	42.6	(4.9)	44.7	(7.5)	39.7	(4.3)
Spain	65.4	(7.3)	61.3	(5.5)	45.2	(10.4)	45.1	(6.5)
United States	66.0	(2.4)	45.1	(3.3)	41.8	(3.2)	43.7	(2.6)
Total	57.1	(1.7)	41.8	(1.6)	36.2	(2.2)	41.2	(1.3)
IV. Total	55.8	(1.6)	39.7	(1.4)	34.7	(1.9)	35.7	(1.2)

[1] See the section on measurement of 12-month disorders in the text for a description of how severity was operationalized and the section on measurement of 12-month service use in the text for a description of how mental health specialty treatment was operationalized. The proportion of all patients who were seen in the mental health specialty sector differs significantly by severity within two of the three overall country income categories, high-income countries (χ^2_3 = 72.5, p <0.001) and upper-middle-income countries (χ^2_3 = 62,3, p <0.001), but not in low/lower-middle-income countries (χ^2_3 = 6.4, p = 0.09). Within-country differences are significant only in Germany, Italy, Japan, New Zealand, Northern Ireland, and the United States (χ^2_3 =8.0–63.0, p = 0.046–<0.001). The proportion of patients within a disorder severity level that received their treatment. In the mental health specialty sector differs significantly across countries within all severity subsamples (χ^2_{24} = 50.4–165.0, p <0.001).

[2] Percents were not reported if the number of cases with any treatment in a level of severity <30. In Nigeria, Lebanon, Japan, China, Romania, Iraq, Shenzhen and Pondicherry (India) combined Severe and Moderate was compared against combined Mild and None categories.

were low/lower-middle-income countries (Colombia, Pondicherry India, Shenzhen, People's Republic of China), in all of which the OR of treatment was highest among people in the highest quartile of the income distribution (highest half in India) with no meaningful gradient below this range and ORs of 2.0 to 4.9. Two others of the seven were lower-middle-income countries (São Paulo Brazil and Lebanon), in both of which the treatment rate was especially low among people in the lowest quartile of the income distribution with no meaningful gradient above this range and ORs of 1.5 to 8.4. The remaining two countries were high income

Table 6.7 The proportions of patients who received follow-up treatment of their 12-month DSM-IV/CIDI disorders by severity of disorder[1]

	Any disorder		Serious disorders[2]		Moderate disorders[2]		Mild disorders[2]		No disorder[2]	
	%	(se)	%	(se)	%	(se)	%	(se)	%	(se)
I. Low/lower-middle-income countries										
Colombia	72.0	(4.3)	92.6	(3.5)	73.1	(7.9)	61.7	(11.3)	63.6	(7.9)
India: Pondicherry	79.6	(6.2)	–	(–)	–	(–)	–	(–)	–	(–)
Iraq	67.4	(7.7)	70.6	(9.5)	70.6	(9.5)	63.8	(10.4)	63.8	(10.4)
Nigeria	76.3	(7.8)	–	(–)	–	(–)	74.6	(8.4)	74.6	(8.4)
PRC: Beijing, Shanghai	77.6	(6.1)	–	(–)	–	(–)	80.8	(6.9)	80.8	(6.9)
PRC: Shenzhen	78.2	(7.5)	87.6	(7.8)	87.6	(7.8)	76.2	(8.4)	76.2	(8.4)
Ukraine	79.1	(3.8)	92.3	(3.6)	82.3	(4.5)	–	(–)	71.8	(7.0)
Total	74.9	(2.3)	85.7	(4.0)	75.8	(4.5)	68.6	(7.6)	72.3	(3.1)
II. Upper-middle-income countries										
Brazil: São Paulo	84.9	(2.3)	92.2	(2.4)	90.6	(3.4)	79.6	(6.9)	75.6	(6.5)
Bulgaria	85.7	(2.0)	97.6	(2.4)	95.3	(3.7)	–	(–)	83.0	(3.5)
Lebanon	78.9	(6.9)	84.1	(4.4)	84.1	(4.4)	75.7	(10.2)	75.7	(10.2)
Mexico	74.5	(4.4)	85.5	(4.2)	76.6	(6.7)	84.3	(6.9)	67.8	(7.7)
Romania	75.7	(5.7)	76.8	(10.8)	76.8	(10.8)	75.1	(7.4)	75.1	(7.4)
South Africa	89.1	(1.7)	93.9	(3.9)	95.7	(3.0)	87.9	(3.6)	87.9	(2.2)
Total	85.3	(1.2)	91.0	(2.0)	89.6	(2.2)	82.2	(3.0)	83.4	(2.0)
III. High-income countries										
Belgium	84.3	(3.9)	84.4	(9.5)	84.3	(10.4)	–	(–)	82.9	(5.3)
France	86.0	(3.9)	87.5	(4.7)	97.3	(1.6)	89.7	(4.4)	79.9	(6.9)
Germany	70.2	(5.1)	89.2	(8.5)	97.2	(0.7)	–	(–)	61.0	(7.4)
Israel	86.1	(1.8)	88.2	(4.1)	89.3	(4.1)	–	(–)	84.3	(2.3)
Italy	94.5	(1.5)	–	(–)	93.5	(3.4)	–	(–)	94.2	(2.5)
Japan	88.3	(2.1)	90.1	(4.4)	90.1	(4.4)	87.8	(2.5)	87.8	(2.5)
Netherlands	85.9	(4.3)	96.6	(2.0)	98.9	(1.2)	–	(–)	78.1	(7.3)
New Zealand	85.7	(1.3)	92.5	(1.4)	88.7	(1.8)	83.5	(3.2)	80.9	(2.9)
Northern Ireland	87.1	(2.2)	97.1	(1.0)	87.3	(4.1)	80.8	(11.7)	79.4	(5.1)
Portugal	87.1	(2.1)	93.3	(2.8)	87.7	(2.9)	91.5	(4.4)	83.5	(3.5)
Spain	88.8	(2.6)	95.3	(1.9)	92.6	(3.0)	91.5	(5.8)	84.6	(4.8)
United States	87.0	(1.4)	93.2	(1.7)	88.8	(2.0)	83.1	(2.9)	83.6	(2.6)
Total	86.2	(0.6)	92.6	(0.9)	89.5	(1.0)	85.5	(1.5)	81.9	(1.1)
IV. Total	84.9	(0.5)	91.7	(0.9)	88.2	(0.9)	82.9	(1.6)	81.3	(1.0)

[1] Missing cell entries indicate that fewer than 30 respondents with the indicated level of disorder severity received treatment in the country.

[2] See the section on measurement of 12-month disorders in the text for a description of how severity was operationalized. See the section on measurement of 12-month service use in the text for a description of how follow-up treatment was operationalized. The proportion of all patients who received follow-up treatment differs significantly by severity within two of the three overall country income categories, high income countries ($\chi^2_3 = 46.4$, p <0.001) and upper-middle-income countries ($\chi^2_3 = 8.4$, p = 0.039), but not in low/lower-middle income countries ($\chi^2_3 = 6.1$, p = 0.11). Within-country differences in the proportion are significant only in Colombia, Ukraine, São Paolo, France, Germany, New Zealand, Northern Ireland, and the United States, ($\chi^2_3 = 7.9$–67.9, p = 0.048–<0.001). The proportion of patients within a disorder severity level that received follow-up care differs significantly across countries within the serious, moderate, and no disorder subsamples ($\chi^2_{24} = 55.4$–85.6, p <0.001) but not in the mild disorder subsample ($\chi^2_{24} = 32.9$, p = 0.08).

countries (Israel and Japan). In Israel, treatment was highest in the highest quartile of the income distribution (OR = 2.1) and there was no meaningful gradient below this range. In Japan, treatment was lowest in the second lowest quartile of the income distribution and there was no meaningful gradient above this range (OR = 2.4–3.5).

Interpretation the survey findings

These results should be interpreted with three limitations in mind. First, response rates in the WMH surveys varied widely and included some surveys where the response rate was below acceptable standards. We attempted to control for differential response

Table 6.8 The proportions of patients who received minimally adequate treatment of their 12-month DSM-IV/CIDI disorders by severity of disorder[1]

	Any disorder		Serious disorders		Moderate disorder		Mild disorders		No disorder	
	%	(se)	%	(se)	%	(se)	%	(se)	%	(se)
I. Low/lower-middle-income countries										
Colombia	14.7	(3.4)	23.1	(8.5)	21.7	(10.5)	6.3	(4.6)	10.1	(3.5)
India: Pondicherry	10.4	(6.3)	–	(–)	–	(–)	–	(–)	–	(–)
Iraq	13.9	(5.5)	23.1	(9.6)	23.1	(9.6)	3.8	(3.0)	3.8	(3.0)
Nigeria	10.4	(9.8)	–	(–)	–	(–)	12.4	(11.7)	12.4	(11.7)
PRC: Beijing, Shanghai	24.1	(7.1)	–	(–)	–	(–)	20.1	(6.2)	20.1	(6.2)
PRC: Shenzhen	–	(–)	–	(–)	–	(–)	–	(–)	–	(–)
Ukraine	–	(–)	–	(–)	–	(–)	–	(–)	–	(–)
Total	15.2	(2.6)	22.2	(7.5)	22.0	(7.7)	6.1	(3.1)	12.2	(3.3)
II. Upper-middle-income countries										
Brazil: São Paulo	36.9	(2.4)	45.5	(5.9)	37.4	(5.6)	30.3	(4.8)	30.3	(5.4)
Bulgaria	23.3	(3.3)	33.3	(8.0)	43.3	(11.1)	–	(–)	16.3	(4.0)
Lebanon	24.5	(7.1)	24.0	(6.2)	24.0	(6.2)	24.8	(10.7)	24.8	(10.7)
Mexico	15.2	(2.7)	11.3	(4.5)	28.6	(6.3)	19.8	(5.8)	11.3	(4.0)
Romania	30.1	(6.0)	30.4	(9.5)	30.4	(9.5)	29.9	(8.3)	29.9	(8.3)
South Africa	–	(–)	–	(–)	–	(–)	–	(–)	–	(–)
Total	28.8	(1.4)	38.4	(3.7)	33.4	(3.6)	26.4	(4.1)	22.3	(2.8)
III. High-income countries										
Belgium	33.6	(5.2)	42.5	(8.5)	35.5	(12.6)	–	(–)	29.2	(6.3)
France	42.3	(5.4)	57.9	(8.5)	37.0	(6.6)	41.5	(9.7)	40.0	(8.3)
Germany	42.0	(6.1)	67.3	(10.7)	53.9	(8.5)	–	(–)	35.2	(8.9)
Israel	35.1	(2.5)	35.2	(5.3)	42.8	(6.8)	–	(–)	33.5	(3.0)
Italy	33.0	(5.1)	–	(–)	33.4	(9.1)	–	(–)	31.0	(7.5)
Japan	37.7	(4.5)	52.8	(8.2)	52.8	(8.2)	33.3	(5.9)	33.3	(5.9)
Netherlands	34.4	(5.0)	67.2	(9.0)	34.1	(10.2)	–	(–)	20.8	(5.1)
New Zealand	–	(–)	–	(–)	–	(–)	–	(–)	–	(–)
Northern Ireland	–	(–)	–	(–)	–	(–)	–	(–)	–	(–)
Portugal	26.8	(2.4)	43.2	(4.7)	25.9	(3.6)	28.0	(9.5)	20.7	(2.9)
Spain	37.3	(3.3)	47.5	(7.5)	43.6	(5.6)	48.5	(9.8)	29.2	(4.6)
United States	25.1	(1.5)	41.8	(2.8)	25.4	(2.3)	22.0	(2.9)	16.2	(1.9)
Total	30.9	(1.1)	43.7	(2.0)	31.6	(1.8)	29.4	(2.5)	25.6	(1.5)
IV. Total	29.0	(0.9)	40.4	(1.7)	31.1	(1.7)	26.1	(2.0)	23.8	(1.2)

[1] Missing cell entries indicate either than that fewer than 30 respondents with the indicated level of disorder severity received treatment in the country or that all the information needed to operationalize minimally adequate treatment was not collected in the survey.

[2] See the section on measurement of 12-month disorders in the text for a description of how severity was operationalized. See the section on measurement of 12-month service use in the text for a description of how minimally adequate treatment was operationalized. The proportion of all patients who minimally adequate treatment differs significantly by severity within two of the three overall country income categories, high income countries (χ^2_3 = 59.8, p <0.001) and upper-middle-income countries (χ^2_3 = 9.3, p = 0.025), but not in low/lower-middle-income countries (χ^2_3 = 7.5, p = 0.06). Within-country differences in the proportion are significant only in Bulgaria, Mexico, Netherlands, Portugal, Spain, and the United States (χ^2_3 = 9.5–71.0, p = 0.023–<0.001). The proportion of patients within a disorder severity level that received minimally adequate treatment differs significantly across countries within each of the disorder severity subsamples (χ^2_{18}= 34.6–63.0, p = 0.011–<0.001).

through post-stratification adjustments, but it is likely that survey response was related to the presence and severity of mental disorders or treatment in ways that were not corrected, leading to biased cross-national comparisons in estimates of prevalence and treatment. Second, some clinically important disorders, most notably non-affective psychoses and dementias, were not assessed in the WMH surveys due to the rarity and complexities associated with assessing these disorders. A related limitation is that individual WMH countries decided not to assess some of the disorders assessed in other countries because of perceived low relevance in their countries. Third, the accuracy of CIDI diagnoses probably varied across countries. Clinical reappraisal studies carried out in conjunction with the WMH surveys in developed Western countries found that CIDI diagnoses had generally good concordance with diagnoses based on independent clinical assessment (Haro et al., 2006), but no comparable studies were carried out in less developed countries and the accuracy of CIDI diagnoses could be worse in those countries due to lower relevance of CIDI symptom descriptions or greater reluctance to endorse emotional problems in countries with shorter traditions of free speech and anonymous public opinion surveying. Given what we know about the nature of these biases, they probably led to an underestimation of the prevalence of mental disorders.

With these limitations in mind, the results reported here reveal high prevalence rates of mental disorders worldwide and disturbingly high levels of unmet need for mental health treatment even among serious cases in high-income countries. The situation appears to be most dire in developing countries where only small proportions of even serious cases received any form of care. Even in the more developed Western nations, only about half of serious cases received any treatment. The fact that study limitations are likely to have led to underestimation of unmet need for treatment, especially in developing countries, means that these troubling findings are likely to be conservative and that the actual situation is worse than suggested here.

We also found that among the minority of cases receiving some services, even fewer were **adequately** treated. Some received non-health care from CAM and human services sectors, despite growing questions over the efficacy and safety of such treatments (Niggemann and Gruber, 2003). In a number of countries, nearly one-quarter of those initiating treatments failed to receive any follow-up care. Consistent with prior studies, only a minority of treatments were observed to meet even minimal standards for adequacy (Agency for Health Care Policy and Research, 1993. American Psychiatric Association 2006; Lehman and Steinwachs, 1998; Wang et al., 2005).

High levels of unmet need worldwide should not be surprising in light of the WHO Project ATLAS findings of much lower mental health expenditures than indicated by the magnitude of the burdens associated with mental illnesses (Lopez et al., 2006; Saxena et al., 2003). Generally greater unmet needs in low/lower-middle-income countries may be due to these nations spending smaller proportions (often less than 1%) of already diminished health budgets on mental health care and relying heavily on out-of-pocket spending by a citizenry ill-equipped to bear these costs (Saxena et al., 2003). Notable exceptions to the rule of greater unmet needs in developing versus developed countries may be explained by higher levels of investment in health care. For example, South Africa's high rates of treatment may reflect its greater spending (8.6% of GDP) on health

care than any low/middle-income country studied. At the other extreme, some high-income countries, most notably Japan and Italy, have very low rates of health care spending relative to other high-income countries (8.0% and 8.4% of GDP, respectively) that may explain their comparatively low rates of treatment (World Health Organization).

Additional research is needed to understand how the limited resources nations invest in mental health treatment can be optimally allocated. An overly simplistic view of our results could be that a meaningful number of services are going to those without apparent needs, as indicated by the fact that a meaningful proportion of patients do not meet criteria for any of the disorders assessed in the WMH surveys and others have only mild disorders. Such potential diversion of limited treatment resources to these individuals with low or no apparent need might be considered concerning in light of the magnitude of unmet needs among cases with clearly defined and serious disorders (Narrow et al., 2002). The weak or lack of relationship between use of specialty sectors and disorder severity could also be evidence of suboptimal allocation. However, before drawing such conclusions, it is critical to identify whether such services are being used appropriately for disorders not assessed in WMH surveys, for sub-threshold symptoms, for secondary prevention of lifetime disorders (e.g. maintenance treatment for lifetime bipolar disorder among patients who were asymptomatic in the past year), or even for primary prevention (Kessler and Price, 1993). Uncovering other factors, beyond clinical severity, disability, or distress, which may motivate use of mental health services, will also be important in the future studies (Mechanic, 2003).

Our finding that the general medical sector is for most countries the largest source of mental health services may reflect conscious attempts by policy makers to broaden access to services rather than concentrating resources on the relatively fewer patients with access to specialty sectors (Rosenheck et al., 1998). It may also reflect 'gatekeeping' by primary care physicians employed in some countries to reserve specialty treatment for serious cases (Forrest, 2003). Whatever the rationale, future research is needed to ensure that mental health care received in general medical sectors is not of low intensity and adequacy, as has been observed in other studies (Wang et al., 2005). This is a source of considerable concern due to the fact that other WMH analyses found that adequacy of treatment is considerably lower in the general medical sector than the mental health specialty sector in most WMH countries (Wang et al., 2008).

Our results concerning predictors of service use are generally consistent with prior research. The consistently higher treatment rates among women than men may be due to a diminished perception of stigma among women compared to men as well as to the greater abilities of women than men to translate non-specific feelings of distress into conscious recognition of having a mental health problem (Kessler et al., 1981). The positive association between income in some countries may reflect the formidable influences of financial barriers to seeking treatment in some countries (Wells et al., 1986). Why this association does not exist in most countries, though, is unclear from the results reported here but deserves further study to determine the ways in which the organization, financing, and delivery of mental health services can achieve equality in access across the income gradient. This has to be done, though, with recognition that this equalization is not due to high use in all socioeconomic sectors in these countries but to unacceptably low use in all socioeconomic sectors.

These results have important practical implications of several sorts. First, alleviating the problem of widespread undertreatment of mental disorders will almost certainly require expansion of treatment resources and governmental as well as private means of financing mental health services. Second, there is also a pressing need to devise rational, transparent, and ethical allocation rules. In many countries it is unclear whether to focus resources on those with the greatest needs or on the larger numbers of people with milder disorders (e.g. to prevent negative sequelae), to deliver services through primary versus specialty sectors or inpatient vs. community settings, or to provide mental health services on parity with those for general medical disorders (Callahan, 1994). These questions should be answered through formal analyses of the burdens from illnesses and the cost-effectiveness of treatments (Gold et al., 1996). Unfortunately rigorous data to compare disease burdens and weigh the costs and benefits of different regimens are largely lacking (Rosenheck et al., 1998). In the absence of such data, decisions regarding resource allocation are often made on the basis of simple cost-minimization and even attitudinal factors such as stigma and desire to punish persons perceived as being personally responsible for their problems (Corrigan and Watson, 2003). It is consequently imperative that research is expanded on the effectiveness of usual treatment practices and on the enhancement of usual care to feasible treatment quality improvement.

Finally, when rational, transparent, and ethical priorities have been set, policy makers need specific designs they can implement to achieve their goals of treatment quality improvement and expansion of treatment. Some techniques employed in managed care systems, such as gatekeeping, increased cost-sharing, utilization review, and prior approval could presumably be brought to bear on the problem of unnecessary use. However, these methods run the serious risk of underuse that may worsen unmet needs for treatment. The impacts of other policies, delivery system features, and means of financing that policy makers could implement are essentially unknown. For these reasons, collection of detailed data on the mental health policies, delivery system features, and means of financing mental health care in different countries is a promising area for future research (Saxena et al., 2003). When merged with WMH surveys on the use and adequacy of treatments, such combined data could shed light on the impacts of policies, delivery system, and financing features and help policy makers choose ones that achieve their desired goals (Mezzich, 2003).

Acknowledgements

This paper is carried out in conjunction with the World Health Organization World Mental Health (WMH) Survey Initiative. We thank the WMH staff for assistance with instrumentation, fieldwork, and data analysis. These activities were supported by the United States National Institute of Mental Health (R01MH070884), the John D. and Catherine T. MacArthur Foundation, the Pfizer Foundation, the US Public Health Service (R13-MH066849, R01-MH069864, and R01 DA016558), the Fogarty International Center (FIRCA R03-TW006481), the Pan American Health Organization, the Eli Lilly & Company Foundation, Ortho-McNeil Pharmaceutical, Inc., GlaxoSmithKline, Bristol-Myers Squibb, and Shire. A complete list of WMH publications can be found at http://www.hcp.med.harvard.edu/wmh/. The São Paulo Megacity Mental Health Survey is supported by the State of São Paulo Research Foundation (FAPESP) Thematic Project Grant 03/00204-3. The Bulgarian Epidemiological Study of common mental disorders EPIBUL is supported by the Ministry of Health and the National Center for Public Health Protection. The Chinese World Mental Health Survey Initiative is supported by the Pfizer Foundation. The Shenzhen Mental Health Survey is supported by the Shenzhen Bureau of Health and the Shenzhen Bureau of Science, Technology, and Information. The Colombian National Study of Mental Health (NSMH) is supported by the Ministry of Social Protection. The ESEMeD project is funded by the European Commission (Contracts QLG5-1999-01042; SANCO 2004123), the Piedmont Region (Italy), Fondo de Investigación Sanitaria, Instituto de Salud Carlos III, Spain (FIS 00/0028), Ministerio de Ciencia y Tecnología, Spain (SAF 2000-158-CE), Departament de Salut, Generalitat de Catalunya, Spain, Instituto de Salud Carlos III (CIBER CB06/02/0046, RETICS RD06/0011 REM-TAP), and other local agencies and by an unrestricted educational grant from GlaxoSmithKline. The WMHI was funded by WHO (India) and helped by Dr R Chandrasekaran, JIPMER. Implementation of the Iraq Mental Health Survey (IMHS) and data entry were carried out by the staff of the Iraqi MOH and MOP with direct support from the Iraqi IMHS team with funding from both the Japanese and European Funds through United Nations Development Group Iraq Trust Fund (UNDG ITF). The Israel National Health Survey is funded by the Ministry of Health with support from the Israel National Institute for Health Policy and Health Services Research and the National Insurance Institute of Israel. The World Mental Health Japan (WMHJ) Survey is supported by the Grant for Research on Psychiatric and Neurological Diseases and Mental Health (H13-SHOGAI-023, H14-TOKUBETSU-026, H16-KOKORO-013) from the Japan Ministry of Health, Labour and Welfare. The Lebanese National Mental Health Survey (LEBANON) is supported by the Lebanese Ministry of Public Health, the WHO (Lebanon), Fogarty International, anonymous private donations to IDRAAC, Lebanon, and unrestricted grants from Janssen Cilag, Eli Lilly, GlaxoSmithKline, Roche, and Novartis. The Mexican National Comorbidity Survey (MNCS) is supported by The National Institute of Psychiatry Ramon de la Fuente (INPRFMDIES 4280) and by the National Council on Science and Technology (CONACyT-G30544- H), with supplemental support from the PanAmerican Health Organization (PAHO). Te Rau Hinengaro: The New Zealand Mental Health Survey (NZMHS) is supported by the New Zealand Ministry of Health, Alcohol Advisory Council, and the Health Research Council. The Nigerian Survey of Mental Health and Wellbeing (NSMHW) is supported by the WHO (Geneva), the WHO (Nigeria), and the Federal Ministry of Health, Abuja, Nigeria. The Northern Ireland Study of Mental Health was funded by the Health & Social Care Research & Development Division of the Public Health Agency. The Romania WMH study projects 'Policies in Mental Health Area' and 'National Study regarding Mental Health and Services Use' were carried out by National School of Public Health & Health Services Management (former National Institute for Research & Development in Health), with technical support of Metro Media Transilvania, the National Institute of Statistics-National Centre for Training in Statistics, SC. Cheyenne Services SRL, Statistics Netherlands and were funded by Ministry of Public Health (former Ministry of Health) with supplemental support of Eli Lilly Romania SRL. The South Africa Stress and Health Study (SASH) is supported by the US National Institute of Mental Health (R01-MH059575) and National Institute of Drug Abuse with supplemental funding from the South African Department of Health and the University of Michigan. The Ukraine Comorbid Mental Disorders during Periods of Social Disruption (CMDPSD) study is funded by the US National Institute of Mental Health (RO1-MH61905). The US National Comorbidity Survey Replication (NCS-R) is supported by the National Institute of Mental Health (NIMH; U01-MH60220) with supplemental support from the National Institute of Drug Abuse (NIDA), the Substance Abuse and Mental Health Services Administration (SAMHSA), the Robert Wood Johnson Foundation (RWJF; Grant 044708), and the John W. Alden Trust.

References

Agency for Health Care Policy and Research (1993). *Depression Guideline Panel, Volume Two: Treatment of Major Depression, Clinical Practice Guideline, No 5*. Rockville, MD: US Department of Health and Human Services, Public Health Service, Agency for Health Care Policy and Research.

American Psychiatric Association (2006). *Practice Guidelines for Treatment of Psychiatric Disorders: Compendium 2006*. Arlington, VA: American Psychiatric Association Press.

Bijl, R.V., de Graaf, R., Hiripi, E., Kessler, R.C., Kohn, R., Offord, D.R., *et al.* (2003). The prevalence of treated and untreated mental disorders in five countries. *Health Affairs (Millwood)*, **22**, 122–33.

Callahan, D. (1994). Setting mental health priorities: problems and possibilities. *Milbank Quarterly*, **72**, 451–70.

Chang, S.M., Hahm, B.J., Lee, J.Y., Shin, M.S., Jeon, H.J., Hong, J.P., *et al.* (2008). Cross-national difference in the prevalence of depression caused by the diagnostic threshold. *Journal of Affective Disorders*, **106**, 159–67.

Corrigan, P.W. and Watson, A.C. (2003). Factors that explain how policy makers distribute resources to mental health services. *Psychiatric Services*, **54**, 501–7.

Demyttenaere, K., Bruffaerts, R., Posada-Villa, J., Gasquet, I., Kovess, V., Lepine, J.P., *et al.* (2004). Prevalence, severity, and unmet need for treatment of mental disorders in the World Health Organization World Mental Health Surveys. *Journal of the American Medical Association*, **291**, 2581–90.

Endicott, J., Spitzer, R.L., Fleiss, J.L., and Cohen, J. (1976). The global assessment sale: a procedure for measuring overall severity of psychiatric disorders. *Archives of General Psychiatry*, **33**, 766–71.

First, M.B., Spitzer, R.L., Gibbon, M., and Williams, J.B.W. (2002). *Structured Clinical Interview for DSM-IV Axis I Disorders, Research Version, Non-patient Edition (SCID-I/NP)*. New York: Biometrics Research, New York State Psychiatric Institute.

Forrest, C.B. (2003). Primary care in the United States: primary care gatekeeping and referrals: effective filter or failed experiment? *British Medical Journal*, **326**, 692–5.

Gold, M.R., Siegel, J.E., Russell, L.B., and Weinstein, M.C. (eds.) (1996). *Cost-effectiveness in Health and Medicine*. New York: Oxford University Press.

Harkness, J., Pennell, B.E., Villar, A., Gebler, N., Aguilar-Gaxiola, S., and Bilgen, I. (2008). Translation procedures and translation assessment in the World Mental Health Survey Initiative. In: Kessler, R.C. and Üstün, T.B. (eds.) *The WHO World Mental Health Surveys: Global Perspectives on the Epidemiology of Mental Disorders*, pp. 91–113. New York: Cambridge University Press.

Haro, J.M., Arbazadeh-Bouchez, S., Brugha, T.S., de Girolamo, G., Guyer, M.E., Jin, R., *et al.* (2006). Concordance of the Composite International Diagnostic Interview Version 3.0 (CIDI 3.0) with standardized clinical assessments in the WHO World Mental Health surveys. *International Journal of Methods in Psychiatric Research*, **15**, 167–80.

Heeringa, S.G., Wells, E.J., Hubbard, F., Mneimneh, Z.N., Chiu, W.T., Sampson, N.A., *et al.* (2008). Sample designs and sampling procedures. In: Kessler, R.C. and Üstün, T.B. (eds.) *The WHO World Mental Health Surveys: Global Perspectives on the Epidemiology of Mental Disorders*, pp. 14–32. New York: Cambridge University Press.

Hu, T.W. (2003). Financing global mental health services and the role of WHO. *Journal of Mental Health Policy and Economics*, **6**, 135–43.

Kessler, R.C., Aguilar-Gaxiola, S., Alonso, J., Angermeyer, M.C., Anthony, J.C., Brugha, T.S., *et al.* (2008). Prevalence and severity of mental disorders in the World Mental Health Survey Initiative. In: Kessler, R.C. and Üstün, T.B. (eds.) *The WHO World Mental Health Surveys: Global Perspectives on the Epidemiology of Mental Disorders*, pp. 534–40. New York: Cambridge University Press.

Kessler, R.C., Brown, R.L., and Broman, C.L. (1981). Sex differences in psychiatric help-seeking: evidence from four large-scale surveys. *Journal of Health and Social Behavior*, **22**, 49–64.

Kessler, R.C., Frank, R.G., Edlund, M., Katz, S.J., Lin, E., and Leaf, P. (1997). Differences in the use of psychiatric outpatient services between the United States and Ontario. *New England Journal of Medicine*, **336**, 551–7.

Kessler, R.C. and Price, R.H. (1993). Primary prevention of secondary disorders: a proposal and agenda. *American Journal of Community Psychology*, **21**, 607–33.

Kessler, R.C. and Üstün, T.B. (2004). The World Mental Health (WMH) Survey Initiative Version of the World Health Organization (WHO) Composite International Diagnostic Interview (CIDI). *International Journal of Methods in Psychiatric Research*, **13**, 93–121.

Lehman, A.F. and Steinwachs, D.M. (1998). Translating research into practice: schizophrenia patient outcomes research team (PORT) treatment recommendations. *Schizophrenia Bulletin*, **24**, 1–10.

Leon, A.C., Olfson, M., Portera, L., Farber, L., and Sheehan, D.V. (1997). Assessing psychiatric impairment in primary care with the Sheehan Disability Scale. *International Journal of Psychiatry in Medicine*, **27**, 93–105.

Lopez, A.D., Mathers, C.D., Ezzati, M., Jamison, D.T., and Murray, C.J.L. (eds.) (2006). *Global Burden of Disease and Risk Factors*. New York: Oxford University Press/World Bank.

Mechanic, D. (1994). Establishing mental health priorities. *Milbank Quarterly*, **72**, 501–14.

Mechanic, D. (2003). Is the prevalence of mental disorders a good measure of the need for services? *Health Affairs (Millwood)*, **22**, 8–20.

Mezzich, J.E. (2003). From financial analysis to policy development in mental health care: the need for broader conceptual models and partnerships. *Journal of Mental Health Policy and Economics*, **6**, 149–50.

Narrow, W.E., Rae, D.S., Robins, L.N. and Regier, D.A. (2002). Revised prevalence estimates of mental disorders in the United States: using a clinical significance criterion to reconcile 2 surveys' estimates. *Archives of General Psychiatry*, **59**, 115–23.

Niggemann, B. and Gruber, C. (2003). Side-effects of complementary and alternative medicine. *Allergy*, **58**, 707–16.

Pennell, B.-E., Mneimneh, Z., Bowers, A., Chardoul, S., Wells, J.E., Viana, M.C., *et al.* (2008). Implementation of the World Mental Health Surveys: In: Kessler, R.C. and Üstün, T.B. (eds.) *The WHO World Mental Health Surveys: Global Perspectives on the Epidemiology of Mental Disorders*, pp. 33–57. New York: Cambridge University Press.

Research Triangle Institute (2002). *SUDAAN: Professional Software for Survey Data Analysis, version 8.0.1*. Research Triangle Park, NC: Research Triangle Institute.

Rosenheck, R., Armstrong, M., Callahan, D., Dea, R., Del Vecchio, P., Flynn, L., *et al.* (1998). Obligation to the least well off in setting mental health service priorities: a consensus statement. *Psychiatric Services*, **49**, 1273–4, 1290.

Saxena, S., Sharan, P., and Saraceno, B. (2003). Budget and financing of mental health services: baseline information on 89 countries from WHO's project atlas. *Journal of Mental Health Policy and Economics*, **6**, 135–43.

Simon, G.E., Goldberg, D.P., Von Korff, M., and Üstün, T.B. (2002). Understanding cross-national differences in depression prevalence. *Psychological Medicine*, **32**, 585–94.

Substance Abuse and Mental Health Services Administration (1993). Final notice establishing definitions for (1) children with a serious emotional disturbance, and (2) adults with a serious mental illness. *Federal Register*, **58**, 29422–5.

Tasman, A., Kay, J., and Lieberman, J.A. (eds.) (2003). *Psychiatry, Second Edition*. Chichester: Wiley.

Üstün, T.B. and Sartorius, N. (eds.) (1995). *Mental Illness in General Health Care: An International Study*. New York: Wiley.

Wang, P.S., Aguilar-Gaxiola, S., Alonso, J., Angermeyer, M.C., Borges, G., Bruffaerts, R., *et al.* (2008). Delay and failure in treatment seeking after first onset of mental disorders in the World Mental Health Survey Initiative. In: Kessler, R.C. and Üstün, T.B. (eds.) *The WHO World Mental Health Surveys: Global Perspectives on the Epidemiology of Mental Disorders*, pp. 522–33. New York: Cambridge University Press.

Wang, P.S., Lane, M., Olfson, M., Pincus, H.A., Wells, K.B., and Kessler, R.C. (2005). Twelve-month use of mental health services in the United States: results from the National Comorbidity Survey Replication. *Archives of General Psychiatry*, **62**, 629–40.

Wells, K.B., Manning, W.G., Duan, N., Newhouse, J.P., and Ware, J.E., Jr. (1986). Sociodemographic factors and the use of outpatient mental health services. *Medical Care*, **24**, 75–85.

World Bank (2003). *World Development Indicators 2003*. Washington DC: The World Bank.

World Health Organization. *Project Atlas: Resources for Mental Health and Neurological Disorders*. Available at: http://www.who.int/globalatlas/dataQuery/default.asp (accessed 6 July 2006).

CHAPTER 7

The global burden of mental disorder

Martin Prince

The World Health Organization's global burden of disease (GBD) estimates provide evidence on the relative impact of health problems worldwide (Murray and Lopez, 1996; World Health Organization, 2006). Patterns of morbidity seem to be globalizing with non-communicable diseases rapidly becoming the dominant causes of ill health in all developing regions except Sub-Saharan Africa (Table 7.1). Within this wider health transition, the GBD report showed for the first time the true scale of the contribution of mental disorders, this revelation attributed to the use of the disability-adjusted life year (DALY), the sum of years lived with disability (YLD), and years of life lost (YLL) as a single integrated measure of disease burden.

Neuropsychiatric conditions (comprising, in descending order of DALY contribution: mental disorders, substance and alcohol use disorders, other neuropsychiatric disorders, dementia, mental retardation, migraine, epilepsy, Parkinson's disease, and multiple sclerosis) account for 14% of all DALYs and 28% of all DALYs attributed to non-communicable disease (Table 7.1) (Murray and Lopez, 1996; World Health Organization, 2006). They are the chief contributor to burden among the non-communicable diseases (Fig. 7.1), more than either cardiovascular disease (22% of non-communicable disease DALYs) or cancer (11%).

Proportionately, mental disorders account for just 9% of the burden in low-income countries, compared with 18% in middle-income and 27% in high-income countries. This is because the burden of communicable, perinatal, and maternal conditions remains high in many low- and low–middle-income countries, swelling the denominator. However, the absolute burden of mental disorder as indicated by per capita DALYs does not vary much between world regions (Fig. 7.2).

Table 7.1 Number ('000s) and proportion of total DALYs contributed by different groups of health conditions by country income level in 2005 and (projected) 2030 (World Health Organization, 2006)

	2005				2030			
	World	HIC	MIC	LIC	World	HIC	MIC	LIC
Total DALYs	1,483,060	119,361	492,549	871,141	1,650,629	118,309	528,066	1,004,236
I: communicable, maternal, perinatal and nutritional conditions	572,292 38.6%	6647 5.6%	99,696 20.2%	465,948 53.5%	49,4384 30.0%	4060 3.4%	79,623 15.1%	410,698 40.9%
II: non-communicable diseases	725,506 48.9%	102,311 85.7%	318,415 64.7%	304,773 35%	938,468 56.9%	105,716 89.4%	380,324 72%	452,416 45.1%
III: injuries	185,262 12.5%	10,403 8.7%	74,439 15.1%	100,420 11.5%	217,777 13.2%	8533 7.2%	68,120 12.9%	141,122 14.1%
Neuropsychiatric conditions	199,606 13.5%[a] 27.5%[b]	32,717 27.4%[a] 32.0%[b]	87,398 17.7%[a] 27.5%[b]	79,490 9.1%[a] 26.1%[b]	237,962 14.4%[a] 25.4%[b]	34,798 29.4%[a] 32.9%[b]	92,590 17.5%[a] 24.3%[b]	110,571 11.0%[a] 24.4%[b]

[a] As a percentage of all DALYs. [b] As a percentage of all non-communicable disease DALYs.
HIC, high-income countries; LIC, low-income countries; MIC, middle-income countries.

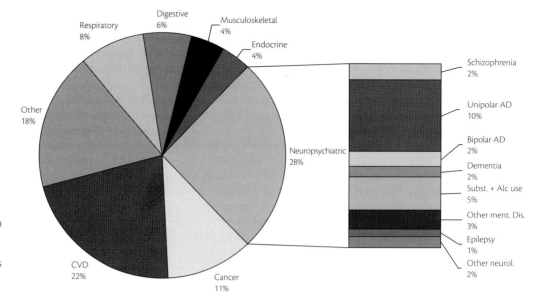

Fig. 7.1 The proportion of disability-adjusted life years (DALYs) arising from non-communicable disease in 2005, attributed to particular disease groups and specific neuropsychiatric disorders (World Health Organization, 2006). AD= affective disoder.

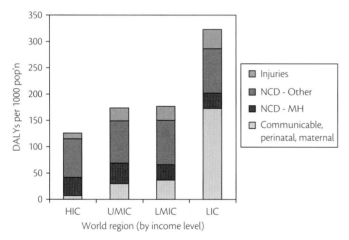

Fig. 7.2 Disability adjusted life years (DALYs) per 1000 population, attributed to different GBD disease categories (I: communicable, perinatal and maternal conditions; II: non-communicable diseases (NCDs), subdivided into neuropsychiatric and other; III: injuries) by country income status. HIC, high-income countries; LIC, low-income countries; LMIC, lower middle-income countries; UMIC, upper middle income countires.

Mental disorders are a leading cause of long-term disability and dependency. According to the GBD, mental disorders account for 31.7% of all years lived with disability, the five major contributors to this total being unipolar depression (11.8%), alcohol-use disorder (3.3%), schizophrenia (2.8%), bipolar depression (2.4%), and dementia (1.6%) (Mathers and Loncar, 2006). Despite an enormous treatment gap, these essentially chronic diseases impose an immense societal burden, particularly in low- and middle-income countries. Depressive and anxiety disorders account for between one-quarter and one-third of all primary-healthcare visits worldwide (Ustun and Sartorius, 1995). Somatization, defined as medically unexplained somatic symptoms coupled with psychological distress and help-seeking is present in around 15% of patients seen in primary care (Escobar et al., 1998; Gureje et al., 1997). Those affected are chronically disabled (Escobar et al., 1998; Gureje et al., 1997;

Kroenke et al., 2002), consult frequently, and account for a high proportion of health care costs (Barsky et al., 2005). By 2030, nearly three-quarters of the estimated 66 million people with dementia worldwide will live in low- or middle-income countries (Alzheimer's Disease International, 2009). The prevalences of mental retardation and epilepsy are three to five times higher in low-income countries than in industrialized countries (Institute of Medicine, 2001). In some low-income countries, up to 90% of patients with epilepsy—a treatable condition for which cost-effective drug therapies are available—do not receive any effective treatment (Scott et al., 2001).

No health without mental health: estimating the full impact of mental disorders

The burden of mental disorders may well have been underestimated in the GBD (Prince et al., 2007), since it is practically impossible to make a neat distinction between the impacts of mental disorders on the one hand, and communicable diseases, maternal and infant disorders, non-communicable diseases, accidents, and injuries on the other.

Mental disorders and mortality

According to the GBD, neuropsychiatric disorders account for 1.2 million deaths per annum and just 1.4% of all years of life lost, the majority arising from dementia, Parkinson's disease, and epilepsy. Only 40,000 deaths are attributed to mental disorder (unipolar and bipolar depression, schizophrenia, and post-traumatic stress disorder) and 182,000 to drug and alcohol use. This is almost certainly a gross underestimate. Each year at least 800,000 people commit suicide, 86% in lower middle-income countries, and over half involve young people (Aaron et al., 2004; Murray and Lopez, 1996; Prasad et al., 2006; World Health Organization, 2006). Mental disorder is overwhelmingly the most important preventable factor (Cavanagh et al., 2003; Phillips et al., 2002; Vijayakumar and Rajkumar, 1999). Non-suicide mortality is also elevated in psychosis (Heila et al., 2005; Kebede et al., 2005), depression (Mogga et al., 2006; Saz and Dewey, 2001), and dementia (Dewey and Saz, 2001). The poor quality of general health care received by those with mental disorders may explain some of the excess mortality (Lawrence et al., 2003).

Interactions between mental and physical health conditions

Much of the burden of mental ill health may be mediated through complex interactions with other health conditions, including infectious disease, reproductive, maternal, and child health (Prince et al., 2007). Mental disorders are risk factors for the development of communicable and non-communicable diseases, and many physical health conditions increase the risk for mental disorder. For example, in population-based studies, depression is a prospective risk factor for cardiovascular diseases including angina, myocardial infarction (Hemingway and Marmot, 1999; Kuper et al., 2002), and stroke (Everson et al., 1998; Jonas and Mussolino, 2000; Larson et al., 2001; Ohira et al., 2001). Living with a disease often increases the risk for mental disorder, through a variety of mechanisms. For example, infection with HIV is consistently associated with a high prevalence of affective disorder (Bing et al., 2001; Ciesla and Roberts, 2001; Maj et al., 1994a), and with neurocognitive impairment particularly in those with symptomatic disease (Maj et al., 1994b; White et al., 1995); apart from the psychological trauma of the diagnosis, HIV infection (Dubé et al., 2005) and highly active antiretroviral treatment (HAART; Cournos et al., 2005) have direct central nervous system effects.

Comorbidity and physical disease management

Comorbidity complicates help-seeking, diagnosis, and treatment, and affects the outcomes of treatment for physical conditions, including disease-related mortality. Comorbid depression predicts reinfarction and death after myocardial infarction (Hemingway and Marmot, 1999; Kuper et al., 2002). Poststroke depression is associated with poor functional outcomes (Chemerinski et al., 2001; Parikh et al., 1990) and increased mortality over 10 years (Morris et al., 1993). In diabetes, depression is associated with poor glycaemic control (Lustman et al., 2000a), complications (de Groot et al., 2001), and death (Katon et al., 2005). In the United States, chronic depressive symptoms were associated with increased AIDS-related mortality (Cook et al., 2004; Ickovics et al., 2001) and more rapid disease progression (Ickovics et al., 2001) independent of receipt of treatment. Cognitive impairment in HIV is associated with greatly increased mortality (Wilkie et al., 1998). Schizophrenia complicates treatment and is associated with worse prognosis (Cournos et al., 2005). A common underlying mechanism may be the poor adherence to treatment regimens that has been demonstrated for behaviour changes in cardiovascular disease (Ziegelstein et al., 2000), for oral hypoglycaemic therapy among people with schizophrenia (Dolder et al., 2003), and for diet (Ciechanowski et al., 2000; Lin et al., 2004), exercise recommendations (Lin et al., 2004), and oral hypoglycaemic medication (Ciechanowski et al., 2000; Lin et al., 2004) among diabetics with depression. Adherence to HAART is adversely affected by depression (Ammassari et al., 2004; Gordillo et al., 1999; Paterson et al., 2000), cognitive impairment (Hinkin et al., 2002, 2004), and alcohol and substance use (Chander et al., 2006).

Mental disorder and women's health

Mental disorders in women are important given associations with reproductive, maternal, and child health. Women are at heightened risk for common mental disorders with a typical female to male gender ratio of 1.5 to 2.0 (Kuehner, 2003; Maier et al., 1999). Abuse, anxiety, depression, substance and alcohol use are all robustly associated with dysmenorrhoea, dyspareunia, and pelvic pain (Latthe et al., 2006). In Asian cultures, explanatory models of reproductive and mental health experiences may enhance these associations; in a study in south India, the complaint of vaginal discharge was associated with common mental disorder rather than reproductive tract infection (Patel et al., 2005). Maternal mental health may also have important implications for infant growth and survival. Maternal schizophrenia is consistently associated with preterm delivery (Bennedsen et al., 1999; Nilsson et al., 2002), low birth weight (Bennedsen et al., 1999; Jablensky et al., 2005; Nilsson et al., 2002), still birth, and infant mortality (Webb et al., 2005). Postpartum depression affects 10% to 15% of women (Cooper et al., 1999; O'Hara 1997; Patel et al., 2003). In developed countries there are adverse consequences for the early mother–infant relationship and for the child's psychological development (Murray and Cooper, 2003). In Asia, two prospective studies suggest an independent association between antenatal common mental disorders and low birth weight (Patel and Prince, 2006; Rahman et al., 2004a), and associations between perinatal common mental disorders and infant undernutrition at 6 months have been consistently demonstrated (Anoop et al., 2004; Patel et al., 2003, 2004; Rahman et al., 2004a,b). Maternal depression reduces adherence to child-health promotion and disease-prevention interventions, e.g. immunization (Rahman et al., 2004a). There is good evidence from developed countries (Paulson et al., 2006) and low- and middle-income countries (Galler et al., 1999) that maternal depression is associated with suboptimal breastfeeding.

Links between mental health, accidents, and injuries

Injury and violence are important causes of death and disability worldwide. According to the 2005 GBD estimates, there were 5.4 million injury deaths globally, accounting for 9% of deaths and 12% of the burden of disease (World Health Organization, 2006). The burden of injury is expected to increase substantially by the year 2030. Mental health problems are both a cause and a consequence of injury. Injury and mental disorder also have many determinants in common, e.g. poverty (Edwards et al., 2006; Patel and Kleinman, 2003), conflict, violence, and alcohol use. Mental health considerations must be integral to any public health approach to injury control.

Implications for the delivery of mental health services

Mental health needs to be recognized as an integral component of primary and secondary health care and mental health awareness needs to be insinuated into all elements of health and social policy, health system planning, and health care delivery. When mental disorders are seen as a distinct health domain, with separate services and budgets, then investing in mental health is perceived as having an unaffordable opportunity cost.

There is ample evidence that treatment of comorbid mental disorder is highly effective in improving mental health and quality of life across a range of disorders including cancer (Osborn et al., 2006), diabetes (Katon et al., 2004), heart disease (Berkman et al., 2003; Rees et al., 2004) and HIV/AIDS (Lechner et al., 2003). The evidence base on whether mental health interventions can improve physical disease outcomes is more mixed. Psychological interventions have been shown to improve diabetic control in type 1 (Winkley et al., 2006) and type 2 diabetes (Ismail et al., 2004). Pharmacological treatments are effective for depression, but do not improve glycaemic control (Katon et al., 2004) or diabetic self-care (Lin et al., 2006; Lustman et al., 1997, 2000b). Antidepressants and cognitive behavioural therapy are safe and moderately effective treatments for depression postmyocardial infarction (Berkman et al., 2003; Glassman et al., 2002; Strik et al., 2000), but do not reduce reinfarction rates or overall mortality. The evidence base for the effectiveness of antidepressants poststroke is weak, both for prevention (Anderson et al., 2004) and treatment (Hackett et al., 2005). A randomized controlled trial of a cognitive behaviour therapy-based intervention for depressed mothers integrated into the routine work of community-based primary health workers in rural Pakistan was effective in increasing immunization rates and reducing diarrhoeal episodes in their infants, as well as much improving the mental health outcome for the mothers, but did not reduce infant stunting (Rahman et al., 2008). Non-randomized evaluations of psychotherapeutic interventions integrated with tuberculosis treatment suggest possible improvements in treatment completion and cure, in Peru (Acha et al., 2007), India (Janmeja et al., 2005), and Ethiopia (Demissie et al., 2003). More research is needed, particularly with regard to HIV, where observational data suggests that antiretroviral adherence might be improved by antidepressant treatment (Yun et al., 2005), but the evidence base for the broad effects of psychosocial interventions is surprisingly limited (Dubé et al., 2005; Prince et al., 2007).

Conclusion

In summary, mental disorders are risk factors for the development of communicable and non-communicable diseases, and a contributory factor to accidental and non-accidental injury. Many health conditions increase the risk for mental disorder, or lengthen episodes of mental illness. The resulting comorbidity complicates help-seeking, diagnosis, and treatment, and affects the outcomes of treatment for physical conditions, including disease-related mortality. Hence, there can be 'no health without mental health'.

Integrated mental health policies will maximize the impact of the small number of mental health professionals, mobilize the forces of public and community health to work for better mental health, and minimize organizational inefficiencies. The strengthening of health care systems to deliver mental health care should focus where possible upon task-shifting to non-specialist health workers within existing programmes and activities (Patel and Thornicroft, 2009); e.g. HIV prevention, the roll-out of antiretroviral treatment, tuberculosis treatment, gender-based violence campaigns, antenatal care, and new chronic disease management programmes.

References

Aaron, R., Joseph, A., Abraham, S., Muliyil, J., George, K., Prasad, J., *et al.* (2004). Suicides in young people in rural southern India. *Lancet*, **363**, 1117–18.

Acha, J., Sweetland, J., Guerra, D., Chalco, K., Castillo, H., and Palacios, E. (2007). Psychosocial support groups for patients with multidrug-resistant tuberculosis: Five years of experience. *Global Public Health*, **2**, 404–17.

Alzheimer's Disease International (2009). *World Alzheimer Report 2009*. London: Alzheimer's Disease International.

Ammassari, A., Antinori, A., Aloisi, M.S., Trotta, M.P., Murri, R., Bartoli, L., *et al.* (2004). Depressive symptoms, neurocognitive impairment, and adherence to highly active antiretroviral therapy among HIV-infected persons. *Psychosomatics*, **45**, 394–402.

Anderson, C.S., Hackett, M.L., and House, A.O. (2004). Interventions for preventing depression after stroke. *Cochrane Database of Systematic Reviews*, 2, CD003689.

Anoop, S., Saravanan, B., Joseph, A., Cherian, A., and Jacob, K.S. (2004). Maternal depression and low maternal intelligence as risk factors for malnutrition in children: a community based case-control study from South India. *Archives of Disease in Childhood*, **89**, 325–9.

Barsky, A.J., Orav, E.J., and Bates, D.W. (2004). Somatization increases medical utilization and costs independent of psychiatric and medical comorbidity. *Archives of General Psychiatry*, **62**, 903–10.

Bennedsen, B.E., Mortensen, P.B., Olesen, A.V., and Henriksen, T.B. (1999). Preterm birth and intra-uterine growth retardation among children of women with schizophrenia. *British Journal of Psychiatry*, **175**, 239–45.

Berkman, L.F., Blumenthal, J., Burg, M., Carney, R.M., Catellier, D., Cowan, M.J., *et al.* (2003). Effects of treating depression and low perceived social support on clinical events after myocardial infarction: the Enhancing Recovery in Coronary Heart Disease Patients (ENRICHD) Randomized Trial. *Journal of the American Medical Association*, **289**, 3106–16.

Bing, E.G., Burnam, M.A., Longshore, D., Fleishman, J.A., Sherbourne, C.D., London, A.S., *et al.* (2001). Psychiatric disorders and drug use among human immunodeficiency virus-infected adults in the United States. *Archives of General Psychiatry*, **58**, 721–8.

Cavanagh, J.T., Carson, A.J., Sharpe, M., and Lawrie, S.M. (2003). Psychological autopsy studies of suicide: a systematic review. *Psychological Medicine*, **33**, 395–405.

Chander, G., Himelhoch, S., and Moore, R.D. (2006). Substance abuse and psychiatric disorders in HIV-positive patients: epidemiology and impact on antiretroviral therapy. *Drugs*, **66**, 769–89.

Chemerinski, E., Robinson, R.G., and Kosier, J.T. (2001). Improved recovery in activities of daily living associated with remission of poststroke depression. *Stroke*, **32**, 113–17.

Ciechanowski, P.S., Katon, W.J., and Russo, J.E. (2000). Depression and diabetes: impact of depressive symptoms on adherence, function, and costs. *Archives of Internal Medicine*, **160**, 3278–85.

Ciesla, J.A. and Roberts, J.E. (2001). Meta-analysis of the relationship between HIV infection and risk for depressive disorders. *American Journal of Psychiatry*, **158**, 725–30.

Cook, J.A., Grey, D., Burke, J., Cohen, M.H., Gurtman, A.C., Richardson, J.L., *et al.* (2004). Depressive symptoms and AIDS-related mortality among a multisite cohort of HIV-positive women. *American Journal of Public Health*, **94**, 1133–40.

Cooper, P.J., Tomlinson, M., Swartz, L., Woolgar, M., Murray, L., and Molteno, C. (1999). Post-partum depression and the mother-infant relationship in a South African peri-urban settlement. *British Journal of Psychiatry*, **175**, 554–8.

Cournos, F., McKinnon, K., and Sullivan, G. (2004). Schizophrenia and comorbid human immunodeficiency virus or hepatitis C virus. *Journal of Clinical Psychiatry*, **66**, 27–33.

de Groot, M., Anderson, R., Freedland, K.E., Clouse, R.E., and Lustman, P. J. (2001). Association of depression and diabetes complications: a meta-analysis. *Psychosomatic Medicine*, **63**, 619–30.

Demissie, M., Getahun, H., and Lindtjorn, B. (2003). Community tuberculosis care through "TB clubs" in rural North Ethiopia. *Social Science & Medicine*, **56**, 2009–18.

Dewey, M.E. and Saz, P. (2001). Dementia, cognitive impairment and mortality in persons aged 65 and over living in the community: a systematic review of the literature. *International Journal of Geriatric Psychiatry*, **16**, 751–61.

Dolder, C.R., Lacro, J.P., and Jeste, D.V. (2003). Adherence to antipsychotic and nonpsychiatric medications in middle-aged and older patients with psychotic disorders. *Psychosomatic Medicine*, **65**, 156–62.

Dubé, B., Benton, T., Cruess, D.G., and Evans, D. L. (2004). Neuropsychiatric manifestations of HIV infection and AIDS. *Journal of Psychiatry & Neuroscience*, **30**, 237–46.

Edwards, P., Roberts, I., Green, J., and Lutchmun, S. (2006). Deaths from injury in children and employment status in family: analysis of trends in class specific death rates. *British Medical Journal*, **333**, 119.

Escobar, J.I., Waitzkin, H., Silver, R.C., Gara, M., and Holman, A. (1998). Abridged somatization: a study in primary care. *Psychosomatic Medicine*, **60**, 466–72.

Everson, S.A., Roberts, R.E., Goldberg, D.E., and Kaplan, G.A. (1998). Depressive symptoms and increased risk of stroke mortality over a 29-year period. *Archives of Internal Medicine*, **158**, 1133–8.

Galler, J.R., Harrison, R.H., Biggs, M.A., Ramsey, F., and Forde, V. (1999). Maternal moods predict breastfeeding in Barbados. *Journal of Developmental & Behavioral Pediatrics*, **20**, 80–7.

Glassman, A.H., O'Connor, C.M., Califf, R.M., Swedberg, K., Schwartz, P., Bigger, J.T., Jr., *et al.* (2002). Sertraline treatment of major depression in patients with acute MI or unstable angina. *Journal of the American Medical Association*, **288**, 701–9.

Gordillo, V., del Amo, J., Soriano, V., and Gonzalez-Lahoz, J. (1999). Sociodemographic and psychological variables influencing adherence to antiretroviral therapy. *AIDS*, **13**, 1763–9.

Gureje, O., Simon, G.E., Ustun, T.B., and Goldberg, D.P. (1997). Somatization in cross-cultural perspective: a World Health Organization study in primary care. *American Journal of Psychiatry*, **154**, 989–95.

Hackett, M.L., Anderson, C.S., and House, A.O. (2004). Management of depression after stroke: a systematic review of pharmacological therapies. *Stroke*, **36**, 1098–103.

Heila, H., Haukka, J., Suvisaari, J., and Lonnqvist, J. (2004). Mortality among patients with schizophrenia and reduced psychiatric hospital care. *Psychological Medicine*, **35**, 725–32.

Hemingway, H. and Marmot, M. (1999). Evidence based cardiology: psychosocial factors in the aetiology and prognosis of coronary heart disease. Systematic review of prospective cohort studies. *British Medical Journal*, **318**, 1460–7.

Hinkin, C.H., Castellon, S.A., Durvasula, R.S., Hardy, D.J., Lam, M.N., Mason, K.I., *et al.* (2002). Medication adherence among HIV+ adults: effects of cognitive dysfunction and regimen complexity. *Neurology*, **59**, 1944–50.

Hinkin, C.H., Hardy, D.J., Mason, K.I., Castellon, S.A., Durvasula, R.S., Lam, M.N., *et al.* (2004). Medication adherence in HIV-infected adults: effect of patient age, cognitive status, and substance abuse. *AIDS*, **18**, S19–25.

Ickovics, J.R., Hamburger, M.E., Vlahov, D., Schoenbaum, E.E., Schuman, P., Boland, R.J., and Moore, J. (2001). Mortality, CD4 cell count decline, and depressive symptoms among HIV-seropositive women: longitudinal analysis from the HIV Epidemiology Research Study. *Journal of the American Medical Association*, **285**, 1466–74.

Institute of Medicine, Committee on Nervous System Disorders in Developing Countries (2001). *Neurological, Psychiatric, and Developmental Disorders. Meeting the Challenge in the Developing World.* Washington DC: National Academy Press.

Ismail, K., Winkley, K., and Rabe-Hesketh, S. (2004). Systematic review and meta-analysis of randomised controlled trials of psychological interventions to improve glycaemic control in patients with type 2 diabetes. *Lancet*, **363**, 1589–97.

Jablensky, A.V., Morgan, V., Zubrick, S.R., Bower, C., and Yellachich, L. A. (2004). Pregnancy, delivery, and neonatal complications in a population cohort of women with schizophrenia and major affective disorders. *American Journal of Psychiatry*, **162**, 79–91.

Janmeja, A.K., Das, S.K., Bhargava, R., and Chavan, B.S. (2004). Psychotherapy improves compliance with tuberculosis treatment. *Respiration*, **72**, 375–80.

Jonas, B.S. and Mussolino, M.E. (2000). Symptoms of depression as a prospective risk factor for stroke. *Psychosomatic Medicine*, **62**, 463–71.

Katon, W.J., Rutter, C., Simon, G., Lin, E.H., Ludman, E., Ciechanowski, P., *et al.* (2004). The association of comorbid depression with mortality in patients with type 2 diabetes. *Diabetes Care*, **28**, 2668–72.

Katon, W.J., Von Korff M., Lin, E.H., Simon, G., Ludman, E., Russo, J., *et al.* (2004). The Pathways Study: a randomized trial of collaborative care in patients with diabetes and depression. *Archives of General Psychiatry*, **61**, 1042–9.

Kebede, D., Alem, A., Shibre, T., Negash, A., Deyassa, N., Beyero, T., *et al.* (2004). Short-term symptomatic and functional outcomes of schizophrenia in Butajira, Ethiopia. *Schizophrenia Research*, **78**, 171–85.

Kroenke, K., Spitzer, R.L., and Williams, J.B. (2002). The PHQ-15: validity of a new measure for evaluating the severity of somatic symptoms. *Psychosomatic Medicine*, **64**, 258–66.

Kuehner, C. (2003). Gender differences in unipolar depression: an update of epidemiological findings and possible explanations. *Acta Psychiatrica Scandinavica*, **108**, 163–74.

Kuper, H., Marmot, M., and Hemingway, H. (2002). Systematic review of prospective cohort studies of psychosocial factors in the etiology and prognosis of coronary heart disease. *Seminars in Vascular Medicine*, **2**, 267–314.

Larson, S.L., Owens, P.L., Ford, D., and Eaton, W. (2001). Depressive disorder, dysthymia, and risk of stroke: thirteen-year follow-up from the Baltimore epidemiologic catchment area study. *Stroke*, **32**, 1979–83.

Latthe, P., Mignini, L., Gray, R., Hills, R., and Khan, K. (2006). Factors predisposing women to chronic pelvic pain: systematic review. *British Medical Journal*, **332**, 749–55.

Lawrence, D.M., Holman, C.D., Jablensky, A.V., and Hobbs, M.S. (2003). Death rate from ischaemic heart disease in Western Australian psychiatric patients 1980-1998. *British Journal of Psychiatry*, **182**, 31–6.

Lechner, S.C., Antoni, M.H., Lydston, D., Laperriere, A., Ishii, M., Devieux, J., *et al.* (2003). Cognitive-behavioral interventions improve quality of life in women with AIDS. *Journal of Psychosomatic Research*, **54**, 253–61.

Lin, E.H., Katon, W., Rutter, C., Simon, G.E., Ludman, E.J., Von Korff M., *et al.* (2006). Effects of enhanced depression treatment on diabetes self-care. *Annals of Family Medicine*, **4**, 46–53.

Lin, E.H., Katon, W., Von Korff, M., Rutter, C., Simon, G.E., Oliver, M., *et al.* (2004). Relationship of depression and diabetes self-care, medication adherence, and preventive care. *Diabetes Care*, **27**, 2154–60.

Lustman, P.J., Anderson, R.J., Freedland, K.E., de Groot, M., Carney, R.M., and Clouse, R.E. (2000a). Depression and poor glycemic control: a meta-analytic review of the literature. *Diabetes Care*, **23**, 934–42.

Lustman, P.J., Freedland, K.E., Griffith, L.S., and Clouse, R.E. (2000b). Fluoxetine for depression in diabetes: a randomized double-blind placebo-controlled trial. *Diabetes Care*, **23**, 618–23.

Lustman, P.J., Griffith, L.S., Clouse, R.E., Freedland, K.E., Eisen, S.A., Rubin, E.H., *et al.* (1997). Effects of nortriptyline on depression and glycemic control in diabetes: results of a double-blind, placebo-controlled trial. *Psychosomatic Medicine*, **59**, 241–50.

Maier, W., Gansicke, M., Gater, R., Rezaki, M., Tiemens, B., and Urzua, R.F. (1999). Gender differences in the prevalence of depression: a survey in primary care. *Journal of Affective Disorders*, **53**, 241–52.

Maj, M., Janssen, R., Starace, F., Zaudig, M., Satz, P., Sughondhabirom, B., *et al.* (1994a). WHO Neuropsychiatric AIDS study, cross-sectional phase I. Study design and psychiatric findings. *Archives of General Psychiatry*, **51**, 39–49.

Maj, M., Satz, P., Janssen, R., Zaudig, M., Starace, F., D'Elia, L., *et al.* (1994b). WHO Neuropsychiatric AIDS study, cross-sectional phase II. Neuropsychological and neurological findings. *Archives of General Psychiatry*, **51**, 51–61.

Mathers, C.D. and Loncar, D. (2006). Projections of global mortality and burden of disease from 2002 to 2030. *PLoS Medicine*, **3**, e442.

Mogga, S., Prince, M., Alem, A., Kebede, D., Stewart, R., Glozier, N., and Hotopf, M. (2006). Outcome of major depression in Ethiopia: population-based study. *British Journal of Psychiatry*, **189**, 241–6.

Morris, P.L., Robinson, R.G., Andrzejewski, P., Samuels, J., and Price, T.R. (1993). Association of depression with 10-year poststroke mortality. *American Journal of Psychiatry*, **150**, 124–9.

#Murray, C.J.L. and Lopez, A.D. (1996). *The Global Burden of Disease. A comprehensive assessment of mortality and disability from diseases, injuries and risk factors in 1990 and projected to 2020.* Cambridge, MA: Harvard University Press.

Murray, L. and Cooper, P.J. (2003). Intergenerational transmission of affective and cognitive processes associated with depression: infancy and the pre-school years. In: Goodyer, I.M. (ed.) *Unipolar Depression: A Lifespan Perspective*, pp. 17–46. Oxford: Oxford University Press.

Nilsson, E., Lichtenstein, P., Cnattingius, S., Murray, R. M., and Hultman, C. M. (2002). Women with schizophrenia: pregnancy outcome and infant death among their offspring. *Schizophrenia Research*, **58**, 221–9.

O'Hara, M. (1997). The nature of postpartum depressive disorders. In: Murray, L. and Cooper, P.J. (eds.) *Postpartum Depression and Child Development*, pp. 3–31. New York: Guilford Press.

Ohira, T., Iso, H., Satoh, S., Sankai, T., Tanigawa, T., Ogawa, Y., *et al.* (2001). Prospective study of depressive symptoms and risk of stroke among Japanese. *Stroke*, **32**, 903–8.

Osborn, R.L., Demoncada, A.C., and Feuerstein, M. (2006). Psychosocial interventions for depression, anxiety, and quality of life in cancer survivors: meta-analyses. *International Journal of Psychiatry in Medicine*, **36**, 13–34.

Parikh, R.M., Robinson, R.G., Lipsey, J.R., Starkstein, S.E., Fedoroff, J.P., and Price, T.R. (1990). The impact of poststroke depression on recovery in activities of daily living over a 2-year follow-up. *Archives of Neurology*, **47**, 785–9.

Patel, V., DeSouza, N., and Rodrigues, M. (2003). Postnatal depression and infant growth and development in low income countries: a cohort study from Goa, India. *Archives of Disease in Childhood*, **88**, 34–7.

Patel, V. and Kleinman, A. (2003). Poverty and common mental disorders in developing countries. *Bulletin of the World Health Organization*, **81**, 609–15.

Patel, V., Pednekar, S., Weiss, H., Rodrigues, M., Barros, P., Nayak, B., *et al.* (2004). Why do women complain of vaginal discharge? A population survey of infectious and pyschosocial risk factors in a South Asian community. *International Journal of Epidemiology*, **34**, 853–62.

Patel, V. and Prince, M. (2006). Maternal psychological morbidity and low birth weight in India. *British Journal of Psychiatry*, **188**, 284–5.

Patel, V., Rahman, A., Jacob, K.S., and Hughes, M. (2004). Effect of maternal mental health on infant growth in low income countries: new evidence from South Asia. *British Medical Journal*, **328**, 820–3.

Patel, V. and Thornicroft, G. (2009). Packages of care for mental, neurological, and substance use disorders in low- and middle-income countries: PLoS Medicine Series. *PLoS Medicine*, **6**, e1000160.

Paterson, D.L., Swindells, S., Mohr, J., Brester, M., Vergis, E.N., Squier, C., *et al.* (2000). Adherence to protease inhibitor therapy and outcomes in patients with HIV infection. *Annals of Internal Medicine*, **133**, 21–30.

Paulson, J.F., Dauber, S., and Leiferman, J.A. (2006). Individual and combined effects of postpartum depression in mothers and fathers on parenting behavior. *Pediatrics*, **118**, 659–68.

Phillips, M.R., Yang, G., Zhang, Y., Wang, L., Ji, H., and Zhou, M. (2002). Risk factors for suicide in China: a national case-control psychological autopsy study. *Lancet*, **360**, 1728–36.

Prasad, J., Abraham, V.J., Minz, S., Abraham, S., Joseph, A., Muliyil, J.P., *et al.* (2006). Rates and factors associated with suicide in Kaniyambadi Block, Tamil Nadu, South India, 2000-2002. *International Journal of Social Psychiatry*, **52**, 65–71.

Prince, M., Patel, V., Saxena, S., Maj, M., Maselko, J., Phillips, M. R., and Rahman, A. (2007). No health without mental health. *Lancet*, **370**, 859–77.

Rahman, A., Iqbal, Z., Bunn, J., Lovel, H., and Harrington, R. (2004a) Impact of maternal depression on infant nutritional status and illness: a cohort study. *Archives of General Psychiatry*, **61**, 946–52.

Rahman, A., Lovel, H., Bunn, J., Iqbal, Z., and Harrington, R. (2004b). Mothers' mental health and infant growth: a case-control study from Rawalpindi, Pakistan. *Child: Care, Health and Development*, **30**, 21–7.

Rahman, A., Malik, A., Sikander, S., Roberts, C., and Creed, F. (2008). Cognitive behaviour therapy-based intervention by community health workers for mothers with depression and their infants in rural Pakistan: a cluster-randomised controlled trial. *Lancet*, **372**, 902–9.

Rees, K., Bennett, P., West, R., Davey, S.G., and Ebrahim, S. (2004). Psychological interventions for coronary heart disease. *Cochrane Database of Systematic Reviews*, 2, CD002902.

Saz, P. and Dewey, M.E. (2001). Depression, depressive symptoms and mortality in persons aged 65 and over living in the community: a systematic review of the literature. *International Journal of Geriatric Psychiatry*, **16**, 622–30.

Scott, R.A., Lhatoo, S.D., and Sander, J.W. (2001). The treatment of epilepsy in developing countries: where do we go from here? *Bulletin of the World Health Organization*, **79**, 344–51.

Strik, J.J., Honig, A., Lousberg, R., Lousberg, A.H., Cheriex, E.C., Tuynman-Qua, H.G., *et al.* (2000). Efficacy and safety of fluoxetine in the treatment of patients with major depression after first myocardial infarction: findings from a double-blind, placebo-controlled trial. *Psychosomatic Medicine*, **62**, 783–9.

Ustun, T.B. and Sartorius, N. (1995). *Mental Illness in General Health Care: an International Study.* Chichester: John Wiley and Sons.

Vijayakumar, L. and Rajkumar, S. (1999). Are risk factors for suicide universal? A case-control study in India. *Acta Psychiatrica Scandinavica*, **99**, 407–11.

Webb, R., Abel, K., Pickles, A., and Appleby, L. (2004). Mortality in offspring of parents with psychotic disorders: a critical review and meta-analysis. *American Journal of Psychiatry*, **162**, 1045–56.

White, D.A., Heaton, R.K., and Monsch, A.U. (1995). Neuropsychological studies of asymptomatic human immunodeficiency virus-type-1 infected individuals. The HNRC Group. HIV Neurobehavioral Research Center. *Journal of the International Neuropsychological Society*, **1**, 304–15.

Wilkie, F.L., Goodkin, K., Eisdorfer, C., Feaster, D., Morgan, R., Fletcher, M.A., *et al.* (1998). Mild cognitive impairment and risk of mortality in HIV-1 infection. *Journal of Neuropsychiatry Clin.Neurosci.*, **10**, 125–32.

Winkley, K., Ismail, K., Landau, S., and Eisler, I. (2006). Psychological interventions to improve glycaemic control in patients with type 1 diabetes: systematic review and meta-analysis of randomised controlled trials. *British Medical Journal*, **333**, 65.

World Health Organization (2006). *WHO Statistical Information System. Working paper describing data sources, methods and results for projections of mortality and burden of disease for 2005, 2015 and 2030.* Geneva: World Health Organization.

Yun, L.W., Maravi, M., Kobayashi, J.S., Barton, P.L., and Davidson, A.J. (2004). Antidepressant treatment improves adherence to antiretroviral therapy among depressed HIV-infected patients. *Journal of Acquired Immune Deficiency Syndromes*, **38**, 432–8.

Ziegelstein, R.C., Fauerbach, J.A., Stevens, S.S., Romanelli, J., Richter, D.P., and Bush, D.E. (2000). Patients with depression are less likely to follow recommendations to reduce cardiac risk during recovery from a myocardial infarction. *Archives of Internal Medicine*, **160**, 1818–23.

CHAPTER 8

Expertise from experience: mental health recovery and wellness

Margaret Swarbrick

Introduction

Persons who were formerly recipients of services (service users) have become architects in the design, delivery, and evaluation of services. This chapter will examine the evolution of the user-led self-help movement, and its impacts on transforming community mental health practice to promote mental health recovery and wellness as a vision and outcome.

Who are service users?

There is no clear consensus regarding how to uniformly define the term 'service user'. There are a variety of terms used to designate a person who lives with a mental disorder who is a past or current recipient of the public mental health service delivery system. Terms include, but are not limited to, a person living with a mental disorder, patient, psychiatric survivor, ex-patient, inmate, client, recipient, mental health consumer, person in recovery, and person living with mental illness. There is much debate regarding terms. For example, many are sceptical about the term 'consumer' because this would imply a person has power and choice when most likely this is not the case. The term 'service user' is the term used internationally and generally applies to identify individuals diagnosed with a mental disorder who have currently, or in the past, used traditional mental health services. This is the term that will be used throughout this chapter.

User-led self-help movement

The self-help user-led movement (also referred to as consumer–survivor–ex-patient movement) has evolved at various paces around the world. Throughout Europe, the United States, as well as Australia and New Zealand, public policy efforts are attempting to include service users in planning and policy and implementation of new transformation endeavours. This movement is underdeveloped in many countries and in others has made significant impacts on transformation of community mental health practice. The following sections will review how the user led self-help

movement emerged. Table 8.1 summarizes key area of focus (social justice, empowerment, recovery, and wellness) and systems change contributions for community mental health practice.

Social justice

Social justice was an important organizing principle. Groups organized because people were being excluded, stigmatized, and subject to practices preventing them from having equal access to reach their full potential, and to contribute equally within society. They faced stigma, discrimination, and were prevented from the same opportunities, freedom, and access other citizens enjoy. People were too often limited in terms of **participation** in the community, as employees, students, volunteers, teachers, carers, parents, advisors, residents; as active citizens (National Social Inclusion Programme (2009). Service users had (and continue to) experience this exclusion in many aspects of life—social, economic, educational, spiritual, recreational/cultural, and health. They encountered higher rates of poverty, unemployment, homelessness, poor health, inadequate access to education, and social isolation.

Social justice through advocacy became the focus to correct violations. Some groups organized around the human rights violations and others act as watchdogs to prevent people from being unnecessarily excluded from society. In the United States the initial advocacy emerged from the user-led 'patient' liberation movement organized by persons who experienced emotional distress, with freedoms denied by the labelling and dehumanizing and stereotypical images propagated by the mental health system and society (Zinman, 1987).

The movement is considered a political paradigm that developed out of societal discrimination based on misunderstanding and misconceptions about service users and disenchantment with the delivery of conventional medical model services. This movement viewed the conventional 'system' as dehumanizing, unresponsive to individual needs, and some factions insisted on complete liberation from psychiatry because they reject the medical models of mental illness, professional control, and forced treatment.

Table 8.1 Key areas of focus and systems change contributions for community mental health practice

Focus	Systems change/contributions
Social justice	◆ Advocacy to uphold human rights, equality and address economic and social inequities ◆ Organized to address injustices service users faced in terms of social, economic, political structures
Empowerment	◆ Access to choices regarding services ◆ Influence the operation and structure of service provision ◆ Participate in system-wide service planning ◆ Participate in decision-making in meaningful roles.
Recovery	◆ Move from symptoms and illness to a vision of mental health recovery ◆ Recovery Vision and 10 Components: 　◆ Hope 　◆ Strengths based 　◆ Peer support 　◆ Self-direction 　◆ Responsibility 　◆ Holistic 　◆ Empowerment 　◆ Respect 　◆ Non-linear 　◆ Individualized and person-centred
Wellness	◆ Recognize and address mortality and morbidity and ill effects of unemployment and lifelong poverty ◆ Holistic view of a person: mental/emotional, physical, intellectual, social, environmental, occupational, financial, and spiritual dimensions

Service users are placing greater attention on issues of social inclusion/exclusion and are helping community health programmes place greater attention to social determinants of health which are formidable barriers to mental health recovery and wellness. A faction of the movement has focused on social justice though advocacy. Mind Freedom (http://www.mindfreedom.org/events_sf) is a lead organization. The Mind Freedom International Vision is to 'Unite in a spirit of mutual cooperation for a nonviolent revolution of mental health human rights and choice'. To find out more about this movement, visit the web page http://www.power2u.org/recovery.htm, which is from the National Empowerment Center's (NEC) Website. The NEC is a peer-run organization that focuses on recovery, self-help, and self-advocacy. For example, the service-user movement has been very active in trying to eliminate the use of seclusion and restraint techniques in psychiatric hospitals (see some articles linked from the website http://www.power2u.org/news.html).

Empowerment

The movement also organized around the belief that service users had limited options, choices, and involvement in their individual services and in the service system as a whole. There was discontent with the traditional system that was viewed as paternalistic and lacking in a range of options and opportunities for meaningful impact on policy planning and decision-making. Empowerment emerged as a means to correct those violations and the pervasive debilitating consequences of individual encounters with the traditional mental health system. Conceptually, **empowerment** is a process by which individuals who generally have lesser power gain control over their lives including the ability to influence the organizational and societal structures within which they live in order to gain mastery over all domains of life, including mental health care (McLean, 1995). Harp (1994), a prominent leader in the United States movement considered empowerment as occurring at four levels: 1) freedom of choice regarding services, 2) influence over

the operation and structure of service provision, 3) participation in system-wide service planning, and 4) participation in decision-making at the community level. Reacting to their experiences of inadequacies with the mental health system and the indignities it engendered, service users organized to empower one another by producing their own service alternatives (Chamberlin, 1978). Types of service alternatives (user-led services) are outlined in Table 8.2.

Mental health recovery

Strong advocacy by the movement (as well as research and strong leadership by prominent leaders) promoted the notion of recovery (Deegan, 1988), now endorsed on an international level (Slade et al., 2008). Service users want the same things that many people in society desire: a sense of belonging, an adequate income, and a decent place to live. They aspire to fulfil various life roles and contribute to their community at large. Recovery is a personal, unique process of (re)gaining physical, spiritual, mental, and emotional balance after one encounters illness, crisis, or trauma. For some, recovery is the ability to work, to live in housing of their own choice, to have friends and intimate relationships, and to become contributing members of their community. Recovery, therefore, is a process of healing and restoring health and wellness during episodes of illness and life stress.

Some debate has occurred regarding a clear definition of **recovery**. For some people, recovery is the ability to live a fulfilling and productive life despite a disability. The Substance Abuse and Mental Health Services Administration (SAMHSA) unveiled a consensus statement outlining the 10 principles necessary to achieve mental health recovery (U.S. Department of Health and Human Services, 2006), which are listed in Table 8.1.

Wellness

In addition to the recovery vision, service users are moving community mental health practice to adopt a focus on wellness.

Table 8.2 Categories of user-led services

Model	Characteristics/benefits	Challenges
Self-help	◆ Systemic costs can be minimal. May be as little as a donation of space, or more extensive involving costs for paid mentoring or training (e.g. GROW) ◆ Presents an open, no-cost venue to access support ◆ Serves as an important source of social, instrumental, and practical support	◆ Self-help may not be well understood or embraced by some professionals and non-professionals ◆ Need an appropriate model and trained facilitators willing to implement model to be effective ◆ Without objective stewardship, self-help groups can become settings where misinformation is spread ◆ May lack resources some people with disabilities may need, such as transportation, sign language interpreters, translated materials or formats
Service user (peer) as employee	◆ Enhances traditional provider agency services through building credibility and empathy with people served ◆ Provides opportunities for peers to share skills through specialized roles, such as navigator, recovery coach, job coach, enhancing service capacity and value	◆ Dual roles (e.g. service provider and service recipient), which can be hard to clarify and can sometimes raise conflict ◆ Feeling isolated, especially if the person is the sole or 'token' service user as provider ◆ Stigmatizing job titles (e.g. consumer case manager, peer advocate) ◆ Self-disclosure: what to disclose and who to disclose to ◆ Job discrimination (e.g. lower salary grades for service user providers)
Service-user led or operated	◆ Can offer the full continuum of support–related services ◆ Builds credibility with service recipients through engaging staff with similar lived experience ◆ Enhances ability to create and maintain a culture with potential to dispel negative experiences service recipients may have had	Limited availability, therefore may require additional inputs: ◆ Funding to develop ◆ Time to grow in strength, and credibility ◆ Systemic effort to create credibility. Being user-led does not guarantee the service employ current best practices
User-led partnership	◆ Invites greater understanding between service users and agency governing bodies ◆ Helps agencies develop and maintain focus on recipient needs and credibility among recipients ◆ Service user volunteers enhance service and systems capacity	◆ Low retention in board roles, unless resources are allocated for mentoring, transportation, etc. as needed ◆ Non-representative peer presence ◆ Relegation of peers to an advisory board or community board status, rather than a governing board ◆ Volunteer services may be devalued, sending mixed messages to volunteers and larger community about importance of their contributions

Wellness is defined as a conscious, deliberate process that requires a person to become aware of, and make choices for, a more satisfying lifestyle (Swarbrick, 1997, 2006). A **wellness lifestyle** includes a balance of health habits, including adequate sleep, rest, and good nutrition; productivity and exercise; participation in meaningful activity; and connections with supportive relationships (Swarbrick, 1997, 2006). Wellness views a person holistically (more than just mental and emotional well-being) and includes physical, intellectual, social, environmental, and occupational, financial, and spiritual dimensions.

In terms of mental health recovery, a person can regain mental and emotional balance by concentrating on the various aspects of overall wellness (e.g. social support, spiritual connections, taking care of one's physical health through rest, sleep, and adequate nutrition). Wellness is so very important because the traditional system has not adequately addressed overall health, especially physical health and the pervasive effects of poverty and unemployment. Of particular concern is the increased morbidity and mortality largely due to treatable medical conditions that are caused by modifiable risk factors such as smoking, obesity, substance abuse, and inadequate access to medical care (NASMHPD, 2006) as well as ill health effects of the medications prescribed for their psychiatric conditions.

In the United States, service users became involved in a national campaign to mobilize action to address this health concern. Many service users have assumed key roles helping the Substance Abuse and Mental Health Services Administration to launch the '10 by 10' Campaign (Manderscheid and del Vecchio, 2008; center for Mental Health Services, 2010). They are mobilizing efforts to address the considerably shortened life expectancy and reduced quality of life associated with living with a serious mental illness (see web site, http://www.bu.edu/cpr/resources/wellness-summit/index.html). They have, and will continue to assume an important lead role advocating for a health promotion and wellness model for community mental health practice, since the lack of a wellness lifestyle has been a powerful contributor to the disability experience and a stimulus to the recovery efforts of service users (Hutchinson et al., 2006). In the US peer wellness coaching and whole health initiatives are new community based work force roles designed to help people modify health risk factors through in strength based focused on wellness (Swarbrick, 2010).

User-led services

Service users have made impacts by defining mental health **recovery** and **wellness** as organizing principles for community mental health services. Additionally they have made strides towards transforming the conventional model of 'care' towards a recovery orientation that includes services developed and delivered by former or current service users (Emerick, 1990; Everett, 1994). User-led services were a natural outgrowth of dissatisfaction with professionally run treatment programmes that were perceived as problem-based rather than focused holistically on mental health recovery and wellness. From mutual support groups, to drop-in centres, to alternative programmes, self-help is essential to mental health recover recovery, either as an adjunct or as an alternative to professionally run community mental health services. There have been a variety of types of services. In the United States the Substance Abuse and Mental Health Service Administration's (SAMHSA's) Center for Mental Health Services (CMHS) funded demonstration projects to examine the feasibility of this model (Van Tosh and del Vecchio, 2000). A range of services evolved including housing programmes, businesses, peer support programmes, case management, and drop-in centres (Salzer, 2001). Services types include: **drop-in** or **self-help centres**, which provide varied services such as meals and housing assistance for members, as well as a place to meet friends and relax; **peer-support programmes**, consisting of self-help groups and services in which users provide services to one another; and **education programmes**, which include training programs during which consumers learn recovery or advocacy skills (Clay, 2005).

Doughty and Tse (2005, 2010) define a service user-run/user-led service as a programme, project, or service planned, administered, delivered, and evaluated by a service-user group based on the needs defined by the group. Operation of the service includes self-governance by the group themselves including staffing, supervision, and control of programme policy and service user responsibility for administrating the programme. Some services are entirely managed by service users; while others incorporate professionals in certain areas of planning, implementation, and evaluation (Solomon, 2004). A variety of methods for categorizing the user-led services have been proposed (Corrigan et al., 2008; Davidson et al., 1999; Doughty and Tse, 2005; Mowbray and Moxley, 1997; Swarbrick et al., 2010).

Two key issues include: **control** of the agency administration (service user vs. non-service user leadership) and the **purpose of the service** (mutual support vs. conventional direct service). An important issue is the degree to which the organization or service is managed and led by service users (wholly, in partnership with non-service users, or by non-service users). Issues of control, governance, who defines the needs and focus of the service, are all factors in terms of defining the service type. The extent to which the role is something that is uniquely performed and controlled by service users distinguishes the category.

User-led services are based on the notion that past and present recipients of services can provide a unique perspective on, and expertise to design and implement services to improve peers' quality of life. Service users develop, control, and provide the services and participation is completely voluntary (members participate of their own volition rather than being required or coerced to attend). There should be an emphasis on strengths and competencies and an important goal is mutuality among members. Services provide opportunities for service users to gain resources or competencies, such as the capacity to help others. Members of the group share responsibilities for operating the services and by design, members have an active role in decisions regarding service and operations. User-led services offer a setting that fosters empowerment by creating opportunities for all members to participate in an inclusive, democratic process of shared decision-making (Swarbrick, 2005).

Historically, the notion of user-led services dates back to Fountain House, founded in 1948 by ex-patients of Rockland State Hospital, New York City, who dubbed themselves WANA (We Are Not Alone) (Beard et al., 1982). Fountain House gave birth to the 'clubhouse' movement, where service users played active roles in the management and operation of the programme (Macias et al., 1999). Over time, this model has evolved such that service users are employees (Salzer, 2001).

Other early user-led services included the work of Howie the Harp, a prominent leader, who pioneered Project Release, a single-room housing service in New York for consumers, based on principles of service delivery, mutual support, and advocacy (Knight, 1997). Judi Chamberlin was another pioneer who started the Ruby Rogers Drop-In Center in Boston (Chamberlin, 1978).

Table 8.2 outlines categories of user-led services.

Self-help

Mutual aid or **self-help** is offered outside the conventional mental health system by and for service users who simply volunteer to help their peers (Swarbrick et al., 2010). The term **self-help group** has also been used to distinguish member-run support groups from professionally-run support groups. Self-help groups are widely available for many different kinds of difficult life experiences. Groups typically held in informal local community settings are a valuable source of ongoing support, education, and connection to a community for current or past service users. These groups are held in-person in informal settings and are increasingly available through the Internet (White and Madara, 2002). They are generally financially accessible because they charge no fees and may have only minimal dues, if any. Groups can serve as bridges to professional treatment through provision of referral information and sharing of experiential knowledge and skills as well as provide ongoing unconditional support.

Self-help groups are facilitated by volunteers, and usually have no formal connection to traditional services. Some are local initiatives though many follow national or international models, and have a relationship to a national organization. Examples of such organizations include: GROW, Recovery International, Double Trouble in Recovery, and the Depression and Bipolar Support Alliance (DBSA). Probably the best-known self-help group, Alcoholics Anonymous (AA), was started in 1935, and has since affected the lives of millions of recovering alcoholics worldwide. AA was the first of what came to be known as 12-step programmes, which came to include groups such as Narcotics Anonymous and Gamblers Anonymous. A tremendous number and variety of member-run self-help groups have evolved since the formation of AA. The first national self-help group for service users was Recovery Inc., started in 1937 by psychiatrist Abraham A. Low. Other self-help groups include Schizophrenics Anonymous, and many local grassroots groups that have been independently initiated by service users.

Over the past decade, people have been participating in online self-help groups, many of which were developed independently over the years by service users. These groups have online message boards, e-mail discussion groups, or scheduled real-time chat meetings. Online self-help networks eliminate many barriers that previously kept people from participating in a community group, including the lack of any local support group or the lack of transportation.

Self-help groups can be a resource for service users who want access to ongoing support. Professionals should be aware of available local self-help groups and clearinghouses. Professionals can advocate for or initiate self-help groups in settings where they most likely are not happening. Additionally they can link people to this resource that can provide an ongoing source of support.

User-led

User-led or operated or delivered (also referred to as peer) services are planned, operated, and evaluated to address social and emotional needs identified by the group. **Services** are managed by former or current service recipients who are paid to serve their peers. Some services are entirely user-managed, while others incorporate the use of non-user professionals in certain areas of planning, implementation, and evaluation. In the user-delivered service category, the inclusion of non-service users or professional involvement is within the control of the service-user operators.

By definition, user-run or operated denotes that service users constitute the majority of the governing board or advisory group that decides policies and procedures. The standard for service user controlled is that more than 51% of the board officers should be self-identified as people who are current or past recipients of the public service delivery system. User-led service agencies may offer multiple services (Collaborative Support Programs of New Jersey administers self-help centres, housing, financial services programs and employment supports: Swarbrick et al., 2009) whereas others operate outside of direct service provision (e.g. user-led programme evaluation agencies such as Consumer Quality Initiatives, Inc. http://www.cqi-mass.org.

User (or peer) partnership, also known as service user initiatives, are different than fully service-user driven services as the partnership model incorporates the use of non-service-user professionals in major aspects of planning, implementation, and evaluation. User partnerships services are offered within a traditional community mental health agency. Decision-making and control is shared by service users and professionals though service users have limited or no direct control in the administration, budgeting, and control of the operation. The executive staff and board of directors are comprised mainly of professionals. **Partnerships** take many forms, ranging from service users who volunteer in support roles, to those who are paid to provide support to peers receiving traditional services. Service users may volunteer to visit peers residing in psychiatric hospitals or serve as an advocate or spokesperson while a participant of a residential programme (Mowbray and Moxley, 1997). Service users bring the unique perspective of having both the service-user experience combined with understanding how to deal with the mental health system. Partnerships programmes generally develop within traditional service settings to fill social or practical needs. An example includes service users providing wellness and recovery education in a locked psychiatric facility (Swarbrick and Brice, 2006) and a peer support model developed by the United States Veterans Administration (Resnick and Rosenheck, 2008).

Service users as employees

Former or current service users have probably always worked in community mental health practice. Recently their personal experience has been recognized as something useful—to actually qualify them for a job. Previously, and in some situations today, people may have felt a need to keep their personal lives private for fear that they would be stigmatized at work or not hired at all. **Service users as employees** is a type of service in which former or current service users are working within the community mental health service system in its usual programmes, operated and administered primarily, but obviously not exclusively by professionals who are not living with a diagnosis of mental illness. There may be designated or specialist positions. Service users who are employed in traditional mental health positions are paid wages for their services. Many are assuming roles (designated peer roles and others not) in a variety of service elements including case management, inpatient, vocational rehabilitation, and crisis outreach. Others occupy an existing mental health position, such as being a doctor, nurse, case manager, staff psychologist, or social worker— they just also happen to be a former or current service user. In some cases, they disclose their experiences as a service user, while in other cases, depending on local culture and the ethics of the profession, they may not.

The prevalence of employment initiatives can be explained by the belief that the experience of service users can possibly impart insight and empathy which can be used to engage in a therapeutic relationship. The lived experience offers a unique perspective that can have positive impacts on the helping relationship. The value of credibility and empathy may outweigh the value of credentials. The expansion of former service users assuming roles and positions can personally enhance mental health recovery by offering a career opportunity and also can impact the 'recovery consciousness' of community mental health practice.

A Pillars of Peer Support Services Summit was convened at the Carter Center in Atlanta, GA. The intent of the summit was to bring together those states (in the US) that currently provide formal training and certification for peer providers working in mental health systems to examine the multiple levels of state support necessary for a strong and vital peer workforce able to engage in state's efforts at system transformation, including recent innovations in Whole Health. A promising role for peer focuses on health and wellness.

There is a growing body of evidence regarding the effectiveness of services provided by service users when compared to employees who are not service users. Studies have demonstrated that service users as employees provide equally effective services when compared to non-peer providers (Schmidt et al., 2008). Other studies have found that there have been positive impacts on the service users themselves (McGill and Patterson, 1990; Sherman and Porter, 1991, Doughty and Tse, 2010, presents a summary of data).

Research

Early research on user-led services has mainly offered descriptive reports that illustrate participant and programme characteristics, service usage, and programme outcomes (Chamberlin et al., 1996; Davidson et al., 1999; Salzer, 2001; Solomon, 2004; Swarbrick, 2007a,b). User-led services seem to offer a tolerant, flexible, and supportive environment. They provide a network of natural supporters, and many people have reported that they provide family-like support and environment (Swarbrick, 2005). Kaufmann and colleagues (1993) identified characteristics of successful services as having: a leader with good organizational skills, a core group of volunteers, an interdependent relationship with the mental health provider system, planned social events, and ongoing recruitment of new members.

The Center for Mental Health Services (CMHS) funded a multisite research study designed to examine the extent to which services by and for service users are effective in improving outcomes of service users when used as an adjunct to traditional mental health services.

The project (the Consumer Operated Services Program—COSP Multisite Research Initiative) used a multisite, random assignment experimental design aimed at generating empirical data meant to provide a more in-depth understanding of peer-operated programmes and services. The study investigated the extent to which user-led programmes are effective in improving empowerment, employment, housing, social inclusion outcomes, and service satisfaction. Over 1800 consumers participated in this study. For details of this study see *On Our Own Together* by Sally Clay (2005).

The CMHS COSP multisite initiative has provided important contributions to help better understand the effectiveness of consumer-operated services on individuals who receive traditional mental health services. Rogers and associates (2007) report that individuals who participated in the consumer-run programme reported higher levels of personal empowerment than individuals who participated in the control intervention (the control condition consisted of an array of traditional mental health services such as pharmacology and medication management, case management, residential services, day services, and psychosocial treatment services). Individuals with greater engagement in and attendance at the consumer-operated service reported higher levels of empowerment. Cross-sectional relationships were examined between participation in consumer-operated services and measures of recovery and empowerment (Corrigan, 2006). Participation in consumer-operated services in the form of peer support was found to be positively associated with recovery and empowerment factors (Corrigan, 2006). Participation in consumer-operated services seems to have a positive effect on empowerment, though the effect is small in magnitude (Corrigan, 2006; Rogers et al., 2007).

Additionally this study has offered some insights into the need for further research needed to better understand the critical ingredients of consumer-operated services that may contribute to positive outcomes. The COSP study was the most rigorous study to date. Randomized control studies are challenging due to the voluntary nature of these services. Funding to conduct such studies is not readily available. In addition, grassroots concerns of the service-user movement have been related to power differentials associated with research. Participatory action research approaches are a viable solution to these concerns as research is greatly needed to better examine and improve this service model.

Programme fidelity is the degree to which a programme contains key ingredients that are connected to core outcomes. Two fidelity measures have been developed, the Fidelity Rating Instrument (FRI; Holter et al., 2004) and the Fidelity Assessment Common Ingredients Tool (FACIT; Campbell and Adkins, 2007; Clay, 2005). The FACIT was developed for the COPP multisite study and the FRI has been used by researchers in Michigan. These fidelity instruments are important tools for further programme development and research endeavours.

Other possibilities

Other mechanisms for systems transformation include involving service users in all aspects of policy development, training, and evaluation. Service users are assuming roles as trainer or educator to prepare a mental health workforce that embraces mental health recovery and wellness. In addition, they can expand roles as auditors, quality improvement or evaluation personnel, as well as meaningful roles as directors or advisors for public policy and programme development. They should continue to be involved in influencing research agendas and funding. It is completely usual to see authorities which serve people who experience other disabling conditions (such as hearing or visual impairments or mobility issues) having directors and leadership teams who have the disability which the organization services. This is not as usual for mental health service users. In fact, there are probably very few people who openly disclose a psychiatric disability managing large community mental health programmes. If we assume that these would be good outcomes, it makes sense for professionals and the service user community to chart a course towards making such leadership happen. Additionally the National Association of State Mental Health Program Directors recently released a report on Consumer Involvement with State Mental Health Authorities (November 2010).

Conclusion

Mosher and Burti (1994) in *Community Mental Health* believed that continued development of a strong user-led movement should be a high priority of every community mental health programme. Further, they stated this would be the most clear and direct statement of a programme's commitment to the principle of preservation and enhancement of power. This chapter has highlighted how a growing movement of people around the world who once were relegated to the 'patient role' are now contributing 'expertise from experience' to inform, reform, and transform community mental health practice. Service users are resilient and capable of leading productive lives. Mental health recovery and wellness are possible, even probable. Empowered service users have become influential leaders who are transforming community mental health practice around the world. They are leading transformation efforts through a social justice advocacy agenda and services focused on wellness and mental health recovery. This chapter has highlighted the philosophical underpinning of the service-user movement and described types of user-led services, impacts both formal and informal, resources, and new and emerging roles. Practitioners are coming to understand the valuable impact the experience of receiving services has in terms of creating responsive community mental health practices that view mental health recovery through the lens of wellness. In order to build new services focused on wellness and recovery and to remodel the current systems into pathways for recovery, service users must play a strong role as architects of services. Professionals, researchers, and policy makers need to move from tokenism, and from mere surprise or acknowledgement, to the assumption that service users have both a right and responsibility to be fully integrated into all aspects and levels of service delivery.

References

Beard, J.H., Propst, R., and Malamud, T.J. (1982). The Fountain House model of psychiatric rehabilitation. *Psychosocial Rehabilitation Journal*, **5**, 47–53.

Campbell, J. and Adkins, R.E. (2007). *Fidelity assessment common ingredients tool e-FACIT workbook users' guide*. St. Louis, MO: Missouri Institute of Mental Health, Behavioral Health Division, Program in Consumer Studies & Training.

Center for Mental Health Services (2010). The 10 by 10 Campaign: a national action plan to improve life expectancy by 10 years in 10 years for people with mental illnesses. A report of the 2007 National Wellness Summit. HHS Publication No. (SMA) 10–4476. Rockville, MD: Center for Mental Health Services, Substance Abuse and Mental Health Service Administration.

Chamberlin, J. (1978). *On our own: Patient controlled alternatives to the mental health system*. New York: McGraw-Hill.

Chamberlin, J., Rogers, S.E., and Ellison, M.L. (1996). Self-help programs: A description of their characteristics and their members. *Psychiatric Rehabilitation Journal,* **19**, 33–42.

Clay, S. (2005). *On our own together: Peer programs for people with mental illness.* Nashville, TN: Vanderbilt Press.

Copeland, M.E. (1997). *Wellness Recovery Action Plan.* West Dummerston, VT: Peach Press.

Corrigan, P. (2006). Impact of consumer-operated services on empowerment and recovery of people with psychiatric disabilities. *Psychiatric Services,* **57**, 1493–96.

Corrigan, P.W., Mueser, K.T, Bond, G.R., Drake, R.E., and Solomon, P. (2008). *Principles and Practices of Psychiatric Rehabilitation: An empirical approach.* New York: Guilford Press.

Daniels, A., Grant, E., Filson, B., Powell, I., Fricks, L., Goodale, L. (eds) (2010). Pillars of peer support: Transforming Mental Health Systems of care through peer support services, www.pillarsofpeersupport.org.

Davidson, L., Chinman, M., Kloos, B., Weingarten, R., Stayner, D., and Tebes, J. (1999). Peer support among individuals with severe mental illness: A review of evidence. *Clinical Psychology: Science and Practice,* **6**, 165–87.

Deegan, P.E. (1988). Recovery: The lived experience of rehabilitation. *Psychosocial Rehabilitation Journal,* **11**, 11–19.

Doughty, C. and Tse, S. (2005). *The effectiveness of service user-run or service user-led mental health services for people with mental illness: A systematic review.* A Mental Health Commission Report. Wellington: Mental Health Commission.

Doughty, C. and Tse, S. (2010) Can consumer-led mental health services be equally as effective? An integrative review of CLMHS in high income countries. *Community Mental Health Journal.* In Press.

Emerick, R. (1990). Self- help groups for former patients: Relations with mental health professionals. *Hospital and Community Psychiatry,* **41**, 401–7.

Everett, B. (1994). Something is happening: The contemporary consumer and psychiatric survivor movement in historical context. *Journal of Mind and Behavior,* **15**, 55–70.

Harp, H. (1994). Empowerment of mental health consumers in vocational rehabilitation. *Psychosocial Rehabilitation Journal,* **17**, 83–90.

Holter, M., Mowbray, C., Bellamy, C., MacFarlane, P., and Dukarski, J. (2004). Critical ingredients of a consumer run services: Results of a national survey. *Community Mental Health Journal,* **40**, 47–63.

Hutchinson, D.S., Gagne, C., Bowers, S., Russinova, Z., Skrinar, G., and Anthony, W.A. (2006). A framework for health promotion services for people with psychiatric disabilities. *Psychiatric Rehabilitation Journal,* **29**, 241–50.

Kaufmann, C., Ward-Colasante, C., and Farmer, J. (1993). Development and evaluation of drop-in centers operated by mental health consumers. *Hospital and Community Psychiatry,* **44**, 675–8.

Knight, E. (1997). A model of the dissemination of self-help in public mental health systems. *New Directions for Mental Health Services,* **74**, 43–51.

McGill, C.W. and Patterson, C.J. (1990). Former patients as peer counselors on locked inpatient units. *Hospital and Community Psychiatry,* **41**, 1017–19.

McLean, A. (1995). Empowerment and the psychiatric consumer/ex-patient movement in the United States: Contradictions, crisis and change. *Social Science Medicine,* **40**, 1053–71.

Macias, C., Jackson, R., Schroeder, C., and Wang, Q. (1999). What is a clubhouse? Report on the ICCD 1996 survey of USA clubhouses. *Community Mental Health Journal,* **35**, 181–90.

Manderscheid, R. and del Vecchio, P. (2008). Moving toward solutions: Responses to the crisis of premature death. *International Journal of Mental Health,* **37**, 3–7.

Mosher, L. and Burti, L. (1994). *Community mental health: A practical guide.* New York: Norton & Company.

Mowbray, C.T. and Moxley, D.P. (1997). A framework for organizing consumer roles as providers of psychiatric rehabilitation. In: Mowbray, C.T., Moxley, D.P., Jasper, C.A., and Howell, L.L. (eds.) *Consumers as Providers in Psychiatric Rehabilitation,* pp. 35–44. Columbia, MD: International Association of Psychosocial Rehabilitation Services.

National Association of State Mental Health Program Directors Council (NASMHPD) (2006). *Morbidity and mortality in people with serious mental illness* (Thirteenth in a Series of Technical Reports). Alexandria, VA: NASMHPD.

National Association of State Mental Health Program Directors (NASMHPD) (2010). Consumer Involvement with State Mental Health Authorities. http://www.nasmhpd.org/general_files/publications/med_directors_pubs/consumer%20involvement%20with%20persons%20with%20SMI%20Final%Part%201.pdf.

National Social Inclusion Programme (2009). *Vision and Progress: Social Inclusion and Mental Health.* Available at: http://www.socialinclusion.org.uk/publications/NSIP_Vision_and_Progress.pdf

Resnick, S. and Rosenheck, R. (2008). Integrating peer provided services: A quasi-experimental study of recovery orientation, confidence, and empowerment. *Psychiatric Services,* **59**, 1307–14.

Rogers, E.S., Teague, G.B., Lichenstein, C., Campbell, J., Lyass, A., Chen, R., *et al.* (2007). Effects of participation in consumer-operated service programs on both personal and organizationally mediated empowerment: results of multisite study. *Journal of Rehabilitation Research and Development,* **44**, 785–800.

Salzer, M. (2001). *Best practice guidelines for consumer-delivered services.* Unpublished Manuscript, Behavioral Health Recovery Management Project.

Schmidt, L.T., Gill, K., Solomon, P., and Pratt, C. (2008). Comparison of service outcomes of case management teams with and without a consumer provider. *American Journal of Psychiatric Rehabilitation,* **77**, 310–29.

Sherman, P.S. and Porter, R. (1991). Mental health consumers as case management aides. *Hospital and Community Psychiatry,* **42**, 494–8.

Slade, M., Amering, M., and Oades, L. (2008). Recovery: An International perspective. *Epidemiologia e Psichiatria Sociale,* **17**, 128–37.

Solomon, P. (2004). Peer support/peer provided services: Underlying process, benefits and critical ingredients. *Psychiatric Rehabilitation Journal,* **27**, 392–401.

Swarbrick, M. (1997). A wellness model for clients. *Mental Health Special Interest Section,* **20**, 1–4.

Swarbrick, M. (2005). Consumer-operated self-help centers: The relationship between the social environment and its association with empowerment and satisfaction. (Doctoral dissertation). New York: New York University.

Swarbrick, M. (2006). A wellness approach. *Psychiatric Rehabilitation Journal,* **29**, 311–14.

Swarbrick, M. (2007a). Consumer-operated self-help centers. *Psychiatric Rehabilitation Journal,* **31**, 76–9.

Swarbrick, M. (2007b). Consumer-operated self-help services. *Journal of Psychosocial Nursing,* **44**, 26–35

Swarbrick, M. and Brice, G. (2006). Sharing the message of hope, wellness and recovery with consumers and staff at psychiatric hospitals. *American Journal of Psychiatric Rehabilitation,* **9**, 101–9.

Swarbrick, M., Bates, F., and Roberts, M. (2009). Peer employment support: A model created through collaboration between a peer-operated service and university. *Occupational Therapy in Mental Health,* **25**, 325–34.

Swarbrick, M. (2010). Wellness Coaching Supervisor manual. Collaborative support programs of New Jersey Inc.

Swarbrick, M., Schmidt, L., and Gill, K. (2010). *Persons in Recovery as Providers: The Wisdom of Experience.* Linthincum, MA: United States Psychiatric Rehabilitation Association.

U.S. Department of Health and Human Services (2006). *National Consensus Statement on Mental Health Recovery.* Rockville, MD: Substance Abuse and Mental Health Services Administration, U.S. Department of Health and Human Services. Available at: http://mentalhealth.samhsa.gov/publications/allpubs/SMA05-4129/ (Accessed 4 January 2010).

Van Tosh, L. and del Vecchio, P. (2000). *Consumer-operated self-help programs: A technical report.* Rockville, MD: U.S. Center for Mental Health Services.

White, B. and Madara, E. (2002). *Self-help group sourcebook,* 7th edn. Denville, NJ: Self-help Clearinghouse.

Zinman, S., Harp, H., and Budd, S. (1987). *Reaching across: Mental health clients helping each other.* CA: California Network of Mental Health Clients.

CHAPTER 9

Measuring the needs of people with mental illness

Mike Slade, Graham Thornicroft, Gyles Glover, and Michele Tansella

Introduction

The importance of needs assessment has been one of the most consistent themes to emerge from the evolution of community mental health services. The term 'need' has become especially influential in European mental health practice. In the United Kingdom, for example, national policy has emphasized the importance of needs assessment underpinning the planning, development, and evaluation of mental health services (Department of Health, 1999).

However, the concept of 'need' is used in different, and sometimes contradictory, ways. At the individual level, all mental health and social care should be provided on the basis of need. At the population level, funding allocation is intended to match the needs of the population, so that whether or not overall resources are adequate, efficiency and equity are achieved. The aim of this chapter is to define needs assessment, to consider different approaches to assessing needs at the individual and at the population levels, and to discuss how needs assessments can be applied in real-world settings in planning and delivering clinical care.

What are needs?

A need involves a lack of something. But of what? The clearest categorization of needs was identified by Brewin (2001), who grouped definitions of need within mental health care into three categories: lack of health, lack of access to services or institutions, and lack of action by mental health workers. Approaches to need within each of these three categories will be reviewed.

Needs for improved health

At the individual level, the concept of need has been grounded in various theories. Maslow put forward a theory of motivation in terms of a hierarchy of needs: physiological; safety; belongingness and love; esteem; and self-actualization (Maslow, 1954). He proposed that people are motivated by the requirement to meet these needs, and that higher-level needs could only be met once the lower and more fundamental needs were met. The clinical relevance of

this theory is that it implies a hierarchy of clinical priorities—interventions to meet basic physiological need (e.g. to ensure adequate food supply) should take priority over interventions to foster, for example, self-esteem.

In practice, health and social care needs are often identified in a widely defined way. In England, for example, the requirement to base the provision of services on level of need was first made explicit in the National Health Service and Community Care Act (Department of Health, 1990), which defined need as 'the requirements of individuals to enable them to achieve, maintain or restore an acceptable level of social independence or quality of life'. This definition equates need with social disablement, which occurs when a person experiences lowered psychological, social, and physical functioning in comparison with the norms of society. Three categories of social functioning measures have been identified: social attainment measures, social role performance measures, and instrumental behaviour measures (Wykes and Hurry, 1991).

Social attainments are achievements in the major life roles, such as marriage and employment. They have the advantage of being easily measurable with relatively high reliability, and so are particularly suited to large-scale, nomothetic studies, and epidemiological research. For example, at a population level significantly higher admission rates are associated with being unmarried, living alone, social deprivation, and drug misuse, and there is a large negative correlation between recovery from schizophrenia and unemployment (Warner, 2004). However, it is difficult to establish whether variables being measured are in a causal or correlative relationship.

Social role performance measures relate to how well a person is coping in their major roles of work, relationships, home, and self-care. They give a more in-depth assessment of a person's performance than social attainment measures, and cover a wide range of subdivided areas, such as instrumental and affective tasks. It can be difficult to take account of the person's social and cultural background, although this has been attempted by using consensual professional judgement (Gurland et al., 1972) or by normative scales (Cochrane and Stopes-Roe, 1977). Definitions of what constitutes pathological lack of function are culture-specific—an issue recognized in current debates about the *Diagnostic and Statistical Manual of Mental Disorders*, 5th edition (DSM-V; Regier et al., 2009).

Instrumental measures record social behaviour, and are more suited to a detailed assessment of individual psychiatric patients, some of whom may not fulfil many life roles. A detailed description of behaviour allows consideration of cultural factors when analysing the data, but do not take account of the context in which behaviour takes place—the person with hygiene problems who does not have access to pleasant washing facilities. They are often designed for use with very disabled people, and so rely on staff reports which may not take account of the person's perceptions of their needs.

Best practice involves **needs-led** care planning: basing the care provided for an individual patient on an assessment of their needs. This approach offers many benefits:

1 The overall level of need gives guidance about which part of the mental health system should treat the patient, e.g. that people with less disabling mental disorders should be seen in primary care settings (Tansella and Thornicroft, 1999).

2 Needs assessment can improve the comprehensiveness of case formulations and care plans by incorporating a broad range of health determinants, such as poor housing or lack of social support.

3 Explicit identification of need can support clinician–patient discussions about care priorities, which is associated with improved treatment satisfaction (Lasalvia et al., 2005) and adherence to treatment (Gray et al., 2006)

4 Identification of needs helps to identify the contribution of services outside the mental health sector.

5 Needs-led care can facilitate more individualized treatment planning than diagnosis-driven approaches, by more closely matching the help offered to patient's needs.

Needs-led care planning can be differentiated from the assessment of **care** needs. Assessing care needs involves identifying whether the patient will benefit from a predefined set of interventions. This will not identify all unmet needs for individual patients. Assessment of need at the patient level should therefore be a separate process from decisions about what care or treatment to provide. There are of course other reasons to consider needs for services, to which we now turn.

Needs for services

The second category of needs assessment schedules suggested by Brewin incorporates those measuring access to mental health services. Underlying these measures is the assumption that an unmet need indicates a lack of access to some form of psychiatric service. This category is used for informing the development of mental health services. It is less appropriate at an individual level, since it assesses needs through the filter of existing services.

At the population level, it is possible to use epidemiological methods to develop prevalence for different disorders, which can be translated into estimates of the need for services. For example, in the United States an epidemiological survey found considerable unmet need of the population level nationwide (Kessler et al., 2005). This study identified that between 1990 to 1992 and 2001 to 2003 the overall annual period prevalence of mental illnesses

remained constant at between 29.4% to 30.5%. Among these cases however there was an increase in the proportion who received any treatment at all, rising from 20.3% to 32.9% between the two times periods. This of course means that 67% of people with mental disorders in the United States receive no treatment. The situation is worse in other countries: a study of depression found that 0% of patients in St Petersburg (Russia) received evidence-based treatment in primary care, and only 3% were referred on to specialist mental health care (Simon et al., 2004). The inability of patients to afford out-of-pocket costs was the primary barrier to care for 75% of people in the study.

International comparisons of population-level needs have also been conducted in recent years. The European Study of the Epidemiology of Mental Disorders (ESEMed), for example, carried out cross-sectional surveys in Belgium, France, Germany, Italy, The Netherlands, and Spain among 8796 representative members of the general population. Individuals with a 12-month mental disorder that was disabling or that had led to use of services in the previous 12 months were considered in need of care. The study found that about 6% of the sample was defined as being in need of mental health care. Nearly half (48%) of these people reported no formal health care use, so that 3.1% of the adult population had an unmet need for mental health care. In contrast, only 8% of the people with diabetes had reported no use of services for their physical condition (Alonso et al., 2007)

Needs for action

Different types of need have been identified: felt (experienced), expressed (experienced and communicated), normative (judgement of professionals), and comparative (based on comparison with the position of other individuals or reference groups) (Bradshaw, 1972). This takes account of the different perceptions of need that can exist. Within health care this approach to need has been used to identify the circumstances when services should provide interventions. Need is taken to mean the ability to benefit in some way from health care, and thus distinguished from demand (what the person asks for) and supply (services given) (Stevens and Gabbay, 1991).

This raises the important topics of coverage and focusing. **Coverage** means the proportion of people who receive treatment who could benefit from it (Habicht et al., 1984). **Focusing** refers to how far those people who actually receive treatment in fact need it: do they have any form of mental illness? (Tansella, 2006) Even in the most well resourced countries one can find both low coverage and poor focusing (World Health Organization 2005a,b). From the public health perspective, therefore, the key issue is to increase both coverage and focus through the optimal use of resources, whatever the level of resources actually available.

Using this definition of need, an Australian study compared current and optimal treatment for 10 high-burden mental disorders in Australia (Andrews et al., 2004). They showed that current levels of treatment at current coverage avert 13% of the overall burden attributable to these disorders. Providing optimal treatment at current coverage would avert 20% of the burden, and optimal treatment at optimal coverage would avert 28%. The development of a more robust treatment evidence base makes this innovative approach to informing public policy more possible, and the approach can be recommended for evidence-based policy initiatives.

Individual-level needs assessment measures

Several standardized approaches to the assessment of patient-level need have been developed, primarily in the United Kingdom. These have shown a transition along a continuum, from an initial focus on assessment of need as an objective state to be defined by experts following careful assessment, towards those which emphasize the subjective nature of needs assessment.

The earliest standardized needs assessment measure was the **Medical Research Council Needs for Care Assessment (NFCAS)** (Brewin et al., 1987). The NFCAS assesses the need for further action by health care professionals, and links identification of a need with a predefined list of actions. A key feature is that the NFCAS is premised on the assumption that need is 'a normative concept which is to be defined by experts' (Bebbington, 1992). There are two problems with the NFCAS. First, the emphasis on identifying available interventions which would be at least partly effective is problematic, given the complexities of deciding that a treatment has not worked. Second, updating the list of actions has proved problematic. However, as Bebbington notes, 'the inevitable value judgements inherent in the procedure have the virtue of being public and consequently accessible to argument' (Bebbington, 1992). An important variation of the NFCAS is the **Cardinal Needs Schedule (CNS)** (Marshall et al., 1995), which also considers patient willingness to accept help and level of carer concern. Training is needed for using both the NFCAS and the CNS, and they are primarily used for research purposes (Kovess-Masféty et al., 2006).

At the other end of this continuum are needs assessment measures which emphasize individual difference and the subjective nature of need. The **AVON Mental Health Measure** was developed by service users, and assesses physical, social, behaviour, access and mental health domains (Markovitz, 1996). It can take up to 20 minutes for completion by the patient and 5 minutes by the staff, and its development has emphasized external validity over other psychometric properties. The **Carers and Users Experience of Services (CUES)** was developed by service users and staff, and assesses 16 domains: the place you live, money situation, the help you get, the way you spend time, your relationships, social life, information/advice, access to services, choice of mental health services, relationship with mental health workers, consultation and contact, advocacy, stigma, any treatment, access to physical health services, and relationship with physical health workers (Lelliott et al., 2001). Completion can take up to 30 minutes. Neither AVON nor CUES have become widely used in mental health services.

The **Client Assessment of Strengths, Interests and Goals (CASIG)** occupies an intermediate point on the continuum. The CASIG is an assessment measure for planning, evaluating and modifying individual and programmatic rehabilitation treatment (Lecomte et al., 2004; Wallace et al., 2001). It covers the service user's goals, current functioning, medication practices, quality of life and treatment, symptoms and unacceptable community behaviours. Two versions have been developed: self-rated and rated by a knowledgeable stakeholder in the person's rehabilitation.

Finally, the **Camberwell Assessment of Need (CAN)** (Phelan et al., 1995) spans both ends of the continuum. It assesses 22 domains of health and social need, and a key development is that it records staff and patient views separately, without giving primacy to either perspective. Research (CAN-R), clinical (CAN-C),

and brief versions (CANSAS) of the CAN have been developed for adults of working age with severe mental health problems (Slade et al., 1999b), and it has been translated in 23 languages. Variants have been developed for people with learning disabilities and mental health problems (CANDID) (Xenitidis et al., 2000, 2003), mentally disordered offenders (CANFOR) (Thomas et al., 2003, 2008), older adults (CANE) (Orrell and Hancock, 2004; Reynolds et al., 2000), and mothers with mental health problems (CAN-M) (Howard et al., 2007, 2008). An updated web resource for the CAN is available at http://www.iop.kcl.ac.uk/prism/can.

The CAN has become the most widely used needs assessment measure internationally (Evans et al., 2000; McCabe et al., 2007), and is the standardized needs assessment measure which is most relevant to routine clinical practice. The short version—CANSAS—can be recommended for routine use in community services. Two specific approaches have been empirically shown to produce patient-level benefit. First, the patient-rated Two-way Communication (2-COM) measure is an amended version of the CAN which gives the patient the opportunity to identify unmet needs and also prioritize those which they wish to discuss with their clinician (van Os et al., 2002). Asking patients to complete 2-COM before an outpatient appointment and then using that information in the appointment was associated with greater patient satisfaction and more likelihood of treatment change (van Os et al., 2004) with improvement sustained at 6-month follow-up (van Os and Triffaux, 2008). Second, a structured approach to collating and feeding back staff and patient ratings for CANSAS and other assessments led to a reduction in psychiatric admissions, probably because of earlier intervention during relapse (Slade et al., 2006b), with improvements in patient-rated unmet need and quality of life for higher premorbid IQ patients (Slade et al., 2006a).

A key feature of the CAN is that staff and patient perspectives on need are assessed and recorded separately. This has contributed to the evidence base on staff-patient agreement on need, which we now review.

Patient and staff perceptions of individual need

There has been a long-standing recognition that differences in perceptions of need can exist, in particular between staff and patient. In the 1990s the importance was identified of acknowledging these differences but prioritizing the staff perspective. For example, United Kingdom policy stated that 'all users…should be encouraged to participate to the limit of their capacity… Where it is impossible to reconcile different perceptions, these differences should be acknowledged and recorded.' (Department of Health Social Services Inspectorate, 1991). Several societal and scientific developments challenge this prioritization of staff over patient perspectives.

First, general societal changes towards consumerism and an emphasis on rights have produced more assertive mental health service users. Easier access by patients to Internet-based information reduces the knowledge disparity. Reduced societal trust in the authoritative expert has eroded the position power of mental health staff. The emphasis put on choice and empowerment raise patient expectations of being more than passive recipients of care (Chamberlin, 2005; Rose et al., 2006).

Second, the prioritization of staff perspectives has been actively challenged by an increasingly vociferous and organized user movement. This opposition has found its voice in the recovery movement, which emphasizes the meaning and values of the patient, and the need for services to foster self-management rather than dependency (Slade, 2009). There has been widespread international policy support for recovery-focussed services (Mental Health Commission of Canada, 2009; New Freedom Commission on Mental Health, 2003) although there can be tensions between what professionals construe as their duty of care and being led by the patient perspective on need (Craddock et al., 2008). Care planning which emphasizes agreement between staff and patients may have additional advantages. A study in Verona showed staff–patient agreement on needs was significantly associated with better treatment outcomes both rated by the patient and by staff (psychopathology, social disability, global functioning, subjective quality of life, and satisfaction with care) (Lasalvia et al., 2008). Similarly, there is robust evidence that crisis plans (advanced statements) which are jointly agreed between staff and patient can be cost-effective in reducing compulsory admission to hospital (Flood et al., 2006; Henderson et al., 2004). These findings indicates that needs assessment and care planning which are based on negotiation and jointly agreed analyses of problems and interventions are likely to become increasingly important in future.

Finally, emerging empirical evidence strongly supports the positioning of the patient perspective at the heart of needs assessment and care planning. Evidence from several studies consistently shows differences between staff and patient perspectives on need (Hansson et al., 2001; Lasalvia et al., 2000), so the two perspectives are not interchangeable. Empirical research suggests two reasons for basing care on the patient rather than staff assessment of need. First the patient rating is more stable than the staff rating (Ochoa et al., 2003; Slade et al., 1999a). Second, longitudinal studies indicate a causal relationship between patient-rated (but not staff-rated) unmet need and quality of life (Lasalvia et al., 2005; Slade et al., 2004, 2005). If the goal of mental health services is to improve quality of life, then best available evidence indicates that the patient's perspective on their unmet needs should drive care planning.

Moving from individual to population levels

In the attempt to move from considering the needs of mentally ill individuals to establishing overall community needs, these complexities are compounded in three ways. First, the needs of a wider range of individuals must be considered. These include immediate carers, people such as neighbours, and local authority staff, e.g. in housing and environmental health. Second, the translation of counts of treatment-amenable problems or service needs into institutional or staff provision requirements raises questions about service design models. What sort of agency should provide particular services, in what type of setting, and how much user choice in service style should be supported by public funding authorities? Third, since reasonable requests for assistance are likely to outstrip available resources, the practical questions which emerge relate to relative rather than absolute need. Thus we need not only to determine the existence and scale of needs, but also their importance in comparison to each other.

The overall level of needs for mental health services varies between places, reflecting differences in the prevalence of disorders. The nature of need has also changed over recent decades, reflecting developments in therapeutic capabilities, particularly in the provision of psychological therapies, changes in the extent to which severely mentally ill peoples service needs have been moulded by institutionalization, and secular trends in the incidence of mental disorders.

Measures to assess population need

Measures to assess population-based need can be classified by the data and by the analytic approaches they use. Three types of data are commonly used. The first type of data describes the use of current mental health services. While this can be criticized as reflecting only current service provision, its ready availability and nationwide coverage mean that is extensively used.

Secondly, direct surveys of population based morbidity, using epidemiological instruments, undertaken at a small or a large scale, offer a perspective independent of service activity. Simple population-based samples are very inefficient in estimating the prevalence of relatively rare conditions such as schizophrenia. Studies thus tend to use two stage procedures, with a relatively brief initial screening process applied to a large number of people followed in-depth interviews for a selected few. 'Booster' samples, perhaps including all the known psychiatric patients for the areas surveyed, may be sought through mental health services (Jenkins et al., 1997). Population surveys depend on the identification of randomly sampled individuals. Some types of mental health problem, notably substance misuse, are commonly associated with socially marginal lifestyles, making it likely that sufferers will be systematically under-represented by traditional population sampling approaches.

The third type of data relates to the views of local people. Local needs assessment studies entail a structured approach to eliciting the views of service users, their carers, interested voluntary sector organizations, and all statutory agencies with responsibilities in the area. Smith has described how this type of study can be integrated into the overall planning process (Smith, 1998).

Government initiatives in England have tried to base the allocation of money between areas on the morbidity as well as the size of their populations. This has led to studies modelling this variation. The first widely used index was developed on the basis of consensus between general practitioners about patient characteristics associated with high use of primary care services (Jarman, 1983). While developed for wider purposes, this was shown to relate reasonably closely to variations in psychiatric admission. Later indices have been established by statistical modelling exercises seeking to quantify the relationship between social variables measured in censuses and either service use (McCrone et al., 2006) or population-based epidemiological findings. The variation between places in the prevalence of the less severe types of mental illness commonly dealt with in primary care is less that that for problems usually managed by specialist mental health services, which again is much less than that observed for forensic services. Thus models developed for one level of care should not be used to estimate patterns of need for other levels.

In practice, no single approach to assessing the needs of a population will suffice. Needs assessment at this level requires the integration of many perspectives. Recent examples of population level needs assessment from the United States, Canada, and New Zealand also reveal that epidemiological studies may not produce data that corresponds directly to needs, and that some sub-populations, e.g. particular ethnic groups, may be less well represented in such approaches, unless considerable methodological care is taken (Hanson et al., 2006; Kumar et al., 2006; Messias et al., 2007).

A newer set of techniques that offer considerable promise are rapid appraisal/rapid assessment techniques. These are methods to undertake brief assessments of population needs which are focussed upon key focused questions, e.g. on how primary care services should be augmented to treat people with depression, and examples of these approaches have been used to positive effect in South Africa (Flisher et al., 2007; Lund, 2002; Lund and Flisher, 2006).

A second emerging new approach involves synthetic estimates of prevalence, which use established national case registers to estimate the prevalence of specific disorders (Martin and Wright, 2009). This approach has not been widely applied in mental health services, but in other areas of health care has been used to identify geographic inequities in service provision (Low et al., 2007).

The relationship between individual- and population-level data

At the level of individuals with mental illness, there is a trend to increasingly involve service users/consumers in assessing needs. We have reviewed evidence that this produces a more comprehensive basis for care planning. In the last decade there has been an important conceptual shift away from the view that professionals defined 'needs' while consumers stated 'demands', to a better appreciation of the many advantages to be gained from identifying, as far as possible, unmet needs in a joint and consensual way as a basis for action. If the provision of care for individual patients should be based on assessment of their health and social needs, can these individual assessments be aggregated to inform service?

For population-level service planning, the key question is what types of interventions to provide, and with what capacity. Therefore data from individual needs assessments cannot simply be aggregated to inform service development decisions. Routinely collected information about individual-level needs will be incomplete in systematic ways (and therefore non-representative), and the sample will comprise people currently using services, so does not represent the needs of the population as a whole. Even if individual needs assessments were nationally aggregated, the principal outcome of population-based needs assessment—resource allocation—is not a neat business. The diversity of views (patient, staff, carer, tax-payer) make a shared interpretation of the data problematic. Any study to identify an equitable new allocation pattern creates winners and losers. Since the results only indicate relative levels of need, losers inevitably argue that their current absolute level of resourcing is already inadequate. Political decisions are thus introduced about how fast resources should be reassigned to achieve the new idea of 'equity', and whether the shift should be achieved by actual transfer, or by differential growth. Indeed, there is an increasingly clear call from service user/consumer groups for involvement in these priority-setting planning exercises (Chamberlin, 2005; Rose et al., 2006).

Shifts of revenue resources are much easier than shifts of capital, but moving the former out of step with the latter may lead to inefficiencies. At the same time, special resources (as always) are likely to be made available to encourage implementation of currently promising service innovations. This process may push the overall distribution of funds away from the point of equity. It is rare for this dimension to be formally considered in the allocation of special allowances. Issues of timeliness, political necessity, expedience, synergy and leadership are all also likely to influence which of the many possible service developments is eventually implemented.

Conclusion

Assessment of need can involve compromises between desirable and attainable information, and value-based judgements about how and what to measure. It is a politically, ethically, and scientifically important concept, and so assessment should be as rigorous and comprehensive as possible. For both individual and population level needs assessment, this means that assessment should cover a wide range of health and social domains, should take account of different perspectives (e.g. patient, staff), and should be a separate process from treatment and resourcing decisions.

Further reading

Andrews, G. and Henderson, S. (eds.) (2000). *Unmet Need in Psychiatry*. Cambridge: Cambridge University Press.

Slade, M., Loftus, L., Phelan, M., Thornicroft, G., and Wykes, T. (1999). *The Camberwell Assessment of Need*. London: Gaskell.

Thornicroft, G. (ed.) (2001). *Measuring Mental Health Needs*, 2nd edn. London: Gaskell.

Thornicroft, G., Becker, T., Knapp, M., Knudsen, H.C., Schene, A.H., Tansella, M., et al. (2006). *International Outcomes in Mental Health. Quality of Life, Needs, Service Satisfaction, Costs and Impact on Carers*. London: Gaskell.

References

Alonso, J., Codony, M., Kovess, V., Angermeyer, M. C., Katz, S. J., Haro, J. M., et al. (2007). Population level of unmet need for mental healthcare in Europe. *British Journal of Psychiatry*, **190**, 299–306.

Andrews, G., Issakidis, C., Sanderson, K., Corry, J., and Lapsley, H. (2004). Utilising survey data to inform public policy: comparison of the cost-effectiveness of treatment of ten mental disorders. *British Journal of Psychiatry*, **184**, 526–33.

Bebbington, P. (1992). Assessing the need for psychiatric treatment at the district level: the need for surveys. In: Thornicroft, G. Brewin, C., and Wing, J. (eds.) *Measuring Mental Health Needs*, pp. 99–117. London: Royal College of Psychiatrists.

Bradshaw, J. (1972). A taxonomy of social need. In: McLachlan, J. (ed.) *Problems and Progress in Medical Care: Essays on Current Research*, pp. 69–82. London: Oxford University Press.

Brewin, C. (2001). Measuring individual needs for care and services. In: Thornicroft, G. (ed.) *Measuring Mental Health Needs*, 2nd edn., pp. 273–90. London: Gaskell.

Brewin, C., Wing, J., Mangen, S., Brugha, T., and MacCarthy, B. (1987). Principles and practice of measuring needs in the long-term mentally ill: the MRC Needs for Care Assessment. *Psychological Medicine*, **17**, 971–81.

Chamberlin, J. (2005). User/consumer involvement in mental health service delivery. *Epidemiologica e Psichiatria Sociale*, **14**, 10–14.

Cochrane, R. and Stopes-Roe, M. (1977). Psychological and social adjustment of Asian immigrants to Britain: a community survey. *Social Psychiatry*, **12**, 195–206.

Craddock, N., Antebi, D., Attenburrow, M.-J., Bailey, A., Carson, A., Cowen, P., et al (2008). Wake-up call for British psychiatry. *British Journal of Psychiatry*, **193**, 6–9.

Department of Health (1990). *National Health Service and Community Care Act*. London: TSO.

Department of Health (1999). *Mental Health National Service Framework*. London: The Stationery Office.

Department of Health Social Services Inspectorate (1991). *Care Management and Assessment: Practice Guide*. London: HMSO.

Evans, S., Greenhalgh, J., and Connelly, J. (2000).Selecting a mental health needs assessment scale: guidance on the critical appraisal of standardized measures. *Journal of Evaluation in Clinical Practice*, **6**, 379–93.

Flisher, A.J., Lund, C., Funk, M., Banda, M., Bhana, A., Doku, V., et al. (2007). Mental health policy development and implementation in four african countries. *Journal of Health Psychology*, **12**, 505–16.

Flood, C., Byford, S., Henderson, C., Leese, M., Thornicroft, G., Sutherby, K., et al. (2006). Joint crisis plans for people with psychosis: economic evaluation of a randomised controlled trial. *British Medical Journal*, **333**, 729.

Gray, R., Leese, M., Bindman, J., Becker, T., Burti, L., David, A., et al. (2006). Adherence therapy for people with schizophrenia. European multicentre randomised controlled trial. *British Journal of Psychiatry*, **189**, 508–14.

Gurland, B., Yorkstone, N., Stone, A., and Frank, J. (1972). The Structured and Scaled Interview to Assess Maladjustment (SSIAM) 1. Description, Rationale and Development. *Archives of General Psychiatry*, **27**, 264–7.

Habicht, J.P., Mason, J.P., and Tabatabai, H. (1984). Basic concepts for the design of evaluations during programme implementation. In: Sahn, D.R., Lockwood, R., and Scrimshaw, N.S. (eds.) *Methods for the Evaluation of the Impact of Food and Nutrition Programmes. Food and Nutrition Bulletin. Suppl. 8*, pp. 1–25. New York: The United Nations University.

Hanson, L., Houde, D., McDowell, M., and Dixon, L. (2006). A population-based needs assessment for mental health services. *Administration and Policy in Mental Health*, **34**, 233–42

Hansson, L., Vinding, H.R., Mackeprang, T., Sourander, A., Werdelin, G., Bengtsson-Tops, A., et al. (2001). Comparison of key worker and patient assessment of needs in schizophrenic patients living in the community: a Nordic multicentre study. *Acta Psychiatrica Scandinavica*, **103**, 45–51.

Henderson, C., Flood, C., Leese, M., Thornicroft, G., Sutherby, K., and Szmukler, G. (2004). Effect of joint crisis plans on use of compulsory treatment in psychiatry: single blind randomised controlled trial. *British Medical Journal*, **329**, 136.

Howard, L., Hunt, K., Slade, M., O'Keane, V., Senevirante, T., Leese, M., et al. (2007). Assessing the needs of pregnant women and mothers with severe mental illness: the psychometric properties of the Camberwell Assessment of Need - Mothers (CAN-M). *International Journal of Methods in Psychiatric Research*, **16**, 177–85.

Howard, L., Slade, M., O'Keane, V., Seneviratne, T., Hunt, K., and Thornicroft, G. (2008). *The Camberwell Assessment of Need for Pregnant Women and Mothers with Severe Mental Illness*. London: Gaskell.

Jarman, B. (1983). Identification of underprivileged areas. *British Medical Journal*, **286**, 1705–9.

Jenkins, R., Bebbington, P., Brugha, T., Farrell, M., Gill, B., and Lewis, G. (1997). The National Psychiatric Morbidity Surveys of Great Britain - strategy and methods. *Psychological Medicine*, **27**, 765–74.

Kessler, R.C., Demler, O., Frank, R.G., Olfson, M., Pincus, H.A., Walters, E.E., et al. (2005). Prevalence and treatment of mental disorders, 1990 to 2003. *New England Journal of Medicine*, **352**, 2515–23.

Kovess-Masféty, V., Wiersma, D., Xavier, M., de Almada, J.M.C., Carta, MG., Dubuis, J., et al. (2006). Needs for care among patients with schizophrenia in six European countries: a one-year follow-up study. *Clinical Practice and Epidemiological Mental Health*, **2**, 22.

Kumar, S., Tse, S., Fernando, A., and Wong, S. (2006). Epidemiological studies on mental health needs of Asian population in New Zealand. *International Journal of Social Psychiatry*, **52**, 408–12.

Lasalvia, A., Ruggeri, M., Mazzi, M.A., and Dall'Agnola, R.B. (2000). The perception of needs for care in staff and patients in community-based mental health services. The South-Verona Outcome Project 3. *Acta Psychiatrica Scandinavica*, **102**, 366–75.

Lasalvia, A., Bonetto, C., Malchiodi, F., Salvi, G., Parabiaghi, A., Tansella, M., et al. (2005).Listening to patients' needs to improve their subjective quality of life. *Psychological Medicine*, **35**, 1655–65.

Lasalvia, A., Bonetto, C., Tansella, M., Stefani, B., and Ruggeri, M. (2008). Does staff-patient agreement on needs for care predict a better mental health outcome? A 4 year follow-up in a community service. *Psychological Medicine*, **38**, 123–33.

Lecomte, T., Wallace, C.J., Caron, J., Perreault, M., and Lecomte, J. (2004). Further validation of the Client Assessment of Strengths Interests and Goals. *Schizophrenia Research*, **66**, 59–70.

Lelliott, P., Beevor, A., Hogman, J., Hohman, G., Hyslop, J., Lathlean, J., et al. (2001). Carers' and Users' Expectations of Services–User version (CUES-U): a new instrument to measure the experience of users of mental health services. *British Journal of Psychiatry*, **179**, 67–72.

Low, A., Unsworth, L., Low, A., and Miller, I. (2007). Avoiding the danger that stop smoking services may exacerbate health inequalities: building equity into performance assessment. *BMC Public Health*, **7**, 198.

Lund, C. (2002). Mental Health Service Norms in South Africa. PhD Thesis. Cape Town: University of Cape Town.

Lund, C. and Flisher, A.J. (2006). Norms for mental health services in South Africa. *Social Psychiatry and Psychiatric Epidemiology*, **41**, 587–94.

Markovitz, P. (1996). *The Avon Mental Health Measure*. Bristol: Changing Minds.

Marshall, M., Hogg, L., Gath, D.H., and Lockwood, A. (1995). The Cardinal Needs Schedule: a modified version of the MRC Needs for Care Schedule. *Psychological Medicine*, **25**, 605–17.

Martin, D. and Wright, J.A. (2009). Disease prevalence in the English population: A comparison of primary care registers and prevalence models. *Social Science and Medicine*, **2**, 266–74.

Maslow, A. (1954). *Motivation and Personality*. New York: Harper and Row.

McCabe, R., Saidi, M., and Priebe, S. (2007).Patient-reported outcomes in schizophrenia. *British Journal of Psychiatry*, **191**, s21–s28.

McCrone, P., Thornicroft, G., Boyle, S., Knapp, M., and Aziz, F. (2006). The development of a Local Index of Need (LIN) and its use to explain variations in social services expenditure on mental health care in England. *Health and Social Care in the Community*, **14**, 254–63.

Mental Health Commission of Canada (2009). *Toward recovery & well-being*. Calgary: Mental Health Commission of Canada.

Messias, E., Eaton, W., Nestadt, G., Bienvenu, O.J., and Samuels, J. (2007). Psychiatrists' ascertained treatment needs for mental disorders in a population-based sample. *Psychiatric Services*, **58**, 373–7.

New Freedom Commission on Mental Health (2003). *Achieving the Promise: Transforming Mental Health Care in America. Final report*. Rockville, MD: U.S. Department of Health and Human Services.

Ochoa, S., Haro, J.M., Autonell, J., Pendas, A., Teba, F., and Marquez, M. (2003). Met and unmet needs of schizophrenia patients in a Spanish sample. *Schizophrenia Bulletin*, **29**, 201–10.

Orrell, M. and Hancock, G. (2004). *The Camberwell Assessment of Need for the Elderly (CANE)*. London: Gaskell.

Phelan, M., Slade, M., Thornicroft, G., Dunn, G., Holloway, F., Wykes, T., et al. (1995). The Camberwell Assessment of Need: the validity and reliability of an instrument to assess the needs of people with severe mental illness. *British Journal of Psychiatry*, **167**, 589–95.

Regier, D.A., Narrow, W. E., Kuhl, E.A., and Kupfer, D.J. (2009). The conceptual development of DSM-V. *American Journal of Psychiatry*, **166**, 645–50.

Reynolds, T., Thornicroft, G., Abas, M., Woods, B., Hoe, J., Leese, M., et al. (2000). Camberwell Assessment of Need for the Elderly (CANE); development, validity, and reliability. *British Journal of Psychiatry*, **176**, 444–52.

Rose, D., Thornicroft, G., and Slade, M. (2006). Who decides what evidence is? Developing a multiple perspectives paradigm in mental health. *Acta Psychiatrica Scandinavica*, 113, 109–14.

Simon, G.E., Fleck, M., Lucas, R., and Bushnell, D.M. (2004). Prevalence and predictors of depression treatment in an international primary care study. *American Journal of Psychiatry*, **161**, 1626–34.

Slade, M. (2009). *Personal recovery and mental illness. A guide for mental health professionals*. Cambridge: Cambridge University Press.

Slade, M., Leese, M., Taylor, R., and Thornicroft, G. (1999a). The association between needs and quality of life in an epidemiologically representative sample of people with psychosis. *Acta Psychiatrica Scandinavica*, **100**, 149–57.

Slade, M., Loftus, L., Phelan, M., Thornicroft, G., and Wykes, T. (1999b). *The Camberwell Assessment of Need*. London: Gaskell.

Slade, M., Leese, M., Ruggeri, M., Kuipers, E., Tansella, M., and Thornicroft, G. 2004). Does meeting needs improve quality of life? *Psychotherapy and Psychosomatics*, **73**, 183–9.

Slade, M., Leese, M., Cahill, S., Thornicroft, G., and Kuipers, E. (2005). Patient-rated mental health needs and quality of life improvement. *British Journal of Psychiatry*, **187**, 256–61.

Slade, M., Leese, M., Gillard, M., Kuipers, E., and Thornicroft, G. (2006a). Pre-morbid IQ and response to routine outcome assessment. *Psychological Medicine*, **36**, 1183–91.

Slade, M., McCrone, P., Kuipers, E., Leese, M., Cahill, S., Parabiaghi, A., *et al.* (2006b).Use of standardised outcome measures in adult mental health services: randomised controlled trial. *British Journal of Psychiatry*, **189**, 330–6.

Smith, H. (1998). Needs assessment in mental health services: the DISC framework. *Journal of Public Health Medicine*, **20**, 154–60.

Stevens, A. and Gabbay, J. (1991). Needs assessment needs assessment. *Health Trends*, **23**, 20–3.

Tansella, M. (2006). Recent advances in depression. Where are we going?. *Epidemiologia e Psichiatria Sociale*, **15**, 1–3.

Tansella, M. and Thornicroft, G. (1999). *Common Mental Disorders in Primary Care*. London: Routledge.

Thomas, S., Harty, M., Parrott, J., McCrone, P., Slade, M., and Thornicroft, G. (2003). *The Forensic CAN: Camberwell Assessment of Need Forensic Version (CANFOR)*. London: Gaskell.

Thomas, S.D., Slade, M., McCrone, P., Harty, M.A., Parrott, J., Thornicroft, G., *et al.* (2008). The reliability and validity of the forensic Camberwell Assessment of Need (CANFOR): a needs assessment for forensic mental health service users. *International Journal of Methods in Psychiatric Research*, **17**, 111–20.

van Os, J., Altamura, A.C., Bobes, J., Owens, D.C., Gerlach, J., Hellewell, J.S.E., *et al.* (2002). 2-com: an instrument to facilitate patient-professional communication in routine clinical practice. *Acta Psychiatrica Scandinavica*, **106**, 446–52.

van Os, J., Altamura, A.C., Bobes, J., Owens, D.C., Gerlach, J., Hellewell, J.S.E., *et al.* (2004). Evaluation of the Two-Way Communication Checklist as a clinical intervention. *British Journal of Psychiatry*, **184**, 79–83.

van Os, J. and Triffaux, J.M. (2008). Evidence that the Two-Way Communication Checklist identifies patient-doctor needs discordance resulting in better 6-month outcome. *Acta Psychiatrica Scandinavica*, **118**, 322–6.

Wallace, C.J., Lecomte, T., Wilde, J., and Libermann, R.P. (2001). CASIG: A consumer-centered assessment for planning individualized treatment and evaluating program outcomes. *Schizophrenia Research*, **50**, 105–9.

Warner, R. (2004). *Recovery from Schizophrenia: Psychiatry and Political Economy*, 3rd edn. New York: Brunner-Routledge.

World Health Organization (2005a). *Mental Health Action Plan for Europe*. Copenhagen: World Health Organization.

World Health Organization (2005b). *Mental Health Declaration for Europe*. Copenhagen: World Health Organization.

Wykes, T. and Hurry, J. (1991). Social behaviour and psychiatric disorders. In: Bebbington, P. (ed.) *Social Psychiatry: Theory, Methodology, and Practice*, pp. 183–208. New Brunswick, NJ: Transaction Press.

Xenitidis, K., Thornicroft, G., Leese, M., Slade, M., Fotiadou, M., Philp, H., *et al.* (2000). Reliability and validity of the CANDID—a needs assessment instrument for adults with learning disabilities and mental health problems. *British Journal of Psychiatry*, **176**, 473–8.

Xenitidis, K., Slade, M., Bouras, N., and Thornicroft, G. (2003). *CANDID: Camberwell Assessment of Need for adults with Developmental and Intellectual Disabilities*. London: Gaskell.

CHAPTER 10

Mental health, ethnicity, and cultural diversity: evidence and challenges

Craig Morgan

Migration is the primary driving force behind increasing ethnic and cultural diversity in many societies around the world. The movement of people across (and within) national boundaries, be it in search of economic prosperity or fleeing war and persecution, has been a central feature of modern history and has accelerated in recent years (Castles and Miller, 2009). Estimates by the United Nations (UN) suggest the total number of migrants (i.e. persons who have lived outside their country of birth for 12 months or more) is around 190 to 200 million or 3% of the world's population (UNDESA, 2004). These estimates do not include settled minority ethnic populations where, increasingly, the majority were born in the countries to which their parents or grandparents migrated. In the United Kingdom (UK), for example, minority ethnic groups now form 12% of the population, with this rising to over 50% in some areas of London (e.g. Newham) (Office for National Statistics: http://www.statistics.gov.uk/census2001/profiles/commentaries/ethnicity.asp). In the most recent edition of their textbook, Castles and Miller (2009) identify a number of trends in migration that are likely to have important ongoing political, economic, and social consequences. These include: the **globalization of migration** (i.e. the tendency for more countries to be affected by migration, both inward and outward); the **acceleration of migration** (i.e. the continued rise in absolute numbers of migrants in most regions of the world); and the **differentiation of migration** (i.e. the increased diversity of types and origins of migrants moving to single countries). These trends are already evident in, for example, many European countries, including Britian which has migrants from over 40 countries (Institute for Public Policy Research: http://news.bbc.co.uk/1/shared/spl/hi/uk/05/born_abroad/html/overview.stm), and the United States (US) where estimates suggest that by 2050 minority ethnic and racial groups will comprise over 50% of the population (U.S. Census Bureau, 2004). What these processes point to is an inexorable rise in ethnic and cultural diversity in many countries. This has major implications for the development and delivery of public services and, in particular, poses an ongoing challenge for mental health policy and service provision.

It is these challenges that are the focus of this chapter. Three specific aspects are critically reviewed, with examples drawn mainly from the US and the UK: 1) the extent of, and variations in, mental health needs in migrant and minority ethnic groups; 2) access to and use of mental health services among these groups; and 3) proposals for ensuring mental health services are more responsive to the needs of ethnically and culturally diverse populations. To begin with, some definitions are necessary.

Culture, ethnicity, and race

There is often confusion and imprecision in use of the terms culture, ethnicity, and race. Culture has been variously defined; for example, as shared patterns of belief, feeling, and adaptation that people carry in their minds (Leighton and Hughes, 1961), as an organized group of ideas, habits, and conditioned responses shared by members of a society (Linton, 1956), and as a blueprint for living (Kluckholm, 1944). Common to most definitions is the idea of culture as a set of socially shared guidelines that shape behaviour, values, and beliefs. These are learned during childhood and adulthood through contacts with, and participation in, core institutions (e.g. education, law, religion, and medicine) and customary events and practices (e.g. rites of passage rituals, funerals, and commemorative events) (Helman, 2007). Cultures are dynamic and heterogeneous, constantly evolving as a consequence of exposure to other beliefs and practices, most notably through migration and, increasingly, global media (Helman, 2007). This ties to further concepts, such as acculturation, assimilation, and biculturalism, which describe the various processes whereby migrants integrate into and become comfortable with the cultural norms of the new society. In turn, migrant populations often bring with them novel traditions and practices which impact on the new society, creating a dynamic interplay in which new and modified cultural forms emerge.

The defining characteristic of ethnicity is a sense of shared identity and group belonging that emerges from, for example, a common heritage, shared language, and physical appearance. Culture, in this definition, is one element that engenders a sense of ethnic identity. What is more, common experiences in host societies, particularly of racism and discrimination, can contribute to the development of a shared identity in migrants from otherwise culturally diverse backgrounds. Fernando (1991), for example, has argued that this is a key factor that has driven the emergence of a Caribbean ethnic identity among migrants to the UK and their children from the culturally diverse islands of the Caribbean. Identity is fluid and those aspects of our heritage and background that we choose to emphasize and which feel prominent at any one point may vary according to context—migrants to the UK from the Caribbean, for example, may identify with their region of origin when in the UK and with their island of origin when in the Caribbean or when socializing with others from the Caribbean (i.e. at one moment, Caribbean; at another, Trinidadian or Jamaican, etc.). Other identities based, for example, on social position, gender, and sexuality overlay and add complexity to any sense of ethnic identity.

In Europe, at least, ethnicity has supplanted race as the primary way of talking about diverse population groups. It is now well established that certain physical characteristics, such as skin colour, do not signify biologically homogenous groups (Jones, 1981). Nevertheless, the perception that this is the case persists and underpins frequent and far-reaching prejudice and discrimination (racism). As Fernando (1991) puts it: '…though a biological myth, race continues to be a social reality' (p. 19). Furthermore, while the language of ethnicity has replaced that of race in much discourse in science and health, skin colour is often used as a short cut to defining ethnic groups (e.g. black vs. white), such that race and ethnicity are frequently conflated.

What this brief discussion emphasizes, then, are the potential pitfalls, both for research and clinical practice, of entangling culture, ethnicity, and race; it further warns against using perceived membership of an ethnic or cultural group as a short cut to acquiring (or assuming) knowledge about an individual's beliefs, values, and needs.

Mental health needs

Epidemiological evidence (1): prevalence and incidence

Studies of the epidemiology of mental disorder in migrant and minority ethnic populations, the majority of which have been conducted in Europe and North America, have produced some varied, some consistent, and, at times, some surprising findings.

To begin with non-psychotic disorders (for which most useable data is of prevalence), examples from the US and the UK illustrate this. A number of recent large-scale epidemiological surveys in the US[1]—which together constitute the Collaborative Psychiatric Epidemiology Surveys with combined samples of over 15,000—have provided a wealth of data on the distribution of mental disorders by ethnic group (Williams et al., 2010). A number of broad patterns emerged. First, the following groups, compared with white Americans, all had lower rates of both lifetime and past-year mental disorders: black American (i.e. African American, black Caribbean), Asian American, and Latino American (with the exception of Puerto Ricans). The prevalence of lifetime disorder for

white Americans was around 37% (Kessler et al., 2005) compared with 28 to 31% for black Americans (Williams et al., 2007), 14% to 18% for Asian Americans (Takeuchi et al., 2007), and 27% to 28% for Latino Americans (excluding Puerto Ricans, with a prevalence similar to white Americans of around 39%) (Alegria et al., 2007). Within the broad black American group, further analyses by Williams et al. (2007) suggest variations by gender, with higher levels of disorder in black Caribbean men compared with African American men. These findings are somewhat surprising, and, in many respects, add to a confusing picture. For example, the earlier Epidemiologic Catchment Area study of 23,000 individuals in five communities found higher rates of both current and lifetime disorder (assessed using the Diagnostic Interview Schedule), particularly phobic and anxiety disorders, in black Americans (26% current; 38% lifetime) compared with white Americans (19% current; 32% lifetime) (Robins and Reiger, 1991). For Hispanic groups, rates similar to those for white Americans were reported (Robins and Reiger, 1991). Other studies, albeit methodologically weaker, have reported higher, lower and similar rates of disorder in minority ethnic groups in the US (for a summary see Williams et al., 2010, pp. 269–77). One group for which there is perhaps more consistency in findings is American Indians. In line with early reports, three recent studies (see Williams et al., 2010, p. 279) found higher rates of mental disorder in these populations.

In the UK, the 2007 Adult Psychiatric Morbidity Survey (McManus et al., 2009a) of over 7000 individuals found no evidence that the prevalence of common mental disorders (CMD) (operationalized as a score of 12 or more on the Clinical Interview Schedule-Revised (CIS-R)) in the week prior to interview was high in minority ethnic populations, with the exception that the prevalence was higher in South Asian women (Deverill and King, 2009). When specific diagnostic groups were considered, some evidence of variations did emerge. These were, compared with other ethnic groups, high rates of lifetime post-traumatic stress disorder (46%) (McManus et al., 2009b) and drug dependence (12%) (Fuller et al., 2009b) in black men and high rates of lifetime suicidal thoughts (15% men; 20% women) (Nicholson et al., 2009) and alcohol dependency (10% men; 4% women) (Fuller et al., 2009a) in white people. There was no evidence of ethnic differences in the prevalence of eating disorders (Thompson et al., 2009). The EMPIRIC study, a cross-sectional survey of 4281 adults, also found few overall differences in the prevalence of CMD between ethnic groups (Weich et al., 2004). However, some variations were evident by age and gender, with the highest rates being in: 1) Irish (rate ratio 2.1) and Pakistani (rate ratio 2.1) men aged 35 to 54 years, and 2) Indian (rate ratio 3.2) and Pakistani (rate ratio 2.8) women aged 55 to 74 years (Weich et al., 2004). Other studies have reported further differences. For example, the Fourth National Survey of Ethnic Minorities (sample n = 8063) found that the weekly prevalence of depression was higher in black Caribbean (6.3%) compared with white British (3.8%) participants (which contrasts with the two surveys noted above) and, broadly, that Asians tended to have lower rates of mental disorder and Irish and white Other groups tended to have higher rates (Nazroo, 1997). Other less robust studies further suggest high rates of self-harm and suicide in young Asian women (Bhugra et al., 1999b, Bhugra et al., 1999a) and high rates of most disorders in the Irish population (Cochrane and Bal, 1989).

The evidence for schizophrenia and other psychoses is more consistent, most of it based on incidence rather than prevalence.

---

[1] These are: the National Comorbidity Survey Replication, the National Survey of American Life, the National Latino and Asian American Study.

There is now strong evidence from studies in the UK, the Netherlands, Sweden, Denmark, Australia, and the US that the incidence of schizophrenia and other psychoses is elevated in migrant and minority ethnic populations (Fearon and Morgan, 2006). In their recent meta-analysis of population-based incidence studies of schizophrenia, Cantor-Graae and Selten (2005) found (from a total of 50 effect sizes) a mean weighted relative risk (RR) for developing schizophrenia among migrant groups of 2.9 compared with indigenous or host populations. The relative risk was particularly high in migrants from developing countries (RR 3.3), in second-generation migrants (RR 4.5), and in migrants from countries where the majority population is black (RR 4.8). This latter finding is intriguing, as we know that it is more visible migrant and minority groups who experience more racism and discrimination. What is more, the degree of increased risk is not consistent across migrant and minority ethnic groups—as hinted at in the meta-analysis conducted by Cantor-Graee and Selten (2005). For example, ÆSOP, a three-centre incidence and case–control study, found that in the UK, compared with white British, the incidence of all psychoses was over six times higher in black Caribbean, around four times higher in black African, and between one-and-a-half and two times higher in Asian and other white (i.e. non-British) populations (Fearon et al., 2006). In a more recent study in east London, the incidence was again found to be higher in most migrant and minority ethnic groups (Kirkbride et al., 2008). However, in Pakistani and Bangladeshi populations, this appeared to be evident for women only. In the Netherlands, the incidence appears to be highest in Moroccan migrants (Veling et al., 2006). The reasons for these variations are unclear; however, speculation has focused on differential exposure to discrimination and the buffering effects of family supports and social networks (Morgan et al., 2010).

There have been fewer studies of the prevalence of psychoses. In the UK, these have tended to report smaller disparities between black Caribbean and white British populations (e.g. Fourth National Survey found an annual prevalence of 0.8% for white British and 1.3% for black Caribbean populations (Nazroo, 1997)). The more recent Adult Psychiatric Morbidity Survey, however, found notable variations by gender. There was a marked increase in yearly prevalence in black men (3%) compared with white men (0.2%), but no differences between women (Sadler and Bebbington, 2009). As in other studies, however, the total number of individuals with a probable psychotic disorder was small and this may explain the variability between studies and the divergence from what is consistently reported in incidence studies.

Asylum seekers and refugees

Most of the data summarized above relates to settled minority ethnic populations. The mental health of asylum seekers and refugees merits particular comment as prior exposure to trauma and stress is likely to be common and, at least initially, legal status and right to remain in the new country may be uncertain. Around 13 million people have refugee status around the world (Fitzpatrick, 2002). Some indication of the likely extent of mental disorder in these populations is provided in Fazel et al.'s (2005) systematic review of 20 studies including over 6000 refugees in seven Western countries. Included studies varied methodologically, but in those with large and more robust samples the overall prevalence of post-traumatic stress disorder was 9%; for major depressive disorder it was 5%, with evidence of considerable comorbidity (Fazel et al.,

2005). The authors note that these rates are lower than in some published studies, but still represent higher levels of disorder than have been reported in several general Western populations (Fazel et al., 2005). In short, there is (not surprisingly) evidence of substantial need for mental health care in refugee populations, particularly related to trauma.

Epidemiological evidence (2): ethnicity, culture, and diagnosis

The epidemiological data on rates of mental disorder in diverse populations have, so far, been presented without consideration of two critical methodological issues: 1) the use of fixed, and often crude, ethnic categories, and 2) the validity of applying diagnostic concepts and measures developed within a particular cultural framework to diverse ethnic and cultural populations. In relation to the first, it is inevitable that large-scale cross-sectional research estimating rates of disorder in populations has to rely on relatively crude variables collected at one point in time. What the definition of ethnicity discussed above suggests is that the findings have to then be treated with caution. One important consideration is that overall estimates for each ethnic group may obscure within group variations, which are hinted at in some of the reported differences by age and gender. It is the second issue, however, which is potentially more important.

All cultures develop beliefs and practices to explain and manage ill health, and these provide socially sanctioned frameworks within which physical and mental distress are experienced, expressed, and made sense of; they influence the responses of others and shape what help is sought, when and from whom. In other words, culture provides us with a language or idiom for expressing and understanding distress. What this means is that the assessments and measures used in epidemiological surveys, based on Western conceptions of mental health and disorder, may not accurately capture expressions of distress that fall outside of this paradigm. A common, perhaps stereotyped, example is the distinction between those cultures that tend to 'somatize' (i.e. express emotional distress through bodily feelings such as headaches, tension, upset stomach, palpitations) and those that tend to 'psychologize' (i.e. express emotional distress in psychological terms such as feeling sad, anxious) (Bhui et al., 2004). In so far as standard assessments (e.g. CIS-R, CIDI) focus on psychological symptoms there is a question about their capacity to accurately measure and capture mental health problems in populations that tend to 'somatize' (e.g. Asian; Lin and Cheung, 1999). In short, and efforts to validate instruments cross-culturally notwithstanding, this raises the possibility that disorder is being over or under diagnosed in some migrant and minority ethnic groups, potentially invalidating reported findings.

To consider a contentious example. Many commentators have forcefully argued that the repeated finding that the incidence of schizophrenia and other psychoses is high in many migrant and minority (particularly black) ethnic groups is a function of misdiagnosis, i.e. of emotional distress arising from difficult life circumstances in black and other minority populations being misconstrued as psychosis by predominantly white psychiatrists unfamiliar with cultural idioms of distress in these populations and/or influenced by negative cultural stereotypes of black people (Fernando, 1991; Morgan and Hutchinson, 2010). There is evidence that misdiagnosis does occur, particularly from studies in the US (Williams et al., 2010). However, studies in the UK that have sought to test this directly in the Caribbean population (which has among the highest reported rates), suggest misdiagnosis alone is not a sufficient explanation. For example, in a study at the Maudsley Hospital in London, where many of the UK studies of migration, ethnicity, and psychosis have been conducted, Hickling et al. (1999) compared diagnoses made independently by British psychiatrists and by a Jamaican psychiatrist in the same group of 66 inpatients. The authors found no difference in the percentage of black inpatients diagnosed with schizophrenia by the British psychiatrists or the Jamaican psychiatrist. In two other UK studies designed to investigate racial stereotyping in psychiatric assessment using case vignettes, there was no evidence that psychiatrists were more likely to diagnose schizophrenia when the ethnicity of the individual in the vignette was black (Lewis and David, 1991, Minnis et al., 2001). What is more, studies conducted in the Caribbean by the same researchers using the same methods do not find high rates (Bhugra et al., 1996; Mahy et al., 1999), a finding which is inexplicable if these methods systematically misdiagnose black people as suffering from psychosis when they are not. This debate highlights a significant point. Important as cultural factors are, and the potential for misdiagnosis notwithstanding, it cannot always and simply be assumed that these underpin ethnic variations in disorder. We know less about the role (or otherwise) of cultural factors and misdiagnosis in explaining the epidemiological findings for non-psychotic disorders.

Epidemiological evidence (3): risk and protective factors

Taken together, the findings summarized above suggest a complicated picture, one which is confused further by the methodological issues that have been noted. What is perhaps most surprising, caveats about methodological problems notwithstanding, is that rates of common mental disorders are not more consistently higher in migrant and minority ethnic groups. There are well-established associations between exposure to adverse social contexts and experiences and all common mental disorders, particularly depression and anxiety (e.g. Karlsen and Nazroo, 2002). Many migrant and minority ethnic groups live in economically and socially deprived areas, have poorer housing, higher rates of unemployment, poorer education, and are exposed to high levels of discrimination and racism (Modood et al., 1997). It may be that counterveiling factors, such as greater access to informal social and community supports, greater resilience, and more effective coping strategies, operate to mitigate the impact of such contexts and experiences on mental health in migrant and minority populations. There is, however, limited research on this, which reflects an imbalance in mental health research in general, where the focus is on risk rather than protective factors. (As an important aside, this is a significant limitation as it may be that knowledge of protective factors is more valuable in developing policies and interventions to prevent mental disorder.)

In contrast, the evidence that rates of serious mental disorder (i.e. psychoses) are higher (to varying degrees) in migrant and minority ethnic groups is substantial and there is now strong evidence that these high rates are largely determined by exposure over the life course to adverse social contexts and experiences (Morgan et al., 2007, 2008, 2010). This apparent paradox (i.e. similar rates of common mental disorders, higher rates of serious mental disorders)

raises a number of intriguing possibilities, including: 1) that emotional distress in certain migrant and minority ethnic groups is more often expressed in the form of perceived threats (paranoia) and distorted perceptions (hallucinations); 2) that exposure to particular types of adverse social experiences involving threat and intrusion (as is common in migrant and minority ethnic groups) more often leads to symptoms of psychosis; and/or 3) that delays in seeking help for emotional distress result in unchecked movement along a continuum of mental ill health, from depression and anxiety through to paranoia, hallucinations, and thought disorder. These possibilities are largely speculative, but certainly merit consideration given the potential implications for intervention. What is more, irrespective of precise aetiological relationships, it is clear that individuals from migrant and minority ethnic populations who present to mental health services will, on average, have greater social and economic needs; these are important targets for intervention both as a basis for improving engagement and promoting recovery.

Access to, and use of, mental health services

There is more consistent evidence on access to and engagement with mental health services among ethnic groups, most of which suggests the needs of individuals from these populations may not always be met to the same extent as the needs of individuals from majority populations. Again, examples from the US and the UK illustrate this.

In the US, the Surgeon General's comprehensive review of research on culture and mental health noted a number of ethnic disparities (U.S. Department of Health and Human Services, 2001). For example, despite apparently similar rates of mental disorder (psychosis notwithstanding), there is evidence that African Americans (compared with white Americans) are less likely to receive treatment (largely because of lower rates of help-seeking) and more likely to use alternative therapies (Robins and Reiger, 1991; Smith Fahie, 1998; Swartz et al., 1998). This may be, partly, related to financial barriers specific to the US health care system (Brown et al., 2000). There is similar evidence that Asian and Latino Americans have very low rates of mental health service utilization (Brown et al., 2000; Chin et al., 2000; Hough et al., 1987). Related to the discussion above, there is some evidence that the likelihood of receiving particular diagnoses varies by migrant and minority ethnic group in the US. Clinically, misdiagnosis matters in so far as it contributes to the receipt of inappropriate care. For example, a study by Minsky et al. (2003) of around 20,000 initial contacts with inpatient and outpatient services, found that Latinos were more likely to be diagnosed with major depression, despite higher levels of self-reported psychotic symptoms. There is further evidence of variations in the type and length of care received. For example, in one study Asian Americans were found to experience longer inpatient stays than white Americans (Snowden and Cheung, 1990) and in another African Americans were found to use emergency psychiatric services more than white Americans (Snowden, 1999), a finding that mirrors research in the UK on the black Caribbean and black African populations (see below). Finally, there is evidence of high drop out rates among minority ethnic groups in the US—one possible important marker of the acceptability and appropriateness of mental health services to the needs of these groups (Walton et al., 2010).

In the UK, similar patterns are evident. For example, a significant number of studies have found that those from black Caribbean and black African ethnic groups, particularly those experiencing psychotic symptoms, access mental health services more often via emergency and coercive routes compared with whites, i.e. fewer GP referrals, more police and court referrals, more compulsory admissions (Morgan et al., 2004). A meta-analysis of 38 studies of compulsory admissions found that, compared with white patients, those of black Caribbean ethnicity were on average around four times more likely to be compulsorily admitted (Bhui et al., 2003). There is evidence from a further review that the likelihood of compulsory admission increases over time, in the event of repeated contacts with services (Singh et al., 2007). There is, however, no evidence of significant delays in seeking treatment (Morgan et al., 2006) and the evidence on satisfaction with mental health care is mixed— some quantitative studies suggest higher levels of dissatisfaction in black groups (Parkman et al., 1997) and some do not (Leavey et al., 1997). This may reflect problems with measurement and there is much anecdotal evidence of dissatisfaction (Keating, 2002). Other migrant and minority ethnic populations in the UK have been less intensively studied. What data there is suggests somewhat different patterns for Asians than for black groups. For example, the limited available data suggests South Asians, compared with other groups, are less likely to be (re-) admitted to hospital (voluntarily or compulsorily) and more likely to have shorter admissions (Bhui et al., 2003). There are, however, reports that South Asians are less likely to have disorder recognized in primary care and are less likely to be referred to specialist care (Bhui et al., 2003)—findings that suggest needs are not being met.

Broadly, and at the risk of over-generalizing, what the data indicate (at least for the US and the UK) is more problematic pathways to, and interactions with, mental health services among migrant and minority ethnic populations. (It is noteworthy that what limited evidence there is for asylum seekers and refugees suggests, not surprisingly, similar problems with access and engagement (McCrone et al., 2005), problems no doubt exacerbated by language barriers and mistrust.) The reasons for these ethnic variations are not fully understood and are likely to differ between groups (Morgan et al., 2004). A lot of attention has focused on cultural factors, particularly beliefs about mental illness, the basic premise being that how individuals and others within their social networks make sense of and understand experiences of distress, will shape how they respond, present complaints and interact with mental health services. There is good evidence that such processes are important (e.g. Kleinman, 1980; Pescosolido, 1999). The example of somatization has already been noted; idioms of distress that are unfamiliar to Western clinicians may lead to under-recognition of disorder and a failure to provide appropriate referral and care—patterns that are evident in Asian and other (e.g. Latino) populations in the West (see above).

This emphasis on cultural beliefs, however, can obscure the role of other important factors that influence how people come into contact and engage with mental health services, including: the nature of symptoms; the range and accessibility of treatment or intervention options; practical barriers; material resources; and prior experiences (including of other family members). Kleinman and Benson (2006), in their discussion of cultural competence (see below), give the example of a Mexican man whose failure to regularly bring his HIV-positive son to clinic was interpreted by clinicians to be the consequence of a different cultural understanding of HIV. Further

exploration, however, revealed that the man had a very good understanding of HIV/AIDS and its treatment; the reason for irregular attendance was that, as a low-paid bus driver who often had to work night shifts, he did not have the time to take his son to the clinic. Such practical and material barriers are more common in migrant and minority ethnic populations who, as noted above, tend to be more socially and economically disadvantaged.

More contentiously, there has been debate about whether the patterns of access, engagement, and satisfaction in migrant and minority ethnic populations reflect institutional racism within mental health services (Norfolk, Suffolk and Cambridgeshire Strategic Health Authority, 2003; Singh and Burns, 2006). Institutional racism (a concept initially developed by Stokely Carmichael) refers to the collective norms and behaviours within organizations that systematically and unwittingly discriminate against those from minority ethnic groups—leading in psychiatry, according to some (e.g. Fernando and Keating, 2009), to the provision of inappropriate care and insensitive practice, which in turn creates dissatisfaction and disengagement. This suggestion has proved controversial and, in the UK, has been vigorously challenged (Singh and Burns, 2006). One problem is a lack of direct evidence; relying on the existence of ethnic disparities alone as evidence of institutional racism becomes somewhat circular. As has been suggested above, other factors outside of psychiatry may be relevant. Nevertheless, there is evidence that some, particularly black, ethnic groups are more dissatisfied with the care they receive (Parkman et al., 1997), and the evidence that differences in rates of compulsory admission between white and black patients in the UK becomes more pronounced over time is an indication that willingness to engage decreases as a consequence of repeated contacts with services (Singh et al., 2007).

Mental health service responses

The question, then, for mental health services in multicultural societies is how to deal effectively with ethnic and cultural complexity; i.e. with how to recognize and respond to the needs of increasingly diverse populations. In response, there have been a multitude of proposals for service development and reform. It is not possible within the scope of this chapter to review these. Nonetheless, two broad and related responses merit particular critical consideration: 1) specialist services for minority ethnic groups, and 1) cultural competence.

In response to the evidence that mainstream mental health services do not adequately meet the needs of diverse ethnic groups, specialist services have been developed targeted at particular populations (especially in Europe and the US). Examples abound (e.g. see Fernando and Keating (2009) for case studies on services for Chinese, African, Caribbean, and South Asian populations in the UK providing specialized forms on intervention including cultural therapy, counselling and day services). It is, however, rare for such services to be rigorously evaluated and effectiveness is consequently unclear. In the US, there is some evidence that ethnic specific programmes for African Americans, Asian Americans, and Mexican Americans do reduce drop-out rates, increase use of outpatient services, reduce reliance on emergency services, and improve outcomes (Walton et al., 2010). Such studies are, however, uncommon and their generalizability to other groups and settings is unclear. It has, moreover, been forcefully argued that the provision of separate services reinforces the perception that ethnic groups are 'other' and, by focusing on cultural difference, the move to separate services indirectly implies that culture is a problem that requires intervention (Bhui and Sashidharan, 2003). What such an approach assumes, moreover, is that ethnicity or culture are always the salient issues for patients from diverse groups (a potential pitfall highlighted in the earlier example of the Mexican man whose son is HIV-positive). A possible exception to this is specialist services for asylum seekers and refugees (e.g. Patel, 2009); it may be that the mental health needs of these groups, and the barriers to engagement with services (e.g. language, mistrust arsing from experiences of persecution and trauma, etc.), are so great that appropriate care can best be delivered through dedicated services, particularly those with expertise in working with survivors of trauma.

Where the focus is on ensuring mainstream services are more able to meet the needs of diverse populations, the overarching aim has been to promote and ensure cultural competence in both individual practitioners and organizations. Indeed, this has become a near ubiquitous guiding concept in the drive to make mental health services more responsive and there can be no doubt that, broadly, ensuring practitioners and organizations are more knowledgeable and skilled in assessing and engaging individuals from a broad range ethnic and cultural groups is a 'good thing'. In practice, there are significant obstacles to achieving this, many related to limitations with the notion of cultural competence itself. There is, for example, no shared definition; this means the concept is difficult to operationalize and apply in such a way that interventions and forms of service delivery can be evaluated. In their review of nine evaluations of cultural competence in mental health care (all from North America), Bhui et al. (2007) found that all had used different definitions. The authors of the review were able to distil from the various definitions some common components, but these remain vague (e.g. '…definitions indicate a common aim, to increase performance and the capabilities of staff when providing service to ethnic minorities' (Bhui et al., 2007: p. 4)). This example begs the question, how is it that performance and capabilities in working with patients from minority ethnic groups are to be increased in staff? The primary mechanism so far advocated is the provision of education and training (Bhui et al., 2007). The problem, however, is that there is no consistency in, or agreement about, the content of such programmes and very few rigorous evaluations of their effectiveness have been conducted (Walton et al., 2010). The result is the piecemeal development of training packages with often widely varying curricula for which, beyond specific case studies and anecdotal accounts, there is no accumulating body of knowledge about what works.

The problems with cultural competence as the guiding principle for ensuring mental health services are responsive to the needs of ethnically and culturally diverse populations may be more fundamental still. Kleinman and Benson (2006: p. 294), for example, argue that the very concept of cultural competence reduces culture to a technical skill; cultural competence, they argue, '…becomes a series of do's and don'ts that define how to treat a patient of a given ethnic background'. What is more, as highlighted above, the emphasis on culture as the primary prism through which to think about the needs of individuals from migrant and minority ethnic groups can blind clinicians to other important factors that may relate more to social position and material resources. Culture and ethnicity are, in effect, conflated, the assumption being that ethnic disparities in need and service use can be resolved by improving

knowledge of cultural diversity. This, to be sure, is not to deny the potential role of culture; it is to suggest a broader response is needed. Kleinman and Benson (2006) propose one such alternative approach, based on ethnography, which seeks a fuller understanding of the local moral worlds of sufferers as a basis for engaging and intervening. Their revised cultural formulation suggests clinicians conduct mini-ethnographies, centred around understanding the following facets of individual's lives and experiences of illness: 1) their ethnic identity (and its importance to the individual); 2) what is at stake (i.e. what is it in the lives of sufferers that is valued and that illness threatens); 3) their illness narrative (to understand how sufferers view their problems); and 4) exposure to psychosocial stressors that may have contributed to onset and hinder recovery. What this approach potentially offers is a broader and more individualized basis on which to negotiate engagement; the importance of culture and ethnic identity are acknowledged, but are set within the wider context of the individual's life—as the authors put it, their approach 'does not ask, for example, "what do Mexicans call this problem"? It asks: "what do you call this problem"?' (Kleinman and Benson, 2006: pp. 293–4).

Conclusion

The evidence to date points to higher rates of some disorders (e.g. psychoses) in migrant and minority ethnic groups and similar rates to those in majority populations of others (e.g. CMD), albeit methodological limitations urge caution in drawing firm conclusions. What is perhaps clearer is that for many of these groups (at least in the US and UK) access to and engagement with mental health services is, for complex reasons, problematic. The select discussions in this chapter serve to highlight a number of key ongoing challenges for mental health services in meeting the needs of migrant and minority ethnic populations. Not least among these is the need to develop conceptually sound and rigorous programmes that can be thoroughly tested and contribute to the development of a sound evidence base for engaging and working with those from diverse groups. Appealing as Kleinman and Benson's (2006) formulation is, for example, the real test comes with attempts to formalize, implement, and evaluate this approach. This may seem demanding (and indeed it is), but it is only through this process that we will generate usable knowledge about how to most effectively organize mental health services and provide care to meet the needs of increasingly diverse populations.

References

Alegria, M., Mulvaney-Day, N., Woo, M., Torres, M., Gao, S., and Oddo, V. (2007). Correlates of past-year mental health service use among Latinos: results from the National Latino and Asian American Study. *American Journal of Public Health*, **97**, 76–83.

Bhugra, D., Hilwig, M., Hossein, B., Marceau, H., Neehall, J., Leff, J., *et al.* (1996). First-contact incidence rates of schizophrenia in Trinidad and one-year follow-up. *British Journal of Psychiatry*, **169**, 587–92.

Bhugra, D., Baldwin, D.S., Desai, M., and Jacob, K.S. (1999a). Attempted suicide in west London, II. Inter-group comparisons. *Psychological Medicine*, **29**, 1131–9.

Bhugra, D., Desai, M., and Baldwin, D.S. (1999b). Attempted suicide in west London, I. Rates across ethnic communities. *Psychological Medicine*, **29**, 1125–30.

Bhui, K. and Sashidharan, S.P. (2003). Should there be separate psychiatric services for ethnic minority groups? *British Journal of Psychiatry*,**182**, 10–2.

Bhui, K., Stansfeld, S., Hull, S., Priebe, S., Mole, F., and Feder, G. (2003). Ethnic variations in pathways to and use of specialist mental health services in the UK. Systematic review. *British Journal of Psychiatry*, **182**, 105–16.

Bhui, K., Bhugra, D., Goldberg, D., Sauer, J., and Tylee, A. (2004). Assessing the prevalence of depression in Punjabi and English primary care attenders: the role of culture, physical illness and somatic symptoms. *Transcultural Psychiatry*, **41**, 307–22.

Bhui, K., Warfa, N., Edonya, P., Mckenzie, K., and Bhugra, D. (2007). Cultural competence in mental health care: a review of model evaluations. *BMC Health Services Research*, **7**, 15.

Brown, E.R., Ojeda, V.D., Wyn, R., and Levan, R. (2000). *Racial and ethnic disparities in access to health insurance and health care*. Los Angeles, CA: UCLA Centre for Health Policy and Research and The Henry J. Kaiser Family Foundation.

Cantor-Graae, E. and Selten, J.P. (2005). Schizophrenia and migration: a meta-analysis and review. *American Journal of Psychiatry*, **162**, 12–24.

Castles, S. and Miller, M.J. (2009). *The age of migration: international population movements in the modern world*. Basingstoke: Palgrave Macmillan.

Chin, D., Takeuchi, D. T., and Suh, D. (2000). Access to health care among Chinese, Korean, and Vietnamese Americans. In: Hogue, C., Hargraves, M.A., and Collins, K.S. (eds.) *Minority Health in America*, pp. 77–98. Baltimore, MD: Johns Hopkins University Press.

Cochrane, R. and Bal, S.S. (1989). Mental hospital admission rates of immigrants to England: a comparison of 1971 and 1981. *Social Psychiatry & Psychiatric Epidemiology*, **24**, 2–11.

Deverill, C. and King, M. (2009). Common mental disorders. In: McManus, S., Meltzer, H., Brugha, T., Bebbington, P., and Jenkins, R. (eds.) *Adult Psychiatric Morbidity in England, 2007: Results of a Household Survey*, pp. 25–52. London: The NHS Information Centre for Health and Social Care.

Fazel, M., Wheeler, J., and Danesh, J. (2005). Prevalence of serious mental disorder in 7000 refugees resettled in western countries: a systematic review. *Lancet*, **365**, 1309–14.

Fearon, P. and Morgan, C. (2006). Environmental factors in schizophrenia: the role of migrant studies. *Schizophrenia Bulletin*, **32**, 405–8.

Fearon, P., Kirkbride, J.B., Morgan, C., Dazzan, P., Morgan, K., Lloyd, T., *et al.* (2006). Incidence of schizophrenia and other psychoses in ethnic minority groups: results from the MRC AESOP Study. *Psychological Medicine*, **36**, 1541–50.

Fernando, S. (1991). *Mental Health, Race and Culture*. London: Macmillan.

Fernando, S. and Keating, F. (2009). *Mental health in a multi-ethnic society: a multidisciplinary handbook*. London: Routledge.

Fitzpatrick, J. (2002). The human rights of refugees, asylum seekers and internally displaced persons: a basic introduction. In: Fitzpatrick, J. (ed.) *Human Rights Protection for Refugees, Asylum Seekers, and Internally Displaced Persons: A Guide to International Mechanisms and Procedures*, pp. 1–22. New York: Transnational.

Fuller, E., Jotangia, D., and Farrell, M. (2009a). Alcohol misuse and dependence. In: McManus, S., Meltzer, H., Brugha, T., Bebbington, P., and Jenkins, R. (eds.) *Adult Psychiatric Morbidity in England, 2007: Results of a Household Survey*, pp. 151–74. London: The NHS Information Centre for Health and Social Care.

Fuller, E., Jotangia, D., and Farrell, M. (2009b). Drug use and dependence. In: McManus, S., Meltzer, H., Brugha, T., Bebbington, P., and Jenkins, R. (eds.) *Adult Psychiatric Morbidity in England, 2007: Results of a Household Survey*, pp. 175–98. London: The NHS Information Centre for Health and Social Care.

Helman, C. (2007). *Culture, health and illness*. London: Hodder Arnold.

Hickling, F.W., Mckenzie, K., Mullen, R., and Murray, R. (1999). A Jamaican psychiatrist evaluates diagnoses at a London psychiatric hospital. *British Journal of Psychiatry*, **175**, 283–5.

Hough, R.L., Landsverk, J.A., Karno, M., Burnam, M.A., Timbers, D.M., Escobar, J.I., *et al.* (1987). Utilization of health and mental health services by Los Angeles Mexican Americans and non-Hispanic whites. *Archives of General Psychiatry*, **44**, 702–9.

Jones, J.S. (1981). How different are human races? *Nature*, **293**, 188–90.

Karlsen, S. and Nazroo, J. (2002). Relation between racial discrimination, social class and health among ethnic minority groups. *American Journal of Public Health*, **92**, 624–31.

Keating, F. (2002). *Breaking the circles of fear: a review of the relationship between mental health services and African and Caribbean communities*. London: Sainsbury Centre for Mental Health.

Kessler, R.C., Berglund, P., Demler, O., Jin, R., Merikangas, K.R., and Walters, E.E. (2005). Lifetime prevalence and age-of-onset distributions of DSM-IV disorders in the National Comorbidity Survey Replication. *Archives of General Psychiatry*, **62**, 593–602.

Kirkbride, J.B., Barker, D., Cowden, F., Stamps, R., Yang, M., Jones, P.B., *et al.* (2008). Psychoses, ethnicity and socio-economic status. *British Journal of Psychiatry*, **193**, 18–24.

Kleinman, A. (1980). *Patients and healers in the context of culture: an exploration of the border land between anthropology, medicine, and psychiatry*. Berkeley; London: University of California Press.

Kleinman, A. and Benson, P. (2006). Anthropology in the clinic: the problem of cultural competency and how to fix it. *PLoS Medicine*, **3**, e294.

Kluckholm, C. (1944). *Mirror for Man*. New York: McGraw-Hill.

Leavey, G., King, M., Cole, E., Hoar, A., and Johnson-Sabine, E. (1997). First-onset psychotic illness: patients' and relatives' satisfaction with services. *British Journal of Psychiatry*, **170**, 53–7.

Leighton, A.H. and Hughes, J.M. (1961). Cultures as causative of mental disorder. *Millbank Memorial Fund Quarterly*, **39**, 446–70.

Lewis, G. and David, A. (1991). Racism and psychiatry. *British Journal of Psychiatry*, **158**, 432–3.

Lin, K.M. and Cheung, F. (1999). Mental health issues for Asian Americans. *Psychiatric Services*, **50**, 774–80.

Linton, R. (1956). *Culture and Mental Disorders*. Springfield, IL: Thomas.

Mahy, G., Mallett, R., Leff, J., and Bhugra, D. (1999). First-contact incidence of schizophrenia in Barbados. *British Journal of Psychiatry*, **175**, 28–33.

McCrone, P., Bhui, K., Craig, T., Mohamud, S., Warfa, N., Stansfeld, S.A., *et al.* (2005). Mental health needs, service use and costs among Somali refugees in the UK. *Acta Psychiatrica Scandinavica*, **111**, 351–7.

McManus, S., Meltzer, H., Brugha, T., Bebbington, P., and Jenkins, R. (eds.) (2009a). *Adult Psychiatric Morbidity in England, 2007: Results of a Household Survey*, London: NHS Information Centre for Health and Social Care.

McManus, S., Meltzer, H. and Wessely, S. (2009b). Posttraumatic stress disorder. In: McManus, S., Meltzer, H., Brugha, T., Bebbington, P., and Jenkins, R. (eds.) *Adult Psychiatric Morbidity in England, 2007: Results of a Household Survey*, pp. 53–70. London: The NHS Information Centre for Health and Social Care.

Minnis, H., Mcmillan, A., Gillies, M., and Smith, S. (2001). Racial stereotyping: survey of psychiatrists in the United Kingdom. *British Medical Journal*, **323**, 905–6.

Minsky, S., Vega, W., Miskimen, T., Gara, M., and Escobar, J. (2003). Diagnostic patterns in Latino, African American, and European American psychiatric patients. *Archives of General Psychiatry*, **60**, 637–44.

Modood, T., Berthoud, R., and Lakey, J. (1997). *Ethnic Minorities in Britain: Diversity and Disadvantage*. London: Policy Studies Institute.

Morgan, C. and Hutchinson, G. (2010). The social determinants of psychosis in migrant and ethnic minority populations: a public health tragedy. *Psychological Medicine*, **40**, 705–9.

Morgan, C., Mallett, R., Hutchinson, G. and Leff, J. (2004). Negative pathways to psychiatric care and ethnicity: the bridge between social science and psychiatry. *Social Science & Medicine*, **58**, 739–52.

Morgan, C., Fearon, P., Hutchinson, G., McKenzie, K., Lappin, J. M., Abdul-Al, R., *et al.* (2006). Duration of untreated psychosis and ethnicity in the AESOP first-onset psychosis study. *Psychological Medicine*, **36**, 239–47.

Morgan, C., Kirkbride, J., Leff, J., Craig, T., Hutchinson, G., Mckenzie, K., *et al.* (2007). Parental separation, loss and psychosis in different ethnic groups: a case-control study. *Psychological Medicine*, **37**, 495–503.

Morgan, C., Kirkbride, J., Hutchinson, G., Craig, T., Morgan, K., Dazzan, P., *et al.* (2008). Cumulative social disadvantage, ethnicity and first-episode psychosis: a case-control study. *Psychological Medicine*, **38**, 1701–15.

Morgan, C., Charalambides, M., Hutchinson, G., and Murray, R.M. (2010). Migration, ethnicity, and psychosis: toward a sociodevelopmental model. *Schizophrenia Bulletin*, **36**, 655–64.

Nazroo, J.Y. (1997). *Ethnicity and mental health: findings from a national community survey*. London: Policy Studies Institute.

Nicholson, S., Jenkins, R. and Meltzer, H. (2009). Suicidal thoughts, suicide attempts and self-harm. In: McManus, S., Meltzer, H., Brugha, T., Bebbington, P., and Jenkins, R. (eds.) *Adult Psychiatric Morbidity in England, 2007: Results of a Household Survey*, pp. 71–88. London: The NHS Information Centre for Health and Social Care.

Norfolk, Suffolk and Cambridgeshire Strategic Health Authority (2003). *Independent inquiry into the death of David Bennett*. Cambridge: Norfolk, Suffolk and Cambridgeshire Strategic Health Authority.

Parkman, S., Davies, S., Leese, M., Phelan, M., and Thornicroft, G. (1997). Ethnic differences in satisfaction with mental health services among representative people with psychosis in south London: PRiSM study 4. *British Journal of Psychiatry*, **171**, 260–4.

Patel, N. (2009). Developing psychological services for refugee survivors of torture. In: Fernando, S. and Keating, F. (eds.) *Mental Health in a Multi-ethnic Society: A Multidisciplinary Handbook.*, pp. 122–135. London: Routledge.

Pescosolido, B.A. and Boyer, C.A. (1999). How do people come to use mental health services? current knowledge and changing perspectives. In: Horwitz, A.V. and Scheid, T.L. (eds.) *A Handbook for the Study of Mental Health: Social Contexts, Theories and Systems*, pp. 392–411. Cambridge: Cambridge University Press.

Robins, L.N. and Reiger, D.A. (eds.) (1991). *Psychiatric Disorders in America: The Epidemiologic Catchment Area Study*. New York: The Free Press.

Sadler, K. and Bebbington, P. (2009). Psychosis. In: McManus, S., Meltzer, H., Brugha, T., Bebbington, P. and Jenkins, R. (eds.) *Adult Psychiatric Morbidity in England, 2007: Results of a Household Survey*, pp. 89–104. London: The NHS Information Centre for Health and Social Care.

Singh, S.P. and Burns, T. (2006). Race and mental health: there is more to race than racism. *British medical Journal*, **333**, 648–51.

Singh, S.P., Greenwood, N., White, S., and Churchill, R. (2007). Ethnicity and the Mental Health Act 1983. *British Journal Psychiatry*, **191**, 99–105.

Smith Fahie, V.P. (1998). Utilization of folk/family remedies by community-residing African American elders. *Journal of Cultural Diversity*, **5**, 19–22.

Snowden, L.R. (1999). African American service use for mental health problems. *Journal of Community Psychology*, **27**, 303–13.

Snowden, L.R. and Cheung, F.K. (1990). Use of inpatient mental health services by members of ethnic minority groups. *American Psychologist*, **45**, 347–55.

Swartz, M.S., Wagner, H.R., Swanson, J.W., Burns, B.J., George, L.K., and Padgett, D.K. (1998). Comparing use of public and private mental health services: The enduring barriers of race and age. *Community Mental Health Journal*, **34**, 133–44.

Takeuchi, D.T., Zane, N., Hong, S., Chae, D.H., Gong, F., Gee, G.C., *et al.* (2007). Immigration-related factors and mental disorders among Asian Americans. *American Journal of Public Health*, **97**, 84–90.

Thompson, J., Brugha, T., and Palmer, B. (2009). Eating disorders. In: McManus, S., Meltzer, H., Brugha, T., Bebbington, P., and Jenkins, R. (eds.) *Adult Psychiatric Morbidity in England, 2007: Results of a Household Survey*, pp. 135–50. London: The NHS Information Centre for Health and Social Care.

UNDESA (2004). *World Economic and Social Survey: International Migration*. New York: United Nations.

U.S. Census Bureau (2004). *US interim projections by age, sex, race and Hispanic origin*. Washington, DC: US Government Printing Office.

U.S. Department Of Health And Human Services (2001). *Mental Health: Culture, Race and Ethnicity – A Supplement to Mental Health: A Report of the Surgeon General*. Rockville, MD, U.S. Department of Health and Human Services.

Veling, W., Selten, J.P., Veen, N., Laan, W., Blom, J.D., and Hoek, H.W. (2006). Incidence of schizophrenia among ethnic minorities in the Netherlands: a four-year first-contact study. *Schizophrenia Research*, **86**, 189–93.

Walton, E., Berasi, K., Takeuchi, D. T., and Uehara, E. (2010). Cultural diversity and mental health treatment. In: Schied, T.L. and Brown, T.N. (eds.) *A Handbook for the Study of Mental Health: Social Contexts, Theories and Systems*, 2nd edn., pp. 439–460. Cambridge, Cambridge University Press.

Weich, S., Nazroo, J., Sproston, K., Mcmanus, S., Blanchard, M., Erens, B., *et al.* (2004). Common mental disorders and ethnicity in England: the EMPIRIC study. *Psychological Medicine*, **34**, 1543–51.

Williams, D.R., Haile, R., Gonzalez, H.M., Neighbors, H., Baser, R., and Jackson, J. S. (2007). The mental health of Black Caribbean immigrants: results from the National Survey of American Life. *American Journal of Public Health*, **97**, 52–9.

Williams, D.R., Costa, M., and Leavell, J.P. (2010). Race and mental health: patterns and challenges. In: Schied, T.L. and Brown, T.N. (eds.) *A Handbook for the Study of Mental Health: Social Contexts, Theories and Systems*, 2nd edn., pp. 268–290. Cambridge: Cambridge University Press.

CHAPTER 11

The mental health challenges of immigration

Richard F. Mollica, Kathia E. Kirschner, and Quyen Ngo-Metzger

The magnitude of mental health and resettlement problems

In 2007 it was estimated that there were 38.1 million foreign-born people living in the United States (U.S. Census Bureau, 2007). Since 1975, the United States has resettled approximately 2.6 million refugees (Office of Refugee Resettlement, 2008). Most immigrants and refugees come to escape poverty, mass violence, and/or political/religious oppression. Since 1960 there has been a continuous increase in immigrants coming from Latin America (from 9.4% in 1960 to 53.6% in 2007) and Asia (from 5.1% in 1960 to 26.8% in 2007). In Europe a similar trend is taking place: the European Union (EU) estimates that 28.8 immigrants currently live in the EU. By the end of 2008, the United Nations High Commissioner for Refugees (UNHCR; 2008) estimated that there were more than 10 million refugees under its mandate and about 26 million conflict-induced displaced persons worldwide. According to the UNHCR, 'The year 2008 saw the mass movement of people within and beyond their borders, uprooted by conflict, calamity or searching for opportunity' (UNHCR, 2008). Patterns of both conflict and human displacement are becoming increasingly more complex. The increase in diversity of immigrant/refugee population from developing countries to the so-called developed countries has increased and poses new challenges to the field of community health and mental health care.

In this chapter we will focus on describing the barriers encountered by highly traumatized immigrants and refugees from culturally diverse backgrounds and provide a model that addresses this population's specific health and mental health problems and barriers to care. Their specific medical problems have been addressed in various previous publications (Ackerman, 1997; Bhuyan and Senturia, 2005; Bikoo, 2007; Cassano and Fava, 2002; Coker et al., 2000; Culpepper, 2002; Durham et al., 2007; Fazel et al., 2005; Gavagan and Brodyaga, 1998; Lifson et al., 2002; Marshall et al., 2005; Miller, 1996; Mollica et al., 1999, 2009; Palinkas et al., 2003; Pottie et al., 2007; Roberts et al., 1998; Schillinger et al., 2002; Southeast Asians in the United States: Southeast Asian Subcommittee of the Asian American/Pacific Islander Work Group, National Diabetes Education Program, 2006; Spiegel and Nankoe, 2004; Tompkins et al., 2006; Yee, 2003). This chapter will therefore focus on the new literature emerging from the areas of health disparities and refugee mental health. Health disparities is here defined as 'a particular type of difference in health (or in the determinants of health that could be shaped by policies) in which disadvantaged social groups systematically experience worse health or more health risks than do more advantaged social groups. Disadvantaged social groups include racial/ethnic minorities, low-income people, women, or others who have persistently experienced discrimination' (Braveman, 2006). Immigrants and refugees as both patients and communities definitely experience health disparities, such as:

- Traumatic life experiences
- Provider-patient communication
- Socioeconomic status
- Cultural differences
- Levels of health literacy
- Limited English Proficiency.

The main setting through which to address these health care barriers is the primary health care (PHC) setting. We will first provide a model for caring for traumatized and culturally diverse patients, and will then focus on an important innovation in their health care: the community health worker.

Health status of immigrant/refugee populations in the United States

Historically, from 1850 until 1960, the predominant immigrants to the United States were from European countries and Canada. In 1965, as part of the civil rights period, the Immigration Act abolished European-origin preferences for immigration, and opened the door to other ethnic/racial groups (Trinh-Shevrin et al., 2009). As a result, the foreign-born population has somewhat diversified in more recent decades. The foreign-born population is defined as those who are not citizens of the United States at birth. After migration to the United States some foreign-born individuals are eligible to become naturalized citizens, usually after a minimum of 5 years of legal residence. In the 2000 census, approximately half of the foreign-born population came from Latin America (14.5 million), and a quarter (7.2 million) came from Asia (Schmidley, 2001). Fourteen per cent were from Europe, and the remaining 8% were from other regions of the world (Schmidley, 2001). Although Mexican immigration to the United States is quite significant in magnitude, it is dissimilar from other migrant populations because of the shared United States–Mexico border. Thus, for the scope of this chapter, we will focus on Asian immigrants to the United States because they are more illustrative of other immigrant groups in Europe and around the world.

Asian Americans are defined according to the United States census (Barnes and Bennett, 2000), as 'people with origins in the Far East, Southeast Asia, or the Indian subcontinent' and in the United States include Chinese (24%), Filipino (20%), Asian Indians (18%), Vietnamese (11%), Korean (10%), and Japanese (8%) and other small subgroups such as Cambodians, Laotians, Pakistanis, Hmong, Thai, Indonesians, and Bangladeshis. Asian Americans are extremely heterogeneous in terms of languages, cultures, and socioeconomic status. The degree of English-language proficiency and acculturation often determines socioeconomic status. For example, Cambodians, Vietnamese, and Hmongs are more likely to be first-generation immigrants, and tend to have much lower socioeconomic status compared to Japanese Americans, who are more likely to have been in the United States for several generations (Trinh-Shevrin et al., 2009). However, data on all Asian Americans are often presented in aggregate, which hides the heterogeneity within the Asian American population. Socioeconomic and health status differ widely by Asian subgroups. In addition, the myth of Asians being 'the model minority' (that all Asians succeed in American society), has hidden the plights of many Asian immigrants who have encountered significant challenges living in the United States (Trinh-Shevrin et al., 2009). For example, proportionately more Asian Americans live in poverty compared to whites and are more likely than whites to have lower-wage jobs that do not provide health insurance (Trinh-Shevrin et al., 2009).

Health disparities among Asian Americans

Currently, a major cause of death among Asian Americans is cancer. Lung and breast cancers are the leading causes of death for men and women, respectively (Trinh-Shevrin et al., 2009). Breast cancer mortality rates have increased among Asian Americans even though they have decreased among all other racial/ethnic groups in the United States (Trinh-Shevrin et al., 2009). This increased mortality may be a consequence of lack of screening, resulting in late-stage diagnosis.

Chronic diseases such as obesity, hypertension, hypercholesterolemia, and diabetes are also increasing among immigrant populations (Trinh-Shevrin et al., 2009). The prevalence of hypercholesterolemia and coronary heart disease are especially high among some Asian subgroups such as South Asians. Asian immigrants have increased risks of being overweight and obesity as they adopt a more sedentary lifestyle and the more calorie-dense Western diet. Higher rates of obesity exist among second-generation immigrant children when compared to first-generation children (Popkin and Mau, 1998). Asian Americans have a 60% increased risk of diabetes compared to whites who are at the same body mass index (McNeely and Boyko, 2004). Compared to non-Hispanic whites, diabetes prevalences are higher among Filipinos and South Asians (Barnes and Bennett, 2002). Furthermore, compared to whites, Asian Americans are more likely to have mental health disorders that are underdiagnosed and untreated (Sorkin et al., 2008, 2009). Post-traumatic stress disorder (PTSD) and depression are especially prevalent among Vietnamese, Cambodian, and Laotian refugees who experienced prior traumas of war, imprisonment, or genocide. A recent population-based study found that 62% of Cambodian immigrants experienced persistent PTSD, and 51% experienced symptoms of depression, two decades after resettlement in the United States (Marshall et al., 2005). Older Asian immigrants, in particular, may experience social and linguistic isolation, increasing their risks for depression (Mui and Kang, 2006). Many remain untreated, or undertreated, because of language barriers and the social and cultural stigma related to mental disorders (Miranda et al., 2002). Problems in communication between patients and their medical providers about mental health issues may exacerbate these disparities (Ngo-Metzger et al., 2007; Sorkin et al., 2009).

The health impact of trauma and immigration

The trauma that people experienced in their country of origin, in addition to the acculturation stress, lead to many social, psychological and physical problems. In a meta-analysis, it was found that, on average, refugees consistently scored lower on indices of mental health than non-refugees, with pre- and postdisplacement contextual factors strongly moderating the effects of trauma on mental health (Porter et al., 2005). Moreover, traumatic life events are associated with not only mental health problems, but increased morbidity, lower life expectancy, and higher risks of medical problems (Friedman and Schnurr, 1995).

While the relationship between traumatic life experiences and mental health has been well established, new research findings are revealing the impact of traumatic life events on physical health (Sareen et al., 2007; Sledjeski et al., 2008). These studies are demonstrating the positive risk for physical health problems directly due to trauma events as well as mediated through trauma-related PTSD and depression.

Exposure to traumatic life events has been demonstrated to be highly correlated with smoking mortality, an increase in alcohol abuse, drug use, and direct physical health problems (i.e. bruising, broken bones, head and organ damage) and long-term physical illnesses (Sareen et al., 2007). It has been well established that cumulative trauma is associated with the psychiatric diagnosis of PTSD and depression in a dose–effect relationship, i.e. increasing levels of trauma lead to higher rates and severity of PTSD and depression (Mollica et al., 1998; Sledjeski et al., 2008).

Over the past 25 years major community studies (Mollica et al., 1998) have demonstrated the high rates of PTSD, depression, and physical disability in highly traumatized refugee populations. A recent RAND Corporation study of the Cambodian community in Long Beach, California, revealed prevalence rates of 62% for

PTSD and 51% for depression 30 years after the Pol Pot genocide in Cambodia (Marshall et al., 2005). Data from the nationwide Canadian community health survey cycle 1.2 conducted in 2002 (N = 36,984) demonstrated that trauma related PTSD is associated with a number of chronic medical disorders (See Table 11.1) (Sareen et al., 2007).

Similarly, a large-scale community study in the United States of mainstream American patients demonstrated the positive relationship between trauma events, PTSD (≥6 months) and physical illness. This study used the data from the National Comorbidity Survey – Replication (NCS-R) to examine the relationship between number of life time traumas, PTSD and 15 self-reported chronic medical conditions (see Table 11.2) (Sledjeski et al., 2008). The NCS-R findings reveal that:

◆ There is a graded relationship between trauma exposure, PTSD, and the majority of major medical conditions

◆ The relationship between PTSD and chronic medical conditions was explained by the number of lifetime traumas experienced.

New evidence increasingly reveals the health impact of depression. The fact that severe depression alone (e.g. suicide) is lethal

Table 11. 1 The association between PTSD and chronic physical health conditions. Community sample n = 36,984, 15 years or more, response rate 77%

	AOR	95% CI
Chronic condition (PTSD ≥ 6months)		
Asthma	1.99	(1.38–2.88)***
Chronic bronchitis, emphysema or chronic obstructive pulmonary disease	3.08	(2.01–4.72)***
Chronic pain conditions		
Fibromyalgia	2.59	(1.50–4.47)**
Arthritis (excluding fibromyalgia)	3.46	(2.49–4.81)***
Back problems (excluding fibromyalgia and arthritis)	2.04	(1.51–2.74)***
Migraine headaches	2.77	(1.99–3.85)***
Cardiovascular diseases		
Hypertension	1.55	(1.09–2.20)*
Heart disease	1.69	(1.08–2.65)*
Neurological diseases		
Stroke	2.31	(0.99–5.36)
Epilepsy	1.69	(0.58–4.94)
Metabolic conditions		
Diabetes	1.58	(0.92–2.73)
Thyroid condition	1.06	(0.68–1.64)
Bowel disorder (Crohn's disease or colitis)	1.85	(1.07–3.21)*
Stomach or intestinal ulcers	1.93	(1.22–3.07)**
Chronic fatigue syndrome	5.78	(3.47–9.65)***
Cancer	2.69	(1.36–5.32)**
Multiple chemical sensitivities	3.95	(2.46–6.35)***

AOR, adjusted odds ratio; 95% CI, confidence interval. * p<0.05; ** p<0.01; *** p<0.001.

is well recognized. However, only recently has it been realized that depression is just as lethal through its effects on chronic diseases (Cassano and Fava, 2003). Those with depression are two to four times more likely to develop hypertension (three-fold risk),myocardial infarction (4-6 fold increase in mortality), diabetes (15% prevalence), and stroke (25% prevalence) (Culpepper, 2002). The high prevalence of depression in resettled refugee communities in the United States is most likely leading to a higher prevalence of chronic medical diseases. For example, there appears to be an epidemic of diabetes facing the Cambodian community and Cambodians are six times more likely to die of this disease if they are depressed (Carlsson et al., 2005).

Communication barriers for immigrant/refugee populations

The foreign born's past trauma, socioeconomic status, and limited understanding of English, the host country's culture, and health care system, puts them at an especially high risk for many health and mental health problems, as well as poor health care access and quality. They are less likely to have a regular doctor, and if ill more likely to delay getting care for over a year (Derose et al., 2009). In the United States, foreign-born individuals are less satisfied with the quality of care received compared to those native-born. Furthermore, those with limited English proficiency (LEP) are less likely to receive mental health services if in need than English-speaking non-citizens (Derose et al., 2009).

Barriers in provider–patient communication

Communicating effectively is a core component of the healthcare encounter, and is the platform on which patients and clinicians make informed treatment decisions. Communication comprises of verbal and non-verbal behaviors that serve as the foundation upon which an effective relationship is built—mutual trust, respect, and partnership. Communication includes not only question-asking and information-giving, but many other dimensions including building rapport, paying attention, and validation of patient's health beliefs (Roter et al., 1988). The United States National Healthcare Disparities Reports have shown that persistent disparities occur in provider-patient communication for Asian Americans (AHRQ, 2008). Asian Americans were more likely than white patients to report that their doctors did not listen, spend as much time, or involve them in decisions as much as they wanted (Ngo-Metzger et al., 2004). They were also more likely than whites to report that their doctors did not understand their backgrounds and values (Ngo-Metzger et al., 2003, 2004). This lack of communication resulted in less health education and more unmet health needs among Asians compared to whites (Ngo-Metzger et al., 2007). In a population-based survey, older Asian Americans were more likely to report mental health needs compared to older whites, but were less likely than whites to have their medical providers discuss their mental health problems with them (Sorkin et al., 2008). Other research has found that Asian American women were less likely to receive cancer screening compared to their white counterparts (De Alba, 2005). Furthermore, Asian American women diagnosed with breast cancer were less likely to receive breast-conserving surgery compared to white women (Goel et al., 2005). Asian Americans with end-stage cancer were also less likely

Table 11.2 The association between lifetime trauma and chronic medical conditions

	No Trauma	Trauma	PTSD	Trauma vs. No trauma		PTSD vs. No trauma		PTSD vs. Trauma		Wald vs. 2, p
	%	%	%	AOR	95% CI	AOR	95%CI	AOR	95% CI	
Arthritis/ Rheumatism	16.9	28.3	38.1	1.9	(1.5–2.5)*	2.8	(1.9–4.1)*	1.5	(1.2–1.8)*	28.7, 0.0001*
Back/Neck pain	17.2	30.2	49.4	1.8	(1.4–2.3)*	3	(2.1–4.2)*	1.7	(1.4–2.0)*	40.9, 0.0001*
Headaches	14.8	22.1	50.3	1.6	(1.1–2.3)+	3.2	(2.1–4.9)*	2	(1.6–2.6)*	41.5, 0.0001*
Chronic pain	1.8	10.1	22.1	5.4	(3.6–7.9)*	10.1	(6.6–15.5)*	1.9	(1.5–2.4)*	113.8, 0.0001*
Heart attack	1.5	3.6	2.7	1.7	(0.6–5.0)	1.5	(0.5–4.9)	0.9	(0.4–1.7)	1.2, 0.56
Heart disease	1.3	4.9	7.5	3.1	(1.3–7.1)*	6.3	(2.3–17.2)*	2.1	(1.5–2.9)*	18.8, 0.0001*
High blood pressure	16.7	24.6	26.7	1.5	(1.0–2.3)	2	(1.3–3.2)	1.3	(1.1–1.7)	10.3, 0.006+
Seasonal allergies	27.6	39	45.2	1.7	(1.3–2.2)*	1.2	(1.1–1.4)*	1.1	(0.9–1.3)	24.7, 0.0001*
Asthma	88.1	11.9	14.1	1.5	(1.0–2.2)	1.4	(0.9–2.0)	0.9	(0.1–1.2)	4.2, 0.12
Lung disease	0.5	2.2	4.6	3.8	(1.0–15.1)	6	(1.3–27.3)	1.6	(0.8–3.0)	5.6, 0.06
Stroke	2	2.6	3.7	1	(0.6–1.9)	2	(0.9–4.6)	1.9	(1.0–3.6)	4.2, 0.12
Epilepsy	0.8	1.8	4.4	2	(0.7–6.0)	3.8	(1.1–13.8)+	1.9	(1.2–3.0)+	7.2, 0.03+
Diabetes	3.1	7.7	7.8	2.6	(1.7–4.1)*	3.1	(1.8–5.3)*	1.2	(0.8–1.7)	19.2, 0.0001*
Ulcer	4.2	9.5	17.5	1.9	(1.2–3.0)+	2.8	(1.7–4.5)*	1.5	(1.1–1.9)*	21.2, 0.0001*
Cancer	1.7	6.4	7.3	3.5	(1.7–7.3)*	4.8	(2.1–10.9)*	1.4	(0.9–2.0)	14.0, 0.0009*

Adjusted for gender, race, age, income, insurance coverage, smoking status, and lifetime diagnoses of MDD, other anxiety disorders, and substance related disorders.
AOR, adjusted odds ratio; 95% CI, confidence interval. * Significant at Bonferroni corrected p <0.003 + marginally significant at p <0.05, n = 9282.

to receive hospice compared to white patients (Ngo-Metzger et al., 2008). These health disparities may be a consequence of communication barriers. A number of barriers to effective provider–patient communication may exist. These barriers include: 1) socioeconomic differences; 2) cultural differences; 3) LEP; and 4) low levels of health literacy.

Socioeconomic differences

Immigrants in the United States are more likely to have lower socioeconomic status (SES) compared to native citizens. Individuals with lower socioeconomic status are more likely to report poor communication with their physicians compared to those with higher SES (AHRQ, 2008; Street, 1991). Research has found that physicians' information giving was positively influenced by patient's communication style, such as question-asking and expressiveness (Street, 1991). Patients' levels of verbal expressiveness were strongly related to their levels of education. After controlling for the patient's communication style, evidence suggested that physicians gave more information to particular types of patients: more educated patients received more health information than their less educated counterparts (Street, 1991). Providers spent a larger proportion of their time in the physical examination of patients with lower education and less time assessing health knowledge and answering patients' questions (Fiscella et al., 2002). These findings persisted across racial/ethnic groups, suggesting that providers associated patients' higher education levels with higher health literacy and competency, and thus gave them more health-related information.

Cultural differences

In addition to socioeconomic differences, providers and patients from different cultural backgrounds may have different explanations of health and illness. Most Western providers belong to a 'biomedical' culture that views diseases as having natural, mechanistic causes that can often be treated by repairing organs or manipulating chemical pathways (Kagawa-Singer et al., 2003). In contrast, patients from different cultures may comprehend their illnesses in other ways. For example, the Western paradigm of the separation of mind and body characteristic of Western biomedicine may be difficult for some patients from different cultures understand (Pang, 2000). Patients may have various explanations for illnesses that may be physical (such as a fall that breaks a bone), supernatural (God's will or evil spirits), or metaphysical (such as bad airs or seasonal changes) (Kagawa-Singer et al., 2003). If the provider insists that the Western biomedical view of disease as the only 'right way,' and discounts the patient's views on her illness, miscommunication may occur. When providers and patients can understand and appreciate each other's perspectives on the illness, they are more likely to communicate effectively and be able to negotiate differences. Effective communication and negotiation are especially important in order to avoid frustration and misunderstanding, and to arrive at an acceptable treatment plan.

Asian cultures encourage showing deference to authority and avoiding conflict in order to 'save face'. Asian people also tend to be less direct and show less emotion compared to individuals from Western cultures; which may lead medical providers to assume that they do not have questions or concerns. Thus, Asian Americans may be less likely to openly question medical professionals, even when they do not understand or disagree. Yet, Asian American patients may leave the medical visit with unresolved questions or unmet expectations. Furthermore, Asian Americans are also more likely to use Eastern herbal or traditional folk medicine, or other Asian complementary and alternative medicine (CAM) (Ahn et al., 2006).These herbs may interact with prescription medications and lead to life-threatening complications (Boullatta et al., 2000). In a national study of 3258 Chinese and Vietnamese American patients seen at 11 community health clinics, two-thirds reported that they used CAM while also receiving Western medical care (Ahn et al., 2006). Yet only 7% reported that their doctors discussed CAM use with them. Patients whose doctors discussed the use of CAM with them were more satisfied compared to those whose doctors failed to understand or discuss their CAM use (Ahn et al., 2006).

Limited English-language proficiency

In the United States, 47 million people speak languages other than English at home, and over 21 million people speak English poorly or not at all (U.S. Census Bureau, 2000). Approximately 4 million Asian Americans have LEP and encounter language barriers when communicating with their medical providers (Trinh-Shevrin et al., 2009). Sixty-one per cent of Vietnamese, 51% of Chinese, and 24% of Filipinos in the U.S. do not speak English well (Barnes and Bennett, 2002). Limited English proficient (LEP) individuals often have problems accessing medical care (Weech-Maldonado et al., 2003); they experience more medical errors (Divi et al., 2007), and receive more medical tests compared to those who speak English well (Hampers et al., 2002). Language barriers result in less health information given to patients (Ngo-Metzger et al., 2007), worse provider–patient communication (Weech-Maldonado et al., 2003), and longer hospital stays (John-Baptiste et al., 2004). Having access to trained, professional interpreters during healthcare visits can alleviate some, but not all, of the health disparities associated with language barriers (Ngo-Metzger et al., 2007). Because of the cultural stigma surrounding mental health issues, Asian Americans may be particularly reluctant to discuss their mental health needs in the presence of an interpreter (Ngo-Metzger et al., 2007). Thus, having a medical or mental health provider who can speak the patient's native language is still optimal.

Even among Asian Americans with higher education who can speak English, those who are non-native English speakers may still encounter serious health literacy challenges. They may lack knowledge about how to navigate the complex and fragmented medical and health insurance systems in the United States. Thus, patients whose native language is not English may encounter obstacles with health literacy (Rudd et al., 2000).

Levels of health literacy

Health literacy is defined as the 'degree to which individuals can obtain, process, and understand the basic health information and services they need to make appropriate health decisions' (Weiss et al., 2003). Health literacy is not confined to just basic reading and writing skills, but is also comprised of listening skills and the ability to understand and use health information. Thus, people with low health literacy tend to have difficulty with both written and oral communication (Goodman, 2001). They have more problems with medication adherence (Kalichman et al., 1999), are more likely to take medications incorrectly, and have worse health outcomes (Schillinger et al., 2002). Health literacy is often associated with individuals' education, income, race, age, and country of birth (Rudd et al., 2000). Immigrants, older individuals, and those who are racial/ethnic minorities are more likely to have lower health literacy compared to whites.

The processes by which health literacy affect health outcomes are still under intense study (Weiss, 2003). However, poor doctor–patient communication may be a fundamental factor. Poor communication impacts all components of the healthcare encounter, from taking an accurate medical history to explanations of diagnoses and treatments. Physicians often use medical jargon that patients do not understand. Furthermore, time pressures created by the 15-minute general medical visit may result in doctors providing information quickly, with little time to answer patients' questions (Williams et al., 2002). This problem can be exacerbated since patients with lower health literacy tend not to ask question (Williams et al., 2002). Previous research has shown that patients with low health literacy are often ashamed to ask for help from providers, even though they do not understand instructions on how to take medications (Weiss, 2003).

The role of primary health care

The Institute of Medicine defines primary health care as 'integrated and accessible care by clinicians who are responsible for addressing a majority of personal health needs through a sustained partnership with patients and practicing in a family and community context' (Institute of Medicine, 1996).

The conceptual model in Fig. 11.1 looks at trauma and health and mental health risks for the traumatized refugee/immigrant patient from diverse cultural backgrounds. In this model, traumatic life events are directly linked to physical health, as well as indirectly

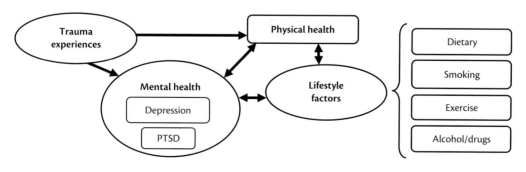

Fig. 11.1 Conceptual model: trauma, PTSD, depression, and physical health.

linked to physical health through the mediation of depression and PTSD. Mental health and physical illness are directly related to major lifestyle factors such as diet, smoking, obesity, lack of exercise, and alcohol/substance abuse that can be directly improved though community-based interventions.

The new focus on trauma as a major health and mental health risk factor highlights the need for a new prevention and intervention strategies in the community-based health care of these populations. In this model, trauma risk assessment is essential to the identification and treatment of major health and mental health problems. Furthermore, treatment must be extended to addressing major life-style through health promotion activities that need to occur in addition to more conventional reliance on medication and/or counseling (Mollica, 2006).

PHC is considered an ideal health care environment for addressing the health and mental health needs of traumatized persons from culturally-diverse communities. PHC serves as the initial point of contact for patients with health-related trauma problems, depression, and PTSD (Barrett et al., 1988). Yet, the usual care by primary care practitioners (PCPs) may be less than optimal with studies indicating the recognition of trauma-related distress as less than 40% (Barrett et al., 1988), diagnosis of PTSD as low as 2% (Taubman-Ben-Ari et al., 2001), and depression less than 50% (Pignone et al., 2002). In PHC veteran clinics where PTSD and depression should be routinely diagnosed, less than 50% of diagnosable patients were identified (Magruder et al., 2005). Under diagnosis and under treatment for historically disadvantaged ethnic groups (e.g. African Americans), those with language barriers (e.g. Hispanics) and special highly traumatized populations (e.g. resettled refugees) may be especially high (Alim et al., 2006; Feldman, 2006; Miranda et al., 2003). For example, Davis et al. (2008) have recently revealed that low-income African Americans in urban primary health care clinics were at a high risk for trauma, with PTSD rates of 22% but only 13.3% of the latter received trauma focused treatment interventions. The identification and treatment of trauma related health and mental health disorders in low income culturally diverse communities in primary health care must be developed and evaluated. Interest of PCPs in a patient's traumatic life history is extremely limited even when the PCPs are caring for patients such as refugees where a history of violence is very common. The fast pace of the PHC visit creates barriers to exploring a patient's traumatic life history and major psychosocial issues. PCPs may also not be aware of the new findings relating traumatic life experiences such as refugee trauma, domestic violence, and history of child abuse to the patient's medical problems.

Although domestic violence is associated with a wide-range of adverse health impact, it is often not identified by PHC providers (Fraser, 2003). A recent study, for example, of 150 women seen consequently in PHC by a female physician revealed that a history of physical and mental abuse (unacknowledged by the PCPs) was associated with an increase in all measures of health care utilization (Sansone et al., 1997). As in the case of all traumatized patients, victims of domestic violence as well as refugees and other traumatized patient groups do not often seek care just for trauma related injuries but for health-related problems which appear unrelated to the trauma events. It is, therefore, essential that there is an adequate risk assessment of trauma events, PTSD and depression in primary health care so that the patient's primary care provider (PCP) can connect the dots between risk and medical illness.

Despite the inherent and current limitations of primary care, it remains the ideal place for diagnosis and treatment of health and mental health problems in the immigrant and refugee population. Firstly, it is their first point of access. For mental health problems, primary health care can be less stigmatizing than special mental health clinics and, despite the many barriers, can meet the immigrants' entire spectrum of mental health and medical needs (Carey et al., 2003). Furthermore, mental health units called Behavioral Health that are staffed by mental health practitioners and are embedded within the primary care setting are in position to maximize the psychosocial treatment of torture survivors.

Some of the barriers that need to be overcome in order to integrate mental health into primary health include the time pressure and lack of knowledge. While it is true that the fast pace of the PHC visit creates barriers to exploring a patient's traumatic life history and major psychosocial issues, it is paramount to take that time. Although the majority of immigrants usually seek help in the primary care setting, most primary care providers (i.e. doctors, nurses, mental health practitioners) still need to be trained in order to effectively identify and treat survivors of mass violence and natural disasters (Henderson et al., 2005). PCPs may not be aware of the new findings relating traumatic life experiences such as refugee trauma, domestic violence, and history of child abuse to the patient's medical problems. Even if the doctor knows of the importance of trauma in the patient's health, they may be lacking the skill necessary to have that discussion with their patients, let alone diagnose and treat in a culturally appropriate manner. Culture- and evidence-based services provided in community clinics are seen as ideal for immigrants who may or may not be survivors of mass violence. Such integrated setting can also improve their quality of life through the management of possible chronic medical and psychiatric conditions. Figure 11.2 demonstrates this new clinical approach at the macro-level (Daniels et al., 2009; Wagner, 1998).

This chronic care model promoted by Wagner (1998) reinforces the conceptual framework described above for the care of immigrants and is consistent with the recent report on American health care by the Institute of Medicine (Institute of Medicine, 2001). Most importantly, an informed active patient and a trained clinical provider team is necessary for improved outcomes. In this model, patient self-management and self-care is essential. For the latter reason, there has been a small but growing movement advancing health promotion, community, and family support, and the enhancement of an immigrant's self-healing, resiliency and coping responses (Mollica, 2006). In addition to training PCPs, the use of community health workers can bring forth Wagner's model of the activated and empowered patient. Community health workers can utilize a community's existing social networks to maximize and facilitate health education, identification and treatment of

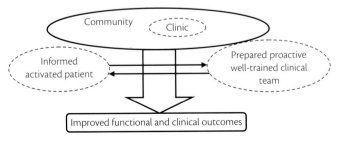

Fig. 11.2 Integrated chronic care model.

common health and mental health problems among immigrant populations.

Use of community health workers as part of healthcare team

For immigrant and minority populations, the use of community health workers (CHWs) is an effective approach for promoting access to health services and increasing health-related knowledge. CHWs have been defined as 'community members who work almost exclusively in community settings and who serve as connectors between…consumers and providers to promote health among groups that have traditionally lacked access to adequate health care' (Norris et al., 2006). They are usually members of the immigrant or minority communities who are lay persons trained to provide advocacy, support, counselling, and information to the target community. A substantial literature suggests that with careful training and monitoring, lay health workers can be extremely effective in health promotion and disease prevention (Norris et al., 2006). For example, the most effective community health workers interventions have been conducted among racial/ethnic minority women (Andrews et al., 2004). The goals of these interventions can often be classified as: 1) increasing access to services; 2) increasing health-related knowledge; or 3) changing health behaviours. For example, Vietnamese-speaking CHWs successfully increased rates of breast and cervical cancer screening among LEP Vietnamese immigrants (Bird et al., 1998). Another intervention using CHWs decreased HIV/AIDS risky behaviours among minority women living in homeless shelters (Nyamathi et al., 2001).

A key component to successful CHW interventions includes cultural tailoring. Cultural tailoring refers to adapting the interventions to reach the target groups' values, beliefs, and practices, but also takes into account individualized personal preferences in order to avoid stereotyping (Fisher et al., 2007). These interventions often rely on the cultural expertise of the community health workers to inform the programmes. The community health workers often address cultural barriers, promote positive health-related behaviour change, and serve as role models in disease management (Lewin et al., 2005).

Community health interventions have been most successful at increasing access to cancer screening, improving maternal and child health in the peripartum period, and improving chronic disease management (Andrews et al., 2004; Lewin et al., 2005). The use of community health workers specifically to address substance abuse has had mixed results. Two interventions among chronic alcohol users have shown non-significant results (Lapham et al., 1995; Leigh et al., 1999). However, other studies have shown that CHWs can decrease depression, encourage positive behaviours, and decrease stress among women with substance abuse (Harris et al., 1998; Washington et al., 2003).

Chronic diseases such as diabetes or hypertension are particularly amenable to CHW interventions. These chronic conditions often require long-term medication adherence as well as lifestyle modifications that include changing one's diet and exercise patterns. The current Reducing Disparities in Diabetes: the Coached Care (R2D2C2) Project focuses on using CHWs to enhance patient–provider communication in order to improve diabetes outcomes. These CHWs function as 'diabetes coaches' who meet with patients for 20 minutes immediately preceding patients' regularly scheduled visits with their healthcare providers. R2D2C2 is unique in its focus (Greenfield et al., 1985) and content (Greenfield et al., 1988) in that it specifically targets the microenvironment of the provider and patient, with the goal of increasing effective participation by patients during office visits. The intervention focuses on: 1) identifying decision options; 2) discussing the alternatives (pros/cons); 3) discussing patient and provider preferences; 4) arriving at a mutual decision; and 5) negotiating conflict. These steps in participating in care are especially crucial and challenging if patients and providers are from discordant cultures or speak different languages. The R2D2C2 project addresses health disparities among Mexican and Vietnamese immigrants in the United States It is an ongoing, 5-year project funded by the United States National Institutes of Health.

During the 2-year intervention period, the 'coaches' focus specifically on improving patients' ability to communicate more effectively with their healthcare providers during the office visits. Coaching sessions occur in the 20 minutes immediately preceding the patient's usual office visit. Patients are coached on skills needed to frame questions, raise issues of concern, participate in treatment decisions, and overcome barriers to effective participation. Because minority and immigrant patients may need additional support to reinforce these skills and overcome barriers to effective participation, the program includes 'debriefing' sessions following the office visits to evaluate how well patients were able to understand the treatment plan. Additionally, coaches telephone patients in between visits to identify problems implementing the treatment decisions made during the visit. The main outcomes in this study will include health outcomes such as serum glucose, blood pressure, and cholesterol levels, as well as depressive symptoms and health-related quality of life. Intermediate outcomes include patient-provider communication, as measured by audiotapes. The R2D2C2, with its goals of enrolling 600 patients in a randomized, controlled trial, will be one of the largest studies using CHWs to reduce health disparities among two vulnerable immigrant groups.

Conclusion

The high risk of health and mental health problems associated with trauma and acculturation stress compounded with low access to care inhibit the recovery of immigrants and refugees and exacerbates existing health disparities. Increasing the knowledge and skills in primary health care is paramount, as is improving outreach efforts that include community-based strategies and partnerships and build upon the already existing social and cultural supports of the community. The use of CHWs can be extremely effective in achieving these goals through a culturally and scientifically-based approach. Only by creating activated doctors and patients working together in a partnership can we make a real change in the way that immigrants/refugees are able to access and receive health and mental health services.

References

Ackerman, L.K. (1997). Health problems of refugees. *Journal of the American Board of Family Practice / American Board of Family Practice*, **10**, 337–48.

Ahn, A.C., Ngo-Metzger, Q., Legedza, A.T., Massagli, M.P., Clarridge, B.R., and Phillips, R.S. (2006). Complementary and alternative medical therapy use among Chinese and Vietnamese Americans: prevalence, associated factors, and effects of patient-clinician communication. *American Journal of Public Health*, **96**, 647–53.

AHRQ (2008). *2007 National Healthcare Disparities Report*. Rockville, MD: U.S. Department of Health and Human Services, Agency for Healthcare Research and Quality. AHRQ Pub. No. 08-0041.

Alim, T., Graves, E., Mellman, T., Aigbogun, N., Gray, E., Lawson, W., et al. (2006). Trauma exposure, posttraumatic stress disorder and depression in an African-American primary care population. *Journal of the National Medical Association*, **98**, 1630–6.

Andrews, J.O., Felton, G., and Wewers, M.E. (2004). Heath J. Use of community health workers in research with ethnic minority women. *Journal of Nursing Scholarship*, **36**, 358–65.

Barnes, J.S. and Bennett, C.E. (2002). *The Asian population: 2000*. C2KBR/01-16. Washington, DC: U.S. Census Bureau.

Barrett, J., Barrett, H., Oxman, T., and Gerber, P. (1988). The prevalence of psychiatric disorders in a primary care practice. *Archives of General Psychiatry*, **45**, 1100–6.

Bhuyan, R. and Senturia, K. (2005). Understanding domestic violence resource utilization and survivor solutions among immigrant and refugee women: introduction to the special issue. *Journal of Interpersonal Violence*, **20**, 895–901.

Bikoo, M. (2007). Female genital mutilation: classification and management. *Nursing Standard*, **22**, 43–9; quiz 50.

Bird, J.A., McPhee, S.J., Ha, N.T., Le, B., Davis, T., and Jenkins, C.N.H. (1998). Opening pathways to cancer screening for Vietnamese-American women: Lay health workers hold a key. *Preventive Medicine*, **27**, 821–9.

Boullatta, J.I. and Nace, A.M. (2000). Safety issues with herbal medicine. *Pharmacotherapy*, **20**, 257–69.

Braveman, P. (2006). Health disparities and health equity: concepts and measurement. *Annual Review of Public Health*, **27**, 167–94.

Carey, P.D., Stein, D.J., Zungu-Dirwayi, N., and Seedat, S. (2003). Trauma and posttraumatic stress disorder in an urban Xhosa primary care population: prevalence, comorbidity, and service use patterns. *Journal of Nervous and Mental Disease*, **191**, 230–6.

Carlsson, J.M., Mortensen, E.L., and Kastrup, M. (2005). A follow-up study of mental health and health-related quality of life in tortured refugees in multidisciplinary treatment. *Journal of Nervous and Mental Disease*, **193**, 651–7.

Cassano, P. and Fava, M. (2002). Depression and public health: an overview. *Journal of Psychosomatic Research*, **53**, 849–57.

Coker, A.L., Smith, P.H., Bethea, L., King, M.R., and McKeown, R.E. (2000). Physical health consequences of physical and psychological intimate partner violence. *Archives of Family Medicine*, **9**, 451–7.

Culpepper, L. (2002). Depression and Chronic Medical Illness: Diabetes As A Model. *Psychiatric Annals*, **32**, 528–34.

Daniels, A., Adams, N., Carroll, C., and Beinecke, R. (2009). A conceptual model for behavioral health and primary care integration: Emerging challenges and strategies for improving international mental health services. *International Journal of Mental Health*, **38**, 100–12.

Davis, R., Kessler, K., and Schwartz, A. (2008). Treatment barriers for low-income, urban African Americans with undiagnosed posttraumatic stress disorder. *Journal of Traumatic Stress*, **2**, 218–22.

De Alba, I., Ngo-Metzger, Q., Sweningson, J.M., and Hubbell, F.A. (2005). Pap smear use in California: are we closing the racial/ethnic gap? *Preventative Medicine*, **40**, 747–55.

Derose, K., Bahney, B., Lurie, N., and Escarce, J. (2009). Immigrants and Health Care Access, Quality, and Cost. *Medical Care Research and Review*, **66**, 355–408.

Divi, C., Koss, R., Schmaltz, S., and Loeb, J. (2007). Language proficiency and adverse events in US hospitals: a pilot study. *International Journal for Quality in Health Care*, **19**, 60–7.

Durham, J., Gillieatt, S., and Ellies, P. (2007). An evaluability assessment of a nutrition promotion project for newly arrived refugees. *Health Promotion Journal of Australia*, **18**, 43–9.

Fazel, M., Wheeler, J., and Danesh, J. (2005). Prevalence of serious mental disorder in 7000 refugees resettled in western countries: a systematic review. *Lancet*, **365**, 1309–14.

Feldman, R. (2006). Primary health care for refugees and asylum seekers: a review of the literature and a framework for services. *Public Health*, **120**, 809–16.

Fiscella, K., Goodwin, M.A., and Stange, K.C. (2002). Does patient educational level affect office visits to family physicians? *Journal of the National Medical Association*, **94**, 157–65.

Fisher, T.L., Burnet, D.L., Huang, E.S., Chin, M.H., and Cagney, K.A. (2007). Cultural leverage: Interventions using culture to narrow racial disparities in health care. *Medical Care Research and Review*, **64**(Suppl. 5), 243S–282S.

Fraser, K. (2003). *Domestic Violence and Women's Physical Health*. Canberra: Australian Domestic & Family Violence Clearinghouse.

Friedman, M.J. and Schnurr, P.P. (1995). The relationship between trauma, post-traumatic stress disorder, and physical health. Neurobiological and clinical consequences of stress: From normal adaptation to post-traumatic stress disorder. In: Friedman, M.J., Charney, D.S., Deutch, A.Y., (eds.) *Neurobiological and clinical consequences of stress: From normal adaptation to post-traumatic stress disorder*. Philadelphia, PA: Lippincott Williams & Wilkins Publishers.

Gavagan, T. and Brodyaga, L. (1998). Medical care for immigrants and refugees. *American Family Physician*, **57**, 1061–8.

Goel, M.S., Burns, R.B., Phillips, R.S., Davis, R.B., Ngo-Metzger, Q., and McCarthy, E.P. (2005). Trends in Breast Conserving Surgery Among Asian Americans and Pacific Islanders, 1992-2000. *Journal of General Internal Medicine*, **20**, 604–11.

Goodman, R. (2001). Psychometric properties of the strengths and difficulties questionnaire. *Journal of the American Academy of Child and Adolescent Psychiatry*, **40**, 1337–45.

Greenfield, S., Kaplan, S., and Ware, J.E., Jr. (1985). Expanding patient involvement in care. Effects on patient outcomes. *Annals of Internal Medicine*, **102**, 520–8.

Greenfield, S., Kaplan, S.H., Ware, J.E., Jr., Yano, E.M., and Frank, H.J. (1988). Patients' participation in medical care: effects on blood sugar control and quality of life in diabetes. *Journal of General Internal Medicine*, **3**, 448–57.

Hampers, L.C. and McNulty, J.E. (2002). Professional interpreters and bilingual physicians in a pediatric emergency department: effect on resource utilization. *Archives of Pediatric & Adolescent Medicine*, **156**, 1108–13.

Harris, R.M., Bausell, R.B., Scott, D.E., Hetherington, S.E., and Kavanagh, K.H. (1998). An intervention for changing high-risk HIV behaviors of African American drug-dependent women. *Research in Nursing & Health*, **21**, 239–50.

Henderson, D.C., Mollica, R.F., Tor, S., Lavelle, J., and Culhane, M.A. (2005). Hayden D. Building primary care practitioners' attitudes and confidence in mental health skills in a post-conflict society: a Cambodian example. *Journal of Nervous and Mental Disease*, **193**, 551–9.

Institute of Medicine (2001). *Crossing the quality chasm: A new health system for the 21st century*. Washington, DC: National Academic Press.

Institute of Medicine (1996). *Primary care: America's health in a new era*. Washignton, DC: National Academy Press.

John-Baptiste, A., Naglie, G., Tomlinson, G., Alibhai, S.M., Etchells, E., Cheung, A., et al. (2004). The effect of English language proficiency on length of stay and in-hospital mortality. *Journal of General Internal Medicine*, **19**, 221–8.

Kagawa-Singer, M. and Kassim-Lakha, S. (2003). A strategy to reduce cross-cultural miscommunication and increase the likelihood of improving health outcomes. *Academic Medicine*, **78**, 577–87.

Kalichman, S.C. Ramachandran, B., and Catz, S. (1999). Adherence to combination antiretroviral therapies in HIV patients of low health literacy. *Journal of General Internal Medicine*, **14**, 267–73.

Lapham, S.C., Hall, M., and Skipper, B. (1995). Homelessness and substance use among alcohol abusers following participation in Project H&ART. *Journal of Addictive Diseases*, **14**, 41–55.

Leigh, G., Hodgins, D.C., Milne, R., and Gerrish, R. (1999). Volunteer assistants in the treatment of chronic alcoholism. *American Journal of Drug and Alcohol Abuse*, **25**, 543–59.

Lewin, S.A., Dick, J., Pond, P., Zwarenstein, M., Aja, G., van Wyk, B.E., et al. (2005). Lay health workers in primary and community health care. *Cochrane Database of Systematic Reviews*, **1**, CD004015.

Lifson, A.R., Thai, D., O'Fallon, A., Mills, W.A., and Hang, K. (2002). Prevalence of tuberculosis, hepatitis B virus, and intestinal parasitic infections among refugees to Minnesota. *Public Health Reports*, **117**, 69–77.

Magruder, K.M. Frueh, B., Knapp, R.G., Davis, L., Hamner, M.B., Martin, R.H., et al. (2005). Prevalence of post-traumatic stress disorder in veterans' affairs primary healthy care clinics. *General Hospital Psychiatry*, **27**, 169–79.

Marshall, G., Schell, T.L., Elliot, M.N., Bethold, S.M., and Chun, C. (2005). Mental health and Cambodian refugees 2 decades after resettlement in the United States. *Journal of the American Medical Association*, **294**, 571–9.

McNeely, M.J. and Boyko, E.J. (2004). Type 2 diabetes prevalence in Asian Americans: Results of a national health survey. *Diabetes Care*, **27**, 66–9.

Miller, B., Kolonel, L., Bernstein, J., and Young, J. (1996). *Racial/ethnic patterns of cancer in the United States 1988-1992. The unequal burden of cancer among Asian Americans*. Bethesda, MD: Asian American Network for Cancer Awareness, Research and Training (AANCART).

Miranda, J., Lawson, W., and Escobar, J. (2002). Ethnic minorities. *Mental Health Services Research*, **4**, 231–7.

Miranda, J., Duan, N., Sherbourne, C., Schoenbaum, M., Lagomasino, I., Jackson-Triche, M., et al. (2003). Improving care for minorities: can quality improvement interventions improve care and outcomes for depressed minorities? Results of a randomized, controlled trial. *Health Services Research*, **38**, 613–30.

Mollica, R.F. (2006). *Healing Invisible Wounds: Paths to Hope and Recovery in a Violent World*. Orlando, FL: Harcourt Press.

Mollica, R.F., McInnes, K., Pham, T., Smith Fawzi, M.C., Murphy, E., Lin, L. (1998). The dose-effect relationships between torture and psychiatric symptoms in Vietnamese ex-political detainees and a comparison group. *Journal of Nervous and Mental Disease*, **186**, 543–53.

Mollica, R.F., Cardozo, B.L., Osofsky, H.J., Raphael, B., Ager, A., and Salama, P. (2004). Mental health in complex emergencies. *Lancet*, **364**, 2058–67.

Mollica, R.F., Lyoo, I.K., Chernoff, M.C., Bui, H.X., Yoon, S.J., et al. (2009). Brain Structural Abnormalities and Mental Health Sequelae in South Vietnamese Ex–Political Detainees Who Survived Traumatic Head Injury and Torture. *Archives of General Psychiatry*, **66**, 1221–32.

Mollica, R.F., McInnes, K., Sarajlic, N., Lavelle, J., Sarajlic, I., and Massagli, M.P. (1999). Disability associated with psychiatric comorbidity and health status in Bosnian refugees living in Croatia. *Journal of the American Medical Association*, **282** 433–9.

Mui, A.C. and Kang, S.Y. (2006). Acculturation stress and depression among Asian immigrant elders. *Social Work*, **51**, 243–55.

Ngo-Metzger, Q., Massagli, M.P., Clarridge, B.R., Manocchia, M., Davis, R.B., Iezzoni, L.I., et al. (2003). Linguistic and cultural barriers to care: Perspectives of Chinese and Vietnamese immigrants. *Journal of General Internal Medicine*, **18**, 44–52.

Ngo-Metzger, Q., Legedza, A.T.R., and Phillips, R.S. (2004). Asian Americans' reports of their health care experiences: Results of a national survey. *Journal of General Internal Medicine*, **19**, 111–19.

Ngo-Metzger, Q., Sorkin, D.H., Phillips, R.S., Greenfield, S., Massagli, M.P., Clarridge, B., et al. (2007). Providing high-quality care for limited English proficient patients: The importance of language concordance and interpreter use. *Journal of General Internal Medicine*, **22**, 324–30.

Ngo-Metzger, Q., Phillips, R.S., and McCarthy, E.P. (2008). Ethnic Disparities in Hospice Use Among Asian-American and Pacific Islander Patients Dying with Cancer. *Journal of the American Geriatrics Society*, **56**, 139–44.

Norris, S.L., Chowdhury, F.M., Van Le, K., Armour, T., Brownstein, J.N., Zhang, X., et al. (2006). Effectiveness of community health workers in the care of persons with diabetes. *Diabetic Medicine*, **23**, 544–56.

Nyamathi, A., Flaskerud, J.H., Leake, B., Dixon, E.L., and Lu, A. (2001). Evaluating the impact of peer, nurse case-managed, and standard HIV risk-reduction programs on psychosocial and health promoting behavioral outcomes among homeless women. *Research in Nursing & Health*, **24**, 410–22.

Office of Refugee Resettlement. (2008). *History*. Washington, DC: Office of Refugee Resettlement.

Palinkas, L.A., Pickwell, S.M., Brandstein, K., Clark, T.J., Hill, L.L., Moser, R.J., et al. (2003). The journey to wellness: stages of refugee health promotion and disease prevention. *Journal of Immigrant Health*, **5**, 19–28.

Pang, K.Y. (2000). Symptom expression and somatization among elderly Korean immigrants. *Journal of Clinical Geropsychology*, **6**, 199–212.

Pignone, M., Gaynes, B., and Rushton, J. (2002). Screening for depression in adults: A summary of the evidence for the U.S. Preventive Services Task Force. *Annals of Internal Medicine*, **136**, 760–4.

Popkin, B.M. and Udry, J.R. (1998). Adolescent Obesity Increases Significantly in Second and Third Generations US immigrants: The National Longitudinal Study of Adolescent of Health. *Journal of Nutrition*, **128**, 701–6.

Porter, M. and Haslam, N. (2005). Predisplacement and Postdisplacement Factors Associated With Mental Health of Refugees and Internally Displaced Persons. *Journal of the American Medical Association*, **294**, 602–12.

Pottie, K., Janakiram, P., Topp, P., and McCarthy, A. (2007). Prevalence of selected preventable and treatable diseases among government-assisted refugees: Implications for primary care providers. *Canadian Family Physician Medecin de Famille Canadien*, **53**, 1928–34.

Roberts, G.L., Williams, G.M., Lawrence, J.M., and Raphael, B. (1998). How does domestic violence affect women's mental health? *Women & Health*, **28**, 117–29.

Roter, D.L., Hall, J.A., and Katz, N.R. (1988). Patient-physician communication: a descriptive summary of the literature. *Patient Education and Counseling*, **12**, 99–119.

Rudd, R.E., Moeykens, B.A., and Colton, T.C. (2000). *Health and Literacy: A Review of Medical and Public Health Literature*.

Sansone, R.A., Wiederman, M., and Sansone, L. (1997). Health care utilization and history of trauma among women in a primary care setting. *Violence and Victims*, **12**, 165–72.

Sareen, J., Cox, B., Stein, M., Afifi, T., Fleet, C., and Asmundso, G. (2007). Physical and mental comorbidity, disability, and suicidal behavior associated with posttraumatic stress disorder in a large community sample. *Psychosomatic Medicine*, **69**, 242–8.

Schillinger, D., Grumbach, K., Piette, J., Wang, C., Wilson, C., Daher, K., et al. (2002). Association of health literacy with diabetes outcomes. *Journal of the American Medical Association*, **288**, 475–82.

Schmidley, A. (2001). *U.S. Census Bureau, Current Population Reports, Series P23-206, Profile of the Foreign-Born Population in the United States: 2000*. Washington, DC: U.S. Census Bureau, U.S. Government Printing Office.

Southeast Asian Subcommittee of the Asian American/Pacific Islander Work Group, National Diabetes Education Program (2006). Hartford, Conn, Khmer Health Advocates. *Silent Trauma: Diabetes, Health Status, and the Refugee. Southeast Asians in the United States* http://www.asianhealth.org/sites/files/794/93238/330887/454445/silenttrauma.pdf

Sledjeski, E.M., Speisman, B., and Dierker, L. (2008). Does number of lifetime traumas explain the relationship between PTSD and chronic medical conditions? Answers from the National Comorbidity Survey-Replication (NCS-R). *Journal of Behavioral Medicine*, **31**, 341–9.

Sorkin, D.H., Pham, E., and Ngo-Metzger, Q. (2009). Racial and ethnic differences in the mental health needs and access to care of older adults in California. *Journal of the American Geriatric Society*, **57**, 2311–17.

Sorkin, D.H., Tan, A., Hays, R.D., Mangione, C.M., and Ngo-Metzger, Q. (2008). Self-reported health status of older Vietnamese and non-Hispanic whites in California. *Journal of the American Geriatric Society*, **56**, 1543–8.

Spiegel, P. and Nankoe, A. (2004). UNHCR, HIV/AIDS and refugees: lessons learned. *Forced Migration Review*, 21–3.

Street, R.L., Jr. (1991). Information-giving in medical consultations: the influence of patients' communicative styles and personal characteristics. *Social Science & Medicine*, **32**, 541–8.

Taubman-Ben-Ari, Rabinowitz, J., Feldman, D., and Vaturi, R. (2001). Post-traumatic stress disorder in the primary care medical setting. *Psychological Medicine*, **31**, 555–60.

UNHCR (2008). *The Year in Review: A world in motion*: Geneva: UNHCR.

Tompkins, M., Smith, L., Jones, K., and Swindells, S. (2006). HIV education needs among Sudanese immigrants and refugees in the Midwestern United States. *AIDS and Behaviour*, **10**, 319–23.

Trinh-Shevrin, C., Islam, N.S., and Rey, M.J. (2009). *Asian American Communities and Health*. San Francisco, CA: John Wiley & Sons

U.S. Census Bureau (2007). *American Community Survey*. Washington, DC: U.S. Census Bureau.

U.S. Census Bureau (2000). *Census 2000 Summary File 3, Matrices P19, P20, PCT13, and PCT14*. Washington, DC: U.S. Census Bureau.

Wagner, E.H. (1998). Chronic disease management: What will it take to improve care for chronic illness? *Effective Clinical Practice*, **1**, 2–4.

Washington, O.G.M. and Moxley, D.P. (2003). Group interventions with low-income African American women recovering from chemical dependency. *Health & Social Work*, **28**, 146–57.

Weech-Maldonado, R., Morales, L.S., Elliott, M., Spritzer, K., Marshall, G., and Hays, R.D. (2003). Race/ethnicity, language, and patients' assessments of care in Medicaid managed care. *Health Services Research*, **38**, 789–808.

Weiss, B.D., Schwartzberg, J., Davis, T., Parker, R., Williams, M., and Wang C. (2003). *Health Literacy, A Manual For Clinicians*. Chicago, IL: AMA Foundation.

Williams MV, Davis T, Parker RM, Weiss BD. (2002). The role of health literacy in patient-physician communication. *Family Medicine*, **34**, 383–9.

Yee, B. (2003). *Health and health care of Southeast Asian American elders: Vietnamese, Cambodian, Hmong and Laotian Elders*. Department of Health Promotion and Gerontology, University of Texas Medical Branch, Galveston, Texas Consortium of Geriatric Education Centers.

SECTION 4

Service components

CHAPTER 12

Organizing the range of community mental health services

Graham Thornicroft, Michele Tansella, and Robert E. Drake

Introduction

In discussing the organization of the full range of community mental health services in this chapter, we shall first consider some important pre-conditions, namely the scale of needs in any given population, the degree of coverage of these needs by existing services, the quantity and quality of available resources, and how far the attitudes of staff and the population at large promote or hinder a service primarily focused upon the needs of service users. We go on to describe a 'balanced care' model, which includes both hospital-based and community-based care, and its application in low-, medium-, and high-resource settings. We then summarize our own experience in developing community care to draw out the key lessons learned, including the need to include a wide range of stakeholder groups. Finally we discuss the key barriers that can impede the implementation of the balanced care model, and methods to overcome these forms of resistance.

The pre-conditions for organizing community mental health services

Population needs, coverage, and focusing

When beginning to plan community mental health services it is usually helpful to understand both the levels of need in the local area, and the available resources. Figure 12.1 shows the relationship between true prevalence and treated prevalence. True prevalence means the total number of cases of a particular condition in a defined area, or population level need. Treated prevalence, by contrast, refers to the fraction of this number who receive care, in other words, the extent of service provision depending upon the available resources. In the National Co-morbidity Replication (NCS-R) Study, for example, a survey of 4319 participants representative of the general population in the United States (A, 100%), the true prevalence of all emotional disorders was 30.5% (B) of those surveyed, while 20.1% of all participants received treatment for any mental disorder (C) (Kessler et al., 2005). Among group C, half of

these individuals did not have an emotional disorder at the time of treatment. Table 12.1 summarizes this information numerically.

In a similar study in six European countries, using the same methods as the NCS-R, among 7731 participants the true prevalence of all emotional disorders was 11.7%, and the treated rate was 6.1% of all respondents (Alonso et al., 2007a). Interestingly, among those who were treated, the majority had no disorder. Therefore in spite of the large differences in total prevalence rates between the United States and Europe, and the methodological differences between these studies, what mental health services share in common is an inability to focus their limited resources upon people who are actually mentally ill.

This raises the important issues of coverage and focusing. **Coverage** means the proportion of people who could benefit from treatment who actually receive it (Alonso et al., 2007b). In Table 12.1, for example, 10.07% of all the population were treated, although 30.50% were prevalent cases, so only one-third of true cases received treatment, indicating poor coverage.

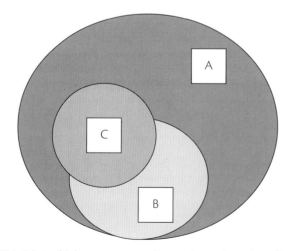

Fig. 12.1 Relationship between true prevalence and treated prevalence. Key: A = total adult population, B = true prevalence, C = treated prevalence.

Table 12.1 National Comorbidity Replication Study (NCS-R) data for true and treated annual prevalence rates of emotional disorders among adults in the general population

	Treated	Not treated	Total
Emotional disorder	10.07%	20.43%	30.50% ⅓ of cases treated: poor coverage[a]
No emotional disorder	10.03% ½ of treated not cases: poor focusing[b]	59.47%	69.50%
Total	20.10%	79.90%	100%

[a] Coverage is the % of people could benefit from treatment who actually receive it
[b] Focusing refers to how far those people actually receiving treatment in fact need it.

Focusing refers to how far those people actually receiving treatment in fact need it. In other words, do they have any form of mental illness (Tansella, 2006)? Even in the best resourced countries we find both low coverage and poor focusing. Within the European Region of the World Health Organization, an Action Plan calls on governments to provide effective care to people with mental illness (Thornicroft and Rose, 2005; World Health Organization, 2005a,b). Yet a comparative international study of depression found that 0% of depressed patients in St Petersburg were treated with antidepressants in primary care, and only 3% were referred on to specialized care. The inability of patients to afford out-of-pocket costs was the reason why 75% of the depressed Russian patients went untreated (Simon et al., 2004). From the public health approach, therefore, the key issue is the appropriate use of resources, whatever the level of resources actually available, namely to increase both coverage and focus. In Table 12.1, for example, 20.1% of the population received treatment but of these half were true cases, and half did not have a diagnosis of a psychiatric condition, and therefore there was poor focusing of the mental health care provided.

Evidence-based practices, implementation, and cultural issues

In addition to the problems of coverage and focus, real-world mental health systems, even in the wealthiest countries, typically fail to assure quality of services (Institute of Medicine, 2006). They do so in three critical ways: by failing to provide effective, or evidence-based, treatments; by failing to implement evidence-based interventions with sufficient fidelity to improve outcomes; and by failing to provide services in culturally sensitive ways that would enhance access and acceptability for people from ethno-racial and other minority backgrounds. The evidence for each of these problems is robust. In the United States, for example, most people with a diagnosis of serious mental illness get no mental health care, and most of those who do receive care get ineffective or harmful interventions (Wang et al., 2002). Probably less than 5% of people with a serious mental illness receive the effective psychosocial services that would benefit them (Drake and Essock, 2009). The reasons are legion: access and acceptability problems for people from minority backgrounds, dropouts due to services that are clinician-centred rather than client-centred, poor alignment between payment systems and evidence-based practices, clinicians' inability or unwillingness to adopt new interventions, inadequate implementation processes, and misinformation from vested interest groups (Drake et al., 2009; Fixsen et al., 2009; Kreyenbuhl et al., 2009; Mojtabai et al., 2009).

Staff attitudes

A further important pre-condition to understand before organizing mental health services is the nature of staff attitudes towards service users and towards models of care. Moving from a mental health system dependent upon hospitals to one which is a balance of hospital and community services implies far more than only a physical relocation of treatment sites. It entails also a fundamental reorientation of perspective. In part this requires new staff attitudes. Table 12.2 shows staff attitudes typical for the two approaches. Within institutions, hierarchical and traditional structures predominate, with a focus on control, order, routine, and the medicalization of treatment and care. Within the balanced care model there is a refocusing upon individualized care, involving service users and family members in care decisions, and upon staff of all disciplines having a greater degree of professional autonomy than is common in traditional hospital settings, within the context of multidisciplinary team work.

Further, therapeutic orientation will vary according to the care setting, as shown in Table 12.3. For example, community-based services will often tend to pay greater attention to assessing and treating people with mental illness in their own home, and will

Table 12.2 Differences in staff attitudes between institutional and community perspectives

Institutional perspective	Community perspective
◆ Seeing service users (usually referred to as patients within institutional settings) within the hospital context	◆ Seeing service user within the home and family context
◆ Focus on symptoms and behavioural control	◆ Focus on needs and goals of the individual and the family
◆ Planned/routine contacts	◆ Flexibility: planned and unplanned contacts
◆ Guidance from set policies and procedures	◆ Responses to changing needs and goals of service users
◆ Hierarchical decision making and authority structure (often biomedical model)	◆ Emphasis on shared decision-making and negotiation (between staff, and between staff and service users)
◆ Stronger belief in pharmacological treatments	◆ Combining pharmacological, psychological and social interventions
◆ View that service users with severe symptoms should remain in hospital	◆ View that symptoms do not necessarily determine the correct care setting for each person
◆ Paternalistic attitude that staff are responsible for the behaviour of service users	◆ Empowering emphasis on the responsibilities of service users along with their choices and consequences
◆ View that service users in hospital are not responsible for their own anti-social behaviour and that these should not be reported to police	◆ Service users assumed to be responsible for their behaviour and to undergo due legal process if committing a crime

Table 12.3 Differences in therapeutic orientation between the institutional and community perspectives

Institutional perspective	Community perspective
◆ Emphasis on symptom relief	◆ Greater focus on service user empowerment
◆ Improved facilities and expertise for physical assessment, investigation, procedures and treatment	◆ Risk of less focused attention on physical health, even to the neglect of this aspect
◆ Seek decision from above in the hierarchy	◆ More autonomy for staff in different disciplines
◆ Focus on control of violent behaviour	◆ Sees behaviour more often within specific contexts
◆ Standardized treatment for groups of individuals	◆ More individualized treatment and care
◆ Regulated timetable	◆ Flexibility in when and where service users are treated
◆ Separated short term treatment and rehabilitation	◆ Integrated therapeutic and social interventions
◆ Culture which tends to avoid risk taking	◆ Culture which will try new approaches to services and to care plans
◆ Commonly clinical and administrative leadership is assumed to be held by medical doctors (which may maintain closer links with other medical specialities)	◆ Leadership can be exercised by any discipline (which may be seen to make mental health services distinct and distant from other medical specialities)

assess a wider range of their clinical and social needs. More fundamentally, the community orientation to a large extent seeks to assist people with mental illness in leading their own lives according to their own specific priorities and goals (putting staff in a facilitatory or supportive role), rather than maintaining the paternalistic view that staff are responsible for virtually all aspects of the lives of those whom they treat.

Implementing the balanced care model

Evidence for a balance of hospital and community care

In this section we shall argue for a balanced care model for adult mental health services and we shall present the evidence for this approach. From a thorough review of the scientific literature, especially focusing upon 'effectiveness' studies (Tansella et al., 2006), we will discuss particular service components, and present the findings in terms of service models which are suitable for areas with low, medium and high levels of resources (Thornicroft and Tansella, 2004). Both the balanced scheme and the three types of resource level are clearly over-simplified, and are solely intended to make complex realities more manageable.

Figure 12.2 indicates that areas with low level of resources (column 1) can only afford to provide most or all of their mental health care in primary health care settings, delivered by primary care staff. The very limited specialist back-up can then offer: training, consultation for complex cases, and inpatient assessment and treatment for cases which cannot be managed in primary care (Mubbashar, 1999; Saxena and Maulik, 2003). Some low-resource countries may in fact be in a pre-asylum stage (Njenga, 2002), in which apparent community care in fact represents widespread neglect or abuse of mentally ill people. Where asylums do exist, policy-makers face difficult choices about whether to upgrade the quality of care they offer (Njenga, 2002), or to convert the resources of the larger hospitals into decentralized services instead (Alem, 2002).

We have deliberately separated the types of care into these three schemes because the differences in mental health care which are possible in low and high resource areas (both between and within countries) are vast. In Europe, for example, there are between 5.5 to 20.0 psychiatrists per 100,000 population, whereas the figure is 0.5 per 100,000 in African countries (Njenga, 2002); the average number of psychiatric beds is 87 per 100,000 population in the European region, and 3.4 in Africa (Alem, 2002), and about 5% to 10% of the total health budget is spent on mental health in Europe

(Becker and Vazquez-Barquero, 2001), whereas in the African continent 80% of countries spend less than 1% of their limited total health budget on mental health, and relevant comparative data available from the WHO Project Atlas website (http://www.who.int/mental_health) (World Bank 2002).

Areas (countries or regions) with a medium level of resources may first establish the service components shown in column 2, and later, as resources allow, chose to add some of the wider range of specialized services indicated in column 3. The choice of which of these more specialized services to develop first depends upon local factors including: services traditions and specific circumstances, consumer, carer, and staff preferences, existing services strengths and weaknesses, and the way in which evidence is interpreted and used.

This balanced care model also indicates that the forms of care relevant and affordable to areas with a high level of resources will be elements from column 3 in addition to the components in columns 1 and 2, which will usually already be present. The model is therefore **additive** and **sequential** in that new resources allow extra levels of service to be provided over time, in terms of mixtures of the components within each step, when the provision of the components in each previous step is complete.

Primary mental health care with specialist back-up

Well-defined psychological problems are common in general health care and primary health care settings in every country, and cause disability in relation to the severity of symptoms. In areas with a low level of resources (column 1) the large majority of cases of mental disorders should be recognized and treated within primary health care (Desjarlais et al., 1995). WHO has suggested that the integration of essential mental health treatments within primary health care in these countries is feasible (World Health Organization, 2001).

General adult mental health care

This refers to a range of service components in areas that can afford more than a primary mental health care system. However, the recognition and treatment of the majority of people with mental illnesses, especially depression and anxiety-related disorders, remains a task which falls to primary care. The elements necessary in such a basic form of a comprehensive mental health service can be called 'general adult mental health care' and this is an amalgam of the following five core components:

1. Low level of resource areas	2. Medium level of resource areas	3. High level of resource areas
(Step A) Primary mental health care with specialist back-up	(Step A) Primary mental health care with specialist back-up *and*	(Step A) Primary mental health care with specialist back-up *and*
	(Step B) General adult mental health care	(Step B) General adult mental health care *and*
		(Step C) Specialized mental health care
Screening and assessment by primary care staff Talking treatments including counselling and advice Pharmacological treatment Liaison and training with mental health specialist staff, when available Limited specialist back-up available for: -training -consultation for complex cases -inpatient assessment and treatment for cases which cannot be managed in primary care, for example in general hospitals	1 Outpatient/ambulatory clinics	1 Specialized clinics for specific disorders or patient groups including: • Eating disorders • Dual diagnosis • Treatment-resistant affective disorders • Adolescent services
	2 Community mental health teams	2 Specialized community mental health teams including: • Early intervention teams • Assertive community treatment
	3 Acute inpatient care	3 Alternatives to acute hospital admission including: • Home treatment/crisis resolution teams • Crisis/respite houses • Acute day hospitals
	4 Long-term community-based residential care	4 Alternative types of long-stay community residential care including: • Intensive 24 hours staffed residential provision • Less intensively staffed accommodation • Independent accommodation
	5 Rehabilitation, occupation and work	5 Alternative forms of rehabilitation, occupation, and work: • Supervised work placements • Cooperative work schemes • Self-help and user groups • Club houses/transitional employment programmes • Vocational rehabilitation • Individual placement and support

Fig. 12.2 Mental health service components in low, medium and high levels of resource areas: a balanced model

Outpatient/ambulatory clinics

Vary according to whether: people can self-refer or need to be referred by other agencies such as primary care; whether there are fixed appointment times or open access assessments; doctors alone or other disciplines also provide clinical contact; direct or indirect payment is made; methods to enhance attendance rates; how to respond to non-attenders; and the frequency and duration of clinical contacts. There is surprisingly little evidence on all of these key characteristics of outpatient care (Becker, 2001), but there is a strong clinical consensus in many countries that such clinics are a relatively efficient way to organize the provision of assessment and treatment, providing that the clinic sites are accessible to local populations. Nevertheless, these clinics are simply methods of arranging clinical contact between staff and patients, and so the key issue is the **content** of the clinical interventions, namely to deliver treatments which are known to be evidence-based (BMJ Books, 2003; Nathan and Gorman, 2002; Roth et al., 2006).

Community mental health teams (CMHTs)

Are the basic building block for community mental health services. The simplest model of provision of community care is for generic (non-specialized) CMHTs to provide the full range of interventions (including the contributions of psychiatrists, community psychiatric nurses, social workers, psychologists, and occupational therapists), usually prioritizing adults with severe mental illness, for a local defined geographical catchment area (Department of Health, 2002; Thornicroft et al., 1999). A series of studies and systematic reviews, comparing CMHTs with a variety of hospital-based services, suggests that there are clear benefits to the introduction of generic community-based multidisciplinary teams: they can improve engagement with services; increase user satisfaction; increase met needs; and improve adherence to treatment; although they do not improve symptoms or social function (Burns, 2001; Simmonds et al., 2001; Thornicroft et al., 1998; Tyrer et al., 1998, 2003). In addition, continuity of care and service flexibility have been shown to be more developed where a CMHT model is in place.

Case management is a method of **delivering** care rather than being a clinical intervention in its own right, and at this stage the evidence suggests that it can most usefully be implemented within the context of CMHTs (Holloway and Carson, 2001). It is a style of working which has been described as the 'co-ordination, integration and allocation of individualized care within limited resources' (Thornicroft, 1991). There is now a considerable literature to show that case management can be moderately effective in improving continuity of care, quality of life, and patient satisfaction, but there is conflicting evidence on whether it has any impact on the use of inpatient services (Mueser et al., 1998; Ziguras and Stuart, 2000; Ziguras et al., 2002). Case management needs to be carefully distinguished from the much more specific and more intensive **assertive community treatment**.

Acute inpatient care

There is no evidence that a balanced system of mental health care can be provided without acute beds. Some services (such as home treatment teams, crisis house, and acute day hospital care, see below) may be able to offer realistic alternative care for some voluntary patients (Howard et al., 2008; Johnson et al., 2005a,b). Nevertheless those who need urgent medical assessment, or those with severe and comorbid medical and psychiatric conditions, severe psychiatric relapse and behavioural disturbance, high levels of suicidality or assaultativeness, acute neuropsychiatric conditions, or elderly people with concomitant severe physical disorders, will usually require high-intensity immediate support in acute inpatient hospital units.

There is a relatively weak evidence base on many aspects of inpatient care, and most studies are descriptive accounts (Szmukler and Holloway, 2001). There are few systematic reviews in this field, one of which found that there were no differences in outcomes between routine admissions and planned short hospital stays (Johnstone and Zolese, 1999). More generally, although there is a consensus that acute inpatient units are necessary, the number of beds required is highly contingent upon which other services exist locally and upon local social and cultural characteristics (Thornicroft and Tansella, 1999). Acute inpatient care commonly absorbs most of the mental health budget (Knapp et al., 1997), therefore minimizing the use of bed-days, e.g. by reducing the average length of stay, may be an important goal, if the resources released in this way can be used for other service components. A related policy issue concerns how to provide acute beds in a humane and less institutionalized way that is acceptable to patients, e.g. in general hospital units (Quirk and Lelliott, 2001; Tomov, 2001).

Long-term community-based residential care

It is important to know whether people with severe and long-term disabilities should be still cared for in larger, traditional institutions, or be transferred to long-term, community-based residential care. The evidence here, for medium- and high-resource level areas, is clear. When deinstitutionalization is carefully carried out, for those who have previously received long-term inpatient care for many years, then the outcomes are more favourable for most people who are discharged to community care (Shepherd and Murray, 2001; Thornicroft and Bebbington, 1989). The TAPS (Team for the Assessment of Psychiatric Services) study in London (Leff, 1997), for example, completed a 5-year follow-up on over 95% of 670 discharged long-stay non-demented people and found that community services were more cost-effective (Knapp et al., 1990).

Rehabilitation, occupation, and work

Rates of unemployment among people with mental disorders are usually much higher than in the general population, and are also higher than among people with severe physical disabilities (Social Exclusion Unit, 2004). Traditional methods of occupation and day care have been day centres or a variety of psychiatric rehabilitation centres (Rosen and Barfoot, 2001). There is little hard evidence about these models of day care, and a recent review of over 300 papers, for example, found no relevant randomized controlled trials. Non-randomized studies have given conflicting results and for areas with medium levels of resources it is reasonable at this stage to make pragmatic decisions about the provision of rehabilitation, occupation, and work services if the specialist and evidence-based options discussed below are not affordable (Catty et al., 2003; Marshall et al., 2001).

Specialized mental health services

The balanced care model suggests that areas with high levels of resources may already provide all or most of the service components in Steps A and B, and are then able to offer additional components from the options shown in Step C in Fig. 12.2.

Outpatient/ambulatory clinics

Specialized outpatient facilities for particular disorders or patient groups are common in many high-resource areas and may include, for example, services dedicated to: people with eating disorders; people with anxiety disorders; people with dual diagnosis (psychotic disorders and substance abuse); cases of treatment-resistant affective or psychotic disorders; those requiring specialized forms of psychotherapy; mentally disordered offenders; mentally ill mothers and their babies; and those with other specific disorders (such as post-traumatic stress disorder). Local decisions about whether to establish such specialized clinics will depend upon several factors, including their relative priority in relation to the other specialized services described below, identified services gaps, and the financial opportunities available.

Community mental health teams

These are by far the most researched of all the components of balanced care, and most randomized controlled trials and systematic reviews in this field refer to such teams (Mueser et al., 1998). Two types of specialized community mental health team have been particularly well developed as adjuncts to generic CMHTs: assertive community treatment (ACT) teams and early intervention (EI) teams.

Assertive community treatment (ACT) teams

These provide a form of specialized mobile outreach treatment for people with more disabling mental disorders, and have been clearly characterized (Killaspy et al., 2006, 2009; Scott and Lehman, 2001; Teague et al., 1998). There is now strong evidence that ACT can produce the following advantages in high level of resource areas: 1) reduce admissions to hospital and the use of acute beds, 2) reduce homelessness, 3) improve accommodation status, and 4) increase service user satisfaction. ACT has not been shown to produce improvements in mental state or social behaviour. ACT can reduce the cost of inpatient services, but does not change the overall costs of care (Latimer, 1999; Marshall and Lockwood, 2003; McCrone et al., 2009; Phillips et al., 2001). Nevertheless, it is not known how far ACT is cross-culturally relevant and indeed there is evidence that ACT may be less effective where usual services already offer high levels of integration and continuity of care, for example in the United Kingdom, than in settings where the treatment-as-usual control condition may offer little to people with severe mental illnesses (Burns, 2009).

Early intervention teams

There has been considerable interest in recent years in the prompt identification and treatment of first or early episode cases of psychosis. Much of this research has focused upon the time between first clear onset of symptoms and the beginning of treatment, referred to as the 'duration of untreated psychosis' (DUP), while other studies have placed more emphasis upon providing family interventions when a young person's psychosis is first identified (Addington et al., 2003; Raune et al., 2004). There is now emerging evidence that longer DUP is a predictor of worse outcome for psychosis; in other words, if patients wait a long time after developing a psychotic condition before they receive treatment, then they may take longer to recover and have a less favourable long-term prognosis.

Few controlled trials have been published of such interventions (Kuipers et al., 2004; Petersen et al., 2005), and a Cochrane systematic review has concluded that there are 'insufficient trials to draw any definitive conclusions…the substantial international interest in early intervention offers an opportunity to make major positive changes in psychiatric practice, but this opportunity may be missed without a concerted international programme of research to address key unanswered questions.' (Marshall and Lockwood, 2004). A more recent Schizophrenia PORT review (Dixon et al., 2010) came to a similar conclusion. It is therefore currently premature to judge whether specialized early intervention teams should be seen as a priority (de Koning et al., 2009; Friis et al., 2003; Harrigan et al., 2003; Larsen et al., 2001; McGorry et al., 2009; Ricciardi et al., 2008).

Alternatives to acute inpatient care

In recent years three main alternatives to acute inpatient care have been developed: acute day hospitals, crisis houses, and home treatment/crisis resolution teams. **Acute day hospitals** are facilities which offer programmes of day treatment for those with acute and severe psychiatric problems, as an alternative to admission to inpatient units. A systematic review of nine randomized controlled trials has established that acute day hospital care is suitable for about 30% of people who would otherwise be admitted to hospital, and offers advantages in terms of faster improvement and lower cost. It is reasonable to conclude that acute day hospital care is an effective option when demand for inpatient beds is high (Marshall et al., 2001).

Crisis houses are houses in community settings which are staffed by trained mental health professionals and offer admission for some people who would otherwise be admitted to hospital. A wide variety of respite houses, havens, and refuges have been developed, but crisis house is used here to mean facilities which are alternatives to non-compulsory hospital admission. The little available research evidence suggests that they are very acceptable to their residents (Szmukler and Holloway, 2001), may be able to offer an alternative to hospital admission for about a quarter of otherwise admitted patients, and may be more cost-effective than hospital admission (Mosher, 1999; Sledge et al., 1996). Nevertheless there is emerging evidence that female patients in particular prefer non-hospital alternatives (such as single sex crisis houses) to acute inpatient treatment, and this may reflect the lack of perceived safety in those settings (Johnson et al., 2009; Killaspy et al., 2000).

Home treatment/crisis resolution teams are mobile community mental health teams offering assessment for people in psychiatric crises and providing intensive treatment and care at home. The key active ingredients appear to be regular home visits, and the combined provision of health and social care (Johnson et al., 2008). A Cochrane systematic review (Catty et al., 2002) found that most of the research evidence is from the United States or the United Kingdom, and concluded that home treatment teams reduce days spent in hospital, especially if the teams make regular home visits and have responsibility for both health and social care (Joy et al., 1998). Indeed a national study in England between 1998 to 2003 found that hospital admissions were reduced by 10% in areas which had crisis resolution teams, and by 23% where these teams offered a 24-hour on-call system (Glover et al., 2006).

Crisis plans and advance directives

A joint crisis plan (JCP) aims to empower the holder and to facilitate early detection and treatment of relapse (Sutherby et al., 1999). It is developed by a patient together with mental health staff. Held by the patient, it contains his or her choice of information, which can include an advance agreement for treatment preferences for any future emergency, when he or she might be too unwell to express coherent views. The JCP format was developed after consultation with national user groups, interviews with organizations and individuals using crisis cards (Sutherby and Szmukler, 1998), and detailed development work with service users in South London. The results of the pilot study (Sutherby et al., 1999) showed that (at 6–12-month follow-up) 57% of participating patients felt more involved in their care, 60% felt more positive about their situation, 51% felt more in control of their mental health problem, and 41% were more likely to continue treatment[1]. The JCP may have direct and indirect effects: family doctors and carers may be able to react earlier to a relapse, while emergency department staff may make better decisions when informed by the JCP. Negotiating the content may clarify treatment issues and build consensus between patients and staff, potentially reducing future compulsion in treatment and care. Recent research has shown that JCPs are able to halve the rates of compulsory treatment in hospital (Henderson et al., 2004), and are cost-effective (Flood et al., 2006).

Alternative types of long-stay community residential care

These are usually replacements for long-stay wards in psychiatric institutions (Shepherd and Murray, 2001). Three categories of such residential care can be identified: 1) **24 hour staffed residential care** (high-staffed hostels, residential care homes or nursing homes, depending on whether the staff have professional qualifications); 2) **day-staffed residential places** (hostels or residential homes which are staffed during the day); and 3) **lower supported accommodation** (minimally supported hostels or residential homes with visiting staff). There is limited evidence on the cost-effectiveness of these types of residential care, and no completed systematic reviews (Chilvers et al., 2003). It is therefore reasonable for policy makers to decide upon the need for such services with local stakeholders (Rosen and Barfoot, 2001; Thornicroft, 2001).

Alternative forms of rehabilitation, occupation, and work

Although vocational rehabilitation has been offered in various forms to people with severe mental illnesses for over a century, its role has weakened because of discouraging results, financial disincentives to work, and pessimism about outcomes for these patients (Cook et al., 2005; Latimer et al., 2006; Lehman et al., 1995). However, recent alternative forms of occupation and vocational rehabilitation have again raised employment as an outcome priority. Consumer and carer advocacy groups have set work and occupation as one of their highest priorities, to enhance both functional status and quality of life (Chamberlin, 2005; Thornicroft et al., 2002).

There are recent indications that it is possible to improve vocational and psychosocial outcomes with supported employment models, which emphasize rapid placement in competitive jobs and support from employment specialists (Drake et al., 1999). Studies of IPS programmes in the United States, Canada, Australia, and other countries have been encouraging in terms of increased rates of competitive employment (Bond et al., 2008; Burns et al., 2007; Cook et al., 2008; Drake and Bond 2008; Howard et al., in press; Lehman et al., 2002; Marshall et al., 2001). At the same time, studies of the IPS model in the United Kingdom have produced conflicting results (Burns et al., 2007; Howard et al., in press), possibly related to weak implementation or the nature of the control group or treatment as usual group used as the comparator (Burns, 2009).

Engagement with local stakeholders

Organizing the range of community-base mental health services effectively requires making links with key local figures and groups in the local community. They will most often include not only family doctors, general hospital, and other health service clinicians, but also the whole range of interests shown in Table 12.4. But a wider array of stakeholders may also wish to have their interests represented and taken into account in decision-making. These constituencies may include: neighbourhood or residents' associations, local school staff, governors and parents, representatives of different cultural and ethnic communities, shopkeepers and members of local business, and church ministers and elders of other faith communities. The importance of these stakeholders emerges particularly at times when plans are being developed to open new mental health facilities, and meaningful consultations at this stage may prevent local opposition which could stop community services from being initiated.

Table 12.4 Key stakeholders at the local level

- Service users/consumers
- Family members/carers
- Health care professionals (mental health and primary care staff)
- Other public services agencies, e.g. police and housing
- Other service provider groups e.g. non-governmental organizations, church, and charitable groups
- Policy makers: politicians, political advisers, and officials
- Service planners and commissioners
- Advocacy groups
- Local media, e.g. newspaper and radio

Lessons learned in organizing community mental health services

What are the overall lessons that we have learned from taking part in the development of community mental health care over the last 20 to 30 years? In our view the following specific issues are common: (Thornicroft et al., 2008):

- Anxiety and uncertainty in the process of change
- Needing to compensate for a possible lack of structure in community services
- Uncertainty about how to initiate new developments
- Managing opposition within the mental health system
- Dealing with opposition from neighbours
- Maximizing and managing a clearly identified budget
- Ensuring that rigidities in the old system are made more flexible
- Creating practical way to minimize the dysfunctional effects of boundaries between different service components
- Maintaining staff morale during periods of change
- Implementing evidence-based practices with sufficient fidelity
- Expecting outside experts to know 'what is the right answer' rather than accepting responsibility for making decisions to suit local circumstances.

Beyond these challenges, we have provisionally concluded that the following overall lessons often apply when developing community care. First, to make service changes robust will take time. Part of the reason for this is that staff will need to be persuaded that change is likely to bring improvements for patients, and indeed their scepticism is a positive asset, to act as a buffer against changes that are too rapid, too frequent, or implausible. The next reason for not rushing change is that to succeed it is likely to need the support of many organizations and agencies, and they need to be identified and included gradually, at the start of each cycle of service changes. Those which are, or which feel, excluded are likely to oppose change, sometimes successfully. Further, in situations where health service changes may be a topic for political debate, then it is usually necessary to build a cross-party consensus on the mental health strategy so that it will continue intact if the government changes. Again this will often take time to achieve.

Time is also needed to progress from the initiation stage of a change to the *consolidation phase*. Typically at the early stages of service reform a charismatic individual or small group will champion the main proposals, and recruit support from stakeholder groups and from others with influence within the healthcare system. In Eastern European countries, for example, the Medical Director/Superintendents of the psychiatric hospital will in practice hold a veto for or against change (Thornicroft and Tansella, 2009). An example of the timescale required is the pattern of services changes in Verona in Italy over the last 30 years, derived from the local case register, as shown in Fig. 12.3. As the number of psychiatric beds has progressively declined, so the provision of day care, residential care, and outpatient and community contacts has steadily increased over many years.

The second overall lesson is that it is essential to listen to users' and families' experiences and perspectives (Thornicroft and

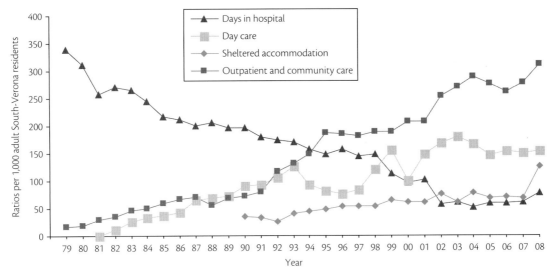

Fig. 12.3 Patterns of mental health service provision in Verona, 1979 to 2008.

Table 12.5 Key barriers and challenges to better mental health care

Barriers	Challenges to overcoming barriers
1 Insufficient funding for mental health services	◆ Inconsistent and unclear advocacy ◆ Perception that mental health indicators are weak ◆ People with mental disorders are not a powerful lobby ◆ Lack of general public interest in mental health ◆ Social stigma ◆ Incorrect belief that care is not cost-effective
2 Mental health resources centralized in and near big cities and in large institutions	◆ Historical reliance on mental hospitals ◆ Fragmentation of mental health responsibilities between different government departments ◆ Differences between central and provincial government priorities ◆ Vested interests of staff in continuing large hospitals ◆ Political risks associated with trade union protests ◆ Need for transitional funding to move to community-based care
3 Complexities of integrating mental health care effectively in primary care services	◆ Primary care workers already overburdened ◆ Lack of training, supervision and ongoing specialized support ◆ Lack of continuous supply of relevant medications in primary care
4 Low numbers and limited types of health workers trained and supervised in mental health care	◆ Poor working conditions in public mental health services ◆ Lack of incentives for staff to work in rural areas ◆ Professional establishment opposes expanded role for non-specialists in mental health workforce ◆ Medical students and psychiatrists trained only in mental hospitals ◆ Inadequate training of general health workforce ◆ Mental health specialists spend more time providing care rather than training and supervising others ◆ Lack of infrastructure to enable community-based supervision
5 Mental health leaders often deficient in public health skills and experience	◆ Those who rise to leadership positions often only trained in clinical management of individuals, not population level needs ◆ Public health training does not include mental health ◆ Lack of training courses in public mental health ◆ Mental health clinical leaders overburdened by clinical and management responsibilities and private practice
6 Fragmentation between mental health advocacy groups	◆ Conceptual and practical differences between consumers and mental health staff, especially about diagnoses and treatments ◆ Divisions between consumer and family member groups ◆ Politicians therefore find it easy to ignore an incoherent message
Information systems	◆ Absence of information systems, implementation standards, and outcomes monitoring. (Drake et al., 2009, 2010)

Adapted from Saraceno et al., 2007.

Tansella, 2009). Everyone involved needs to keep a clear focus on the fact that the primary purpose of mental health services is to improve outcomes that are valued by people with mental illnesses themselves. The intended beneficiaries of care therefore need to be—in some sense—in the driving seat when planning and delivering treatment and care. This a profound transformation, changing from a traditional and paternalistic perspective, in which staff were expected to take all important decisions in the 'best interests' of patients, to an approach in which people with mental illness work, to a far greater extent, are in partnership with care providers.

The third lesson is that the team managing such a process needs clear expertise to manage the whole **budget** and that the risks are high that services changes will be used as an occasion for budget cuts. Having a protected budget is necessary but not sufficient as it is also vital to be able to exercise flexibility within the overall budget, typically to re-use money saved by reducing the use of inpatient beds for community mental health teams, or occupational or residential services. When such a financial boundary (sometimes called a 'ring fence') for mental health funds is not established and fiercely maintained, then money can easily be diverted to other areas of health care. In other words, financial mechanisms need to be created which ensure that money will follow the patients into the community.

The next key point is something of a paradox: as mental health care is progressively deinstitutionalized, so some aspects of the mental health system need to be institutionalized! For example, pre-qualification level professional teaching and training curricula will need to be redesigned to include theoretical and practical aspects of delivering care in community settings, and codified in training curricula. Similarly, post-qualifying training courses need to be taught on a regular basis, particularly in the early stages for staff making the transition from hospital to community clinical duties. A further aspect of new forms of institutionalization is the need for some new legal arrangements, such as mental health or legal capacity laws which may need to be revised or recreated to ensure that their provisions still make sense in the new context, where most clinical contacts between staff and people with mental illnesses take place outside hospitals. Even more important, standards of quality in regard to the implementation of evidence-based practices must be instituted in ways that are perceived as helpful guides, rather than burdens, by clinicians and users.

Understanding barriers to change

We have argued that serious, but surmountable, barriers face those who wish to develop a balanced care model. To enact such a vision means eroding, quickly or slowly, forms of resistance that have often prevented meaningful improvement in mental health care across the globe. The key barriers have been identified as shown in Table 12.5 (Saraceno et al., 2007).

Finally, we reaffirm the central importance of learning from experience—primarily the experience of people with mental illness and their family members. Our central contention in this book is that the primary aim of mental health care is to achieve better outcomes for individuals with mental illness. As the intended beneficiaries, therefore, people with mental illness need to have a central say in what services are planned, how they are provided, how their impact is assessed: in short—in every aspect of care (Chamberlin 2005; Rose 2001). If there is one defining characteristic that we wish

to see embodied in the future, it is that service users are actually included as full partners in directly contributing to better mental health care.

References

Addington, J., Coldham, E.L., Jones, B., Ko, T., and Addington, D. (2003). The first episode of psychosis: the experience of relatives. *Acta Psychiatrica Scandinavica*, **108**, 285–9.

Alem, A. (2002). Community-based vs. hospital-based mental health care: the case of Africa. *World Psychiatry*, **1**, 99–100.

Alonso, J., Lépine J.P., and the ESEMeD/MHEDEA 2000 Scientific Committee (2007a). Overview of the key ESEMeD data. *Journal of Clinical Psychiatry*, **68**(Suppl 2), 3–9.

Alonso, J., Codony, M., Kovess, V., Angermeyer, M.C., Katz, S.J., Haro, J.M., *et al.* (2007b). Population level of unmet need for mental healthcare in Europe. *British Journal of Psychiatry*, **190**, 299–306.

Becker, T. 2001). Out-patient psychiatric services. In: Thornicroft, G. and Szmukler, G. (eds.) *Textbook of Community Psychiatry*, pp. 277–82. Oxford: Oxford University Press.

Becker, T. and Vazquez-Barquero, J.L. (2001). The European perspective of psychiatric reform. *Acta Psychiatrica Scandinavica*, **410**, 8–14.

BMJ Books (2003). *Clinical Evidence, Volume 9*. London: BMJ Books.

Bond, G.R., Drake, R.E., and Becker, D.R. (2008). An update on randomized controlled trials of evidence-based supported employment. *Psychiatric Rehabilitation Journal*, **31**, 280–90.

Burns, T. (2001). Generic versus specialist mental health teams. In: Thornicroft, G. and Szmukler, G. (eds.) *Textbook of Community Psychiatry*, pp. 231–41. Oxford: Oxford University Press.

Burns, T. (2009). End of the road for treatment-as-usual studies? *British Journal of Psychiatry*, **195**, 5–6.

Burns, T., Catty, J., Becker, T., Drake, R.E., Fioritti, A., Knapp, M., *et al.* (2007). The effectiveness of supported employment for people with severe mental illness: a randomised controlled trial. *Lancet*, **370**, 1146–52.

Catty, J., Burns, T., and Comas, A. (2003). Day centres for severe mental illness. *Cochrane Library*, 1. Oxford: Update Software.

Catty, J., Burns, T., Knapp, M., Watt, H., Wright, C., Henderson, J., *et al.* (2002). Home treatment for mental health problems: a systematic review. *Psychological Medicine*, **32**, 383–401.

Chamberlin, J. (2005). User/consumer involvement in mental health service delivery. *Epidemiologica e Psichiatria Sociale*, **1**, 10–14.

Chilvers, R., Macdonald, G., and Hayes, A. (2003). *Supported housing for people with severe mental disorders (Cochrane Review)*. Oxford: Update Software.

Cook, J.A., Leff, H.S., Blyler, C.R., Gold, P.B., Goldberg, R.W., Mueser, K.T., *et al.* (2005). Results of a multisite randomized trial of supported employment interventions for individuals with severe mental illness. *Archives of General Psychiatry*, **62**, 505–12.

Cook, J.A., Blyler, C.R., Leff, H.S., McFarlane, W.R., Goldberg, R.W., Gold, P.B., *et al.* (2008). The employment intervention demonstration program: major findings and policy implications. *Psychiatric Rehabilitation Journal*, **31**, 291–5.

de Koning, M.B., Bloemen, O.J., van Amelsvoort, T.A., Becker, H.E., Nieman, D.H., van der Gaag, M., *et al.* (2009). Early intervention in patients at ultra high risk of psychosis: benefits and risks. *Acta Psychiatrica Scandinavica*, **119**, 426–42.

Department of Health (2002). *Community Mental Health Teams, Policy Implementation Guidance*. London: Department of Health.

Desjarlais, R., Eisenberg, L., Good, B., and Kleinman, A. (1995). *World Mental Health. Problems and Priorities in Low Income Countries*. Oxford: Oxford University Press.

Dixon, L.B., Dickerson, F., Bellack, A.S., Bennett, M., Dickinson, D., Goldberg, R.W., *et al.* (2010). The 2009 schizophrenia PORT psychosocial treatment recommendations and summary statements. *Schizophrenia Bulletin*, **36**, 48–70.

Drake, R. E. and Bond, G. R. (2008). Supported employment: 1998 to 2008. *Psychiatric Rehabilitation Journal*, **31**, 274–6.

Drake, R.E. and Essock, S.M. (2009). The science to service gap in real world schizophrenia treatment. *Schizophrenia Bulletin*, **35**, 677–8.

Drake, R.E., McHugo, G.J., Bebout, R.R., Becker, D.R., Harris, M., Bond, G.R., *et al.* (1999). A randomized clinical trial of supported employment for inner-city patients with severe mental disorders. *Archives of General Psychiatry*, **56**, 627–33.

Drake, R.E., Essock, S.M., Bond, G.R. (2009). Implementing evidence-based practices for the treatment of schizophrenia patients. *Schizophrenia Bulletin*, **35**, 704–13.

Drake, R.E., Deegan, P., Woltmann, E., Haslett, W., Drake, T., and Rapp, C. (2010). Comprehensive electronic decision support systems. *Psychiatric Services*, **61**, 714–7.

Fixsen, D., Naoom, S., blasé, K., Friedman, R., and Wallace, F. (2009). *Implementation research: a synthesis of the literature*. Tampa, FL: University of South Florida.

Flood, C., Byford, S., Henderson, C., Leese, M., Thornicroft, G., Sutherby, K., *et al.* (2006). Joint crisis plans for people with psychosis: economic evaluation of a randomised controlled trial. *British Medical Journal*, **333**, 729–32.

Friis, S., Larsen, T.K., Melle, I., Opjordsmoen, S., Johannessen, J.O., Haahr, U., *et al.* (2003). Methodological pitfalls in early detection studies – the NAPE Lecture 2002. Nordic Association for Psychiatric Epidemiology. *Acta Psychiatrica Scandinavica*, **107**, 3–9.

Glover, G., Arts, G., and Babu, K.S. (2006). Crisis resolution/home treatment teams and psychiatric admission rates in England. *British Journal of Psychiatry*, **189**, 441–5.

Harrigan, S.M., McGorry, P.D., and Krstev, H. (2003). Does treatment delay in first-episode psychosis really matter?. *Psychological Medicine*, **33**, 97–110.

Henderson, C., Flood, C., Leese, M., Thornicroft, G., Sutherby, K., and Szmukler, G. (2004). Effect of joint crisis plans on use of compulsory treatment in psychiatry: single blind randomised controlled trial. *British Medical Journal*, **329**, 136.

Holloway, F. and Carson, J. (2001). Case management: an update. *International Journal of Social Psychiatry*, **47**, 21–31.

Howard, L., Heslin, M., Leese, M.N., McCrone, P., Rice, C., Jarrett, M., *et al.* (2010). Supported employment: randomised controlled trial. *Br J Psychiatry*, **196** (5), 404–411.

Howard, L.M., Rigon, E., Cole, L., Lawlor, C., and Johnson, S. (2008). Admission to women's crisis houses or to psychiatric wards: women's pathways to admission. *Psychiatric Services*, **59**, 1443–9.

Institute of Medicine (U.S.) (2006). *Committee on Crossing the Quality Chasm: Adaptation to Mental Health and Addictive Disorders). Improving the quality of health care for mental and substance-use conditions*. Washington, DC: National Academy Press.

Johnson, S., Nolan, F., Hoult, J., White, I. R., Bebbington, P., Sandor, A., *et al.* (2005a). Outcomes of crises before and after introduction of a crisis resolution team. *British Journal of Psychiatry*, **187**, 68–75.

Johnson, S., Nolan, F., Pilling, S., Sandor, A., Hoult, J., McKenzie, N., *et al.* (2005b). Randomised controlled trial of acute mental health care by a crisis resolution team: the north Islington crisis study. *British Medical Journal*, **331**, 599.

Johnson, S., Needle, J., Bindman, J., and Thornicroft G. (2008). *Crisis Resolution and Home Treatment in Mental Health*. Cambridge: Cambridge University Press.

Johnson, S., Gilburt, H., Lloyd-Evans, B., Osborn, D.P., Boardman, J., Leese, M., *et al.* (2009). In-patient and residential alternatives to standard acute psychiatric wards in England. *British Journal of Psychiatry*, **194**, 456–63.

Johnstone, P. and Zolese, G. (1999). Systematic review of the effectiveness of planned short hospital stays for mental health care. *British Medical Journal*, **318**, 1387–90.

Joy, C., Adams, C., and Rice, K. (1998). *Crisis intervention for people with severe mental illness. (The Cochrane Library)*. Oxford: Update Software.

Kessler, R.C., Demler, O., Frank, R.G., Olfson, M., Pincus, H.A., Walters, E.E., *et al.* (2005). Prevalence and treatment of mental disorders, 1990 to 2003. *New England Journal of Medicine*, **352**, 2515–23.

Killaspy, H., Dalton, J., McNicholas, S., and Johnson, S. (2000). Drayton Park, an alternative to hospital admission for women in acute mental health crisis. *Psychiatric Bulletin*, **24**, 101–4.

Killaspy, H., Bebbington, P., Blizard, R., Johnson, S., Nolan, F., Pilling, S., *et al.* (2006). The REACT study: randomised evaluation of assertive community treatment in north London. *British Medical Journal*, **332**, 815–20.

Killaspy, H., Kingett, S., Bebbington, P., Blizard, R., Johnson, S., Nolan, F., *et al.* (2009). Randomised evaluation of assertive community treatment: 3-year outcomes. *British Journal of Psychiatry*, **195**, 81–2.

Knapp, M., Beecham, J., Anderson, J., Dayson, D., Leff, J., Margolius, O., *et al.* (1990). The TAPS project. 3: Predicting the community costs of closing psychiatric hospitals. *British Journal of Psychiatry*, **157**, 661–70.

Knapp, M., Chisholm, D., Astin, J., Lelliott, P., and Audini, B. (1997). The cost consequences of changing the hospital-community balance: the mental health residential care study. *Psychological Medicine*, **27**, 681–92.

Kreyenbuhl J., Buchanan R.W., Dickerson F.B., Dixon, L.B. (2009). The schizophrenia patient outcomes research team (PORT): updated treatment recommendations. *Schizophrenia Bulletin*, **36**, 94–103.

Kuipers, E., Holloway, F., Rabe-Hesketh, S., and Tennakoon, L. (2004). An RCT of early intervention in psychosis: Croydon Outreach and Assertive Support Team (COAST). *Social Psychiatry and Psychiatric Epidemiology*, **39**, 358–63.

Larsen, T.K., Friis, S., Haahr, U., Joa, I., Johannessen, J.O., Melle, I., *et al.* (2001). Early detection and intervention in first-episode schizophrenia: a critical review. *Acta Psychiatrica Scandinavica*, **103**, 323–34.

Latimer, E.A. (1999). Economic impacts of assertive community treatment: a review of the literature. *Canadian Journal of Psychiatry*, **44**, 443–54.

Latimer, E.A., Lecomte, T., Becker, D.R., Drake, R.E., Duclos, I., Piat, M., *et al.* (2006). Generalisability of the individual placement and support model of supported employment: results of a Canadian randomised controlled trial. *British Journal of Psychiatry*, **189**, 65–73.

Leff, J. (1997). *Care in the Community. Illusion or Reality?* Wiley, London.

Lehman, A.F., Carpenter, W.T., Jr., Goldman, H.H., and Steinwachs, D.M. (1995). Treatment outcomes in schizophrenia: implications for practice, policy, and research. *Schizophrenia Bulletin*, **21**, 669–75.

Lehman, A.F., Goldberg, R., Dixon, L.B., McNary, S., Postrado, L., Hackman, A., et al. (2002). Improving employment outcomes for persons with severe mental illnesses. *Archives of General Psychiatry*, **59**, 165–72.

Marshall, M., Crowther, R., Almaraz-Serrano, A., Creed, F., Sledge, W., Kluiter, H., *et al.* (2001). Systematic reviews of the effectiveness of day care for people with severe mental disorders: (1) acute day hospital versus admission; (2) vocational rehabilitation; (3) day hospital versus outpatient care. *Health Technology Assessment*, **5**, 1–75.

Marshall, M. and Lockwood, A. 2003). Assertive community treatment for people with severe mental disorders. *Cochrane Database of Systematic Reviews*, **2**, CD001089.

Marshall, M. and Lockwood, A. (2004). Early intervention for psychosis. *Cochrane Database of Systematic Reviews*, **2**, CD004718.

McCrone, P., Killaspy, H., Bebbington, P., Johnson, S., Nolan, F., Pilling, S., *et al.* (2009). The REACT study: cost-effectiveness analysis of assertive community treatment in north London. *Psychiatric Services*, **60**, 908–13.

McGorry, P.D., Nelson, B., Amminger, G.P., Bechdolf, A., Francey, S.M., Berger, G., *et al.* (2009). Intervention in individuals at ultra high risk for psychosis: a review and future directions. *Journal of Clinical Psychiatry*, **70**, 1206–12.

Mojtabai R., Fochtmann L., Chang S., Kotov R., Craig T.J., Bromet, E. (2009). Unmet need for mental health care in schizophrenia: an overview of literature and new data from a first-admission study. *Schizophrenia Bulletin*, **35**, 679–95.

Mosher, L.R. (1999). Soteria and other alternatives to acute psychiatric hospitalization: a personal and professional review. *Journal of Nervous and Mental Disease*, **187**, 142–9.

Mubbashar, M. (1999). Mental health services in rural Pakistan. In: Tansella, M. and Thornicroft, G. (eds.) *Common Mental Disorders in Primary Care*, pp. 67–80. London: Routledge.

Mueser, K.T., Bond, G.R., Drake, R.E., and Resnick, S.G. 1998). Models of community care for severe mental illness: a review of research on case management. *Schizophrenia Bulletin*, **24**, 37–74.

Nathan, P. and Gorman, J. (2002). *A Guide to Treatments that Work*, 2nd edn. Oxford: Oxford University Press.

Njenga, F. (2002). Challenges of balanced care in Africa. *World Psychiatry*, **1**, 96–8.

Petersen, L., Jeppesen, P., Thorup, A., Abel, M.B., Ohlenschlaeger, J., Christensen, T.O., *et al.* (2005). A randomised multicentre trial of integrated versus standard treatment for patients with a first episode of psychotic illness. *British Medical Journal*, **331**, 602.

Phillips, S.D., Burns, B.J., Edgar, E.R., Mueser, K.T., Linkins, K.W., Rosenheck, R.A., *et al.* (2001). Moving assertive community treatment into standard practice. *Psychiatric Services*, **52**, 771–9.

Quirk, A. and Lelliott, P. (2001). What do we know about life on acute psychiatric wards in the UK? A review of the research evidence. *Social Science and Medicine*, **53**, 1565–74.

Raune, D., Kuipers, E., and Bebbington, P.E. (2004). Expressed emotion at first-episode psychosis: investigating a carer appraisal model. *British Journal of Psychiatry*, **184**, 321–6.

Ricciardi, A., McAllister, V., and Dazzan, P. (2008). Is early intervention in psychosis effective?. *Epidemiologica e Psichiatrica Sociale*, **17**, 227–35.

Rose, D. (2001). *Users' Voices, The perspectives of mental health service users on community and hospital care*. London: The Sainsbury Centre.

Rosen, A. and Barfoot, K. (2001). Day care and occupation: structured rehabilitation and recovery programmes and work. In: Thornicroft, G. and Szmukler, G. (eds.) *Textbook of Community Psychiatry*, pp. 296–308. Oxford: Oxford University Press.

Roth, A., Fonagy, P., Parry, G., Target, M., and Woods, R. (2006). *What Works for Whom?* London: Guildford Press.

Saraceno, B., van Ommeren, M., Batniji, R., Cohen, A., Gureje, O., Mahoney, J., *et al.* (2007). Barriers to improvement of mental health services in low-income and middle-income countries. *Lancet*, **370**, 1164–74.

Saxena, S. and Maulik, P. (2003). Mental health services in low and middle income countries: an overview. *Current Opinion in Psychiatry*, **16**, 437–42.

Scott, J. and Lehman, A. (2001). Case management and assertive community treatment. In: Thornicroft, G. and Szmukler, G. (eds.) *Textbook of Community Psychiatry*, pp. 253–64. Oxford: Oxford University Press.

Shepherd, G. and Murray, A. (2001). Residential care. In: Thornicroft, G. and Szmukler, G. (eds.) *Textbook of Community Psychiatry*, pp. 309–320. Oxford: Oxford University Press.

Simmonds, S., Coid, J., Joseph, P., Marriott, S., and Tyrer, P. (2001). Community mental health team management in severe mental illness: a systematic review. *British Journal of Psychiatry*, **178**, 497–502.

Simon, G.E., Fleck, M., Lucas, R., and Bushnell, D.M. (2004). Prevalence and predictors of depression treatment in an international primary care study. *American Journal of Psychiatry*, **161**, 1626–34.

Sledge, W.H., Tebes, J., Rakfeldt, J., Davidson, L., Lyons, L., and Druss, B. (1996). Day hospital/crisis respite care versus inpatient care, Part I: Clinical outcomes. *American Journal of Psychiatry*, **153**, 1065–73.

Social Exclusion Unit (2004). *Mental Health and Social Exclusion*. London: Office of the Deputy Prime Minister.

Sutherby, K. and Szmukler, G. I. (1998). Crisis cards and self-help crisis initiatives. *Psychiatric Bulletin*, **22**, 4–7.

Sutherby, K., Szmukler, G. I., Halpern, A., Alexander, M., Thornicroft, G., Johnson, C., *et al.* (1999). A study of "crisis cards" in a community psychiatric service. *Acta Psychiatrica Scandinavica*, **100**, 56–61.

Szmukler, G. and Holloway, F. (2001). In-patient treatment. In: Thornicroft, G. and Szmukler, G. (eds.) *Textbook of Community Psychiatry*, pp. 321–37. Oxford: Oxford University Press.

Tansella, M. (2006). Recent advances in depression. Where are we going? *Epidemiologia e Psichiatria Sociale*, **15**, 1–3.

Tansella, M., Thornicroft, G., Barbui, C., Cipriani, A., and Saraceno, B. (2006). Seven criteria to improve effectiveness trials in psychiatry. *Psychological Medicine*, **36**, 711–20.

Teague, G.B., Bond, G.R., Drake, R.E. (1998). Program fidelity in assertive community treatment: Development and use of a measure. *American Journal of Orthopsychiatry*, **68**, 216–32.

Thornicroft, G. (1991). The concept of case management for long-term mental illness. *International Review of Psychiatry*, **3**, 125–32.

Thornicroft, G. (2001). *Measuring Mental Health Needs*, 2nd edn. London: Royal College of Psychiatrists, Gaskell.

Thornicroft, G. and Bebbington, P. (1989). Deinstitutionalisation from hospital closure to service development. *British Journal of Psychiatry*, **155**, 739–53.

Thornicroft, G. and Rose, D. (2005). Mental health in Europe. *British Medical Journal*, **330**, 613–614.

Thornicroft, G. and Tansella, M. (2004). Components of a modern mental health service: a pragmatic balance of community and hospital care: overview of systematic evidence. *British Journal of Psychiatry*, **185**, 283–90.

Thornicroft, G. and Tansella, M. (2009). *Better Mental Health Care*. Cambridge: Cambridge University Press.

Thornicroft, G. and Tansella, M. (1999). *The Mental Health Matrix: a Manual to Improve Services*. Cambridge: Cambridge University Press.

Thornicroft, G., Wykes, T., Holloway, F., Johnson, S., and Szmukler, G. (1998). From efficacy to effectiveness in community mental health services. PRiSM Psychosis Study. 10. *British Journal of Psychiatry*, **173**, 423–27.

Thornicroft, G., Becker, T., Holloway, F., Johnson, S., Leese, M., McCrone, P., *et al.* (1999). Community mental health teams: evidence or belief?. *British Journal of Psychiatry*, **175**, 508–13.

Thornicroft, G., Rose, D., Huxley, P., Dale, G., and Wykes, T. (2002). What are the research priorities of mental health service users? *Journal of Mental Health*, **11**, 1–5.

Thornicroft, G., Tansella, M., and Law, A. (2008). Steps, challenges and lessons in developing community mental health care. *World Psychiatry*, **7**, 87–92.

Tomov, T. (2001). Central and Eastern European Countries. In: Thornicroft, G. and Tansella, M. (eds.) *The Mental Health Matrix. A Manual to Improve Services*, pp. 216–27. Cambridge: Cambridge University Press.

Tyrer, P., Evans, K., Gandhi, N., Lamont, A., Harrison-Read, P., and Johnson, T. (1998). Randomised controlled trial of two models of care for discharged psychiatric patients. *British Medical Journal*, **316**, 106–9.

Tyrer, S., Coid, J., Simmonds, S., Joseph, P., and Marriott, S. (2003). Community mental health teams (CMHTs) for people with severe mental illnesses and disordered personality. *Cochrane Database of Systematic Reviews*, **2**, CD000270.

Wang, P.S., Demler, O. Kessler, R.C. (2002). Adequacy of treatment for serious mental illness in the United States. *American Journal of Public Health*, **92**, 92–8.

World Bank (2002). *World Development Report 2002. Building Institutions for Markets*. Washington DC: World Bank.

World Health Organization (2001). *World Health Report 2001. Mental Health: New Understanding, New Hope*. Geneva: World Health Organization.

World Health Organization (2005a). *Mental Health Declaration for Europe*. Copenhagen: World Health Organization.

World Health Organization (2005b). *Mental Health Action Plan for Europe*. Copenhagen: World Health Organization.

Ziguras, S.J. and Stuart, G.W. (2000). A meta-analysis of the effectiveness of mental health case management over 20 years. *Psychiatric Services*, **51**, 1410–21.

Ziguras, S.J., Stuart, G.W., and Jackson, A.C. (2002). Assessing the evidence on case management. *British Journal of Psychiatry*, **181**, 17–21.

CHAPTER 13

Crisis and emergency services

Sonia Johnson, Jonathan Totman, and Lorna Hobbs

Introduction: acute care outside the inpatient unit

Our primary focus in this chapter is people with significant mental illnesses who are experiencing an exacerbation of their mental health or social problems of such severity that they reach the threshold for inpatient admission, or else seem likely very soon to reach this threshold unless pre-emptive action is taken. This is a relatively restrictive definition, excluding, for example, many crisis intervention services that have aimed to optimize the psychological adjustment of people experiencing difficult transitions in their lives. However, a focus on acute care at the threshold of admission is readily justified in economic, pragmatic, and policy terms. From the perspective of service users and carers, easy and prompt access to helpful and acceptable crisis services to help them at the times when they are most distressed is consistently rated as very important, with avoiding inpatient admission whenever possible also often identified as an important priority (Rose, 2001). From an economic and policy point of view, acute care, especially in hospital, consumes a large share of the mental health budget in most countries (Holloway and Sederer, Chapter 19, this volume), making it very desirable that optimal outcomes are achieved as efficiently as possible.

Given these major reasons for regarding acute care as a priority, the evidence base is surprisingly weak. For example, none of the 2009 recommendations of the Schizophrenia Patient Outcomes Research Team (PORT) (Dixon et al., 2010) related to models of acute care delivery, and the National Institute of Health and Clinical Excellence (NICE) guidelines on schizophrenia and bipolar disorder make in relation to acute care only the general recommendations that crisis resolution and home treatment teams should be available. Despite this lack of robust evidence, mental health crises and, in particular, models aimed at diverting people from hospital admission, have been the focus of considerable innovative service development in the past few decades. In this chapter we complement Holloway and Sederer's discussion of inpatient care by reviewing four other main types of care: two aimed mostly at initial triage of people experiencing crises (stand-alone emergency services and emergency department services in the general hospital), one combining assessment and provision of a community alternative to acute admission (crisis resolution and home treatment teams), and one mainly aimed at providing an alternative (community residential crisis services). Acute day care is also excluded from our discussion as it is covered elsewhere, but, as the final section suggests, it should also be seen as a potentially important element in integrated care pathways.

Emergency clinics

An early innovative model for management of mental health crises was the walk-in clinic offering assessment combined with triage and, in some cases, brief treatment to people experiencing mental health crises. In the United States in the 1950s and 1960s, these clinics were closely allied to crisis intervention theory (Caplan, 1964), in which a crisis was regarded not as a manifestation of psychiatric illness but a general human response to severe psychosocial stress, presenting challenges but also opportunities for growth if the crisis was negotiated in an adaptive way. In the heyday of the theory in the 1950s and 1960s in the United States, walk-in crisis clinics proliferated in casualty departments and, later, community mental health centres. Failure to recruit many otherwise mentally healthy individuals to brief crisis interventions, a concern that the needs of the severely mentally ill were not being addressed and funding restrictions contributed to the waning of this model in the United States in the 1970s and 1980s (Goldfinger and Lipton, 1985).

As walk-in crisis intervention services declined in the United States, similar services proliferated in Europe, especially in the Netherlands and German-speaking countries (Häfner, 1977; Katschnig et al, 1993). As in the United States, European services tended not to attract the generally healthy population originally envisaged (Katschnig et al, 1993), and doubts were in any case increasing about the extent to which they, as opposed to the severely mentally ill, were an appropriate target group. Dissatisfaction also grew with the capacity of these services to prevent hospital admission. In Holland, for example, ambulatory mental health services providing walk-in emergency care to a wide range of people were believed to have caused a marked increase in psychiatric admissions during the 1980s (Gersons, 1996).

Following disenchantment with these early walk-in services, this form of service has not generally been in the spotlight again as a significant innovative model, although walk-in facilities continue to be an element of crisis services in many areas. An advantage of such services is in reducing the burden on casualty department mental health services and the need for distressed individuals with mental health problems to wait for attention in these hectic settings (see below). Current mental health policies often advocate access and early intervention as key priorities: a re-examination of the activities and potential value of walk-in mental health facilities would be a useful research focus.

Acute psychiatry in the casualty department/emergency department

While the stand-alone walk-in clinic has declined in prominence as a service model, the general hospital emergency department (ED), also known in the United States as the emergency room and in the United Kingdom as the Accident and Emergency (A&E) or casualty department, has remained a mainstay of emergency psychiatry. Increasing use of EDs by mental health patients has been documented in the United States and Europe, and has been attributed both to reductions in inpatient bed numbers and to lack of other readily accessible treatment settings, making it a default setting for accessing out-of-hours help in particular (e.g. Bruffaerts et al. 2008). Data from hospital audits suggest that a high proportion of patients attending EDs with mental health problems are not in contact with mental health services, even though their problems may be severe (Callaghan et al. 2001).

The rise in presentations by mentally ill people has prompted research into the challenges faced by ED staff and the experiences of service users (Clarke et al. 2007). Based on action research in a London hospital, Crowley (2000) suggests there is a 'clash of cultures' between the ED, with its focus on immediate stabilization, and the needs of psychiatric patients for more individualized care, with time needed to pinpoint the principal issues that need attention. Multiple logistical factors contribute to further delays in assessment and treatment, including: availability of on-call psychiatric liaison staff, communication with other teams, lack of inpatient beds and (in the case of Mental Health Act assessments) legal directives (Crowley, 2000; Henderson et al. 2003). In the hectic environment of the A&E department, where speed and timeliness are central, psychiatric emergencies may be seen as difficult and burdensome. Patients who are uncooperative, aggressive, or very distressed may be especially unacceptable. Further, the casualty department environment may exacerbate problems (Johnson and Baderman, 1995): stigmatizing and punitive attitudes (especially towards repeat attenders following self-harm (Simpson, 2006)), the noisy and hectic environment, and the distressing sights and sounds sometimes experienced may all contribute. Similar findings have been reported in Australia (Broadbent et al. 2004), Canada (Clarke et al. 2007), and the United States (e.g. Allen et al. 2002).

Findings from various countries converge to suggest a general lack of confidence amongst non-psychiatrically trained nurses and doctors in assessing mental health problems (Clarke et al., 2006; Crowley, 2000). This may well be due in part to the constraints imposed by the ED environment itself; indeed, there is evidence that assessments carried out by psychiatrically trained personnel are compromised in this setting (Taggart et al. 2006), and that patients assessed in these settings are more likely to be admitted to hospital than if assessed elsewhere (Cotton et al., 2007).

Given these problems with quality and appropriateness of care in relation to the environment, it is not surprising that many patients with mental health problems find the experience of attending the ED aversive (Clarke et al. 2007). In the United Kingdom, these difficulties may have been exacerbated by Department of Health guidelines advising that all patients attending A&E should be discharged within 4 hours (2001a). Hospitals failing to meet this target incur financial penalties. Henderson et al. (2003) argue that this mandate has particular implications for emergency psychiatry, where assessment and treatment are notoriously time-consuming. Thus a stringent focus on targets may increase casualty staff's impatience with people with mental health problems.

These issues are far from new and methods for addressing them have been developed at several levels within the health care system. The most obvious strategy is to try to avoid assessments in this setting: alternative forms of crisis care that may allow this are discussed below. However, in most areas, hospital A&E departments continue to play a vital role within the mental health care system. Most strategies for service improvement in this setting involve employing specialist psychiatric personnel (Wand and White, 2007). Most frequently this takes the form of a consultation-liaison service, whereby an on-call psychiatrist (and/or other specialist mental health professional) receives referrals from the ED.

In the United Kingdom, provision of consultation-liaison services from mental health professionals varies greatly (Ruddy and House, 2003). A 2008 report by the Academy of Medical Royal Colleges is highly critical of mental health care in the ED, stressing its disparity with physical health care and the urgent need to bring standards in line (Academy of Medical Royal Colleges, 2008). The report calls for the expansion of liaison services, mental health training for ED staff, and national standards for service provision. The Royal College of Psychiatrists (RCP) has also published guidelines on the care of people attending A&E following deliberate self-harm (DSH), one of the top five reasons for emergency hospital admission in the United Kingdom (NICE, 2004). It recommends that all such patients receive psychosocial assessment by a trained member of staff (RCP, 2004). Again, actual service availability may fall short of recommendations. In an audit of DSH presentations to a modern hospital A&E department, Hughes and Kosky (2007) report 'substandard' service provision, particularly around risk assessment and arrangement of aftercare.

In the United States, difficulties in sustaining a network of comprehensive community services in many areas (Allen, 2007) have meant that hospitals have increasingly taken on responsibility for managing psychiatric emergencies, as well as playing a central role in the triage and follow-up of psychiatric admissions (Allen et al. 2002). One response to this has been an upsurge in dedicated psychiatric emergency services (PESs) in general hospitals, returning to some extent to the Emergency Clinic model described above. These services vary in structure and organization but essentially operate on the principle that more effective care is provided by separating, to some degree, physical and mental health services. A 2002 report by the American Psychiatric Association (APA) Task Force on Psychiatric Emergency Services recommends the provision of an independent PES in hospitals with over 3000 visits per year (Allen et al. 2002). The report outlines advantages of a separate PES facility, both for patient care and economic efficiency: 'In a separate space and with appropriate staff, a controlled and supportive milieu can develop despite high levels of disturbance and rapid turnover.' The provision of dedicated and well-staffed PESs in larger hospitals may be a way of reducing the volume of inpatient admissions (Allen et al. 2002). Currier and Allen (2003) documented the increasingly large range of services provided by PESs in major centres, including assessment, diagnosis, treatment initiation and arrangement of aftercare. They emphasize the concomitant need for—and current absence of—guidelines and standards for best practice. Others have also championed the drive towards more elaborate hospital-based PESs. Woo et al. (2007) evaluated the impact of a dedicated PES service on a range of outcome measures. Compared to the previous, consultation-based service, the new PES led to shorter waiting times, improved access to thorough assessment, reduced use of seclusion and fewer absconsions. The independent PES model does, however, have its critics: Wand and White (2007), for example, argue that segregating the mentally and physically ill in this way may increase the likelihood that the physical problems of the mentally ill are not attended to appropriately and may perpetuate the stigma associated with mental illness.

Wand and White (2007) support the increasing utilization by EDs of mental health liaison nurses (MHLNs). This role is now well established in Australia, Canada, and the United Kingdom, though its scope varies between hospital settings (Wand and White, 2007). A growing body of international research suggests numerous benefits of employing MHLNs within the ED, close to the point of triage. Patients may be assessed without the need for initial medical screening and subsequent referral, thereby streamlining mental health care and reducing service delays. Studies evaluating the impact of MHLNs in the ED have reported reduced patient waiting times, improved access to thorough assessment, and (more tentatively) reduced readmission rates (Callaghan et al. 2003; Wand and White, 2007). Medical staff also value the expertise brought to the emergency department by the psychiatric liaison nurse, with the potential for support and education around mental health (Wand and White, 2007).

Clinical practice and working relationships may be further enhanced by direct training and clear practice guidelines (Broadbent et al. 2004; Clarke et al. 2006). Mental health training for ED and ambulance staff is a key mandate in 2004 Department of Health guidelines and has been identified as a priority by the Academy of Royal Colleges (2008). As well as improving patient care, training may help dispel stigma (Hughes and Kosky, 2007). However, some expresses scepticism; Simpson (2006) suggests that for patients who self-harm, a more radical revision of services is needed, perhaps with a more user-led focus.

If the ED is to continue acting as a last resort for those in crisis and an access point into mental health services, it is essential for it to work collaboratively with other organizations. Effective communication is particularly important for the ED, which straddles mental health and acute care trusts and sees such a diverse range of patients. Ensuring better continuity of care is a central aim of United Kingdom health policy (Healthcare Commission, 2008) and a key challenge for acute mental health systems in all countries. Where crisis resolution teams (CRTs) and other forms of community-based crisis assessment and home treatment services are available, the relationship between these services and the ED is crucial for continuity: one potential model is the integration of the CRT and liaison service as in Hackney, East London, where a single acute service incorporating both has operated since 2001 (Nolan and Tang, 2008). Cassar et al. (2002) draw attention to a key consideration regarding the population served by A&E departments, which suggests high quality service provision needs to be maintained in this setting: studies have found that A&E departments see high numbers of young, male, unemployed, and homeless patients. These groups may be less likely to seek help from primary care settings and often have no ongoing contact with mental health services (Cassar et al. 2002), so that their use of this setting may provide the sole opportunity for engaging them with continuing mental health care.

Home-based acute services

Services that provide some combination of acute assessment outside a hospital context and intensive treatment based in patients' homes have been an element in deinstitutionalization from the beginning: terms used to describe them have included crisis resolution team (CRT), intensive home treatment team, crisis assessment and treatment team, and mobile crisis service. The first such service to be widely written about and discussed was that established by Arie Querido in Amsterdam in the 1930s (Querido, 1935). Querido was influenced by ideas about the importance of social environment arising from the mental hygiene movement in the United States in the early 20th century (Salmon, 1916). Responding also to economic pressure during the Depression to save on hospital costs, he instituted a city-wide system of home visiting by a psychiatrist and a social worker whenever a patient was referred for admission. An alternative treatment plan, sometimes involving further home visits, was implemented whenever possible. In the United Kingdom, community visits in crises were instituted in some areas as early as the 1950s, as in the Worthing experiment: initiated in 1956, this involved home visits by a psychiatrist and a social worker to all those referred for acute admission, and was reported to result in falls in admission of 55% and 79% to two local hospitals (Carse et al., 1958).

Very early home-visiting initiatives such as the Worthing experiment tended to form part of a shift throughout a catchment-area's services towards greater community working: they were not distinct specialist teams. In the 1960s and early 1970s, specialist acute community teams with a focus on preventing admissions were established and evaluated in various countries. One of the most extensive of these initiatives was the network of services developed by Paul Polak in Denver, Colorado, in the 1970s (Polak and Kirby, 1976). Polak's innovations included a team which assessed all individuals referred for admission at home and offered 24-hour home treatment whenever feasible, integration of hospital and community treatment teams, and a network of family sponsor homes, in which families were paid to accommodate up to two patients in crisis, supported by the home treatment team

Some of the working practices of current CRTs can be traced back to two services that share the somewhat confusing distinction of being cited in support of two major innovative models: assertive outreach teams (AOTs) and CRTs (see chapter 15). The Training in Community Living service established by Leonard Stein and colleagues in Madison, Wisconsin in the late 1970s (Stein and Test, 1980), and the service established by John Hoult and his colleagues in Sydney in 1979 (Hoult, 1991) resembled current CRTs in recruiting patients at the point of acute admission during a crisis and diverting them wherever possible to home treatment. However, like AOTs and unlike CRTs, the initial Madison and Sydney teams continued to treat people intensively in the community once the initial crisis had resolved, with the long-term goals of improving their stability in the community and their social functioning. Following these initial experiments, Leonard Stein and John Hoult both concluded that the crisis treatment function would be better split off from continuing care, as it seemed to them difficult for a single team to have both functions (Johnson and Thornicroft, 2008a). The subsequent 30 years have seen such specialist services for crisis assessment and intensive home treatment introduced in a variety of settings, ranging from individual model services to nationwide implementations, such as in the United Kingdom and in Norway. In the following we give an overview of these implementations, focusing especially on the United Kingdom experience as so far the most extensive and thoroughly tested version of the model.

Specialist crisis assessment and home treatment teams: the Australian experience

England may lay claim to the most wholesale recent implementation of specialist crisis teams, but Australian pioneers have been responsible for much development of the model, and the Australian history of such services is now relatively long. Following budget cuts, John Hoult's initial Sydney home treatment team was integrated with two existing case management teams, in order to provide an intensive home treatment capacity within these teams. This service continues to this day to provide an assessment and intensive treatment service to people in crisis which is integrated into a community mental health team, a model that presents a significant, though almost unevaluated, alternative to specialist crisis resolution and home treatment teams (Rosen, 1997).

Subsequent policy reviews resulted in the introduction of specialist crisis and home treatment services first in New South Wales in the 1980s, and then in the 1990s in the state of Victoria. Victoria has since 1994 had a relatively prescriptive policy prefiguring the English National Health Service (NHS) modernization in requiring that a particular service configuration be adopted everywhere. This includes so-called crisis assessment and treatment teams (CATTs), which operate 24 hours and serve adults of working age during office hours and the whole population out of hours (Carroll et al., 2001). These teams resemble in most respects the CRT model subsequently introduced throughout England and described below.

The national CRT policy in England

Most early United Kingdom experiments with home-based care in crises involved a service delivered as part of the range of functions of a community mental health team, as in the Worthing Experiment described above. In the 1990s, concern grew that community mental health teams operating in office hours 5 days a week could not offer an effective alternative to admission, and experimentation

with specialist team models of crisis assessment and home treatment began in a few centres, notably Birmingham (Dean et al. 1993). In 1995, John Hoult, recently arrived from Australia, established the Yardley Psychiatric Emergency Team (Minghella et al. 1998). This can be seen as the first full United Kingdom implementation of the crisis resolution (CRT) model, in which Hoult drew on his observations regarding the organizational features associated with greatest effectiveness in Australian teams. The model was replicated in a variety of centres including Bradford and Islington, London.

Early implementations of the CRT model were seen as successful, and, against the background of a perceived 'crisis in acute care' (Appleby, 2003), with unmet demand for inpatient beds and considerable user dissatisfaction with hospital care, CRT introduction was adopted as national policy in the NHS Plan for England (Department of Health, 2000). This and the subsequent Mental Health Policy Implementation Guide (Department of Health, 2001b) mandated the development of 335 CRTs across England. Each was expected to carry a caseload of 20 to 30 at a time, to see around 300 people a year in total, and to be available 24 hours a day, 7 days a week. This policy has resulted in an an extensive change in the national community mental health care system. In 2000, very few areas had CRTs. Now they are available in every Trust in the country, several thousand mental health professionals have migrated into them (Glover and Johnson, 2008), and in 2008/9, the annual expenditure on CRTs was around £239 million (Department of Health, 2009).

Acute home treatment in continental Europe

Until recently, no European country apart from the United Kingdom had adopted specialist crisis teams as a national model, with many countries favouring integration of crisis management and home treatment with continuing care in generic community teams serving small local areas (Katschnig and Konieczna, 1990). However, some teams designated as crisis intervention teams seem to be providing assessment in crisis and subsequent intensive home treatment somewhat resembling the CRT model. For example, four mental health catchment areas in Paris are served by the Equipe Rapide d'Intervention de Crise (ERIC), which operates 24 hours and provides home assessments and interventions lasting up to a month. ERIC resembles CRTs in aiming to assess patients referred for acute admission and to prevent this wherever possible by providing care at home instead (Robin et al., 2001). Another example comes from Austria, where crisis intervention teams that work to a substantial extent in patients' homes and aim to prevent admission have been established in several regions (Haberfellner et al., 1997). Norway is now the second country to follow England in adopting CRTs as national policy, with all areas mandated to establish such services by 2008: ongoing research there will yield a further perspective on the experience of widespread implementation of this model (Gråwe et al., 2005).

Mobile crisis services in North America

Of the earliest evaluated services offering treatment at home rather than in hospital several were in the United States (Langsley et al., 1971; Pasamanick et al. 1964; Polak and Jones, 1973) and one in Canada (Fenton et al., 1979); these pioneering services often do not seem to have been sustained. Since the 1980s, the term mobile crisis service has been used in the United States to describe a very wide range of services in which home visits in crisis are an element (Heath, 2005). At their simplest, these are triage services, often based in general hospital emergency rooms with the role of visiting patients at home when assessment in the emergency room is not feasible to assess whether admission is required or whether some other care plan can be made. Mobile crisis teams in this basic form do not continue management of the crisis, but refer to other services which can undertake this (Allen, 1996). However, some more extended models have been described (Geller et al. 1995, Heath, 2005), where services offer some further home visits before referring on to other services. A shared characteristic of all variants of the mobile crisis service is a lack of published data on their activities and outcomes (Geller et al., 1995).

Principles and practice of crisis resolution and home treatment teams

Thus services combining the functions of crisis assessment and short-term intensive home treatment have been described in various parts of the developed world. A feature of their development is that they have tended to be established by energetic pioneers as a pragmatic response to difficulties they identified in the service systems in which they worked rather than on the basis of a well-defined theoretical model. As well as a view that psychiatric admission is often best avoided both on economic grounds and for patients' well-being, autonomy and good social functioning, core working principles have tended to be that home treatment allows a greater focus on social milieu than is possible in hospital, with services aiming to engage social networks and to address the social triggers and perpetuating factors for crises (Johnson and Needle, 2008).

The relatively loosely defined nature of the model, which might be seen as more a vehicle for delivering care than a distinct form of treatment, accommodates a range of treatment styles and philosophies. However, a substantial consensus supports a set of core organizational characteristics and interventions for CRTs. Box 13.1 summarizes these organizational characteristics. The focus exclusively on severe crises that would otherwise result in admission is seen as crucial if the CRT is to have the resources to divert patients from hospital: these guidelines are influenced by previous experiences of community crisis intervention services that have tended to drift towards mainly recruiting a 'worried well' population who might not otherwise be seen by secondary mental health services (Katschnig and Cooper, 1991). In practice, most CRTs are also likely to be carrying out a certain amount of pre-emptive work, accepting patients who appear very likely to meet the threshold for hospital admission in the very near future unless another highly intensive intervention, such as intensive home treatment by a CRT, is instituted.

A gatekeeping role, with patients admitted to acute beds only if the CRT has assessed and agreed that this is necessary, is important if admissions are to be effectively reduced (Glover et al., 2006). Twenty-four hour availability is also important if severely ill people are to be managed at home, as carers need to be confident that help is available at any time. Keeping a community office open 24 hours a day may, however, be impractical if the volume of night-time work is low: CRTs sometimes base themselves close to the hospital casualty department at night, or staff may be on call from home. A full multidisciplinary team seems desirable if a full range of psychological,

---

Box 13.1 Key organizational characteristics of CRTs

- A multidisciplinary team capable of delivering a full range of emergency psychiatric interventions in the community

- Senior psychiatrists work within the team alongside members of the other main mental health professions

- Target group is people who, in the absence of the CRT, would require admission to an acute hospital bed

- Rapid assessment is offered in the community, with a response within an hour when this is needed

- Intensive home treatment offered rather than hospital admission whenever initial assessment indicates this is feasible

- When patients are admitted, contact maintained and early discharge to home treatment takes place whenever feasible

- Low patient:staff ratios allow visits two or three times daily when required.

- 24-hour availability (though staff may be on call from home during the night)

- For patients already on the caseload of other community services (e.g. community mental health teams), the team works in partnership with these services

- Team approach, with caseload shared between clinicians and at least daily handover meetings for review of patients

- Gatekeeping role: team controls access to all local acute inpatient beds

- Intensive home treatment programme is short term, with most patients discharged to continuing care services (if needed) within 6 weeks.

---

social, and biological perspectives on assessment and interventions is to be available, though in practice some professions (nurses and doctors) seem to be much better represented than others (occupational therapists and psychologists) (Glover and Johnson, 2008). Many of the skills required by CRT staff are in any case specific to the CRT worker role rather than to a specific profession.

Core interventions

Expert consensus and various guidelines on CRTs identify a core range of interventions to be delivered by CRTs, although the details of many of these are not highly specified (Crompton and Daniel, 2007; Department of Health, 2001b; Johnson and Needle, 2008). Box 13.2 summarizes these interventions.

Assessment is necessarily a core task for CRT practitioners: all need to feel confident in assessing and re-assessing risk, suitability for home treatment, symptoms and their response to treatment, substance misuse, social difficulties that may have triggered or be perpetuating the crisis, and psychological and social resources for coping with the crisis. Other core interventions include engaging and supporting social networks, helping address immediate practical difficulties that are an obstacle to recovery, prescribing and managing medication, often key to trying to reduce quickly the severity of initial symptoms and disturbance so that home treatment remains feasible. Beyond these simple but essential activities

Box 13.2 Core CRT interventions

- Comprehensive initial assessment, including risk, symptoms, social circumstances, stressors and relationships, substance use, and physical health status

- Opportunities to talk through current problems with staff, brief interventions aimed at increasing problem-solving abilities, and daily living skills

- Education about mental health problems for patients and social network

- Engagement—intensive attempts to establish a relationship and negotiate a treatment plan which is acceptable to patients

- Symptom management, including starting or adjusting medication

- Medication administered to patients in the community and their adherence encouraged and supervised, twice daily if needed

- Practical help—support with pressing financial, housing, or childcare problems, getting home into a habitable state, obtaining food

- Identification and discussion of potential triggers to the crisis, including difficulties in family and other important relationships. May include 'systems' work

- Discharge planning beginning at an early stage, so that continuing care services are available as soon as the crisis has resolved

of engaging, assessing, monitoring, supporting, educating, and ensuring appropriate medication is received, a standard array of CRT interventions has not been established, and practice is likely to vary depending on the skills, interests and approaches of clinicians and managers in each team. As already discussed, the idea that the antecedents to crises are often social and can more readily be addressed in patients' own homes has been important in the development of CRTs. Many CRTs thus aim to intervene with patients' social networks in some way, identifying and addressing some of these social triggers. Bridgett and Polak (2003a,b) describe a relatively structured approach to social systems intervention, involving the early use of social systems meetings at which problems in the system are identified and the participants encouraged to find solutions. Other forms of intervention that may be useful within CRTs include brief psychological interventions focusing on symptoms or substance use, structured work on relapse prevention or developing crisis plans to be implemented in any future crisis, and interventions focusing on problem solving or medication adherence. More evidence on what interventions and ways of working are most effective within a CRT framework would be very useful.

Current evidence on community-based crisis assessment and home treatment

When CRTs first became national policy in the United Kingdom, they were criticized for their scanty evidence base (Pelosi and Jackson, 2000), derived mainly from older studies in which neither experimental nor control group were very comparable with current models (Johnson and Thornicroft, 2008b). What do we now know about their impact? Some positive findings can be reported. When the model is implemented with relatively high fidelity, including 24-hour cover and gatekeeping, we now have congruent evidence from national bed use data (Glover et al. 2006), naturalistic investigations of the effects of implementing the model within catchment areas (Jethwa et al. 2007; Johnson et al., 2005a; Keown et al. 2007), and a randomized controlled trial (Johnson et al., 2005b) that reductions in numbers of admissions occur. This effect probably relates more to voluntary than compulsory admissions (Furminger and Webber, 2009; Johnson et al., 2005a,b; Keown et al. 2007), and appears to be associated with lower overall healthcare costs (McCrone et al., 2009a,b). Some limited evidence also supports the idea that service users are more satisfied with acute care when CRTs are available, but we do not know what the views of carers are about the current UK model and other outcomes, such as symptoms and social functioning, appear similar after an episode of acute care with or without a CRT (Johnson et al., 2005a,b). The workforce implications of this reorganization of the acute care system are also important: a survey of London CRT staff was reassuring, suggesting fairly good satisfaction and low burnout (Nelson, et al., 2009).

Some reservations about the implementation of the model have also emerged, especially in two recent reports by the National Audit Office (2007) and the Healthcare Commission (2005). Implementation of gatekeeping appears to vary greatly between Trusts, with many admissions taking place without CRT assessment in many trusts, and both ward managers and crisis team leaders still view a significant minority of hospital admissions as unnecessary. Discontinuities of care seem to be occurring at various points in the acute care system, and service users and carers, whilst in the main positive about the possibility of receiving care in their own homes, also report some unsatisfactory experiences of CRT care. These relate especially to relationships to staff, with reports that contacts are fleeting and superficial and too many staff are involved in each episode of care, and to the range of interventions offered, with complaints that these are limited beyond the prescribing and dispensing of medication. There is thus considerable scope for further service development and evaluative research with the aim of attaining and sustaining mature and effective teams that are closely integrated with the remainder of the care system. Getting the model right is important for the NHS if this is to remain the predominant way of delivering acute care in the community. Given its effects on admissions, costs and service user satisfaction, the model is also a promising one for implementation elsewhere in the developed world, making it all the more important to achieve an understanding of how to implement and optimize it.

Community-based crisis residential services

Staying at home during a crisis is preferred by many service users, but not always practical or desirable. The risk of harm to self or others is too great for some patients to be left alone for extended periods of time without supervision. Others may be severely functionally impaired, have no fixed abode, or live in environments that exacerbate their difficulties (e.g. those in abusive relationships). A further impediment to home treatment is that some carers may feel unable to sustain their role in supporting someone at home. Where these difficulties are severe hospital may be indicated: however, where they are available, residential services outside hospital provide a further potential solution to unmet needs for containment, company, or respite.

Residential alternatives have a history spanning many decades, but have yet to become a standard component in catchment area services in any country. This is despite strong advocacy from service user groups and a view that they may provide a recovery environment that is less stigmatizing, coercive, and institutionalized than inpatient hospital care (Howard et al., 2009). Models of residential crisis service provision in the community include freestanding crisis houses, family sponsor homes, and hybrid services in which acute beds are combined with another service type in the community.

Crisis houses

Crisis houses are usually unlocked, stand alone community units that are based in converted residential premises (Davies et al. 1994). They typically serve up to 15 patients at a time. A comprehensive United Kingdom survey carried out as part of the Alternatives Study identified several sub-types of free-standing community residential service (Johnson et al., 2009). Clinical crisis houses included mental health professionals among their staff and overlapped considerably with acute wards in the types of care provided. Crisis team beds were small clusters of beds very closely linked to a CRT, which usually managed the service and controlled admission to the beds. The final group of services identified were non-clinical alternatives, characteristically managed by voluntary sector organizations and aiming to offer a range of interventions significantly different from those provided in hospital, though most services were closely integrated into local catchment area service systems and little evidence of radically different treatment models was found.

In the United States, crisis houses also vary in the degree to which they adhere to conventional clinical practices and staffing patterns, but some more distinctive models, including user-led services, have been described (Greenfield et al., 2008). One of the earlier and more radical crisis house alternatives was Loren Mosher's Soteria service, which operated from 1971 to 1983. The service aimed to manage first- or second-episode psychosis in a crisis house setting with minimal reliance on antipsychotic medication. A small randomized controlled trial suggested similar or better outcomes for Soteria patients as compared to hospitalized patients, including lower subsequent use of antipsychotic medication. Furthermore, 43% of Soteria patients reported being well after 2 years without ever having received medication (Bola and Mosher, 2002). Despite these encouraging results, uptake of the Soteria model has been minimal in the United States, but similar services have been established in Switzerland, Germany, Sweden, Hungary, and Finland (Ciompi et al., 1992).

Other United States crisis house alternatives adhere to more conventional clinical models, and Warner (2010) suggests that this has led in some places to a pressure to establish relatively large facilities that admit compulsorily detained patients and provide a low cost alternative to scarce and expensive acute beds: this may make it difficult to meet the aspiration to provide care that is tranquil and domestic in atmosphere and individualized in character.

Can crisis houses act as a substitute for admission?

Two types of evidence are available regarding the extent to which crisis houses are a true substitute for acute admission. Randomized controlled trial evidence on the extent to which patients referred for acute admission can instead be treated in to a crisis house setting is available from two trials. Fenton et al. (1998) found in such a trial that around two-thirds of patients destined for acute psychiatric hospital wards could be managed in a community residential alternative, with outcomes similar to hospital admission. More recently, Greenfield et al. (2008), also in the United States, compared admission to a consumer-run crisis residential programme with inpatient hospital admission. Their report from the study documents no instances in which patients randomized to the crisis residential programme had to be admitted instead to hospital, but dangerousness to others was a pre-randomization exclusion criterion. Other evidence comes from observational studies comparing crisis residential service and hospital users. In the Alternatives Study (Johnson et al., 2010) similarities outweighed differences in a comparison between users of four community crisis residential services and local acute hospital wards, but users of the community services were more like to be help-seekers, more often already known to mental health services and less likely to pose a risk to others. Qualitative interviews with local managers, clinicians and service users indicated that they saw the roles of community alternatives as distinct but overlapping, with community alternatives able to provide acute care for some, but not all, potential acute inpatients and also to relieve pressure on acute wards through early discharge and by admitting pre-emptively some patients who at a later stage would be likely otherwise to require hospitalization.

Do community residential alternatives have any advantages over acute wards?

As in most areas of acute care, the evidence comparing community residential alternatives with hospitals in terms of outcomes is relatively insubstantial. However, most findings indicate greater service user satisfaction with the community alternatives, accompanied by relatively few differences on other measured outcomes (Fenton et al., 1998; Gilburt et al., 2010; Howard et al., 2010; Lloyd-Evans et al., 2009; Osborn et al., 2010; Slade et al., 2010). Greenfield et al. (2008) are unusual in reporting greater symptomatic improvement as well as greater service satisfaction: the relatively large size of their trial and distinctive consumer-led nature of their model are potential explanations for this. Given the relative equipoise on other outcomes and the advantages in terms of service user acceptability, cost becomes a very important consideration: community residential crisis services vary widely in cost, but are often reported to be less expensive than hospital, especially because of their shorter length of stay (Byford et al., 2010; Greenfield et al., 2008; Warner, 2010). This may help ensure that this continues to be a model of interest, even in straitened economic circumstances, although more robust evidence regarding more clearly defined models is still needed before a definite recommendation can be made as to whether services of this kind should be a standard part of all catchment area mental health service systems.

Family sponsor homes

In family sponsor homes, families are selected and trained to provide short-term crisis accommodation and support (Brook, 1980). Supported by community mental health services, family sponsor homes aim to prevent hospitalization and facilitate community reintegration by offering a safe and normative family environment in which patients can recover from immediate crisis (Brook, 1980). Like crisis houses, family sponsor homes have a long history. However, the model seems currently to be used relatively little. Polak's original Denver acute service network (see above) included family sponsor homes, and a United States survey indicated that family sponsor homes were the most widely available form of residential alternative crisis care during the 1970s (Stroul, 1988). Family sponsor homes have continued to operate in Madison, Wisconsin (Bennet, 1995; Warner, 2010), but there have been no published evaluations of such services in the United States since the original Denver study.

In the United Kingdom, the only published description of such a service is of the Accredited Accommodation Scheme in Powys, Wales (Readhead et al., 2002). Initially, the scheme aimed to provide crisis care, but in practice it was expanded to provide planned periods of respite and rehabilitative social care. The Alternatives Study survey (Johnson et al., 2009) identified no current acute family sponsor home schemes in England. Elsewhere in Europe, Denmark has a long history of placing adults in family care as an alternative to hospitalization. Small naturalistic studies of Danish family sponsor homes, modelled on United States programmes, provide some level of support for their effectiveness in terms of patient/family satisfaction and reductions in readmissions and bed days (Aagaard et al., 2008). Thus despite its long history and the appealing normalization principles on which it is based, the capacity of this form of care to substitute for acute hospital admission remains unknown.

Conclusion: towards an integrated and evidence-based acute care system

The current chapter and Holloway and Sederer's on inpatient services delineate the key components of local acute care systems. Some, like acute inpatient beds and services in the casualty departments, are apparently indispensable and inescapable elements in all areas; others are additional components introduced to achieve better quality of care. Holloway and Sederer describe inpatient care as 'from the research perspective, the Cinderella of contemporary mental health services': this description can readily be extended to acute psychiatry in general. The ethical and practical difficulties of doing research with severely ill individuals at the time of a crisis are considerable (Howard et al., 2009). A lack of clearly defined models of care in this area has both contributed to and been perpetuated by the limited research base. Whereas in other areas of mental health service provision such as assertive community treatment, supported employment and early intervention for psychosis there are theory-driven and clearly defined models of care, with fidelity measures often available to evaluate them, in acute care most approaches to care have been pragmatic and ad hoc. Large variations in service models such as crisis houses, home treatment teams, and indeed acute inpatient wards impede evaluative research.

With regard to service delivery, a strong emphasis in recent policy making in the NHS has been on the concept of integrated care pathways (Healthcare Commission, 2008), guided by a clear vision of which service elements most effectively meet individual patients' needs at each stage in the crisis and characterized by smooth transitions and coordination between components of the service system. Continuity of care is especially crucial within the acute care system as needs must be assessed and the right services mobilized rapidly to support acutely distressed service users and their social networks, while periods of treatment with particular acute services are brief, making it necessary to organize coordination between services and planning of the next stage in the patient's journey very quickly. While most of the relevant literature focuses on single components in the acute care pathway, mechanisms for achieving effective coordination and continuity of care between them need to be major foci for future service planning and research. In this context, models of care that integrate two or more elements in the acute system are of particular interest for their capacity both to enhance continuity and for the synergy that may be achieved between services. For example, models of care integrating home treatment teams with crisis beds (Lloyd-Evans et al. 2009) and with acute day services have been described in the NHS. Such a combination may enhance the capacity of home treatment teams to manage people outside hospital by allowing the needs of people whose homes are an unsuitable setting for treatment or who need activity and social contact outside the home to be met. Crisis residential services may also be integrated with community mental health teams, as in the study described by Boardman et al. (1999), which made a naturalistic comparison between two 24-hour staffed residential units attached to and integrated with community mental health centres and acute hospital wards. This suggested superior symptomatic and social outcomes, a reduction in unmet need, and greater patient satisfaction in patients receiving treatment in the residential units. Thus a goal for further research and service planning in this area is to progress towards an integrated acute care pathway, aiming to establish clearly defined and evidence-based models of care that include mechanisms for maximizing continuity of care. There is no shortage of work still to be done to achieve this.

References

Aagaard, J., Freiesleben, M., and Foldager, L. (2008). Crisis homes for adult psychiatric patients. *Social Psychiatry and Psychiatric Epidemiology*, **43**, 403–9.

Academy of Medical Royal Colleges (2008). Managing urgent mental health needs in the acute trust: a guide by practitioners, for managers and commissioners in England and Wales. London: Academy of Medical Royal Colleges.

Allen, M.H. (1996). Definitive treatment in the psychiatric emergency service. *Psychiatric Quarterly*, **67**, 247–62.

Allen, M.H. (2007). The organization of psychiatric emergency services and related differences in restraint practices. *General Hospital Psychiatry*, **29**, 467–9.

Allen, M., Forster, P., Zealberg, J., and Currier, G. (2002). *Report and recommendations regarding psychiatric emergency services*. Washington, DC: American Psychiatric Association Taskforce on Psychiatric Emergency Services.

Appleby, L. (2003). So, are things getting better? *Psychiatric Bulletin*, **27**, 441–2.

Bennett, R. (1995). The crisis home program of Dane County. In: Warner, R. (ed.) *Alternatives to the Hospital for Acute Psychiatric Treatment*, pp. 213–23, Washington, DC: American Psychiatric Press.

Boardman, A.P., Hodgson, R.E., Lewis, M., *and Allen, K* (1999). North Staffordshire Community Beds Study: longitudinal evaluation of psychiatric in-patient units attached to community mental health centres. I. Methods, outcome and patient satisfaction. *British Journal of Psychiatry*, **175**, 70–8.

Bola, J.R. and Mosher, L.R. (2002). Predicting drug-free treatment response in acute psychosis from the Soteria project. *Schizophrenia Bulletin*, **28**, 559–75.

Bridgett, C. and Polak, P. (2003a). Social systems intervention and crisis resolution. Part 1: Assessment. *Advances in Psychiatric Treatment*, **9**, 424–31.

Bridgett, C. and Polak, P. (2003b). Social systems intervention and crisis resolution. Part 2: Intervention. *Advances in Psychiatric Treatment*, **9**, 432–8.

Broadbent, M., Jarman, H., and Berk, M. (2004). Emergency department mental health triage scales improve outcomes. *Journal of Evaluation in Clinical Practice*, **10**, 57–62.

Brook, B.D. (1980). Community families: A seven-year program perspective. *Journal of Community Psychology*, **8**, 147–51.

Bruffaerts, R., Sabbe, M., and Demyttenaere, K. (2008). Emergency psychiatry in the 21st century: critical issues for the future. *European Journal of Emergency Medicine*, **15**, 276–8.

Byford, S., Sharac, J., Lloyd-Evans, B., Gilburt, H., Osborn, D.P.J., Leese, M., *et al.* (2010) Alternatives to standard acute inpatient care in England: readmissions, service use and costs after discharge. *Accepted by British Journal of Psychiatry*, 197(Suppl. 53), s20–s25.

Callaghan, P., Eales, S., Leigh, L., Smith, A., and Nichols, J. (2001). Characteristics of an Accident and Emergency liaison mental health service in East London. *Journal of Advanced Nursing*, **35**, 812–18.

Callaghan, P., Eales, S., Coates, T., and Bowers, L. (2003). A review of research on the structure, process and outcome of liaison mental health services. *Journal of Psychiatric and Mental Health Nursing*, **10**, 155–65.

Caplan, G. (1964) *Principles of Preventive Psychiatry*. New York: Basic Books.

Carroll, A., Pickworth, J., and Protheroe, D. (2001). Service innovations: An Australian approach to community care-the Northern Crisis Assessment and Treatment Team. *Psychiatric Bulletin*, **25**, 439–41.

Carse, J., Panton, N.E., and Watt, A. (1958). A district mental health service. The Worthing Experiment. Lancet, 39–41.

Cassar, S., Hodgkiss, A., Ramirez, A., and Williams, D. (2002). Mental health presentations to an inner-city accident and emergency department. *Psychiatric Bulletin*, **26**, 134–6.

Ciompi, L., Dauwalder, H.P., Maier, C., Aebi, E., Trutsch K., Kupper Z., *et al.* (1992). The pilot project 'Soteria Berne'. Clinical experiences and results. *British Journal of Psychiatry*, **161**, 145–53.

Clarke, D.E., Brown, A.M., Hughes, L., and Motluk, L. (2006). Education to improve the triage of mental health patients in general hospital emergency departments. *Accident and Emergency Nursing*, **14**, 210–18.

Clarke, D.E., Dusome, D., and Hughes, L. (2007). Emergency department from the mental health client's perspective. *International Journal of Mental Health Nursing*, **16**, 126–31.

Cotton, M.A., Johnson, S., Bindman, J., Sandor, A., White, I.R., Thornicroft, G., *et al.* (2007). An investigation of factors associated with psychiatric hospital admission despite the presence of crisis resolution teams. *BMC Psychiatry*, **7**, 52.

Crompton, N. and Daniel, D. (2007). Guidance statement on fidelity and best practice for crisis services. London: Department of Health/Care Services Improvement Partnership.

Crowley, J.J. (2000). A clash of cultures: A&E and mental health. *Accident and Emergency Nursing*, **8**, 2–8.

Currier, G.W. and Allen, M. (2003). Organization and function of academic psychiatric emergency services. *General Hospital Psychiatry*, **25**, 124–9.

Davies, S., Presilla, B., Strathdee, G., and Thornicroft, G. (1994). Community beds: the future for mental health care? *Social Psychiatry and Psychiatric Epidemiology*, **29**, 241–3.

Dean, C., Phillips, J., Gadd, E., Joseph, M., and England, S. (1993). Comparison of community based service with hospital based service for people with acute, severe psychiatric illness. *British Medical Journal*, **307**, 473–6.

Department of Health (2000). *The NHS Plan*. London: The Stationery Office.

Department of Health. (2001a). *Reforming Emergency Care: First Steps of a New Approach*. London: Department of Health.

Department of Health (2001b). *Crisis Resolution/Home Treatment Teams. The Mental Health Policy Implementation Guide*. London: Department of Health.

Department of Health (2009). *The 2008/09 National survey of Investment in Mental Health Services*. London: Department of Health.

Dixon, L., Dickerson, L. Bellack, A., Bennett., M., Dickinson, W., Goldberg, R.W., *et al.* (2010). The 2010 Schizophrenia PORT Psychosocial Treatment Recommendations and Summary Statements. *Schizophrenia Bulletin*, **36**, 48–70.

Fenton, F.R., Tessier, L., and Struening, E.L. (1979). A comparative trial of home and hospital psychiatric care. One year follow-up. *Archives of General Psychiatry*, **36**, 1073–9.

Fenton, W.S., Mosher, L.R., Herrell, J.M., and Blyler, C.R. (1998). Randomized trial of general hospital and residential alternative care for patients with severe and persistent mental illness. *American Journal of Psychiatry*, **155**, 516–22.

Furminger, E. and Webber, M. (2009). The effect of crisis resolution and home treatment on assessments under the 1983 Mental Health Act: An increased workload for approved social workers? *British Journal of Social Work*, **39**, 901–17.

Geller, J.L., Fisher, W.H., and Mc Dermeit, M. (1995). A national survey of mobile crisis services and their evaluation. *Psychiatric Services*, **46**, 893–7.

Gersons, B.P. (1996). From emergency to social psychiatric service centers; the Amsterdam experience. *European Psychiatry*, **11**, 192.

Gilburt, H., Slade, M., Rose, D., Lloyd-Evans, B., Johnson, S., and Osborn, D.P.J., *et al.* (2010). Service users' experiences of residential alternatives to standard acute wards: qualitative study of similarities and differences. Accepted by *British Journal of Psychiatry* 197(Suppl. 53), s26–s31.

Glover, G., Arts, G., and Babu, K.S. (2006). Crisis resolution/home treatment teams and psychiatric admission rates in England. *British Journal of Psychiatry*, **189**, 441–5.

Glover, G. and Johnson, S. (2008). The crisis resolution team model: recent developments and dissemination. In: Johnson, S., Needle, J., JBindman, J., and Thornicroft, G. (eds) *Crisis Resolution and Home Treatment in Mental Health*, pp. 23–34. Cambridge: Cambridge University Press.

Goldfinger, S.M. and Lipton, F.R. (1985) Emergency psychiatry at the crossroads. *New Directions for Mental Health Services*, **28**, 107–10.

Gråwe, R.W., Ruud, T., and Bjørngaard, H. (2005). Alternative interventions in acute mental health care. *Tidsskrift for Den norske lægeforening*, **125**, 3265–8.

Greenfield, T.K., Stoneking, B.C., Humphreys, K., Sundby, E., and Bond, J. (2008). A randomized trial of a mental health consumer-managed alternative to civil commitment for acute psychiatric crisis. *American Journal of Community Psychology*, **42**, 135–44.

Haberfellner, E.M., Hallermann, G., and Schwarz-Traunmuller, B. (1997). Mobile crisis intervention and emergency psychiatry – Experience over three years. *Psychiatrische Praxis*, **24**, 235–6.

Häfner, H. (1977) Psychiatric crisis intervention – a change in psychiatric organization. Report on developmental trends in the Western European countries and in the USA. *Psychiatria Clinica*, **10**, 27–63.

Healthcare Commission (2005). *Count me in: results of a national census of inpatients in mental health hospitals and facilities in England and Wales*. London: Commission for Healthcare Audit and Inspection.

Healthcare Commission (2008). *The Pathway to Recovery: a review of acute inpatient mental health services*. London: The Healthcare Commission.

Heath, D.S. (2005) *Home Treatment for Acute Mental Disorders*. New York: Brunner-Routledge.

Henderson, M.J., Hicks, A.E., and Hotopf, M.H. (2003). Reforming emergency care: implications for psychiatry. *Psychiatric Bulletin*, **27**, 81–2.

Hoult J. (1991). Home treatment in New South Wales. In: Hall, P., and Brockington, I.F. (eds.) *The Closure of Mental Hospitals*, pp. 107–14. London: Gaskell/Royal College of Psychiatrists.

Howard, L., Flach, C., Leese, M., Byford, S., Killaspy, H., Cole, L., *et al.* (2010). The effectiveness and cost effectiveness of admissions to women's crisis houses compared with traditional psychiatric wards–a pilot patient preference randomized controlled trial. *British Journal of Psychiatry*, **197**(Suppl. 53), s32–40.

Howard, L.M., Leese, M., Byford, S., Killaspy, H., Cole, L., Lawlor, C., *et al.* (2009). Methodological challenges in evaluating the effectiveness of women's crisis houses compared with psychiatric wards. *Journal of Nervous Mental Disorders*, **197**, 722–7.

Hughes, L. and Kosky, N. (2007). Meeting NICE self-harm standards in an accident and emergency department. *Psychiatric Bulletin*, **31**, 255–8.

Jethwa, K., Galappathie, N., and Hewson, P. (2007). Effects of a crisis resolution and home treatment team on in-patient admissions. *Psychiatric Bulletin*, **31**, 170–2.

Johnson, S., and Baderman, H. (1995) Psychiatric emergencies in the casualty department. In: Phelan, M., Strathdee G., and Thornicroft, G. (eds.) Emergency mental Health Services in the Community, pp. 213–32. Cambridge: Cambridge University Press.

Johnson, S., Nolan, F., Hoult, J., White, I.R., Bebbington, P., McKenzie, N., *et al.* (2005a) Outcomes of crises before and after introduction of a crisis resolution team. *British Journal of Psychiatry*, **187**, 68–75.

Johnson, S., Nolan, F., Pilling, S., Sandor, A., Hoult, J., McKenzie, N., *et al.* (2005b) Randomised controlled trial of acute mental health care by a crisis resolution team: the north Islington crisis study. *British Medical Journal*, **331**, 599.

Johnson, S., and Needle, J. (2008). Crisis resolution teams: rationale and core model. In: Johnson, S., Needle, J., JBindman, J., and Thornicroft, G. (eds.) *Crisis Resolution and Home Treatment in Mental Health*, pp. 67–84. Cambridge: Cambridge University Press.

Johnson, S., and Thornicroft, G. (2008a). The development of crisis resolution and home treatment teams. In: Johnson, S., Needle, J., JBindman, J., and Thornicroft, G. (eds.) *Crisis Resolution and Home Treatment in Mental Health*, pp. 9–22. Cambridge: Cambridge University Press.

Johnson, S., and Thornicroft, G. (2008b). The classic home treatment studies. In: Johnson, S., Needle, J., JBindman, J., and Thornicroft, G. (eds.) *Crisis Resolution and Home Treatment in Mental Health*, pp 37–50. Cambridge: Cambridge University Press.

Johnson, S., Gilbert, H., Lloyd-Evans, B. *et al.* (2009). Inpatient and residential alternatives to standard acute wards in England. *British Journal of Psychiatry*, **194**, 456–63.

Johnson, S. Lloyd-Evans, B., Morant, N., Gilburt, G. Shepherd, M. Slade, D., *et al.* (2010). Alternatives to standard acute inpatient care in England: roles and populations served. *British Journal of Psychiatry*, **197**(Suppl. 53), s6–s13.

Katschnig, H., and Cooper, J. (1991). Psychiatric emergency and crisis intervention services. In: Bennett, D.H. and Freeman, H.L. (eds.), *Community psychiatry: the principles*, pp. 517–42. Edinburgh, Churchill Livingstone.

Katschnig, H., and Konieczna, T. (1990). Innovative approaches to delivery of emergency services in Euope. In: Marks, I.M. and Scott, R.L. (eds.), *Mental Health Care Delivery*, pp. 85–103. Cambridge: Cambridge University Press.

Katschnig, H., Konieczna, T., and Cooper, J. (1993) *Emergency psychiatric and crisis intervention services in Europe: a report based on visits to services in seventeen countries*. Geneva: World Health Organization.

Keown, P., Tacchi, M.J., Niemiec, S., and Hughes J. (2007). Changes to mental healthcare for working age adults: impact of a crisis team and an assertive outreach team. *Psychiatric Bulletin*, **31**, 288–92.

Langsley, D. G., Machotka, P., and Flomenhaft, K. (1971). Avoiding mental hospital admission: a follow-up study. *American Journal of Psychiatry*, **127**, 1391–4.

Lloyd-Evans, B., Slade, M., Jagielska, D., and Johnson, S. (2009). Residential alternatives to acute psychiatric hospital admission: systematic review. *British Journal of Psychiatry*, **195**, 109–17.

McCrone, P., Johnson, S., Nolan, F. *et al.* (2009a) Economic evaluation of a crisis resolution service: a randomised controlled trial. *Epidemiologia e Psichiatria Sociale*, **18**, 54–8.

McCrone, P., Johnson, S., Nolan, F. *et al.* (2009b) Impact of a crisis resolution team on service costs in the UK. *Psychiatric Bulletin*, **33**, 17–19.

Minghella, E., Ford, R., Freeman, T., Hoult, J., McGlynn, P., and O'Halloran, P. (1998). *Open All Hours: 24-hour Response for People with Mental Health Emergencies*. London: Sainsbury Centre for Mental Health.

National Audit Office (2007). *Helping People through Mental Health Crisis: the Role of Crisis Resolution and Home Treatment Teams*. London: National Audit Office.

National Institute for Clinical Excellence (NICE). (2004). *Self- Harm: The Short Term Physical and Psychological Management and Secondary Prevention of Self-Harm in Primary and Secondary Care* (Guideline 16). London: National Collaborating Centre for Mental Health.

Nelson, T., Johnson, S., and Bebbington, P. (2009). Satisfaction and burnout among staff of crisis resolution, assertive outreach and community mental health teams. *Social Psychiatry and Psychiatric Epidemiology*, **44**, 541–9.

Nolan, F. and Tang, S. (2008) Early discharge and joint working between CRT and hospital service. In: Johnson, S., Needle, J., Bindman, J., and Thornicroft, G. (eds.) *Crisis Resolution and Home Treatment in Mental Health*, pp. 187–96. Cambridge: Cambridge University Press.

Osborn, D.P.J., Lloyd-Evans, B, Johnson, S., Gilburt, H., Byford, S., Leese, M., *et al.* (2010). Residential alternatives to hospital: a comparison of satisfaction, ward atmosphere and service user experiences. *British Journal of Psychiatry*, **197**(Suppl. 53), s41–s45.

Pasamanick, B., Scarpitti, F. R., Lefton, M., Dinitz, S., Wernet, J. J. and McPheeters, H. (1964). Home versus hospital care for schizophrenics. *Journal of the American Medical Association*, **187**, 177–81.

Pelosi, A.J., and Jackson, G.A. (2000). Home treatment-engimas and fantasies. *British Medical Journal*, **320**, 308–9.

Polak, P. R. and Jones, M. (1973). The psychiatric nonhospital: a model for change. *Community Mental Health Journal*, **9**, 123–32.

Polak, P.R. and Kirby, M.W. (1976). A model to replace psychiatric hospitals. *Journal of Nervous and Mental Disease*, **162**, 13–22.

Querido, A. (1935). Community mental hygiene in the city of Amsterdam. *Mental Hygiene*, **19**, 177–95.

Readhead, C., Henderson, R., Hughes, G., and Nickless, J. (2002). Accredited accommodation: an alternative to inpatient care in rural north Powys. *Psychiatric Bulletin*, **26**, 264–5.

Robin, M., Pochard, F., Ampelas, J. -F., Kannas, S., Bronchard, M., Mauriac, F., *et al.* (2001). Psychiatric emergency and crisis services in France. *Therapie Familiale*, **22**, 153–68.

Rose, D. (2001). *Users' Voices: The Perspectives of Mental Health Service Users on Community and Hospital Care*. London: The Sainsbury Centre for Mental Health.

Rosen, A. (1997). Crisis management in the community. *Medical Journal of Australia*, **167**, 633–8.

Ruddy, R. and House, A. (2003). A standard liaison psychiatry service structure? : A study of the liaison psychiatry services within six strategic health authorities. *Psychiatric Bulletin*, **27**, 457–60.

Royal College of Psychiatrists (2004). *Assessment Following Self-Harm in Adults*. London: Royal College of Psychiatrists.

Salmon, T.W. (1916). Mental Hygiene. In J. Milton and J. Rosenau (eds.), *Preventive Medicine and Hygiene*, pp 331–61. New York: D. Appleton and Co. [*As reprinted in the American Journal of Public Health, 2006, 96:, 1740–2.*]

Simpson, A. (2006). Can mainstream health services provide meaningful care for people who self-harm? A critical reflection. *Journal of Psychiatric and Mental Health Nursing*, **13**, 429–36.

Slade, M. Byford, S. Barrett, B., Lloyd-Evans, B., Osborn, D.P.J., Skinner, R., *et al.* (2010) Alternatives to standard acute inpatient care in England: short term clinical outcomes and cost-effectiveness. *British Journal of Psychiatry*, **197**(Suppl. 53), s14–s19

Stein, L.I., and Test, M.A. (1980). Alternative to mental hospital treatment. Conceptual model, treatment program, and clinical evaluation. *Archives of General Psychiatry*, **37**, 392–7.

Stroul, B.A. (1988). Residential crisis services: a review. *Hospital and Community Psychiatry*, **39**, 1095–9.

Taggart, C., O'Grady, J., Stevenson, M., Hand, E., McClelland, R., and Kelly C. (2006). Accuracy of diagnosis at routine psychiatric assessment in patients presenting to an accident and emergency department. *General Hospital Psychiatry*, **28**, 330–5.

Wand, T. and White, K. (2007). Examining models of mental health service delivery in the emergency department. *Australian and New Zealand Journal of Psychiatry*, **41**, 784–91.

Warner, R. (2010). The roots of hospital alternative care (Editorial). *British Journal of Psychiatry*, **197**(Suppl. 53), s4–s5.

Woo, B.K.P., Chan, V.T., Ghobrial, N., and Sevilla, C.C. (2007). Comparison of two models for delivery of services in psychiatric emergencies. *General Hospital Psychiatry*, **29**, 489–91.

CHAPTER 14

Early interventions for people with psychotic disorders

Paddy Power and Pat McGorry

Introduction

Early intervention (EI) in psychosis has established itself as a cornerstone of service provision in psychosis over the last two decades. It is the latest in a line of key developments in the management of psychotic disorders over the last 60 years, following the introduction of antipsychotic medication, de-institutionalization, community care, and more effective psychosocial interventions. It borrows from principles that have emerged over the last few decades in other areas of medicine, social care, and education. Its focus is on early detection, prevention, and intervention in young people with emerging first-episode psychosis. It has become a social movement in its own right, developing its own national and international associations (e.g. the International Early Psychosis Association: http://www.iepa.org.au) World Health Organization-endorsed principles (Bertolote and McGorry, 2005), and attracting considerable political, media, and community support.

This explosion of interest in EI over the past two decades has prompted governments in many developed countries to adopt the EI model, with some promoting it as a top priority for mental health service planning (Appleby, 2009). Countries such as United Kingdom, Canada, Australia, and New Zealand have committed to national roll-outs of these services. This has been further supported by recent economic evaluations highlighting the substantial health savings involved (McCrone et al., 2008; Mihalopoulos et al., 2009).

The field is now moving into other forms of serious mental illness, not only in conditions typically affecting young people but even into old age psychiatry (Naismith et al., 2009). However, questions remain regarding the long-term benefits of a focus on early intervention (Bertelsen et al., 2008; Craig, 2003; Gafoor et al., 2010; Pelosi, 2009) and there is much to discover about the true extent of its merits. There is still uncertainty about the ideal model. EI services wrestle with the dilemma of whether they are for all age groups or specifically for young people, whether they are extensions of child and adolescent mental health services, or young adult services, or both, whether they are limited to non-affective psychoses or all forms of serious mental illness, and whether they are best provided independently of generic services or embedded as subcomponents of these services.

What is the aim of EI?

The aim of EI is not only to focus on early detection, intervention, and prevention at an age when people are most likely to develop psychosis, but also on maintaining this approach throughout the 'critical period' of the first 2 to 3 years of recovery from a first episode (Birchwood et al., 1998). The peak age of onset is in late adolescence and early adulthood (Kessler et al., 2005). Putting more appropriate resources into this early phase of illness will not only ameliorate and prevent unnecessary suffering but it will also maximize the chances of a full recovery, minimize the risk of relapse, thereby reducing the overall burden and costs for individuals, families, and society (McCrone et al., 2008; Mihalopoulos et al., 2009).

Why does EI in psychosis matter?

There is now a substantial body of evidence highlighting the damaging delays that individuals with first-episode psychosis routinely experience in accessing help and treatment (mean duration of untreated illness of 2–3 years). These delays significantly reduce the potential for the illness to respond to treatment as well as patients' capacity to return to normal functioning (Marshall et al., 2009; Perkins et al., 2005). This is made all the more imperative because these disorders typically develop when people are beginning to establish their own independence and consolidate their educational, social, and vocational trajectories. Prolonged periods of illness have a capacity to seriously disrupt and dislocate individuals from these developmental trajectories making it very difficult to regain their premorbid functioning even if treatment is effective. The high rates of suicide (approximately 1% per year during the first 5 years) and depression attest to the extent of suffering individuals experience in their early years of illness (Power and Robinson, 2009).

At a neurobiological level, there is evidence to suggest that neuronal connectivity and glial cell function may be disrupted in a dynamic way during the emergence of psychosis, compromising the brain's 'information processing' systems and leading to restricted cognitive capacity and functioning (McGlashan, 2006). Associated changes in brain structure and volume emerge early and reach a plateau within several years of onset (Cahn et al., 2002; Ho et al., 2003; Velakoulis et al., 1999). A similar plateau is reached as symptoms and cognitive deficits become entrenched. The earlier one intervenes the greater the potential to reverse this process. Antipsychotic medication and psychosocial interventions may operate by extinguishing the 'chemical firestorm' of psychosis and allowing a return to the normal processes of neuronal plasticity and connectivity. Through relearning and reconnectivity, a gradual return to normal functioning can be achieved (McGlashan, 2006). Neuroprotective strategies may ultimately have an important role to play in future therapeutics (Berger et al., 2003).

What do EI services look like?

Although there is a rich amount of variation, most EI services are clinic-based and composed of specialist community-based multidisciplinary mental health teams focusing on young adults with emerging first-episode psychosis (Pinfold et al., 2007). A small number of EI services also provide specialist youth-focused hospital services. Individual EI teams generally cater for relatively large catchment areas (e.g. greater than 250,000 population), encouraging new referrals and providing the mainstay of community mental health services needed over the first 2 to 3 years of follow-up. Staff-to-patient ratios are typically relatively high (e.g. 1:15) so more time can be given to home-based psychosocial interventions and assertive follow-up. At the end of this 'critical period', those making a good recovery return to primary care while those requiring ongoing mental health follow-up are transferred to generic services. EI has an established tradition since it emerged in the early 1990s of close ties with research and evaluation, hence there is now a strong evidence base supporting EI in psychosis (McGorry et al., 2010).

Who are these EI services for?

Most EI services focus on emerging adults presenting with a first episode of psychosis, and many include adolescents as young as 14 or 15 years, the age from which the incidence of first-episode psychosis begins to rise rapidly (Edwards and McGorry, 2002; Pinfold et al., 2007). A minority of services also include clients at ultra-high risk (UHR) of psychosis (see below). Virtually all EI services target those with non-affective psychoses (schizophrenia, schizoaffective disorder, schizophreniform psychosis, brief psychotic episodes, delusional disorders), most include affective psychoses (manic psychosis, depressive psychosis), some include organic psychoses, and few will include reactive psychosis (e.g. post-traumatic stress disorder) or psychoses complicating personality disorders (Fig. 14.1 describes the diagnostic distribution).

Psychotic disorders affect about 3% of the population and have an annual inception rate of just over 1 in 3000 (Reay et al., 2010). Most psychotic disorders emerge between the mid-teens and late twenties (Kessler et al., 2005) during a critical phase of neurobiological and psychosocial maturation when the accumulating effects of predisposing and precipitating factors (such as genetics, brain maturation,

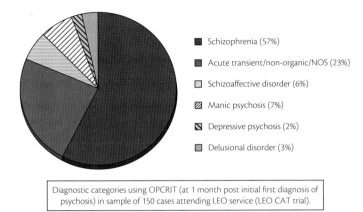

- ■ Schizophrenia (57%)
- ■ Acute transient/non-organic/NOS (23%)
- ▨ Schizoaffective disorder (6%)
- ▨ Manic psychosis (7%)
- ▨ Depressive psychosis (2%)
- ▨ Delusional disorder (3%)

Diagnostic categories using OPCRIT (at 1 month post initial first diagnosis of psychosis) in sample of 150 cases attending LEO service (LEO CAT trial).

Fig. 14.1 ICD 10 Diagnostic distribution in first episode psychosis population aged 16 to 35 years.

drugs, stress) come to a head. Almost a half of all first-episode psychosis presentations to mental health services are 16 to 35-years-olds (Reay et al., 2010). At this stage in life, psychosis is twice as common in males (Power et al. 1998) and this is reflected in EI team caseloads (Pinfold et al., 2007; Power et al., 2007b). Non-affective psychosis accounts for about two,thirds of presentations in this age group (Power et al., 1998, Reay et al., 2010). Affective disorder accounts for about a fifth and the rest include a rather diverse collection of relatively rare conditions including organic psychoses etc. In the developing world organic factors (e.g. AIDS and other illnesses) contribute to a much greater proportion (Mbewe et al., 2006).

In older adult populations of first-episode psychosis, aged 36 to 65 years old, psychotic depression becomes the most common disorder (Reay et al., 2010). A further peak in psychosis emerges later in life in the over 65-year-olds with the aging brain and the involutional phase of life when dementia, physical illnesses, depression, alcohol-related psychoses (accounting for 54%, 15%, 12%, 6% respectively), become much more prevalent than schizophrenia spectrum disorders (4%) (Reimann and Hafner, 1973). In these late-onset populations, the gender disparity seen in younger populations is reversed, even in the schizophrenia-like psychoses (Reeves et al., 2002).

What actually is first-episode psychosis?

The rather broad inclusion of disorders under the rubric of 'psychosis' begs the question what exactly is 'psychosis'? Traditionally, 'psychosis' is defined as a syndrome characterized by either hallucinations, delusions, or thought disorder. However, as these are ubiquitous experiences even in normal healthy adult populations they would generally only be considered pathological when they become persistent, severe, distressing, or disabling. In simple terms, they might be viewed along a continuum with 'normality' in much the same way as one might view depression, anxiety, and a host of other syndromes. Psychotic disorders might be at one extreme of that continuum and the UHR group might be one stage earlier with attenuated or fleeting features of psychosis and comorbid depression and anxiety features (Fig. 14.2).

However, defining when psychotic experiences actually become pathological is a rather more dynamic and challenging process, particularly when one considers that the subjective appraisal and reaction of an individual and his/her social milieu plays a significant role in whether the experiences become distressing or disabling.

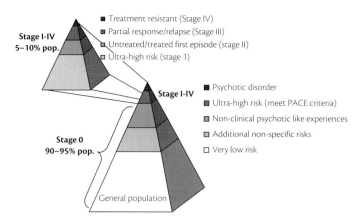

Fig. 14.2 General population risk of psychosis and clinical staging I–IV.

For some individuals such experiences might even be experienced as life-affirming. In certain cultural or social settings transient psychotic experiences are actively sought as a rite of passage or experimentation deliberately induced by mind-altering substances or sensory stimulation/deprivation

Large surveys reveal that almost a fifth of the general adult population admit to lifetime experiences of psychotic symptoms (van Os et al., 2001), with about 5% population having such experiences in the last year (Johns et al., 2004). When clinically assessed, only about 1.5% to 2% actually meet clinical criteria for a 'psychotic disorder'. For those that do not, there are interesting correlations with age, gender, ethnicity, IQ, urbanicity, victimization, recent stress, substance use, and 'neurotic disorders' (Johns et al., 2004). Follow-up identifies them to be at higher risk of emerging psychotic disorders (Krabbendam et al., 2005). Nonetheless, despite the apparent 'normality' of fleeting psychotic experiences, there is good evidence that their presence indicates a heightened risk of subsequent psychotic as well as other disorders. Subgroups within the general population appear to be at greater risk when exposed to additional factors (stress, drugs, mood changes) which can precipitate into a disabling and persistent psychotic disorder. Hence these psychotic-like experiences can be genuinely viewed as warning signs of future mental disorder, either psychotic or otherwise. While there are undoubtedly some who will never require or even be adversely affected by treatment, others will gain the most benefit from interventions at this early stage.

Until the 1990s, there have been few, if any, consistent diagnostic definitions of when someone has crossed the boundary from the prodromal phase to full-threshold psychosis (Breitborde et al., 2009). This posed a considerable dilemma in the past for practitioners working in early psychosis, not only when faced with trying to detect who is actually at highest risk but also knowing when to start treatments and, if refused, when legal compulsions might be warranted.

For the purposes of early intervention services an internationally agreed definition has been pragmatically derived to define the point at which a psychotic prodrome ends and an **'acute psychotic episode'** begins. This point of 'transition to psychosis' is based on the upper cut-off of the CAARMS measure, designed to assess 'at risk mental states' (Yung et al., 2005). In approximate terms this is when someone has experienced unremitting frank psychotic symptoms for more than a week. Prior to this 'transition' point, the evidence suggests that the condition is more likely than not to either remit spontaneously or fail to progress (Yung et al., 2009). It is also the point when one would routinely advise antipsychotic

medication and might begin to consider compulsory treatment if the risks were high. Researchers in the United States have modified this definition of the 'transition' slightly and extended the duration criterion to one month of persistent and severe psychotic symptoms (Woods et al., 2009).

However, this definition of an acute psychotic episode still does not sit particularly well with our international diagnostic criteria e.g. a Brief Psychotic Episode (ICD 10) requires 2 weeks' duration (World Health Organization, 1992). A manic or depressive episode with psychosis accepts any duration of psychosis, however fleeting. Earlier stages of the emerging psychoses e.g. the 'at risk mental state' are also not well covered by existing international diagnostic systems, though DSM V may address this by including a set of criteria for the 'psychosis risk syndrome' (Carpenter, 2009; Miller and Holden, 2010). Furthermore, the presence alone of psychotic symptoms does not provide a wholly satisfactory set of criteria for 'psychotic disorder' either. It is limited to the functional realms of perception, cognitive appraisal, and verbal expression. It takes no account of disturbances of mood, motor, and executive functions that are also central to acute psychotic episodes e.g. catatonia, affective disturbances, negative symptoms and cognitive deficits.

Distinguishing the type of first-episode psychosis

Once a **'psychotic episode'** is confirmed, the question remains what kind of psychosis is the person experiencing? In EI, the approach to diagnosis challenges the traditional and deterministic views of psychotic disorders such 'schizophrenia' and opens the doors to a better understanding of the gene-environment interactions underpinning the onset and course of the illness (McGorry et al., 2006). No longer is a simplistic dichotomy made between schizophrenia, brief psychotic episodes, drug-induced psychosis, and stress-induced psychosis. Substance use and stress are seen as just one of many predisposing and precipitating environmental factors that interact in a dynamic way with other underlying genetic or developmental vulnerabilities to precipitate an episode of psychosis in much the same way as cigarette smoking, stress, and diet might contribute with other underlying risk factors that 'cause' a heart attack. The severity of the episode depends largely on the interaction of these factors as well as well as how quickly the condition is caught. The essential treatment of psychoses remains the same except in adjusting for stage of illness (see stages below) and mood. If any diagnostic distinction is to be made, it is between the affective, non-affective, and organic psychoses. The others (e.g. drugs, stress) are viewed as complicating comorbidities with the potential to worsen prognosis rather than reasons for withholding treatment. Recent evidence of the higher rates of relapse of psychosis with first-episode patients with substance use disorders (Jonnson et al., 2004) confirms this view.

The clinical staging model of psychosis

To overcome some of the above difficulties, a clinical staging model for psychosis has been developed, similar in principle to the staging categories for cancers and other medical illnesses (McGorry et al., 2006). This allows for more appropriate assessment of the levels of uncertainty regarding diagnosis in the early stages and for a more suitable range of interventions to be introduced at different stages in the illness.

As in other medical conditions, there is an explicit assumption that a certain percentage of individuals will naturally progress from a more benign stage to a more severe stage of illness if untreated. The effectiveness of treatments/interventions at different stages can be measured by their ability to reduce this percentage or by the numbers needing treatment in order to prevent one progression to the next stage. In recent years major advances have been made in identifying who will progress or who will benefit most from treatments at different stages. Nonetheless, prognostic indicators at the individual level remain crude and there is still considerable scope for refinement using biomarkers and other measures of prognosis.

How can the stages be identified and what is their prognosis?

Stage 0: asymptomatic at-risk group

Unfortunately, as yet there are no accurate 'universal' screening tools for identifying who is most likely to develop psychosis within the asymptomatic general population. At the individual level, genetic vulnerability is clearly one of the most important predisposing risks (Weinberger and Berger 2009). However, the interactive effects of developmental and environmental factors play a major role (Barnett and Jones, 2008; Van Os and Poulton, 2009). Highlighting this is the fact that only a fifth of individuals with psychosis report an affected first-degree relative (Faridi et al., 2009). Accurately attributing risk to all these factors in any individual remains a considerable challenge and the dangers of falsely attributing risk are very high. However, non-invasive preventative strategies for those with two first-degree relatives with psychosis may have some merit given the transition rate is about 10% over a 10-year period (Johnstone et al., 2005). Improving mental health literacy and education about drug use would be recommended.

At a group level, certain populations are at much greater risk of psychosis. 'Hot spots' of psychosis exist in inner city areas, particularly in neighbourhoods with high levels of social disintegration (Kirkbride et al., 2007; Boydell and McKenzie, 2008). This appears to be partially independent of culture and ethnicity and possibly limited to the non-affective psychoses. Again at a public health level, it may be possible to reduce the risk of psychosis by targeting high risk subgroups but the danger of large numbers being stigmatized may outweigh the benefits.

Stage 1a: mild symptomatic (non-specific) group

This includes mild subclinical populations with mild or non-specific symptoms including neurocognitive deficits or mild functional decline. The likelihood of spontaneous remission is high and only a small proportion progress to the next stage of illness. Interventions at this stage should be benign and non-specific, e.g. information, support, and general counselling services, etc.

Stage 1b: UHR group with subthreshold/prodromal symptoms

It is now possible to specify the degree of predictive accuracy of UHR criteria to between 20% and 60% (i.e. the percentage of individuals that will develop psychosis within 1 year of being assessed) (Yung et al., 2009). There are now several well-developed assessment and case-finding tools that include the CAARMS (Yung et al., 2005), SIPS and SOPS (Miller et al., 2003), and SPIA (Gross 1989). The former expand the mild-end psychosis ratings of the BPRS (Overall and Gorham, 1962) and CASH (Andreasen, 1987) together with trait risk factors, while the Basic Symptoms criteria rely on a broad scatter of symptoms and neurocognitive features, dividing the prodrome into early and late stages.

The UHR group can be identified by the PACE criteria using the CAARMS (Yung et al., 2005). In summary, this describes a clinical population of young people (aged 14–30) with one or more of the following features: 1) attenuated positive psychotic features in the last year, 2) brief limited intermittent psychotic symptoms (self-remitting psychotic symptoms lasting less than a week), and 3) trait and state risk factor group (schizotypal personality disorder or first-degree relative with psychosis) plus a significant deterioration in functioning (greater than 30 point drop in GAF score) in the last year. On average, between 20% and 40% of young clinical populations with these 'at risk mental state' characteristics will progress to a frank psychotic disorder within 12 months, if untreated (Yung et al., 2009). Interventions are discussed in the treatment section later in this chapter.

Stage 2: clinical populations who have made the transition to psychosis

For clinical populations presenting with suspected first-episode psychosis, the accuracy of clinical acumen in recognizing psychosis is much better though still limited. At the primary health care level, general practitioners (GPs) will recognize and refer about 50% of first-episode psychosis patients presenting to them with untreated first episode psychosis. With specific GP education training this proportion can be increased to 80% (Power et al., 2007a). Still, about 15% of people with schizophrenia in developed countries are never detected or treated by health services even though some might be known to social services and homeless agencies (Link and Dohrenwend, 1980). These figures are higher (up to a half of cases of schizophrenia are never treated) in developing countries (Padmavathi et al., 1998; Kurihara et al., 2005). At the next level of secondary care, detection of psychosis by mental health clinicians is much closer to 100% but engagement in treatment still falls well short of this, with at least 10% failing to engage even in well-resourced early detection teams (Power et al., 2007a). For those that do engage, initial diagnostic dilemmas are common and changes in diagnosis (even to non-psychotic disorders) are not unusual. For this reason, clinicians generally limit diagnostic distinctions to 'affective' and 'non-affective' psychosis rather than more specific diagnostic categories such as schizophrenia waiting then until the diagnosis becomes clearer during follow-up.

Once individuals with psychosis engage in treatment with antipsychotic medication, the prospect of remission from the first episode is good. About 60% of first-episode patients will achieve full remission from psychosis within the first 18 months of follow-up and another 30% will achieve partial remission (Craig et al., 2004). Treatment resistance is relatively uncommon in the first episode and affects about 10% of first-episode populations (Huber and Lambert, 2009). Factors that predict a good response to treatment include female gender, later age of illness onset, good pre-morbid functioning, short duration of untreated psychosis (DUP), absence of abnormalities on magnetic resonance imaging, and adherence to medication (Addington et al., 2009; Lieberman et al., 2003).

Stage 3: incomplete/partial remission and relapse

As noted earlier, about 40% of patients will only achieve partial or no remission with treatment. Even for those who do remit completely, about two-thirds will relapse within 5 years with traditional interventions, giving an overall rate of relapse of 80% for all first-episode patients (Robinson et al., 1999). Few (16%) relapse within the first year and the majority (60%) relapse between the end of the first year and the third year. Up to 80% of patients who relapse will relapse again during the first 5 years of follow-up. Remission is generally slower and less complete with each relapse. Predictors of relapse include non-adherence to treatment, poor pre-morbid functioning, long DUP, substance use, stress, life events, and high expressed emotion (Gleeson et al., 2009; Robinson et al., 1999). Relapse rates are significantly lower for those attending EI services (Craig et al., 2004).

Stage 4: severe, persistent unremitting illness

Less than 10% of patients are treatment-resistant within the first year. However, with each subsequent relapse, resistance rates accumulate so that by the fifth year most patients with non-affective psychosis end up with persistent psychotic symptoms. This suggests that in the initial years psychotic disorders are usually episodic and for most patients only becoming enduring after several relapses. One of the cornerstones of good long-term treatment therefore is sustaining initial recovery and preventing relapse in the critical initial years of follow-up.

Duration of untreated psychosis and delays in the pathways to care

One of the central concepts in EI is the duration of untreated psychosis (DUP). It is essentially the time from the onset of psychosis to the start of evidence-based treatment (Marshall et al., 2009).

The mean DUP in most first-episode psychosis populations is 1 year and the median 3 months. If the prodrome is included, then the mean duration of untreated illness (DUI) is 3 years. These periods are a measure of the delays in accessing treatment and can be viewed as the sum of the delays in the steps in the pathways to care (Fig. 14.3).

Intervening to reduce these delays in one of the core aims of EI. Depending on the extent of delay in each step in the 'pathways to care' certain interventions (e.g. public health campaigns, GP education, early detection teams) will be more effective in impacting on these delays and therefore the overall DUP/DUI (Power et al., 2007a).

Interventions and services

Health education programmes

The goal in health education is to raise awareness and understanding of what constitutes psychosis and to facilitate prompt access to appropriate services. These campaigns can be targeted at different tiers in the pathways to care starting with the general population, school-based programmes, non-health professionals, health professionals, and mental health professionals. Such health education programmes do need to be carefully designed for the specific needs of their audience in order to maximize the potential for appropriate referrals.

One of the drawbacks of broad generalist campaigns is their potential to generate a high proportion of inappropriate referrals from the general public (as high as 8:1) (Johannessen et al., 2005). However, they have the benefit of encouraging referrals early in the pathways to care and thereby a greater potential to impact on the overall DUP. On the other hand, specialist campaigns targeting health professionals generate far fewer inappropriate referrals to mental health services (less than 2:1) but because they intervene in the final steps in the pathways to care their capacity to impact on the overall DUP is quite limited (Power et al., 2007a).

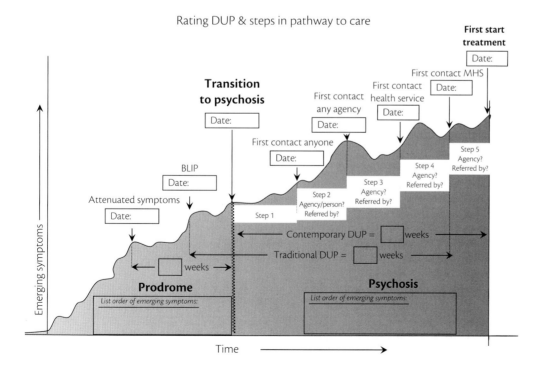

Fig. 14.3 Duration of untreated psychosis and steps in the pathways to care.

One of the most well-evaluated public health campaigns is the TIPS (Early Identification and Treatment of Psychosis) programme in Norway (Johannessen et al., 2005). This included TV, cinema, and newspaper advertisements highlighting the early signs of psychosis and encouraging affected individuals to contact a local early intervention service. The TIPS programme evaluation revealed a significantly shorter DUP (median 5 weeks) in the area with the campaign compared with the comparison area (median DUP 16 weeks) as well as significantly lower symptom ratings (Melle et al., 2004). However, it was not clear where in the pathway to care the campaign had most impact and to what extent the receiving early intervention service made a difference.

Several other campaigns have been evaluated showing varying degrees of impact. Public health education programmes include Compass Melbourne (Wright et al., 2006), PEPP in London, Ontario (http://www.pepp.ca), and EPIP in Singapore (http://www.epip.org.sg). Primary care training programmes include OASIS & LEO CAT (Power et al., 2007b) in south London, England, and DETECT in Dublin, Ireland (http://www.detect.ie).

Improving the accessibility and appeal of 'front end' mental health services

Mapping local pathways to care for first-episode patients is a very revealing exercise and helps expose the common barriers to assessment and treatment for first-episode populations. Some of these barriers can be easily remedied by simple promotion of front-end services and better linkage with referrers such as education, primary care, social services, correctional services, etc. Others are more complicated and steeped in cultural obstacles and prejudices. One of the common obstacles is the perception by communities of front end mental health clinics. This can be partially addressed by relatively simple investment into the visual appeal and reception of these clinics or locating them in primary health care settings or youth-friendly facilities. Providing extended hours services and capacity for outreach assessments can also go a long way to minimizing the risk of contact with traditional emergency services, police, and hospital. However, it is essential that these front-end services are well resourced with properly trained clinicians experienced in the complex subtleties and risks of presentations of patients with early psychosis.

Some interesting examples include:

Youth health clinics

A national programme of youth mental health clinics (headspace) has been in operation in all states in Australia since 2006 (http://www.headspace.org.au). These 30 centres combine health, mental health, and social and vocational services under the same roof and allow rapid access internally to young people aged 12 to 25 years requiring specialist assessments by specially trained mental health staff located within the clinic. The clinics are located in shopping precincts, high streets, near schools, or areas traditionally occupied by primary health centres. These centres are an integral part of broader EI and youth services and one of a range of entry options into these services. Similar initiatives are being developed in Ireland (http://www.headstrong.ie) and England (http://wheres-your-head-at.org).

Early detection and assessment teams

These specialist mental health EI teams combine local health promotion with rapid access to specialist mental health assessment.

Some target the UHR group alone on the basis that combining them with the FEP group might risk prejudicing the UHR group and inappropriately mix them with established cases. In practice, UHR clinics only manage to attract a minority of those truly at risk and have a significant false positive rate of 60–80% (Yung et al., 2009). Most other detection teams specifically target the FEP population alone (e.g. DETECT, Ireland) while others work alongside UHR detection teams (e.g. LEO CAT. London). Finally, most EI services combine the UHR and FEP group with more generalist crisis assessment and home-based treatment teams. This typically results in major challenges in triaging and fast-tracking of potential early psychosis cases.

First-episode inpatient units

Dedicated first-episode units are relatively rare but there are a few notable examples designed to cater for young people with first-episode psychosis (Craig and Power, 2010). They include the EPPIC Unit (originally opened in 1984), the LEO unit in south London, England (opened in 2001), and the Early Psychosis Unit in Toronto, to name a few. It is surprising that there are not more, given that most first-episode patients require hospitalization and these units are generally no more expensive to operate than generic acute wards. What is particularly concerning is that general adult wards are likely to fall well short in meeting the needs of young people presenting for the first time and that accommodating them in these wards can be very traumatizing in itself.

First-episode units incorporate facilities and programmes designed for young people with psychosis and their families. Ideally, they include intensive care areas within their units so that any acutely disturbed patients can be cared for by the same team rather than transferred out to an adult psychiatric intensive care unit for extended periods. The emphasis of these units is to provide specialist comprehensive assessments, containment of risk, collaborative engagement in treatments, and promotion of hope and recovery. These units are usually closely integrated with local community-based EI teams, providing continuity of care throughout the hospitalization process and post-discharge.

As yet, there have been virtually no evaluations of these units (Craig and Power, 2010). However, early evidence suggests that use of mental health detention and intensive care is relatively low, that low-dose antipsychotic medication is the norm, and the numbers of serious untoward incidents are low (Power and McGorry, 2008).

Initial assessment, formulation, diagnosis, and initial treatment plan

Regardless of location, rapid access to comprehensive mental health assessment is critical for EI. This forms the basis of a clinical formulation and collaborative development of an individually tailored package of interventions with the patient and their carers. Ideally, incorporating elements of an adolescent assessment is preferable with its developmental perspective, involvement of families, and agencies such as education for collateral information. Biopsychosocial assessments can be greatly enhanced by including a life-story or developmental timeline from both the patient and his or her family, understanding the quality and extent of personal psychosocial development and emotional maturity as well as the onset and course of the illness, tying in pivotal life events along the way (see Fig. 14.4). It is vital to elicit risk behaviours at this early

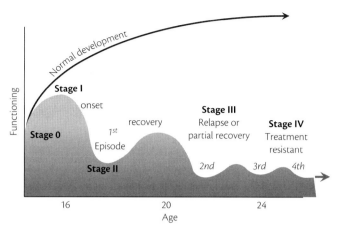

Fig. 14.4 Developmental timelines/trajectories and clinical staging of psychosis.

Table 14.1 Standard list of investigations during initial assessment

Type of test	Test
Routine bloods	Haemotology Erythrocyte sedimentation rate Liver function tests Urea & electrolytes Thyroid function test Serum calcium & phosphate Fasting blood glucose Fasting lipid profile
Blood tests if indicated	Prolactin Autoantibody screen Hepatitis screen HIV
Urine	Drug screen Pregnancy test
Imaging and neurophysiology	Electrocardiogram MRI or CT scan
Extra tests if indicated	Electroencephalogram Lumbar puncture

stage given the high prevalence of suicidality and aggression during the first episode. This should include more general risk behaviours typically seen in this age group, especially risk behaviours which might contribute to psychosis or impede engagement and recovery.

The initial screening and assessment can be best undertaken by specially trained clinicians who have an affinity and understanding both of young people and families as well as a comfort and empathy with people who are experiencing psychosis. Core details include: 1) the onset, nature, course, severity, and duration of the prodrome and psychosis, 2) aggravating and precipitating factors, e.g. stress and drugs, 3) protective factors, 4) preliminary responses to any treatments, 5) underlying and pre-existing vulnerabilities, 6) level of maturity, personality, coping skills, and extent of premorbid functioning, 7) presence of comorbidities, 8) the patient's reaction and degree of distress, disturbance, dysfunction and risk behaviours, 9) understanding, extent of help sought, and willingness to engage in treatment, 10) responsibilities e.g. parenting, work, etc., 11) understanding, reactions, and needs of significant others e.g. parents, siblings, partners, friends, work colleagues etc., and 12) the level and type of services available.

Once first-episode psychosis patients have been identified it is essential to undertake a complete psychiatric medical assessment, including a physical examination and biological investigations (see Table 14.1), so that an initial diagnostic and risk formulation can be completed. Investigations should also provide a baseline for future reference for medication side effects such as the metabolic syndrome etc. Broader assessments should also provide a baseline for future reference, e.g. 1) premorbid and current lifestyle/ health factors such as diet, weight, sleep, exercise, daily routine, 2) premorbid neurodevelopmental problems and degree of current neurocognitive deficits, 3) extent of personal psychological, emotional and social development including vocational/educational/ social/recreational activities, 4) lifetime goals and aspirations, 5) the potential psychological and social impact of the illness, 6) the potential for risk such as disengagement, neglect, exploitation, suicide and violence. Families should always be interviewed as early as possible to obtain collateral details, provide explanations, communicate risk, and assess needs.

The assessment should routinely involve a prompt evaluation by the responsible consultant psychiatrist, ideally before the diagnosis is given to the patient and his or her family and a treatment plan

agreed upon. If undertaken in a sensitive and collaborative manner it is surprising how many patients and carers will engage well with treatment even if their understanding of psychosis is limited (in the LEO CAT study 147 out of 150 cases commenced on antipsychotic medication). Many will already suspect the diagnosis and will need time to work through their fears and be reassured about the prospects for recovery. Counselling about treatment options and recovery should be provided in a hopeful manner with anticipated time course, obstacles, and expected outcomes over the 1 to 2 years of follow-up. Advice about the duration treatment and follow-up is important to outline at this early stage as patients will hold on to one's 'promises' later. The risk of relapse should be highlighted and it is also important to be frank and honest about the prognosis with and without treatment.

Patients and carers benefit greatly from a personalized orientation to services with an explanation of the interventions and roles of different health professionals on the team. Information resources (pamphlets, websites, staff photo charts, information evenings, etc.) enhance the professional standing of the service and encourage respect for the involvement of clients and carers. Additional resources can then be targeted for the remaining patients or carers with special needs or difficulties.

Interventions in the ultra high risk (UHR) group

This area remains controversial partly because of unease about defining the boundaries of what constitutes a 'need for care' on the one hand, and when specific interventions are warranted (e.g. antipsychotic medication) on the other. One thing is clear, people who meet the UHR criteria and are help-seeking have a demonstrable need for clinical care. Typically they present with distress, impaired functioning (GAF scores in the 50s) and generally meet criteria for non-psychotic mental disorders, typically blends of anxiety and depression. So the key issue is what to offer in treatment, not whether to treat. Clearly one needs to treat what is already manifest on its merits. This may in itself reduce the risks of persistence or progression to more severe clinical states, including psychosis. In addition, there is a legitimate role in this group for research trials that focus on preventing progression or the evolution of the clinical phenotype of psychosis. Here treatments effective in more advanced psychosis such as low dose antipsychotics, cognitive behavioural therapy (CBT), and potentially neuroprotective interventions may have a place depending on risk-benefit considerations and patient preference.

Several placebo randomized control trials (in patients meeting the PACE criteria for UHR) highlight the benefit of low dose antipsychotic medications in the context of comprehensive psychosocial care in the short term (McGlashan et al., 2006; McGorry et al., 2002; Phillips et al., 2007). Transition rates to psychosis were significantly lower (e.g. 10%) in the samples randomized to medication compared to placebo (e.g. 35%). However, there is still considerable debate about the ethics, and drop-out and refusal rates are high with antipsychotic medication. Also, once medication was withdrawn, the rates of transition returned to levels seen in the placebo group. Estimates suggest that four UHR patients would need to be treated in order to prevent one from developing psychosis (McGorry et al., 2002). While this indicates a potent therapeutic effect, the adverse effects of antipsychotic medications and the availability of more benign alternatives at this stage mean that antipsychotic medication should be withheld until the person has developed sustained psychosis above the threshold for 'transition to psychosis' or at least until either there has been a failure to respond to simpler interventions or a worsening of the clinical risk. A recent placebo-controlled randomized controlled trial (n = 80) of the omega 3 fatty acid eicosapentanoic acid (EPA) in an UHR group demonstrated a significantly lower transition rate (2.6% vs. 21%, p = 0.028), comparable with that seen in response to antipsychotic medication. In contrast to antipsychotics, the benefit seen with EPA was maintained throughout the 12-month follow-up period, well beyond the 12-week treatment phase (Amminger et al., 2010). EPA is less effective in later stages of psychosis perhaps illustrating the clinical staging principle outlined above.

In keeping with this idea, psychological interventions such as CBT appear to have their own independent benefits and should be offered as first line. In the EDIE trial (n = 58) patients randomized to CBT were significantly less likely to progress to psychosis (6% vs. 26%, p <0.05) and symptom scores improved at 12 months (p <0.02) (Morrison et al., 2004). Drop-out rates were also much lower than with the above medication trials. Therefore, sequential use of CBT followed by adding medication for non-responders may be the best strategy. Alternatively, it is possible that the situation is analogous to the best practice guidelines recommended in depression, i.e. that pharmacotherapy and psychological interventions have independent benefits, that combined therapy is best in the short term and that the addition of psychological interventions provides more sustained benefits in the long term (International Early Psychosis Writing Group, 2005).

Interventions in the first episode of psychosis

Pharmacotherapy

Treatment guidelines in first-episode psychosis recommend antipsychotic medication as soon as a diagnosis of an acute episode of psychosis is confirmed. Ideally, the choice of antipsychotic medication should be based on patient preference, determined by the side-effect profile. A recent meta-analysis confirms that there is virtually no significant difference between the efficacy of the first-generation and second-generation antipsychotics (FGAs and SGAs) in the first episode (Crossley et al., 2010). However, there are clear differences in side-effect profiles: the main difference being neurological/extrapyramidal side effects with the FGAs versus metabolic factors with some of the SGAs. Certain SGAs (risperidone and olanzapine) may protect against grey matter changes commonly seen in the emerging first episode (Girgis et al., 2006; Lieberman et al., 2005). Low-dose risperidone is also more effective than haloperidol in preventing relapse (Schooler et al., 2005). For these reasons the SGAs are preferable in most cases (Kahn et al., 2008).

Young patients and their carers need plenty of opportunity to talk through these pros and cons before starting medication. They are particularly prone to extrapyramidal side effects at standard doses, especially with FGAs (Kahn et al., 2008). This commonly leads to non-compliance (Fleischhacker et al., 2003) so low doses are preferable. Low doses (e.g. risperidone 2 mg/day) are effective and safe in the majority of first-episode patients (McGorry et al., 2011; Merlo et al., 2002). The advice is to 'start low and go slow' increasing every 2 to 3 weeks if no therapeutic response is seen. If no response is seen after the third increment, the medication should be switched to another atypical agent starting at a mid-range dose and increasing also if no response is seen. In cases of treatment resistance by the fourth month, serious consideration should be given to clozapine once a formal multidisciplinary team case review has addressed all contributing factors (Fig. 14.5). Benzodiazepines are recommended in the short-term for anxiety, agitation and insomnia. Given the recent benefits observed with the omega-3 fatty acids in the UHR there is no good reason why EPA should not be offered as a supplement in the first episode. Indeed, two studies have shown it to be partially effective in recent-onset psychosis (Emsley et al., 2002; Berger et al., 2007).

If the episode is primarily affective then the advice is to promptly add a mood stabilizer in acute manic psychosis and an antidepressant in acute depressive psychosis to the above antipsychotic regimen unless the psychotic features are very mild and fleeting. Doses of mood stabilizers and antidepressants need to be titrated up to relatively high doses given that affective psychosis represents the more severe end of the affective spectrum. Doses of antimanic

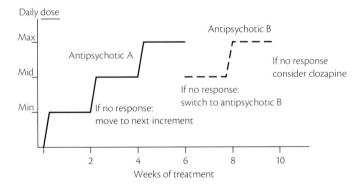

Fig. 14.5 Antipsychotic medication regimen in first episode psychosis. In depressive psychosis: add antidepressant at start and titrate upwards until response. In manic psychosis: add mood stabilizer at start and titrate upwards to antimanic dose.

agents and antidepressants need to be adjusted downwards after the acute episode to prophylactic levels to minimize the risk of side effects during the recovery. Though lithium is the gold standard, valproate is usually preferred because of its tolerability, particularly in atypical manic presentations. However, both should be used with caution in female patients given their teratogenic effects. Folate should be routinely prescribed with valproate.

Unfortunately, there are no clear guidelines about the duration of treatment after the first episode. Standard practice in uncomplicated non-affective psychosis is to continue antipsychotic medication for at least a year after remission though some EI services routinely advise 18 months or longer. It is important to remember that relapse is most likely to occur between the first and third years of follow-up and that perhaps a longer period of prophylaxis would be far more protective (Chen et al., 2008: Wunderink et al., 2007). This is particularly important in those with adverse prognostic indicators (e.g. family history, younger age of onset, long DUP, etc.) or high levels of risk behaviours when unwell.

For typical affective psychoses, common practice is to gradually withdraw the antipsychotic several months after remission but to continue the mood stabilizer or antidepressant for a minimum of 18 months depending on the duration of the history.

Psychological interventions

There is now a wealth of modularized CBT and psychosocial packages, catering for different aspects of the first episode and comorbidities. Ideally, all first-episode patients should be offered individual sessions. However, timing is crucial as many patients are not able to benefit from formal sessions until they have recovered sufficiently from the acute episode. Initial sessions during the acute episode are best tailored towards engagement, support, and psychoeducation, withholding more formal CBT interventions until the individual can make more rational appraisals of their psychotic experiences (Jackson et al., 2005, 2008). Interventions for comorbid conditions such as anxiety, depression, and suicidality, and drug use may be just as legitimate but in contrast to CBT in other disorders, longer courses of therapy may be appropriate (Haddock and Lewis, 2005; Penn et al., 2005).

Some interventions do not require formal training in CBT and should be provided as a matter of routine by all clinicians involved in patient care. Relapse prevention counselling is one such intervention requiring limited extra training and resources. This assists patients to develop their own early warning signs/relapse signatures and care plans to manage relapses (Gleeson, 2005; Gleeson et al., 2009).

Unfortunately, results have been disappointing from the limited number of trial of psychological interventions in first episode psychosis. The large SoCRATES trial did demonstrate some significant advantages with CBT over routine care and supportive therapy but at only 5 weeks, the intervention was very brief (Lewis et al., 2002). Other trials of interventions such as COPE (facilitating adjustment after the first episode) (Jackson et al., 2005), ACE (active cognitive therapy for early psychosis) (Jackson et al., 2008), LifeSPAN (addressing suicidality during the first episode) (Power et al., 2003), CAP (cannabis and psychosis) (Edwards et al., 2006), and relapse prevention therapy (the Prevention of Relapse in Psychosis trial; http://www.controlled-trials.com/ISRCTN83557988) so far have yielded limited findings. At this stage the evidence in favour of family interventions is stronger.

Family interventions

The needs of carers are often overlooked during the first episode despite the high levels of stress and burden reported. Even minimal attention to their needs and an explanation by professionals can have a major impact on relieving carers' uncertainties and supporting the often fragile fractured relationships induced by the illness. Being dependent on carers again at an age when young individuals would be expected to be increasingly independent can be a source of extreme tension and frustration for all concerned. High expressed emotion is well known to influence outcome and for some families formal family work is essential. Most families, however, manage with limited need for formal family interventions and most services limit this to psychoeducation sessions and regular care planning sessions (McNab and Linszen, 2009).

Vocational/educational/psychosocial interventions

As many patients with first-episode psychosis are already disadvantaged by both their pre-morbid circumstances and the effects of the illness on their education and work histories, vocational strategies can go a long way to reversing this and rebuilding self-esteem and resilience. Recovery-style group interventions with a focus on healthy living, lifestyle issues, diet, stress management, parenting, and recreational activities all have their place. Individual Placement and Support (IPS), not just with work but also education, appears to be the most appropriate and effective approach with young first-episode patients (Killackey et al., 2008, 2009). It is also adaptable to different socio-political settings and appears to have better outcomes than other models of vocational rehabilitation.

Discharge and long-term follow-up

Most EI services are time limited to 3 years as a maximum, some even as short as 18 months. Adequate time needs to be given to preparing patients for discharge, equipping them and their carers with the knowledge that they need to carry with them into the future about their condition, its treatment, and how to minimize the risk of relapse. This should include advice about genetic counselling, childbirth, and practical advice about what to say to future health professionals, prospective employers, insurers, partners, and friends. Patients should be given copies of service discharge summaries with their relapse prevention plans and recommendations for future management. These recommendations and risks should be made explicit at formal handovers to follow-up services.

At the end of EI service provision, about 40% of cases i.e. those in 'stages 1–2' (see above) and in remission can be followed up by primary care alone (Power et al., 2007b). However, for the rest (stages 3–4) ongoing follow-up with mental health services would be advisable.

Long-term outcomes

Though there is consistent evidence that outcomes during EI services contact are significantly better than those obtained in standard services, this differential effect does not appear to be sustained after leaving EI services when assessed at the 5-year point. This raises the question of whether EI services should be continued for longer, e.g. 5 years, or up to a certain age. Perhaps this should be the case for some patients but it may not be necessary for all. The difficulty at the moment is that prognostic indicators are still quite crude, poorly validated, and untested in differentiating who might or might not benefit from EI interventions beyond the traditional 2 to 3 years of follow-up. Regardless of whether this is possible, it's clear that the patients fair better when in EI services than in generic services.

Models of EI services

There are at least eight main service components in EI services: health/community education and links, early detection and assessment, UHR interventions, acute inpatient care, acute home-based treatment, recovery psychosocial interventions, relapse prevention strategies, and service evaluation/research/training/promotion. What is fascinating about the evolution of different models of EI services is that no one service is exactly the same and there is a considerable degree of individual innovation to local circumstances (Table 14.2). In England, most are stand-alone specialist community mental health teams with case manager caseloads of 15 and medical case loads of 80 supported by additional psychology,

Table 14.2 Useful sources of further information

Type	Source
Associations	International (http://www.iepa.org.au) United Kingdom (http://www.iris-initiative. co.uk)
United Kingdom EI Networks	First Episode Research Network (http:// www.frenonline.org) London EI Research & Services Networks
Fact sheets	http://www.mentalhealthfirstaid.csip.org. uk/~earlydetection/factsheets/ http://www.orygen.org.au
Patient Booklets	Compton, M. and Broussard, B. (2009). *The First Episode of Psychosis: A Guide for Patients and Their Families.* Oxford: Oxford University Press.
Textbooks	Aitchison, K., Meehan, K., and Murray, R. (eds.) (1999). *First Episode Psychosis.* London: Martin Dunitz. Birchwood, M., Fowler, D., and Jackson, C. (2004). *Early Intervention in Psychosis: A Guide to Concepts, Evidence and Interventions.* Chichester: John Wiley & Sons. Edwards, J. and McGorry, P. (eds.) (2002). *Implementing Early Intervention in Psychosis: A Guide to Establishing early intervention services.* London: Martin Dunitz. French, P., Smith, J., Shiers, D., Reed, M., and Rayne, M. (eds.) (2010). *Promoting Recovery in Early Psychosis: A Practice Manual.* Oxford: Blackwell Publishing. Jackson, H. and McGorry, P.D. (eds.) (2009). *The Recognition and Management of Early Psychosis: A Preventative Approach,* Cambridge: Cambridge University Press.
Journal	*Early Intervention in Psychiatry*

family and vocational input. Case loads vary widely in other countries with ratios of up to 50:1 in some EI services. To some extent higher caseloads are appropriate if certain functions are acquired by other teams, e.g. Early Detection and Crisis Assessment or Home Treatment teams, leaving the EI team with a focus on specific components of EI. Conversely, some EI teams do not case manage at all and provide purely supplementary psychosocial interventions on the back of generic teams. There are very few comparisons of these interesting variations in EI service provision, despite the cost differentials involved. One such study is near completion in Camden and Islington, London.

The future of EI services

EI services are now an integral part of many national mental health strategies even in countries where resources are traditionally very limited. EI has proven its worth in the short-term despite its critics. It has captured the imagination and sustained enthusiasm of health service managers, clinicians, academics, and community agencies. It well received by young people, their families, and referrers. There is now clear evidence of better outcomes with EI and that it is more cost-effective that generic care. EI has successfully driven reform and extra investment in mental health care. There is no legitimate premise to support 'late intervention' with older models of care. However, as with any new emerging model, EI is a work in progress and there are a number of challenges to be faced. This includes overcoming the obstacles of providing EI to older adults (Reay et al., 2010) and whether EI can be sustained over the longer term. In the area of early detection, there is the prospect soon of discovering biomarkers and more refined clinical measures that can better differentiate a person's risk of progression and treatment responses at different stages of psychosis. For other disorders in psychiatry, there is the opportunity to extend the EI concept. As in medicine generally, the principle is almost certain to be equally applicable to most if not all domains of mental health care where persistent and disabling disorders may develop. Meeting these challenges will be a test of the capacity of mental health reform and EI in particular in the years to come.

The field of early intervention has already moved beyond the realm of psychosis into other areas of mental health (Insel, 2007). Its vision of providing **personalized**, **participatory**, **pre-emptive** and **predictive** care echoes developments in other fields of medicine. New models of youth mental health with these principles as their premise are rapidly establishing themselves in a number of countries (Australia, Ireland, Canada, and England). They provide an exciting new challenge to mental health care and, given the extent of morbidity in our youth population, one to which a response is long overdue.

References

Addington, J., Lambert, T., and Burnett, P. (2009). Complete and incomplete recovery from first-episode psychosis. In: Jackson, H. and McGorry, P.D. (eds.) *The Recognition and Management of Early Psychosis: A Preventative Approach*, pp. 201–21. Cambridge: Cambridge University Press.

Amminger, G.P., Schafer, M.R., Papageorgiou, K., Klier, C.M., Cotton, S.M., Harrigan, S.M., *et al.* (2010). Long-chain omega-3 fatty acids for indicated prevention of psychotic disorders: a randomized, placebo-controlled trial. *Archives of General Psychiatry*, **67**, 146–54.

Andreasen, N. (1987). *The Comprehensive Assessment of Symptoms and History (CASH) Interview.* Iowa City, IA: The University of Iowa.

Appleby, L. (2009). *Executive summary. New Horizons: Towards a shared vision for mental health.* London: Department of Health.

Barnett, J. and Jones, P. (2008). Genes and the social environment. In: Morgan, C., McKenzie, K., and Fearon, P. (eds.) *Society and Psychosis*, pp. 58–74. Cambridge: Cambridge University Press.

Berger, G.E., Proffitt, T.M., McConchie, M., Yuen, H., Wood, S.J., Amminger, G.P., *et al.* (2007). Ethyl-eicosapentaenoic acid in first-episode psychosis: a randomized, placebo-controlled trial. *Journal of Clinical Psychiatry*, **68**, 1867–75.

Berger, G.E., Wood, S., and McGorry, P.D. (2003). Incipient neurovulnerability and neuroprotection in early psychosis. *Psychopharmacology Bulletin*, **37**, 79–101.

Bertelsen, M., Jeppesen, P., Petersen, L., Thorup, A., Ohlenschlaeger, J., le Quach, P., *et al.* (2008). Five-year follow-up of a randomized multicenter trial of intensive early intervention vs standard treatment for patients with a first episode of psychotic illness: the OPUS trial. *Archives of General Psychiatry*, **65**, 762–71.

Bertolote, J. and McGorry, P. (2005). Early intervention and recovery for young people with early psychosis: consensus statement. *British Journal of Psychiatry, 187(Suppl. 48)*, s116–119.

Birchwood, M., Todd, P., and Jackson, C. (1998). Early intervention in psychosis. The critical period hypothesis. *British Journal of Psychiatry*, **172**(Suppl. 33), s53–s59.

Boydell, J. and McKenzie, K. (2008). Society, place and space. In: Morgan, C., McKenzie, K., and Fearon, P. (eds.) *Society and Psychosis*, pp. 78–94. Cambridge: Cambridge University Press.

Breitborde, N.J.K., Srihari, V.H., and Wood, S.W. (2009). Review of the operational definition for first-episode psychosis. *Early Interven Psychiatry*, **3**, 259–65.

Cahn, W., Hulshoff Pol, H.E., Lems, E.B., van Haren, N.E., Schnack, H.G., van der Linden, J.A., *et al.* (2002). Brain volume changes in first-episode schizophrenia: a 1-year follow-up study. *Archives of General Psychiatry*, **59**, 1002–10.

Carpenter, W.T. (2009). Anticipating DSM-V: should psychosis risk become a diagnostic class? *Schizophrenia Bulletin*, **35**, 841–3.

Chen, Y.H., Hui, L.M., Lam, M., Law, C.W., Chiu, P.Y., Chung, W.S., *et al.* (2008). A double-blind randomized placebo-controlled relapse prevention study in remitted first-episode psychosis patients following one year of maintenance therapy. *European Journal of Psychiatry, 23*, S107–S108.

Craig, T.K. (2003). A step too soon or a step too far? *Journal of Mental Health*, **12**, 335–59.

Craig, T.K., Garety, P., Power, P., Rahaman, N., Colbert, S., Fornells-Ambrojo, M., *et al.* (2004). The Lambeth Early Onset (LEO) Team: randomised controlled trial of the effectiveness of specialised care for early psychosis. *British Medical Journal*, **329**, 1067.

Craig, T.K. and Power, P. (2010). In patient provision in psychosis. In: French, P., Shiers, D., Smith, J., Reed, M., and Rayne, M. (eds.) Promoting Recovery in Early Psychosis: A practical manual.

Crossley, N., Constante, M., Power, P., and McGuire, P. (2010). Efficacy of atypical v. typical antipsychotics in the treatment of early psychosis: meta-analysis. *British Journal of Psychiatry*, **196**, 434–9.

Edwards, J., Elkins, K., Hinton, M., Harrigan, S.M., Donovan, K., Athanasopoulos, O., *et al.* (2006). Randomized controlled trial of a cannabis-focused intervention for young people with first-episode psychosis. *Acta Psychiatrica Scandinavica* **114**, 109–117.

Edwards, J. and McGorry, P.D. (2002). *Implementing Early Intervention in Psychosis: A Guide to Establishing Early Psychosis Services.* London: Martin Dunitz.

Emsley, R., Myburgh, C., Oosthuizen, P., and van Rensburg, S.J. (2002). Randomized, placebo-controlled study of ethyl-eicosapentaenoic acid as supplemental treatment in schizophrenia. *American Journal of Psychiatry*, **159**, 1596–8.

Faridi, K., Pawliuk, N., King, S., Joober, R., Malla, A.K. (2009). Prevalence of psychotic and non-psychotic disorders in relatives of patients with a first episode psychosis. *Schizophrenia Research*, **114**, 57–63.

Fleischhacker, W.W., Oehl, M.A., and Hummer, M. (2003). Factors influencing compliance in schizophrenia patients. *Journal of Clinical Psychiatry*, **64**(Suppl. 16), 10–13.

Gafoor, R., Nitsch, D., McCrone, P., Craig, T., Garety, P., Power, P., and McGuire, P. (2010). Effect of early intervention on 5 year outcome in non-affective psychosis. *British Journal of Psychiatry, in* **196**, 372–6.

Girgis, R.R., Diwadkar, V.A., Nutche, J.J., Sweeney, J.A., Keshavan, M.S., and Hardan, A.Y. (2006). Risperidone in first-episode psychosis: a longitudinal, exploratory voxel-based morphometric study. *Schizophrenia Research*, **82**, 89–94.

Gleeson, J. (2005). Preventing EPISODE II: relapse prevention in first-episode psychosis. *Australas Psychiatry*, **13**, 384–7.

Gleeson, J., Linszen, D., and Wiersma, D. (2009). Relapse prevention in early psychosis. In: Jackson, H. and McGorry, P.D. (eds.) *The Recognition and Management of Early Psychosis: A Preventative Approach*, pp. 349–64. Cambridge: Cambridge University Press.

Gross, G. (1989). The 'basic' symptoms of schizophrenia. *British Journal of Psychiatry*, 155(Suppl. 7), s21–s25; discussion 37–40.

Haddock, G. and Lewis, S. (2005). Psychological interventions in early psychosis. *Schizophrenia Bulletin*, **31**, 697–704.

Ho, B.C., Andreasen, N.C., Nopoulos, P., Arndt, S., Magnotta, V., and Flaum, M. (2003). Progressive structural brain abnormalities and their relationship to clinical outcome: a longitudinal magnetic resonance imaging study early in schizophrenia. *Archives of General Psychiatry*, **60**, 585–94.

Huber, C.G. and Lambert, M. (2009). Treatment resistance in first-episode psychosis. In: Jackson, H. and McGorry, P.D. (eds.) *The Recognition and Management of Early Psychosis: A Preventative Approach*, pp. 365–81. Cambridge: Cambridge University Press.

Insel, T.R. (2007). The arrival of pre-emptive psychiatry. *Early Intervention in Psychiatry*, **1**, 5–6.

International Early Psychosis Writing Group (2005). International clinical practice guidelines for early psychosis. *British Journal of Psychiatry*, **187**(Suppl. 48), s120–s124.

Jackson, H., McGorry, P., Edwards, J., Hulbert, C., Henry, L., Harrigan, S., *et al.* (2005). A controlled trial of cognitively oriented psychotherapy for early psychosis (COPE) with four-year follow-up readmission data. *Psychological Medicine* 35, 1295–306.

Jackson, H.J., McGorry, P.D., Killackey, E., Bendall, S., Allott, K., Dudgeon, P., *et al.* (2008). Acute-phase and 1-year follow-up results of a randomized controlled trial of CBT versus Befriending for first-episode psychosis: the ACE project. *Psychological Medicine*, **38**, 725–35.

Johannessen, J.O., Larsen, T.K., Joa, I., Melle, I., Friis, S., Opjordsmoen, S., *et al.* (2005). Pathways to care for first-episode psychosis in an early detection healthcare sector: part of the Scandinavian TIPS study. *British Journal of Psychiatry*, **187**(Suppl. 48) s24–s28.

Johns, L.C., Cannon, M., Singleton, N., Murray, R.M., Farrell, M., Brugha, T., *et al.* (2004). Prevalence and correlates of self-reported psychotic symptoms in the British population. *British Journal of Psychiatry*, **185**, 298–305.

Johnstone, E.C., Ebmeier, K.P., Miller, P., Owens, D.G., and Lawrie, S.M. (2005). Predicting schizophrenia: findings from the Edinburgh High-Risk Study. *British Journal of Psychiatry*, **186**, 18–25.

Jonnson, F., Freeman, J., Hinton, M., Towle, L., O'Donnell, J., and Power, P. (2004). Cannabis and psychosis: a clinical audit of the prevalence and persistence of cannabis use in first-episode psychosis patients attending the Lambeth Early Onset (LEO) service in London. *Schizophrenia Research*, **70**(Suppl. 1), 72.

Kahn, R.S., Fleischhacker, W.W., Boter, H., Davidson, M., Vergouwe, Y., Keet, I.P., *et al.* (2008). Effectiveness of antipsychotic drugs in first-episode schizophrenia and schizophreniform disorder: an open randomised clinical trial. *Lancet*, **371**, 1085–97.

Kessler, R.C., Berglund, P., Demler, O., Jin, R., Merikangas, K.R., and Walters, E.E. (2005). Lifetime prevalence and age-of-onset distributions of DSM-IV disorders in the National Comorbidity Survey Replication. *Archives of General Psychiatry*, **62**, 593–602.

Killackey, E., Jackson, H.J., and McGorry, P.D. (2008). Vocational intervention in first-episode psychosis: individual placement and support v. treatment as usual. *British Journal of Psychiatry, 193*, 114–20.

Killackey, E., Jackson, H., Fowler, D., and Neuchterlein, K.H. (2009). Enhancing work function in early psychosis. In: Jackson, H. and McGorry, P.D. (eds.) *The Recognition and Management of Early Psychosis: A Preventative Approach*, pp. 331–48. Cambridge: Cambridge University Press.

Kirkbride, J.B., Morgan, C., Fearon, P., Dazzan, P., Murray, R.M., and Jones, P.B. (2007). Neighbourhood-level effects on psychoses: re-examining the role of context. *Psychological Medicine 37*, 1413–25.

Krabbendam, L., Myin-Germeys, I., Bak, M., and van Os, J. (2005). Explaining transitions over the hypothesized psychosis continuum. *Australian and New Zealand Journal of Psychiatry, 39*, 180–6.

Kurihara, T., Kato, M., Reverger, R., Tirta, I.G.R., and Kashima, H. (2005). Never-treated patients with schizophrenia in the developing country of Bali. *Schizophrenia Research, 79*, 307–13.

Lewis, S., Tarrier, N., Haddock, G., Bentall, R., Kinderman, P., Kingdon, D., et al. (2002). Randomised controlled trial of cognitive-behavioural therapy in early schizophrenia: acute-phase outcomes. *British Journal of Psychiatry, 181*(Suppl. 43), s91–s97.

Lieberman, J.A., Tollefson, G., Tohen, M., Green, A.I., Gur, R.E., Kahn, R., et al. (2003). Comparative efficacy and safety of atypical and conventional antipsychotic drugs in first-episode psychosis: a randomized, double-blind trial of olanzapine versus haloperidol. *American Journal of Psychiatry, 160*, 1396–404.

Lieberman, J.A., Tollefson, G.D., Charles, C., Zipursky, R., Sharma, T., Kahn, R.S., et al. (2005). Antipsychotic drug effects on brain morphology in first-episode psychosis. *Archives of General Psychiatry, 62*, 361–70.

Link, G. and Dohrenwend, B.P. (1980). Formulation of hypotheses about the ratio of untreated cases of true prevalence studies of functional psychiatric disorders in adults in the United States. In: Dohrenwend, B.P., Dohrenwend, B.S., Gould, M.S., Link, B., Neugebauer, R., and Wunsch-Hitzig, R. (eds.) *Mental illness in the United States: Epidemiological estimates*, pp. 113–48. New York: Praeger:

Marshall, M., Harrigan, S.M. and Lewis, S. (2009). Duration of untreated psychosis: definition, measurement and association with outcome. In: Jackson, H. and McGorry, P.D. (eds.) *The Recognition and Management of Early Psychosis: A Preventative Approach*, pp. 125–45. Cambridge: Cambridge University Press.

Mbewe, E., Haworth, A., Welham, J., Mubanga, D., Chazulwa, R., Zulu, M.M., et al. (2006). Clinical and demographic features of treated first-episode psychotic disorders: a Zambian study. *Schizophrenia Research, 86*, 202–7.

McCrone, P., Dhanasiri, S., Patel, A., Knapp, M., and Lawton-Smith, S. (2008). *Paying the price: The cost of mental health care in England to 2026*. London: The King's Fund.

McGlashan, T.H. (2006). Is active psychosis neurotoxic? *Schizophrenia Bulletin, 32*, 609–13.

McGlashan, T.H., Zipursky, R.B., Perkins, D., Addington, J., Miller, T., Woods, S.W., et al. (2006). Randomized, double-blind trial of olanzapine versus placebo in patients prodromally symptomatic for psychosis. *American Journal of Psychiatry, 163*(5): 790–9.

McGorry, P.D., Yung, A.R., Phillips, L.J., Yuen, H.P., Francey, S., Cosgrave, E.M., et al. (2002). Randomized controlled trial of interventions designed to reduce the risk of progression to first-episode psychosis in a clinical sample with subthreshold symptoms. *Archives of General Psychiatry, 59*, 921–28.

McGorry, P.D., Hickie, I.B., Yung, A.R., Pantelis, C., and Jackson, H.J. (2006). Clinical staging of psychiatric disorders: a heuristic framework for choosing earlier, safer and more effective interventions. *Aust N Z J Psychiatry, 40*, 616–22.

McGorry, P., Johanessen, J.O., Lewis, S., Birchwood, M., Malla, A., Nordentoft, M., et al. (2010). Early intervention in psychosis: keeping faith with evidence-based health care. *Psychological Medicine 40*, 399–404.

McGorry, P., Cocks, J., Power, P., Burnett, P., Harrigan, S., and Lambert, T. (2011). Very low dose risperidone in first episode psychosis a safe and effective way to initiate treatment. *Schizophrenia Research and Treatment, in* press.

McNab, C. and Linszen, D. (2009). Family intervention in early psychosis. In: Jackson, H. and McGorry, P.D. (eds.) *The Recognition and Management of Early Psychosis: A Preventative Approach*, pp. 305–29. Cambridge: Cambridge University Press.

Melle, I., Larsen, T.K., Haahr, U., Friis, S., Johannessen, J.O., Opjordsmoen, S., et al. (2004). Reducing the duration of untreated first-episode psychosis: effects on clinical presentation. *Archives of General Psychiatry, 61*, 143–50.

Merlo, M.C., Hofer, H., Gekle, W., Berger, G., Ventura, J., Panhuber, I., et al. (2002). Risperidone, 2 mg/day vs. 4 mg/day, in first-episode, acutely psychotic patients: treatment efficacy and effects on fine motor functioning. *Journal of Clinical Psychiatry, 63*, 885–91.

Mihalopoulos, C., Harris, M., Henry, L., Harrigan, S., and McGorry, P. (2009). Is early intervention in psychosis cost-effective over the long term? *Schizophrenia Bulletin, 35*, 909–18.

Miller, G. and Holden, C. (2010). Psychiatry. Proposed revisions to psychiatry's canon unveiled. *Science 327*, 770–1.

Miller, T.J., McGlashan, T.H., Rosen, J.L., Cadenhead, K., Cannon, T., Ventura, J., et al. (2003). Prodromal assessment with the structured interview for prodromal syndromes and the scale of prodromal symptoms: predictive validity, interrater reliability, and training to reliability. *Schizophrenia Bulletin, 29*, 703–15.

Morrison, A.P., French, P., Walford, L., Lewis, S.W., Kilcommons, A., Green, J., et al. (2004). Cognitive therapy for the prevention of psychosis in people at ultra-high risk: randomised controlled trial. *British Journal of Psychiatry, 185*, 291–7.

Naismith, S.L., Glozier, N., Carter, P.E., Scott, E., and Hickie, I.B. (2009). Early intervention or cognitive decline: Is there a role for multiple behavioural interventions? *Early Intervention in Psychiatry, 3*, 19–27.

Overall, J.E. and Gorham, D.R. (1962). The Brief Psychiatric Rating Scale. *Psychological Reports, 10*, 799–812.

Padmavathi, R., Rajkumar, S., and Srinivasan, T.N. (1998). Schizophrenic patients who were never treated a study in an Indian urban community. *Psychological Medicine, 28*, 1113–17.

Pelosi, A. (2009). Is early intervention in the major psychiatric disorders justified? No. *British Medical Journal, 337*, a710.

Penn, D.L., Waldheter, E.J., Perkins, D.O., Mueser, K.T., and Lieberman, J.A. (2005). Psychosocial treatment for first-episode psychosis: a research update. *American Journal of Psychiatry, 162*, 2220–32.

Perkins, D.O., Gu, H., Boteva, K., and Lieberman, J.A. (2005). Relationship between duration of untreated psychosis and outcome in first-episode schizophrenia: a critical review and meta-analysis. *American Journal of Psychiatry, 162*, 1785–804.

Phillips, L.J., McGorry, P.D., Yuen, H.P., Ward, J., Donovan, K., Kelly, D., et al. (2007). Medium term follow-up of a randomized controlled trial of interventions for young people at ultra high risk of psychosis. *Schizophrenia Research, 96*, 25–33.

Pinfold, V., Smith, J., and Shiers, D. (2007). Audit of early intervention service development in England in 2005. *Psychiatric Bulletin,31*, 7–10.

Power, P. and McGorry, P. (2008). First episode psychosis inpatient services: a comparison of the EPPIC and LEO inpatient units. *Early Intervention in Psychiatry, 2*(Suppl 1), A14.

Power, P. and Robinson, J. (2009). Suicide prevention in first-episode psychosis. In: Jackson, H. and McGorry, P.D. (eds.) *The Recognition and Management of Early Psychosis: A Preventative Approach*, pp. 257–82. Cambridge: Cambridge University Press.

Power, P., Elkins, K., Adlard, S., Curry, C., McGorry, P., and Harrigan, S. (1998). Analysis of the initial treatment phase in first-episode psychosis. *British Journal of Psychiatry, 172*(**Suppl. 33**), 71–6.

Power, P.J., Bell, R.J., Mills, R., Herrman-Doig, T., Davern, M., Henry, L., Yuen et al. (2003). Suicide prevention in first episode psychosis: the development of a randomised controlled trial of cognitive therapy for acutely suicidal patients with early psychosis. *Australian and New Zealand Journal of Psychiatry,* **37**, 414–20.

Power, P., Iacoponi, E., Reynolds, N., Fisher, H., Russell, M., Garety, P., *et al.* (2007a). The Lambeth Early Onset Crisis Assessment Team Study: general practitioner education and access to an early detection team in first-episode psychosis. *British Journal of Psychiatry,* **191**(Suppl. **51**), s133–s139.

Power, P., McGuire, P., Iacoponi, E., Garety, P., Morris, E., Valmaggia, L., *et al.* (2007b). Lambeth Early Onset and Outreach and support in South London services. *Early Intervention in Psychiatry,* **1**, 97–103.

Reay, R., Mitford, E., McCabe, K., Paxton, R., andTurkington, D. (2010). Incidence and diagnostic diversity in first-episode psychosis. *Acta Psychiatrica Scandinavica,* **121**, 315–19.

Reeves, S., Stewart, R., and Howard, R. (2002). Service contact and psychopathology in very-late-onset schizophrenia-like psychosis: the effects of gender and ethnicity. *International Journal of Geriatric Psychiatry,* **1**, 473–9.

Reimann, H. and Hafner, H. (1973). Mental disorders of the elderly in Mannheim: An investigation of incidence rate. *Social Psychiatry,* **7**, 53–69.

Robinson, D., Woerner, M.G., Alvir, J.M., Bilder, R., Goldman, R., Geisler, S., *et al.* (1999). Predictors of relapse following response from a first episode of schizophrenia or schizoaffective disorder. *Archives of General Psychiatry,* **56**, 241–7.

Schooler, N., Rabinowitz, J., Davidson, M., Emsley, R., Harvey, P.D., Kopala, L., *et al.* (2005). Risperidone and haloperidol in first-episode psychosis: a long-term randomized trial. *American Journal of Psychiatry,* **162**, 947–53.

van Os, J., Hanssen, M., Bijl, R.V., and Vollebergh, W. (2001). Prevalence of psychotic disorder and community level of psychotic symptoms: an urban-rural comparison. *Archives of General Psychiatry,* **58**, 663–8.

Van Os, J. and Poulton, R. (2009). Environmental vulnerability and genetic-environmental interactions. In: Jackson, H. and McGorry, P.D. (eds.) *The Recognition and Management of Early Psychosis: A Preventative Approach,* pp. 47–59. Cambridge: Cambridge University Press.

Velakoulis, D., Pantelis, C., McGorry, P.D., Dudgeon, P., Brewer, W., Cook, M., *et al.* (1999). Hippocampal volume in first-episode psychoses and chronic schizophrenia: a high-resolution magnetic resonance imaging study. *Archives of General Psychiatry,* **56**, 133–41.

Weinberger, D. and Berger, G. (2009). Genetic vulnerability. In: Jackson, H. and McGorry, P.D. (eds.) *The Recognition and Management of Early Psychosis: A Preventative Approach,* pp. 32–46. Cambridge: Cambridge University Press.

Woods, S.W., Addington, J., Cadenhead, K.S., Cannon, T.D., Cornblatt, B.A., Heinssen, R., *et al.* (2009). Validity of the prodromal risk syndrome for first psychosis: findings from the North American Prodrome Longitudinal Study. *Schizophrenia Bulletin,* **35**, 894–908.

World Health Organization (1992). *The ICD-10 classification of mental and behavioural disorders – clinical descriptions and diagnostic guidelines.* Geneva: World Health Organization.

Wright, A., McGorry, P.D., Harris, M.G., Jorm, A.F. and Pennell, K. (2006). Development and evaluation of a youth mental health community awareness campaign – The Compass Strategy. *BMC Public Health* **6**, 215.

Wunderink, L., Nienhuis, F.J., Sytema, S., Slooff, C.J., Knegtering, R., and Wiersma, D. (2007). Guided discontinuation versus maintenance treatment in remitted first-episode psychosis: relapse rates and functional outcome. *Journal of Clinical Psychiatry,* **68**, 654–61.

Yung, A.R., Yuen, H.P., McGorry, P.D., Phillips, L.J., Kelly, D., Dell'Olio, M., *et al.* (2005). Mapping the onset of psychosis: the Comprehensive Assessment of At-Risk Mental States. *Australian and New Zealand Journal of Psychiatry,* **39**, 964–71.

Yung, A.R., Klosterkotter, J., Cornblatt, B., and Schultze-Lutter, F. (2009). At-risk mental state and prediction. In: Jackson, H. and McGorry, P. (eds.) *The Recognition and Management of Early Psychosis: A Preventative Approach,* pp. 83–105. Cambridge: Cambridge University Press.

CHAPTER 15

Case management and assertive community treatment

Helen Killaspy and Alan Rosen

Introduction

Recent decades have seen the relocation of psychiatric care from hospital-based settings to community-based services. The initial phases of deinstitutionalization led to a replication of the general hospital outpatient clinic model for review of community patients by psychiatrists, but gradually services began to expand the support available to people with more severe mental health problems. Over time, the addition of nurses, psychologists, occupational therapists, and social workers led to the establishment of community mental health teams. As community health and social care provision expanded, it became an increasingly complex system to navigate. Case management was developed to address this by assigning individual staff to assess service users' needs and coordinate their treatment and care. Contemporary mental health services use a variety of models of case management of which assertive community treatment (ACT) is the most intensive and clearly defined form. This chapter explores these models of community mental health care, the evidence for them, and the possible explanations for the discrepancies in their effectiveness reported in the international literature.

Types of case management

Case management is the process of drawing together and ensuring coordinated delivery of all the services and interventions required to address service users' various needs (e.g. treatment, social, accommodation, financial, employment, leisure, cultural needs). Various models of case management have been described and categorized according to the main expected outcomes of the work (e.g. clinical, social networks, strengths, rehabilitation) or the type of support offered (e.g. passive response/brokerage or active response models) (see Table 15.1 and Rosen and Teesson, 2001). Case management has also been developed for specific groups of service users (e.g. those receiving care from forensic services, older people, those in the first episode of psychosis and, in the United States, children and adolescents). The brokerage model historically comprised an administrative approach from relatively junior and generic, office-based staff that involved little more than referring service users to appropriate resources. Over time it has become much more clinically orientated with assessments and interventions being led by more highly qualified and experienced mental health professionals working together in community mental health teams and holding individual case loads. The approach in many countries has become more proactive and many contacts are made in the client's home. The main aims are to improve clinical and social outcomes and to intervene to avoid relapse and hospital admission wherever possible. In addition, increasingly, all mental health services are encouraged to use a 'Recovery' orientation that engages clients in a collaborative 'doing with' partnership rather than a didactic 'doing to' approach (Roberts and Wolfson, 2004), regardless of the model of case management used. The analogy of evolution from a 'travel agent' to a 'travel companion' to a 'travel guide' has also been used to describe the increasingly proactive, supportive, collaborative, and expert role of the case manager (Rosen and Teesson, 2001).

Evidence for case management

A systematic review of seven randomized controlled trials of case management (excluding ACT) found that it was efficacious at maintaining contact with service users but not at improving clinical outcomes including quality of life, symptoms, and social functioning (Marshall et al., 1998). A more recent national study in Australia showed that case management reduced the chances of hospital admission for people with serious mental health problems by threefold (Morgan et al., 2006). However, a systematic review of studies of case management, found it to be only moderately effective for service users with the most severe and complex mental health needs, especially when case loads were high (Mueser et al., 1998). More intensive models with lower case loads have been developed to address this. Intensive case management has been defined as case management where the case load is less than 20 and ACT has been considered a specific form of intensive case

Table 15.1 Models of case management. Adapted from Rosen and Teesson (2001) as modified from Harris and Bergman (1993) and Bergman and Harris (1988)

Case management model	(A) Clinical (Stein and Test) (Harris and Bergman) (Lamb) (Kantor)	(B) Networking (Harris and Bergman) (Bachrach) (Drake)	(C) Strengths (Rapp)	(D) Rehabilitation (Anthony and Farkas)
1. Focus	INDIVIDUAL PERSPECTIVE i.e. dyad - Intensive Outreach	SOCIAL SYSTEMS - Enhance impoverished networks	OPTIMISM - Empowerment - Mastery - Collaboration	EDUCATION/ TRAINING - Brokerage - Skills - Support
2. Aims	1. To support individual clients': - best functioning - developing sense of self - more mature relationships and interests	1. To increase the capacity of client's natural or devised network to provide: - emotional support - tangible aid - advice - information - companionship	1. To help client achieve EMPOWERMENT AND MASTERY (Midwest US Utopian Strain)	1. To BROKER or negotiate for all services they need or want
	2. Outreach into community	2. To enhance impoverished networks (e.g. of homeless dually diagnosed) to increase client's social margin	2. Achievements and opportunities more important than failures and limitations	2. To develop clients' SKILLS & SUPPORTS to maintain satisfaction in chosen environment
	3. Intensive high frequency contact at times of crisis		3. To foster COLLABORATION	3.... with least amount of ongoing professional intervention
3. Initial motivation required	Requires LOW initial engagement/cooperation/motivation		Requires HIGH initial engagement/education/cooperation/motivation	
4. Case manager role	Therapist/Clinician (as well as securing resources)	Facilitator Conductor Network member	Collaborator and Companion	Manager Broker of resources Teacher guide
5. Training	Clinical professional background	Professional or para-professional group or system training	BA level lay person (doesn't require extensive clinical knowledge)	BA with technical training in rehabilitation
6. Who benefits?	Clients who are difficult to engage Clients with a potential for insight.	Clients with large networks, e.g. drug culture Clients with no networks e.g. homeless.	Engaged, cooperative clients (not those with high resistance, e.g. substance misusers and homeless).	Educated and goal driven individuals.

management (Burns et al., 2007). Conversely, intensive case management could be considered a diluted form of ACT since studies of the efficacy and effectiveness of ACT preceded those of intensive case management.

Development of ACT

One of the first models of community-based treatment was Stein and Test's (1980) 'Training in Community Living', an alternative approach to admission to psychiatric hospital in Madison, Wisconsin that involved moving ward staff out of the hospital to work with service users in their own homes. The model was tested in a randomized controlled trial and it was found to be able to prevent admissions (Stein and Test, 1980). It was successfully replicated in Sydney, Australia where substantially better outcomes for the subsample with schizophrenia were found (Hoult, 1986; Hoult et al., 1984) and it gradually evolved into two specific home treatment models, ACT and 24-hour mobile crisis resolution. Crisis resolution aims to treat people at home during a period of acute mental health crisis and avoid the need for hospital admission. It is an intensive, time-limited (usually to a few weeks or months) approach used for service users with any of the full range of mental health problems. This model proved inadequate to keep individuals with severe and persistent disability from recurrent admissions to hospital and ACT developed in response to this, to focus on patients with longer-term mental health problems such as schizophrenia, schizoaffective disorder, and bipolar affective disorder who have complex clinical problems (including functional and cognitive impairment and comorbidities such as substance misuse) and social needs (such as homelessness and social isolation) and who have difficulties in engaging with standard community mental health services. These service users have sometimes been called 'revolving door patients' due to their recurrent cycle of relapse in the community, readmission (often involuntarily), treatment, improvement in symptoms and functioning, discharge from hospital, failure to engage with community services, discontinuation of medication, relapse, and readmission. The ACT approach therefore addresses the needs of service users with severe problems and complex needs for whom standard case management and crisis intervention is inadequate. Stein, one of the cofounders of the ACT model, described it as a completely new class of intervention to case management to emphasize these critical differences in practice. However, these days a broadening consensus would consider ACT to be the 'gold standard' of case management with a capacity to incorporate useful elements of other models (Rosen et al., 2007; Rosen and Teesson, 2001). It has gradually evolved into an internationally accepted model (McGrew et al., 1994) that attempts to intervene in the 'revolving door' cycle to prevent readmission by maintaining therapeutic engagement and improving functioning through supporting adherence to treatment and care. The fidelity of ACT teams to this model can be assessed using the Dartmouth ACT Scale (DACTS; Teague et al., 1998).

Differences between standard case management and ACT

A number of books and guidelines have detailed ACT staffing and practice (Allness and Knoedler, 1998; Department of Health, 2002a; Stein and Santos, 1998). Differences in ACT and standard case management by community mental health services are summarized in Table 15.2. The ACT team takes full responsibility for its clients when in the community and in hospital. ACT teams should be staffed with a full complement of the different mental health professional disciplines (psychiatry, nursing, occupational therapy, psychology, social work) and non-professional staff should also be represented, such as support workers. There are growing indications that some staff should be service users in recovery, operating as peer support workers (Rosen et al., 2007) and there should be at least one vocational rehabilitation expert and one dual diagnosis expert (for service users with substance misuse and mental health problems) within the team. The team should have their own inpatient beds and be responsible for their own clients' admissions and discharges. Staff work with smaller case loads (maximum 10 per worker) than standard community mental health services (around 30–35 per worker) and the maximum total case load for an ACT team of 10 mental health workers is around 100 compared to 300 to 350. They also share their case work with other team members, so that over time all staff get to know all the team's clients. This is facilitated by working shifts to provide an extended hours service (usually around 12 hours per day including weekends) and by having daily team meetings where clients are discussed and the work for each day is planned. This sharing of cases is known as 'the team approach' or 'team case management'. Although some ACT teams use only team case management, there is no evidence to suggest that clients should not also have an individual case manager to coordinate their care by other team members and to coach and advocate for them (Rosen et al., 2007).

Table 15.2 Differences between assertive community treatment and standard community mental health services (after Killaspy et al., 2006)

Assertive community treatment team	Standard community mental health team
Total team client numbers: 80–100	Total team client numbers: 300–350
Extended hours (0800–2100 every day)	Office hours only (0900–1700, Mon–Fri)
'In vivo' work, i.e. meet client at home or in café, park, etc.	Office-based appointments and home visits
Assertive engagement: multiple attempts, flexible and various approaches, e.g. befriending, offering practical support	Offer appointments at office and/or home visits
'No drop-out' policy, i.e. commitment to continue to try to engage in long term	Discharge if unable to make or maintain contact
Maximum individual staff:client ratio = 1:12	Maximum individual staff:client ratio =1:35
Team-based approach i.e. all team members work with all clients	Case management very little sharing of work with individual clients between team members
Frequent (daily) team meetings to discuss clients and daily plans	Weekly team meetings
Use skills of team rather than outside agencies as much as possible	'Brokerage', i.e. referral to outside agencies for advice and services on, e.g. social security benefits, housing, employment, substance misuse

In the standard case management model, there may be very little sharing of work between team members (other than covering each other's caseloads when a team member is away), with the exception of the psychiatrist and junior doctor who are likely to work alongside case managers with all the team's clients. The small caseloads mean that ACT teams can provide a more intensive service, with around three times the number of face to face contacts of standard services (Killaspy et al., 2006). The bulk of these take place in the patient's home or elsewhere in the community whereas in standard case management, the majority of appointments are arranged at the team's office (except when the person is in crisis when the crisis resolution home treatment service may be employed). Seeing clients at home or in another community location away from the office is known as 'in vivo' work. The ACT teams focus on social needs, providing practical assistance with housing to support clients to maintain their tenancy, support with finances (such as assistance with banking and ensuring the client is receiving the benefits they are entitled to) and support with every day living tasks (such as shopping, cooking, and cleaning). They use a collaborative approach to facilitate engagement and try to provide as much support as they can from the expertise of the ACT team members, rather than brokering out to other services. Both standard case management and ACT provide individual and family/carer support, psychological interventions, and other evidence-based interventions including support with medication, but ACT teams have the flexibility, because of their smaller case loads and extended hours, to provide more support including delivering and administering prescribed medications where necessary. This also means that if a client is relapsing, the ACT team can increase their level of support, recalibrate medication rapidly, and hopefully avoid the need for admission, where standard services would need to make a referral to the crisis resolution service (where it exists) for more intensive home-based support. The ACT teams can also ensure that service users attend medical appointments and complete required investigations and interventions to improve and maintain their general health. If the service user has difficulties organizing themselves to attend these appointments, the ACT team can also attend these appointments with them. The support and education that ACT can provide to families and informal carers is also more intensive than standard case management as they are more likely to meet due to the higher frequency of home visits and their ability to visit out of office hours (Killaspy et al., 2009a). This has been shown to result in greater client and family satisfaction with services than standard case management (Hoult et al., 1984).

Evidence for ACT

The ACT model is one of the most extensively evaluated mental health interventions and there is good evidence for its efficacy (Mueser et al., 1998; Bond et al., 2001). A Cochrane review published in 1998 identified 75 randomized controlled trials comparing ACT to some form of standard care such as an outpatient clinic or community mental health service. It included 17 of these in a meta-analysis that concluded that when targeted at high users of inpatient services, ACT reduced the costs of care by decreasing the frequency and length of admissions. Other positive outcomes included increased engagement with services, more stability in accommodation, and improved satisfaction for patients and their carers (Marshall and Lockwood, 1998). Its cost-effectiveness was further established by a subsequent review (Latimer, 1999).

However, it has been difficult to appraise the efficacy of ACT in England and other countries with similar service systems that include well established community mental health teams. The Cochrane meta-analysis (Marshall and Lockwood, 1998) included only two European trials (Aberg-Wistedt, 1995; Audini et al., 1994), the rest being from the United States or Canada. A randomized controlled trial of intensive case management/ACT in Australia showed modest advantage over standard case management for participants in social functioning but not in inpatient service use (Issakidis et al., 1999). However, this study was not funded to assess outcomes beyond 12 months follow-up and so further potential gains from longer-term ACT could not be reported. A number of randomized controlled trials of intensive case management for people with severe and enduring mental health problems in the United Kingdom have also shown somewhat less impressive gains from ACT than the United States trials (Burns et al., 1999; Harrison-Read et al., 2002; Holloway and Carson, 1998; Thornicroft et al., 1998). However, none of these studies were designed specifically to investigate the ACT model (McGrew et al., 1994) and they have been heavily criticized for their methodological limitations (Marshall et al., 1999) and the conflation of their conclusions that ACT showed no advantage over standard care when the experimental intervention bore limited resemblance to ACT (Rosen and Teesson, 2001). In order to understand the discrepancies in the international evidence it is worthwhile to explore these studies in more detail.

Evidence for intensive case management in the United Kingdom

The PRiSM project (Thornicroft et al., 1998) was a large, naturalistic study that compared outcomes for patients with a diagnosis of a psychotic illness in two areas of London, one of which had developed a more intensive community service including an extended hours service for longer-term clients that provided both day care and home-based treatment and a crisis resolution service, and the other area provided standard outpatient and community mental health teams operating within office hours. The PRiSM study was particularly criticized for the lack of fidelity to the ACT model that the intensive service provided (although none of the teams assessed in the study were set up as ACT teams and the results were not reported as relating to ACT, the study was editorialized and commented on as though they were), the lack of targeting on 'hard to engage' clients (over a third had no measurable psychiatric symptoms or functional disabilities), some differences between the psychiatric morbidity in the two geographical areas that made comparisons more difficult to interpret, and its conclusions that it had uniquely tested 'real world' effectiveness over efficacy (Marshall et al., 1999; Rosen et al., 2001). The UK700 Study (Burns et al., 1999) was a randomized controlled trial of over 700 service users case managed by community mental health teams in four regions of England. They were randomly allocated to case management with staff with a caseload maximum of either 15 or 30 to 35. Similarly, Holloway and Carson's (1998) randomized controlled trial investigated outcomes for community mental health service users when the caseload size was eight or 30. Neither of these studies were trials of ACT. Harrison-Read et al. (2002) carried out a randomized controlled trial to evaluate an enhanced community mental health service that focused on patients who were high users of inpatient care and had small caseloads (8–15). The service had no dedicated psychiatrist, no inpatient beds, and used individual case management only rather than the team approach.

All these studies found that the more intensive community mental health service achieved a higher frequency of contacts with service users, and service users were more satisfied with it than the standard service. However none found evidence of any advantage over the standard service in reduced inpatient service use or improvements in other clinical and social outcomes. The Cochrane review (Marshall and Lockwood, 1998) concluded that there was a case for a randomized trial of the ACT model in the United Kingdom.

ACT in England

Given the strength of the international evidence in favour of ACT at the time, it was incorporated into the National Service Framework for Mental Health in England (Department of Health, 1999) and by 2004, 263 ACT teams had been set up (Department of Health, 2005). This provided an opportunity for a definitive randomized controlled trial to compare clinical outcomes and cost-effectiveness of ACT with standard treatment from community mental health teams for clients identified as difficult to engage and who were high users of inpatient care. Evaluating the effectiveness of ACT as teams developed had the advantage that professionals were enthusiastic and prepared for scrutiny of their work and there was less ethical concern about randomization to a service that was not available previously.

The 'REACT' (Randomised Evaluation of Assertive Community Treatment in North London) study (Killaspy et al., 2006) involved 251 patients with a diagnosis of a severe and enduring mental health problem (such as schizophrenia, schizoaffective disorder, or bipolar affective disorder) who had high use of inpatient services in the previous 2 years and were identified by community mental health teams as difficult to engage. They were randomly allocated to receive ACT from one of two local teams or to continue with their community mental health team. All the teams were independently assessed for their model fidelity: one of the ACT teams was assessed as high fidelity and the other as 'ACT-like' (Wright et al., 2003) and all the community mental health teams scored as having low ACT model fidelity. The features of the model that were missing for the two ACT teams were not having a substance misuse worker, not employing service users and not offering a 24-hour service (although both operated in the evenings and weekends). These components were commonly missing across ACT teams in London at the time (Wright et al., 2003). The primary outcome was inpatient service use assessed 18 months after randomization and secondary outcomes included patient satisfaction, engagement, social functioning, symptoms, needs, attitudes towards medication, adverse events, substance misuse, and quality of life. At follow-up there were no differences in any measure of inpatient service use, clinical, or social functioning between ACT and the standard community mental health teams' case management (Killaspy et al., 2006). This had not changed at 36-month follow-up when data on inpatient service use, adverse events and use of supported accommodation were examined (Killaspy et al., 2009b). However, ACT clients were better engaged, less likely to drop-out of contact, and more satisfied with services (Killaspy et al., 2006). Nevertheless, the REACT study did not find that ACT was more cost-effective than standard case management, mainly because the bulk of health care costs are in inpatient service use (McCrone et al., 2009). Latimer (1999) found that higher fidelity ACT reduced inpatient service use by nearly one-quarter more than lower fidelity programmes and cautioned that as service systems become less dependent on inpatient units the cost advantages of ACT would become harder to achieve.

Possible reasons for international differences in effectiveness of ACT

The reasons why ACT does not appear to be as effective in the United Kingdom as the United States and Australia require further examination and are summarized in Table 15.3. One possible explanation is that the services against which ACT has been compared in the United Kingdom were more community-based than those in the earlier American trials and may have shared some aspects of the ACT approach. There is considerable evidence for this since although home treatment teams in the United States and Australia have been reported to make more 'in vivo' contacts than United Kingdom teams, community mental health teams in the United Kingdom make more 'in vivo' contacts than standard care comparison teams in the United States (Burns et al., 2002), though there is no evidence that standard community mental health teams in the United Kingdom make any more 'in vivo' contacts than similar teams in Australia. Since 'in vivo' work has been found to be one of the most effective components of home treatment (Catty et al., 2002) this difference may be of particular importance in understanding the international research findings.

Table 15.3 Factors that may influence the effectiveness of ACT

Factor	Description
Evolution and variability of treatment as usual	Services that ACT has been compared with vary and 'standard' community mental health care has evolved and may replicate key aspects of the ACT model such as 'in vivo' working and sharing caseloads
Evolution of the ACT model	ACT now often incorporates specific evidence-based interventions, expertise, and services (such as supported employment) but the delivery of these varies from team to team
Variability of the ACT model	Incorporation of ACT into other specialist mental health services (e.g. homeless services, early intervention services, forensic services, dual diagnosis services etc.) may have introduced further variation in the approach.
Failure to specify some aspects of the approach	Some aspects of ACT have not been clearly specified (the use or avoidance of coercion is an example) and may be of particular relevance in terms of effectiveness.
Variability of social and economic context	In many areas, low-income housing and hospital-based care are severely restricted such that people with severe mental health problems are vulnerable to homelessness, incarceration, addiction, victimization, and other negative outcomes, but not high rates of hospitalization
Variability in quality of ACT	The quality of ACT teams varies, fidelity assessment only captures some of the variance, and some teams are poorly implemented, supervised, and monitored for outcomes.

Morse and McKasson (2005) noted that outcomes from studies investigating the effectiveness of ACT were influenced by the degree to which comparison services offered ACT features. In the REACT study (Killaspy et al., 2006), although ACT model fidelity was low for the comparison community mental health services, they shared with the ACT teams four of seven features subsequently identified as important for the success of intensive case management: primary clinical responsibility; based in the community; team leader doing clinical work; time-unlimited service (Burns et al., 2007). The other three 'critical' factors were that the team meets daily, shares responsibility for caseloads, and is available 24 hours a day. However, in the Australian trial of ACT (Issakidis et al., 1999) the comparison service had greater ACT fidelity than the intensive case management of the PRiSM study, yet greater benefit for ACT was still shown.

Another possible explanation for the research findings in the United Kingdom is that inpatient mental health services in inner cities are operating at a very high admission threshold and interventions aimed at reducing admissions are therefore unlikely to succeed (Burns, 2007). Although the focus on inpatient service use as the main outcome for assessing efficacy and effectiveness of ACT has been criticized as outdated (Rosen et al., 2008), nevertheless, the participants in the REACT study who received ACT made no gains in any of the measures of clinical or social function above those of standard care patients. This suggests that community mental health teams in the United Kingdom are providing a service which, with fewer face to face contacts and higher case loads, is able to support patients and prevent admissions as effectively as a well resourced ACT team (Killaspy et al., 2006, 2009b).

Another possible explanation therefore is that although ACT services in the United Kingdom are succeeding in engaging 'hard to reach' clients, they are not operating with adequate ACT model fidelity to build on this to deliver the evidence-based interventions likely to improve clinical outcomes. This appears likely since a survey of ACT teams in England carried out in 2003 found that only 12% of the 222 teams who participated scored as having high model fidelity on the DACTS (Teague et al., 1998). Many did not provide an extended hours service, few had dedicated inpatient beds and few were adequately staffed to provide appropriate medical and psychosocial interventions: only half had a psychiatrist, only one-fifth had a psychologist and very few had a substance misuse or vocational rehabilitation specialist. A recent postal survey of ACT team managers suggests that this situation has not improved (Ghosh and Killaspy, 2010).

Inadequate implementation of the ACT model may therefore explain at least some of the differences in its effectiveness reported in the international literature. A recent study that compared ACT in London and Melbourne, Australia, found that: the London teams had around one-quarter the amount of input from a psychiatrist compared to the Melbourne teams (0.6 full-time equivalents per team caseload of 100, compared to 1.9 full-time equivalents); only half the London teams operated outside of office hours compared to all the Melbourne teams; the majority of Melbourne teams made the bulk of their contact *in vivo* whereas this was the case for only a third of the London teams' contacts; and the Melbourne teams scored higher for using the team approach (Harvey et al., in press). These differences in delivery of the 'critical ingredients' of ACT are likely to influence its effectiveness.

Active engagement or coercion in ACT

A consistent finding in the international literature is that ACT is more acceptable to 'hard to engage' clients than standard case management (Killaspy et al., 2006; Marshall and Lockwood, 1998; Mueser et al., 1998). This appears to be related to the particular style of the ACT approach that engages clients as partners in agreeing their care plans rather than directing them to accept treatment and support (Killaspy et al., 2009a). Although, conversely, it has been postulated that ACT is a coercive, intrusive, and paternalistic approach (Gomory, 2001), the cofounders of ACT have clearly stated that coercion is not part of the model (Test and Stein, 2001). A qualitative study of staff contacts with 45 clients of one ACT in Madison, Wisconsin found very few instances of coercive interactions and a wide range of collaborative approaches to increase clients' engagement (Angell et al., 2006). Similarly, Davidson and Campbell (2007) found that fewer coercive strategies were used by ACT staff in Northern Ireland than other community mental health service staff. In the REACT study (Killaspy et al., 2006) ACT clients' ratings of intrusiveness of the service were lower than community mental health teams' clients, despite having three times the number of contacts, most of which were in their own homes.

Evidence-based interventions and ACT

It seems reasonable to expect that a period of time to engage and implement effective treatment plans is required before improved clinical outcomes are likely to be seen. This may even involve an increase in the admission rates of ACTs in the first instance, which could clearly influence the primary outcome of inpatient service use chosen in most studies of ACT. An Australian evaluation of ACT with homeless people led to improved social function and housing stability but increased inpatient service use initially, possibly because improved engagement meant clients were locatable when acutely unwell. Admissions gradually reduced considerably in later years of treatment to a similar level as a comparison ACT team in another catchment of the same city without such a concentration of homeless clients (Teeson, 1995; Teeson and Hambridge, 1992). It seems logical to suppose that after the initial engagement period, delivery of evidence-based interventions would be required to effect positive clinical outcomes. These interventions include medication review and management (prescribing, delivering, and administration), cognitive behavioural therapy and family interventions (NICE, 2009). Combining ACT with various specialist psychosocial interventions that are delivered from within the service has been shown to be effective in improving clinical outcomes. Examples include reduced admissions with multiple family psychoeducation groups (McFarlane, 2002), reduction in co-occurring substance misuse when specialist substance misuse workers are employed in the team (Drake et al., 1998) and successfully attaining competitive employment when vocational rehabilitation workers are employed in the team particularly when the 'individual placement and support' model is used (Gold et al., 2006). These kinds of specialist interventions are likely to be limited in ACT teams in the United Kingdom since they do not appear to be adequately staffed to deliver them. This could further explain the lack of effectiveness reported in United Kingdom studies of ACT.

Evidence for ACT from elsewhere in Europe

Elsewhere in Europe less research on ACT has been carried out as it has been implemented more recently. However, it appears that a similar picture to the United Kingdom is emerging. In the Netherlands a randomized trial of ACT for clients with longer-term mental health problems and high levels of clinical need failed to find any clinical advantage for ACT over standard community care, although engagement and satisfaction were greater for ACT clients (Sytema et al., 2007). This finding is particularly interesting since the authors specifically stated that there was no shortage of inpatient beds in the rural area where the study was carried out and therefore it might have been expected, given Burns' argument (2007) that ACT shows most impact on inpatient service use in areas with the highest use, that that it would have been associated with a reduction in inpatient service use. However, conversely one could argue that perhaps the easy availability of inpatient beds may have reduced the impetus on the ACT teams to reduce admissions.

Potentially more promising results have been found for 'Function-ACT' (FACT), a Dutch hybrid or diluted variation on ACT which combines within the same team the delivery of intensive case management and standard care for patients requiring differing levels of support (van Veldhuizen, 2007). Drukker et al. (2008) have reported beneficial effects of FACT in one region with regard to remission amongst individuals with unmet needs related to psychosis and no comorbid alcohol problem, but to date there have been no trials comparing FACT with ACT or reports of its effectiveness across sites, despite widespread implementation in the Netherlands. Robust studies of its effectiveness are required since similar, diluted ACT approaches are being suggested in England as part of service redesign in the context of the economic recession. Such reconfigurations also risk disrupting the collaborative partnerships that many ACT services have with mental health rehabilitation services (Royal College of Psychiatrists, 2009).

In Denmark, a randomized controlled trial of ACT enhanced by family intervention and social skills training for patients experiencing their first episode of psychosis was associated with marginally greater improvements in positive and negative psychotic symptoms than patients who received standard community mental health team care, but no difference in inpatient service use. It is of note that the 'ACT' service was office-based and rarely carried out home visits (Petersen et al., 2005) and therefore its classification as ACT is highly questionable.

Some United Kingdom and European experts consider that ACT fails to show much advantage over standard case management in the United Kingdom compared to the United States because the standard community mental health and social services in the United Kingdom provide a background 'safety net' that is considered more established and more effective than the United States equivalent (Burns et al., 2007). However this does not explain the more encouraging results from studies of ACT in Australia where well-established and well-resourced standard community mental health and social care services exist. There is also some controversy over whether consumer and carer groups in the United Kingdom consider their 'safety net' to be adequate (A. Rosen, personal communication). In some countries with well-established primary care services, transfer of case management from secondary mental health services to general practitioners and other primary care workers can provide an alternative to standard case management that is, arguably, a better 'safety net'. An example is the 'CLIPP' (consultation liaison in primary care psychiatry) programme in operation in Victoria, Australia where a detailed, collaborative, individualized care plan is drawn up with the service user that includes early warning signs of relapse and a crisis intervention plan.

Shared care workers liaise across the primary and secondary care interface and intervene at times of crisis to provide more intensive support and avoid admission to hospital where possible, as well as providing assessment and advice for new referrals from primary care to secondary mental health care services (Meadows, 1998). Similar models exist in many other countries but robust evaluations of their efficacy with regard to those with more severe and enduring mental health problems are needed.

Summary

The evidence from studies of case management suggests that its most intensive form, ACT is the most clinically effective and, when focused on high users of inpatient care it is cost-effective. Findings from studies of ACT in the United States strongly support its effectiveness when compared with less well developed standard community mental health services, and in Australia when compared with well established community mental health services. However,

in the United Kingdom and other European countries with highly developed community mental health services that replicate key components of the ACT model (such as 'in vivo' working and having full clinical responsibility for the team's clients), the implementation of ACT has not been found to be cost-effective. This may be because other active components of the ACT model (the team-based approach, offering a time-unlimited service, making the bulk of contacts 'in vivo' and offering extended hours of operation) have not been as well implemented in the United Kingdom as in Australia and parts of the United States. In addition, the United Kingdom teams do not appear to be adequately staffed with the specialists necessary to deliver evidence-based interventions that can improve clinical outcomes for clients. Despite inadequate implementation, policy makers and service planners in the United Kingdom have begun to consider whether the elements of the ACT model that encourage engagement and appear to be popular with service users can be incorporated into the work of standard community mental health services. The results of trials such as the UK700 study have shown that this cannot be achieved through a simple reduction in case loads and further research to establish the effectiveness of diluted ACT models should be carried out before such reconfigurations take place. Adequate investment in ACT teams to operate with key components and to be staffed to deliver evidence-based approaches is needed to enable them to improve clinical outcomes for their clients.

Case management systems may be employed effectively at different levels of intensity to meet the individual needs of different service users. At the lower end of intensity, support needs may simply involve regular medication review and general supportive counselling, mentoring or coaching. Whether this level of case management can be successfully devolved to primary care liaison services is open to further evaluation. Service users with higher levels of need and recurrent complex mental health problems require more intensive support from mobile teams able to provide flexible and proactive response at times of crisis. For those with the most severe and persistent problems, ACT is still likely to be the most effective mode of service delivery.

References

Aberg-Wistedt, A., Cressell, T., Lidberg, Y., Liljenberg, B., and Osby, U. (1995). Two-year outcome of team-based intensive case management for patients with schizophrenia. *Psychiatric Services*, **46**, 1263–6.

Allness, D.J., and Knoedler, W.H. (1998). *The PACT model of community-based treatment for persons with severe and persistent mental illness. A manual for PACT start-up*. Arlington, VA: National Alliance for the Mentally Ill.

Angell, B., Mahoney, C.A., and Martinez, N.I. (2006). Promoting treatment adherence in assertive community treatment. *Social Service Review*, **80**, 485–526.

Audini, B., Marks, I.M., Lawrence, R.E., Connolly, J., and Watts, V. (1994). Home-based versus out-patient/in-patient care for people with serious mental illness. Phase II of a controlled study. *British Journal of Psychiatry*, **165**, 204–10.

Bergman, H.C. and Harris, H. (1988). '*Clinical Case Management for the Chronically Mentally Ill: A Conceptual Analysis*'. Lecture, Institute on Psychiatric Services, New Orleans, Louisiana, American Psychiatric Association, October, 1988.

Bond, G.R., Drake, R.E., Mueser, K.T., and Latimer, E. (2001). Assertive community treatment for people with severe mental illness: Critical ingredients and impact on patients. *Disease Management and Health Outcomes*, **9**, 141–59.

Burns., T., Creed, F., Fahy, T., Thompson, S., Tyrer, P., White, I. for the UK 700 Group (1999). Intensive versus standard case management for severe psychotic illness: a randomised trial. *Lancet*, **353**, 2185–9.

Burns, T., Catty, J., Watt, H., Wright, C., Knapp, M., and Henderson, J. (2002). International differences in home treatment for mental health problems: results of a systematic review. *British Journal of Psychiatry*, **181**, 375–82.

Burns, T., Catty, J., Dash, M., Roberts, C., Lockwood A., and Marshall, M. (2007). Use of intensive case management to reduce time in hospital in people with severe mental illness: systematic review and meta-regression. *British Medical Journal*, **335**, 336.

Catty, J., Burns, T., Knapp, M., Watt, H., Wright, C., Henderson, J., *et al* (2002). Home treatment for mental health problems: A systematic review. *Psychological Medicine*, **32**, 383–401.

Davidson, G. and Campbell, J. (2007). An examination of the use of coercion by assertive outreach and community mental health teams in Northern Ireland. *British Journal of Social Work*, **37**, 537–55.

Department of Health (1999). *The National Service Framework for Mental Health*. London: DH.

Department of Health (2002a). *Policy Implementation Guide. Assertive Community Treatment Teams*. London: DH.

Department of Health (2002b). *Mental Health Policy Implementation Guide. Community Mental Health Teams*. London: DH.

Department of Health (2005). *National Service Framework for Mental Health, Five Years On*. London: DH.

Drake, R., McHugo, G., Clark, R., Teague, G. Xie, H., Miles, K. Ackerson, T. (1998). Assertive community treatment for persons with co-occurring severe mental illness and substance misuse disorder. *A clinical trial. American Journal of Orthopsychiatry*, **68**, 201–15.

Drukker, M., Maarschalkerweerd, M., Bak, M., Driessen, G., à Campo, J., de Bie, A., *et al.* (2008). A real-life observational study of the effectiveness of FACT in a Dutch mental health region. *BMC Psychiatry* 2008, **8**, 93.

Ghosh, R. and Killaspy, H. (2010). A National Survey of Assertive Community Treatment Services in England. *Journal of Mental Health* [ePub September 28, 2010.]

Gold, P., Meisler, N, Santos, A, Carnemolla, M., Williams, O, Kelleher, J. (2006). Randomised trial of supported employment integrated with assertive community treatment for rural adults with severe mental illness. *Schizophrenia Bulletin*, **32**, 378–95.

Gomory, T. A critique of the effectiveness of assertive community treatment. *Psychiatric Services*, 2001, **52**, 1394–5.

Harris, M. and Bergman, H.C. (eds.) (1993). *Case management for mentally ill patients*. Langhorne, PA: Harwood Academic.

Harrison-Read, P., Lucas, B., Tyrer, P., Ray, J., Shipley, K., Simmonds, S., *et al.* (2002). Heavy users of acute psychiatric beds: randomised controlled trial of enhanced community management in outer London, *Psychological Medicine*, **32**, 403–16.

Harvey, C., Killaspy, H., Martino, S., White, S., Priebe, S., Wright, C., *et al.* (2011). A comparison of the implementation of assertive community treatment in Melbourne, Australia, and London, England. *Epidemiology and Psychiatric Sciences*, **20**, 1–11.

Holloway, F. and Carson, J. (1998). Intensive case management for the severely mentally ill. *British Journal of Psychiatry*, **172**, 19–22.

Hoult, J., Rosen, A., and Reynolds, I. (1984). Community orientated treatment compared to hospital orientated treatment. *Social Science and Medicine*, **18**, 1005–10.

Hoult, J. (1986). Community care of the acutely mentally ill. *British Journal of Psychiatry*, **149**, 337–44.

Issakidis, C., Sanderson, K., Teesson, M., Johnston, S., and Bulrich, N. (1999). Intensive case management in Australia: a randomized controlled trial. *Acta Psychiatrica Scandinavica*, **99**, 360–7.

Killaspy, H., Johnson, S., Pierce, B., Bebbington, P., Pilling, S., Nolan, F., and King, M. (2009a). A mixed methods analysis of interventions delivered by assertive community treatment and community mental health teams in the REACT trial. *Social Psychiatry and Psychiatric Epidemiology*, **44**, 532–40.

Killaspy, H., Kingett, S., Bebbington, P., Blizard, R., Johnson, S., Nolan, F., *et al.* (2009b). Three year outcomes of participants in the REACT (Randomised Evaluation of Assertive Community Treatment in North London) study. *British Journal of Psychiatry*, **195**, 82–3.

Killaspy, H., Bebbington, P., Blizard, R., Johnson, S., Nolan, F., Pilling, S., *et al.* (2006). REACT: A Randomised Evaluation of Assertive Community Treatment in North London. *British Medical Journal*, **332**, 815–19.

Latimer, E. (1999). Economic impacts of assertive community treatment: A review of the literature. *Canadian Journal of Psychiatry*, **44**, 443–54.

Marshall, M., Gray, A., Lockwood, A., and Green, R. (1998). Case management for people with severe mental disorders. *Cochrane Database of Systematic Reviews*, **2**, CD000050.

Marshall, M. and Lockwood, A. (1998). Assertive community treatment for people with severe mental disorders (Cochrane Review). *Cochrane Library*, **4**. Oxford: Update Software.

Marshall, M., Bond, G., Stein, L., Shepherd, G., McGrew, J., Hoult, J., *et al.* (1999). PRiSM Psychosis Study: Design limitations, questionable conclusions, *British Journal of Psychiatry*, **175**, 501–3.

McCrone, P., Killaspy, H., Bebbington, P., Johnson, S., Nolan, F., Pilling, S., *et al.* (2009). The REACT Study: Cost-Effectiveness of Assertive Community Treatment in North London. *Psychiatric Services*, **60**, 908–13.

McFarlane, W. (2002). *Multifamily groups in the treatment of severe psychiatric disorders*. New York: Guildford Press.

McGrew, J.H., Bond, G.R., Dietzen, L., Salyers, M. (1994). Measuring the fidelity of implementation of a mental health program model. *Journal of Consulting and Clinical Psychology*, **62**, 670–8.

Meadows, G. (1998). Establishing a collaborative service model for primary mental health care. *Medical Journal of Australia*, **168**, 162–5.

Morgan, V., Korten, A., and Jablensky, A. (2006). Modifiable risk factors for hospitalization among people with psychosis: Evidence from the National Study of Low Prevalence (Psychotic) Disorders. *Australian and New Zealand Journal of Psychiatry*, **40**, 683–90.

Morse, G. and McKasson, M. (2005). Assertive community treatment. In: Drake, R.E., Merrens, M.R., and Lynde, D.W. (eds.) *Evidence based mental health practice: A textbook*, pp. 317–47. New York: Norton.

Mueser, K.T., Bond, G.R., Drake, R.E., and Resnick, S.G. (1998). Models of community care for severe mental illness: A review of research on case management. *Schizophrenia Bulletin*, **24**, 37–74.

NICE (2002 updated 2009). *Schizophrenia: core interventions in the treatment and management of schizophrenia in primary and secondary care. Clinical Guideline No. 1.* London: National Institute for Health and Clinical Excellence.

Petersen, L., Jeppesen, P., Thorup, A., Maj-Britt A., Øhlenschlæger, J., Torben Østergaard., C., *et al.* (2005). A randomised multicentre trial of integrated versus standard treatment for patients with a first episode psychotic illness, *British Medical Journal*, **331**, 602.

Roberts, G. and Wolfson, P. (2004). The rediscovery of recovery: open to all. *Journal of Mental Health*, **10**, 37–49.

Rosen, A and Teesson, M.(2001). Does case management work? The evidence and the abuse of evidence based medicine. *Australian and New Zealand Journal of Psychiatry*, **35**, 731–46.

Rosen, A., Mueser, K., and Teesson, M. (2007). Assertive community treatment–issues from scientific and clinical literature with implications for practice. *Journal of Rehabilitation Research and Development*, **44**, 1–13.

Rosen, A., Bond, G.R., and Teesson, M. (2008). Commentary on Burns T, et al.'s "Use of intensive case management and meta-regression". *British Medical Journal*, **335**, 336. Evidence based mental health *British Medical Journal*, **11**, 2.

Royal College of Psychiatrists, Rehabilitation and Social Faculty (2009). *Enabling recovery for people with complex mental health needs: a template for rehabilitation services in England*. London: Royal College of Psychiatrists.

Stein, L.I. and Santos, A.B. (1998). *Assertive community treatment of persons with severe mental illness*. New York: Norton.

Stein, L.I. and Test, M.A. (1980). Alternatives to mental hospital treatment. *Archives of General Psychiatry*, **37**, 392–7.

Sytema, S., Wunderink, L., Bloemers, W., Roorda, L., and Wiersma, D. (2007). Assertive community treatment in the Netherlands: a randomized controlled trial. *Acta Psychiatrica Scandinavica*, **116**, 105–12.

Teague, G.B., Bond, G.R., and Drake, R.E. (1998). Program fidelity in assertive community treatment: Development and use of a measure. *American Journal of Orthopsychiatry*, **68**, 216–32.

Teesson, M. (1995). 'Evaluation of mental health service delivery in an inner city area' (Thesis). Sydney (Australia): University of New South Wales.

Teesson, M. and Hambridge, J. (1992). Mobile community treatment in inner city and suburban Sydney. *Psychiatric Quarterly*, **63**, 119–27.

Test, M. and Stein, L. (2001). Critique of the effectiveness of assertive community treatment. *Psychiatric Services*, **52**, 1396–7.

Thornicroft, G., Wykes, T., Holloway, F., Johnson, S., and Smuzkler, G. (1998). From efficacy to effectiveness in community mental health services. PRiSM Psychosis Study10. *British Journal of Psychiatry*, **173**, 423–7.

Van Veldhuizen, J.R. (2007). FACT: a Dutch version of ACT. *Community Mental Health Journal*, **43**, 421–33.

Wright, C., Burns, T., James, P., Billings, J., Johnson, S., Muijen, M., et al. (2003). Assertive outreach teams in London: Models of Operation. Pan London Assertive Outreach Study Part 1. *British Journal of Psychiatry*, **183**, 132–8.

CHAPTER 16

Psychiatric outpatient clinics

Thomas Becker and Markus Koesters

Introduction

Specialist psychiatric outpatient services have not, in recent years, been a priority of either the conceptual development or the study of community mental health care. General (or psychiatric) hospitals or community mental health team bases—at all of which outpatient clinics are held—can be considered community based as they are all located 'in the community'. However, there may have been an implicit assumption that services should be considered community based only if conceptually they have moved away from hospitals or other institutions. Also, the outpatient clinic model, in its traditional form, has been 'single-handed'. As such, outpatient clinics lack multidisciplinary input. A recent review of the community-based United Kingdom mental health care system, however, suggests that outpatient clinics are reported by more than two-thirds of so-called local implementation teams (Glover, 2007). There may also be a current trend towards specialized clinics for subgroups of patients, e.g. people with affective disorders, mentally disordered offenders, young adults, new mothers, patients with neuroses and eating disorders. Also, there may be a degree of under-reporting of outpatient clinics in surveys of local mental health services (Glover, 2007). Historically, these services have been a core element in the provision of psychiatric treatment, and it is likely that outpatient care continues to be a service element meeting important clinical needs in a large number of people with mental disorders.

History of outpatient care

In Europe, outpatient care started in the second half of the 19th century with charitable organizations that aimed at the implementation of postdischarge care in a period when mental health care was dominated by large asylums (Shorter, 2007). In the 20th century, outpatient care was a key element in the mental health care reform movement that occurred in England between the 1930s through to the 1960s (Freeman and Bennett, 1991). After the era of deinstitutionalization the developments in mental health care systems aimed at achieving a system of 'balanced care' (Thornicroft and Tansella, 1999), where outpatient treatment, more and more specialized and provided by multiprofessional teams, plays still a major role, supplemented by alternative community services and programmes (Becker and Vazquez-Barquero, 2001).

Functions of outpatient clinics

In this chapter, we review the literature on outpatient clinics. A systematic literature search including EMBASE, Medline, PsycInfo, and the Cochrane databases of controlled trials (CCTR) and systematic reviews (CDSR) was conducted, with the terms 'outpatient clinics' and 'mental health' or 'psychiatry' combined with comprehensive search strategies for controlled trials (The Cochrane Collaboration, 2009) and systematic reviews (Shojania and Bero, 2001). Although the search was intentionally broad with a high false positive rate, just about 1000 references were revealed and only 53 publications remained for detailed evaluation after abstract screening. For further improvement of the literature search, a backward citation search of relevant key papers was conducted. The term **psychiatric outpatient clinics**, as used in this text, refers to facilities providing office-based support and therapy for people with mental disorders. It is important to bear in mind that the conceptual boundaries with other ambulatory settings such as (crisis intervention and) home treatment, day hospital care, case management, or assertive community treatment which are covered in other chapters of this book are sometimes blurred. Furthermore, there is substantial variety between outpatient clinics both across countries and within countries. While in Italy outpatient services are delivered mainly by outpatient clinics organized in mental health care centres, most having a multidisciplinary team (de Girolamo et al., 2007), psychiatrists ('Nervenärzte'), psychologists, and general practitioners in office practice, the majority of whom are single-handed, provide most of the outpatient care services in Germany (Salize et al., 2007). Similarly, most outpatient clinics in England are staffed by doctors alone (Glover, 2007), whereas in France the availability and organization of the health service heavily depends on the region (Verdoux, 2007). Furthermore, outpatient clinics vary with respect to (Thornicroft and Tansella, 2004):

◆ Referral (self-referral vs. referral by primary care)

◆ Appointment times (fixed appointment times vs. open access)

◆ Clinical contact (doctors alone or other disciplines)

◆ Payment

◆ Methods to enhance attendance rates

◆ Response to non-attenders

◆ Frequency and duration of appointments

Evaluation of outpatient services

Outpatient treatment compared to other settings

Despite outpatient treatment being a standard component in most mental health care systems, there is only little evidence on the effectiveness of outpatient treatment as an element of the health care system as compared with other service components. However, the vast majority of treatment trials have been conducted within outpatient settings, and their results suggest that this setting is able to deliver effective treatment.

Outpatient versus day hospital treatment

A recent Cochrane review summarized the evidence of day hospital versus outpatient care for people with schizophrenia (Shek et al., 2009). The review included only four randomized controlled trials that were conducted between 1966 and 1986 and concluded that there is insufficient evidence to draw a definite conclusion as to whether day hospital treatment (with higher treatment intensity) has an advantage over outpatient care. An older version of that review (Marshall et al., 2001a) included an additional group of four studies of people with depression, anxiety, personality, and neurotic disorders, and it drew similar conclusions. Two trials in this latter review suggested that day treatment might be superior to outpatient care in patients 'refractory to outpatient treatments', but data from these trials could not be combined due to differences in the reporting of data. On the basis of these reviews and all other studies reviewed, the conclusion was that it was not possible to draw further conclusions regarding differential effects of the two treatment modalities (Marshall et al. 2001b). In line with this review, a recent study comparing the efficacy of short-term day hospital with outpatient psychotherapy in patients with personality disorders (Arnevik et al., 2009) showed improvement in both groups, but there were no significant differences between day hospital and outpatient treatment. In contrast, a South Korean study (Kong, 2005) found an advantage of a day treatment programme compared to the usual outpatient clinic care. In this study, 50 adult patients with eating disorders were randomized to a day treatment or standard outpatient care. There was significantly more improvement in most outcome measurements in people who were treated in the day treatment condition.

Outpatient versus inpatient treatment

One fairly old and small trial compared specialized outpatient treatment as an alternative to full-time hospitalization (Levenson et al., 1977). A sample of 20 patients with acute schizophrenia were randomly assigned to the two groups. There were no significant differences between the two groups in terms of treatment efficacy, but 'cost per remission' was about six times higher ($3330 vs. $565) in the hospital group, although patients in the outpatient treatment group were given daily appointments and a regimen of pharmacotherapy, psychotherapy, and family counselling.

In a recent pilot study patients were randomized to home treatment or hospital-based outpatient treatment (Dewa et al., 2009). Both treatment modalities were part of a first-episode psychosis programme and provided care through a multidisciplinary team. The primary difference between both treatment modalities was where the care was delivered (home vs. hospital setting). In both treatment groups, patients showed significant clinical improvement, but there was no difference in improvement rates between the groups. However, the results are based on a small sample of 29 completers.

Gowers et al. (2007) compared clinical effectiveness of three treatment settings for anorexia nervosa in adolescents. They randomized 170 adolescents to inpatient, specialist outpatient treatment, or treatment as usual in the general community. The clinical outcomes of the three treatment groups did not differ significantly at 1- and 2-year follow-up.

Outpatient versus community mental health teams

Tyrer et al. (1998) randomized 155 patients to community multidisciplinary teams or hospital-based outpatient care. The authors compared clinical outcomes and cost of care 1 year after discharge from inpatient care. Clinical outcomes were similar between the two groups, but readmission to hospital was more likely in the hospital-based care programme.

Limitations of studies

Most of the studies mentioned above failed to show a significant difference in clinical efficacy between mental health care components, but in a randomized controlled trial Sellwood et al. (1999) showed that, as compared with outpatient treatment alone, an additional home-based rehabilitation intervention significantly improved interpersonal functioning and social behaviour although there were no differences in positive or negative symptoms of psychosis. Given that there are effective pharmacological treatment options for most of the conditions studied, differences in the efficacy between service components might be negligible. However, there may be differences in other patient relevant outcomes beyond clinical efficacy (e.g. patient/user and carer satisfaction). Furthermore, there is a lack of evidence regarding the issue of what contributes to an effective outpatient clinic. Our literature search failed to reveal any trials comparing types of outpatient clinic with respect to clinical outcomes.

Costs

There is a general consensus that outpatient and community care are generally cheaper than care in hospital settings. There are, in fact, trials indicating that community treatment is also more cost-effective (Goldberg, 1991), but there are only a few randomized controlled trials comparing cost-effectiveness of outpatient clinics compared to other service components. Byford (2007) published the economic evaluation of a trial comparing inpatient psychiatric treatment, specialist outpatient treatment, and general outpatient treatment (Gowers et al., 2007, see above). In terms of a broad service provision perspective, specialist outpatient treatment was the cheapest, whereas the general outpatient group was the most expensive treatment option, although the difference in costs between the three groups was not statistically significant. In cost-effectiveness analyses, specialist outpatient treatment had the highest probability of being cost-effective and combined outpatient treatments (specialist and general) also showed a greater probability of being more cost-effective than inpatient services.

The Cochrane review (Shek et al., 2009, see above) that compared day treatment with outpatient care concludes that the suggestion of day hospitals being more expensive than outpatient treatment is offset by the suggestion of savings in inpatient care. Thus, it has remained unclear whether day hospitals are cost-effective as compared with outpatient treatment. Tyrer et al. (1998) concluded that in their trial the hospital-based outpatient treatment was more expensive than community care, mainly because of the lower readmission rate in the latter group.

Conclusions

It is fair to conclude that the evidence on efficacy (and effectiveness) of psychiatric outpatient clinics, in comparison with other treatment settings, is insufficient. There is a lack of clarity as to whether 'packages of care' (outpatient clinic, community mental health team) are distinct with clearly defined, 'unique' borders delineating one from the other. Also, the body of evidence on distinct treatment modules, e.g. psychotropic drug treatment and psychotherapeutic interventions, applies to mental health care provision irrespective of the locus of care, and many treatment studies have found clinical improvement in pre–post, placebo, or head-to-head comparisons of patients many or most of whom were seen in outpatient and community settings. It is likely that outpatient clinic work is 'hidden' in the comparator condition of 'treatment as usual' in many studies of non-hospital-based psychiatric treatment. There is a clinical consensus in many countries that such clinics are an efficient way of organizing assessment and treatment of people with mental disorders, provided that clinic sites are accessible to local populations. Nevertheless, outpatient clinics are simply methods of arranging clinical contact between staff and patients. The key issue is the content of the clinical interventions and the evidence of their efficacy (Thornicroft and Tansella, 2004). Outpatient clinics can be considered one valuable element of mental health care systems but settings of outpatient care may vary.

References

Arnevik, E., Wilberg, T., Urnes, Ø., Johansen, M., Monsen, J.T., and Karterud, S. (2009). Psychotherapy for personality disorders: short-term day hospital psychotherapy versus outpatient individual therapy—a randomized controlled study. *European Psychiatry*, **24**, 71–8.

Becker, I. and Vazquez-Barquero, J. L. (2001). The European perspective of psychiatric reform. *Acta Psychiatrica Scandinavica*, **104**, 8–14.

Byford, S., Barrett, B., Roberts, C., Clark, A., Edwards, V., Harrington, R., et al. (2007). Economic evaluation of a randomised controlled trial for anorexia nervosa in adolescents. *British Journal of Psychiatry*, **191**, 436–40.

de Girolamo, G., Bassi, M., Neri, G., Ruggeri, M., Santone, G., and Picardi, A. (2007). The current state of mental health care in Italy: problems, perspectives, and lessons to learn. *European Archives of Psychiatry and Clinical Neuroscience*, **257**, 83–91.

Dewa, C.S., Zipursky, R.B., Chau, N., Furimsky, I., Collins, A., Agid, O., et al. (2009). Specialized home treatment versus hospital-based outpatient treatment for first-episode psychosis: a randomized clinical trial. *Early Intervention in Psychiatry*, **3**, 304–11.

Freeman, H.L. and Bennett, D.H. (1991) Origins and development. In: Freeman, H.L. and Bennett, D.H. (eds.), *Community Psychiatry*, pp. 40–70. Edinburgh: Churchill Livingstone.

Glover, G. (2007). Adult mental health care in England. *European Archives of Psychiatry and Clinical Neuroscience*, **257**, 71–82.

Goldberg, D. (1991). Cost-effectiveness studies in the treatment of schizophrenia: a review. *Social Psychiatry and Psychiatric Epidemiology*, **26**, 139–42.

Gowers, S.G., Clark, A., Roberts, C., Griffiths, A., Edwards, V., Bryan, C., et al. (2007). Clinical effectiveness of treatments for anorexia nervosa in adolescents: randomised controlled trial. *British Journal of Psychiatry*, **191**, 427–35.

Kong, S. (2005). Day treatment programme for patients with eating disorders: randomized controlled trial. *Journal of Advanced Nursing*, **51**, 5–14.

Levenson, A.J., Lord, C.J., Sermas, C.E., Thornby, J.I., Sullender, W., and Comstock, B.S. (1977). Acute schizophrenia: an efficacious outpatient treatment approach as an alternative to full-time hospitalization. *Diseases of the Nervous System*, **38**, 242–5.

Marshall, M., Crowther, R., Almaraz-Serrano, A., Creed, F., Sledge, W., and Kluiter, H. (2001a). Systematic reviews of the effectiveness of day care for people with severe mental disorders: (1) Acute day hospital versus admission; (2) Vocational rehabilitation; (3) Day hospital versus outpatient care. *Health Technology Assessment Database*, **5**, 1–75.

Marshall, M., Crowther, R., Almaraz-Serrano, A., and Tyrer, P. (2001b). Day hospital versus out-patient care for psychiatric disorders. *Cochrane Database of Systematic Reviews*, **2**, CD003240.

Salize, H.J., Rossler, W., and Becker, T. (2007). Mental health care in Germany: current state and trends. *European Archives of Psychiatry and Clinical Neuroscience*, **257**, 92–103.

Sellwood, W., Thomas, C.S., Tarrier, N., Jones, S., Clewes, J., James, A., et al. (1999). A randomised controlled trial of home-based rehabilitation versus outpatient-based rehabilitation for patients suffering from chronic schizophrenia. *Social Psychiatry and Psychiatric Epidemiology*, **34**, 250–3.

Shek, E., Stein, A.T., Shansis, F.M., Marshall, M., Crowther, R., and Tyrer, P. (2009). Day hospital versus outpatient care for people with schizophrenia [Systematic Review]. *Cochrane Database of Systematic Reviews*, 4, CD003240.

Shojania, K.G. and Bero, L.A. (2001). Taking advantage of the explosion of systematic reviews: An efficient MEDLINE search strategy. *Effective Clinical Practice*, **4**, 157–62.

Shorter, E. (2007). The historical development of mental health services in Europe. In: Knapp, M., McDaid, D., Mossialos, E., and Thornicroft, G. (eds.) *Mental Health Policy and Practice Across Europe*, pp.15–33. Milton Keynes: Open University Press.

The Cochrane Collaboration (2009). *Cochrane Handbook for Systematic Reviews of Interventions* Version 5.0.2 Available at: http://www.cochrane-handbook.org

Thornicroft, G. and Tansella, M. (1999). *The Mental Health Matrix. A Manual to Improve Services*. Cambridge: Cambridge University Press.

Thornicroft, G. and Tansella, M. (2004). Components of a modern mental health service: a pragmatic balance of community and hospital care: Overview of systematic evidence. *British Journal of Psychiatry*, **185**, 283–90.

Tyrer, P., Evans, K., Gandhi, N., Lamont, A., Harrison-Read, P., and Johnson, T. (1998). Randomised controlled trial of two models of care for discharged psychiatric patients. *British Medical Journal*, **316**, 106–9.

Verdoux, H. (2007). The current state of adult mental health care in France. *European Archives of Psychiatry and Clinical Neuroscience*, **257**, 64–70.

CHAPTER 17

Day hospital and partial hospitalization programmes

Aart H. Schene

Introduction

Partial hospitalization (PH) as a treatment modality for psychiatric disorders has evolved over more than 60 years now. PH fills the wide gap between inpatient or full-time hospitalization (FTH) on the one hand and outpatient or community mental health care on the other. For patients, carers, and professional staff, PH has the potential to offer more than low-frequency outpatient visits while at the same time it prevents the disadvantages of a hospital admission.

In this chapter I discuss some of the main issues regarding the current status and the future development of PH: history, development, conceptual issues and definition, different types of PH programmes, (cost-)effectiveness of PH in comparison with FTH and outpatient treatment, selection criteria, treatment models, and therapeutic factors. In the last section I review the place of this component in the total of psychiatric services.

History

The history of PH goes back to the 1930s. Shortage of money urged Dzagharov (1937) in Moscow to open a hospital without beds in 1932. Next, Adams House started in Boston (1935), and Lady Chichester Hospital in Hove (1938) was the first in the United Kingdom After these pre-war pioneers, the post-war period saw at first a slow further development: Marlborough Day Hospital in London (1946), Allan Memorial Institute in Montreal (1946), Yale University Clinic (1948), Menninger Clinic (1949), Bristol Day Hospital (1951), Massachusetts Mental Health Center (1952), and the Maudsley Day Hospital (1953).

Two post-war PH-pioneers, Bierer and Cameron, deserve mention. Bierer (1951) initiated a Social Psychotherapy Centre (later Marlborough Day Hospital) in London in 1946. In his view, the day hospital was the predecessor of the era of social psychiatry. Later, he described the day hospital as a treatment centre independent of the hospital, with preventive, outpatient, and temporary inpatient services, and based on the principles of the therapeutic community (Bierer, 1961). The main focus was to keep patients in contact with their normal living environment.

Cameron (1947) introduced the term 'day hospital' in 1946 when he opened such a service as part of the Allan Memorial Institute of Psychiatry, being part of a large general hospital. Cameron described it as an extension and addition to FTH. In comparison with Bierer, whose ideas very much resemble the later philosophy of the United States community mental health centres, Cameron had a more medical view on psychiatry. Without knowing it, these two pioneers represented two distinct visions on the later development of PH: the day hospital and day treatment.

Further development of PH differed much between different countries. For the United Kingdom, Farndale (1961) described the rapid increase of day hospital settings in the late fifties as a 'day hospital movement'. Between 1959 and 1979 the number of day hospitals increased from 58 to 303 (Brocklehurst, 1979). *Better Services for the Mentally Ill* (Department of Health and Social Security, 1975) had mentioned a ratio of day hospital places of 30 per 100,000 and of day centre places of 60 per 100,000. Between 1974 and 1982, day hospital places rose from 9400 to 15,300. For day care centres the rise in that period was from 3600 to 5000 places. The United States saw the growth of PH in the sixties mainly as a result of the 1963 Community Mental Health Center Construction Act, while countries such as the Netherlands and Germany started to develop PH as late as the 1970s and 1980s (Bosch and Veltin 1983; Schene, 1985; Schene et al., 1986).

Development and further growth

During its first decades, the development of PH was initiated and stimulated by different motives. First, the post-war period saw a growing optimism about the possibilities of treating mental disorders. Not only by biological methods but also by individual and group psychotherapeutic techniques as well as occupational, family, and social psychiatric methods. Secondly, PH pioneers saw the hospital setting with its strong boundaries towards the outside world as a less adequate structure to use this new type of treatment. Thirdly, the sixties showed that PH could have an important and specific role in the run-down of large mental hospitals and in the further development of community-oriented psychiatry. Finally, effectiveness studies like those of Kris (1960), Zwerling and Wilder (1962), Meltzhoff and Blumenthal (1966), and Herz et al. (1971) contributed to a scientific support of this new type of treatment and gradually decreased the prejudices of hospital-oriented clinicians and other staff.

Also related to the process of deinstitutionalization was the rise in day care centres. When patients with long-term psychiatric disabilities have to live in the community, staff and services once located within the hospital should be redistributed within the community. Day hospitals fulfilled the acute service while day care centres started as maintenance programmes and in many places developed into psychosocial rehabilitation centres.

Comparison with inpatient and outpatient services

To understand its inherent qualities, we compare PH with inpatient and outpatient services. In comparison with the former, PH has the advantages that the disruption to life's normal routine (finances, housemaking, social contacts, hobbies, etc.) is less pronounced. Scapegoating the patient is less severe, as is the rejection by family members and other relatives. Contact with children and partner can be continued. Daily interaction with the outside world gives the patient good opportunities to develop skills and to generalize those from the therapeutic environment to the normal living situation (DiBella et al., 1982; Schene, 1985).

There also is a constant interplay in the way in which the patient and family or support system interact with each other. Because patients have to travel each day they expect to get an active treatment and not just to 'hang around on the ward'. The change from inpatient to PH to outpatient can be more gradual. PH is accepted more easily by patient and carers, providing the opportunity to intervene in an earlier stage of the illness or decompensation. The therapeutic climate gives fewer opportunities for regression, stimulates healthy behaviour, and produces less loss of self-esteem (Davidson et al., 1996). Stigmatization of patients might be lower as well as costs.

The disadvantages of PH, in comparison with FTH, for patients, are the daily travelling, the fact that they get less structure, support, and care, and mostly have no 24-hour availability of staff. They do not have the opportunity to be free of family or network contacts for a period of time, which in certain cases can be healing. For professionals the control of aggression and other disturbing behaviours is less easy and therefore more distressing. They have to decide each day anew if patients can go home. Involuntary admissions are not possible.

In comparison with outpatient treatment, PH has the advantage to give more intensive, more differentiated, and mostly multidisciplinary treatment. Medical diagnostics, assessments, observations, and certain therapeutics are more easily given. PH also provides more structure, more support, and more contact and learning opportunities with other patients. The disadvantages of PH in comparison with outpatient treatment are more stigmatization, more opportunity for regression, and more travelling.

Definition

A Task Force on Partial Hospitalization of the American Psychiatric Association (Casarino et al., 1982) was first to define PH as an ambulatory treatment programme, which includes the major diagnostic, medical, psychiatric, psychosocial, and prevocational treatment modalities, designed for patients with serious mental disorders, who require coordinated intensive, comprehensive, and multidisciplinary treatment not provided in an outpatient setting.

DiBella et al. (1982) defined psychiatric PH more quantitatively as a psychiatric treatment programme of eight or more waking hours per week, designed for improvement of a group of six or more ambulatory patients, provided by two or more multidisciplinary clinical staff, and consisting of carefully coordinated, multimodality interconnected therapies within a therapeutic milieu. Patients participate regularly in the entire programme, which occurs almost always during at least 2 days per week for at least 3 weeks, with most of the treatment periods of at least 3 hours but less than 24 hours.

Later Block and Lefkovitz (1991) restricted the definition of PH to a time-limited, ambulatory, active treatment programme that offers therapeutically intensive, coordinated, and structured clinical services within a stable therapeutic milieu. Programmes are designed to serve individuals with significant impairment resulting from a psychiatric, emotional or behavioural disorder.

In summary, PH means multidisciplinary, multimodality, and comprehensive programmes, available to several or groups of patients with severe mental illness, with regular opening hours and patient participation of at least 2 days per week, with most of the participation periods of at least 3 hours but less than 12 hours. It may be an acute (admission within 48–72 hours) or non-acute service; patients can participate somewhere in the range between low (2 half-days per week) and high intensity (4–5 days per week) and the length of participation can be a few weeks to indefinite.

Typology of partial hospitalization

In the field of PH an amalgam of terms and terminology is being used including day services, day hospital, partial hospital, day treatment, day centre, and day care. In different countries these terms may have different meanings. This confusion has to do with the wish to categorize and characterize PH services for which many criteria could be used; target population, type of treatment, duration of treatment or care, staff composition, organizational structure, and connection with other mental health services, etc.

Looking at specific target populations (Farndale, 1961), we can distinguish age groups (young children, adolescents, adults, old people), diagnostic categories (Bystritsky et al., 1996; Gerlinghoff et al., 1998; Lussier et al., 1997; Rosie et al., 1995) or combinations like elderly and infirm old people, mentally defective patients, handicapped persons, young patients with schizophrenia, and others.

Considering the connection with the mother institution, we find services that are freestanding and organizationally independent, freestanding but organizationally connected with other mental health services, freestanding on the terrain of a psychiatric or general hospital, units where patients use the same facilities as inpatients, and PH integrated on a psychiatric unit, which also contains inpatient and outpatient services.

Considering the part of the day, a distinction in day treatment, evening treatment, evening and night treatment, and weekend treatment can be made (De Hert et al., 1996; DiBella et al., 1982; Schene 1985). With regard to programmes, we can distinguish short-term, medium-term, and long-term services. The therapeutic orientation can be medical psychiatric, psychotherapeutic, or more rehabilitative. PH has to be distinguished from psychosocial rehabilitation programmes (self-help houses, Fountain House, therapeutic social clubs, and lounge programmes).

Four functions of partial hospitalization

In the United Kingdom, a distinction is made between day hospitals and day centres. Day hospitals offer: 1) active treatment, including medication and a range of professional interventions (psychological, social, occupational), aimed at people who need more intensive treatment than could be given on an outpatient basis, or 2) rehabilitation for those for whom day treatment is a step in the transition process from inpatient treatment towards the community (Shepherd 1991). Day centres, on the other hand, meet clients' long-term needs for support and social contact, assisting them in adjusting or re-adjusting to the demands of work and trying to relieve the strain on the family.

In the United States, a distinction is made between day hospital, day treatment, and day care (Rosie 1987) as well as between the intensive care model, rehabilitation model, and chronic care model (Klar et al., 1982). The day hospital/intensive care model provides diagnostic and treatment services for acutely ill patients who would otherwise be treated on traditional psychiatric inpatient units. The typical length of stay is between 4 to 8 weeks.

The day treatment programme/rehabilitation model provides an alternative to outpatient care for patients who have severe impairments in vocational or social performance. These programmes strive for symptom reduction and improved functioning and have a length of stay between 3 and 12 months.

The day care centre/chronic care model is indicated for patients who would otherwise require custodial care, for patients who might deteriorate in the community, and for patients who require regular treatment but cannot tolerate a more active treatment programme. It has modest expectations of patient improvement, high symptom tolerance, and a supportive, practical treatment approach. It offers maintenance care and social programming for individuals who require daily structure and supervision to prevent relapse. The length of stay is more than 1 year (Catty et al., 2007; Holloway 1991).

To summarize and integrate these different classifications, Schene and colleagues (1988) described PH in terms of the distinct functions it could fulfil in the total mental health care system and distinguished four types:

1 Alternative to acute inpatient: a medically oriented staff with high staff/patient ratio offers PH in or close to a general hospital for patients with acute illnesses who would otherwise be treated as inpatients.

2 Continuation of acute inpatient: transition to outpatient care can be organized on or close to the inpatient unit; staff, patients, and treatment resemble those of the first function.

3 Extension to outpatient care: either for specialized intensive treatment or rehabilitation for patients who do not require inpatient care but who benefit from more intensive care than is possible on an outpatient basis.

4 Day care or rehabilitation: long-term maintenance or rehabilitation of patients with chronic, debilitating mental disorders.

Evaluative research

The main questions researchers have tried to answer considered the (cost-)effectiveness of PH in comparison with FTH as well as with outpatient treatment. The evaluative research on PH has been reviewed extensively, first in non-systematic reviews (Creed et al., 1989a; DiBella et al., 1982; Herz 1982; Mason et al., 1982; Parker and Knoll 1990; Rosie 1987; Schene, 2004; Schene and Gersons 1986) but more recent systematic ones have been published as well (Catty et al., 2007; Horvitz-Lennon 2001; Marshall et al., 2003;). However the underlying questions of all reviews are comparable:

1 For what percentage of patients otherwise hospitalized, PH is a good alternative?

2 What is the (cost-)effectiveness of PH in comparison with FTH?

3 What is the (cost-)effectiveness of PH in comparison with outpatient treatment or day care?

Effectiveness of partial versus full-time hospitalization

Acute day hospital treatment as an alternative for inpatient treatment has been studied in randomized controlled trials (RCTs) in the United States (Herz et al., 1971; Sledge et al., 1996a,b; Washburn et al., 1976; Zwerling and Wilder 1962, 1964), the United Kingdom (Creed et al., 1989b, 1990, 1997; Dick et al., 1985a,b; Priebe et al., 2006), and the Netherlands (Kluiter et al., 1992; Schene et al., 1993). Three non-randomized controlled trials give some additional information (Fink et al., 1978; Michaux et al., 1972; Penk et al., 1978).

The aim of most studies was to randomize the patient population admitted to acute psychiatric wards towards FTH or PH in order to find how many patients could be treated by PH just as well as by FTH. However, in most studies not all admitted patients could actually be randomized. Only Zwerling and Kluiter did a randomized study on an unselected group of patients referred to FTH. All other studies suffered from design violation between admission and randomization, mostly because patients were 'too ill' to be randomized. This pre-randomization attrition influences the percentage of the population randomized to PH that after randomization had to be admitted to FTH: the smaller the selection before randomization, the higher the percentage of patients who failed in PH and had to be admitted to FTH. Zwerling, for instance, randomized 100% of admitted patients but had to admit 34% of those randomized to PH. For the other studies these percentages were respectively: 100% and 39.2% (Kluiter), 55% and 12% (Creed), 42% and 12% (Schene), 22% and 0% (Herz), 22% and 0% (Dick), and 15% and 0% (Washburn).

Earlier studies were less stringent and sophisticated in their methodology. Later studies had more differentiated outcome measures, made better descriptions of their patient selection, also measured family burden, costs and satisfaction with services, and calculated the use of medication. In their Cochrane review Marshall et al. (2003) concluded that for between 18.4% and 39.1% of otherwise FTH-patients PH is a feasible alternative. Both PH and FTH are just as effective (on social functioning, burden on carers, deaths (suicide, homicide, all causes), number unemployed at follow-up and readmission) but PHP has three main advantages: a more rapid improvement in mental state, a higher satisfaction with services, and lower costs.

The overall conclusion must be that PH can be a good alternative for about 20% to 40% of patients in need of acute psychiatric admission. For that population there are no differences between PH and FTH in the reduction of symptoms while there is some tendency that social functioning has a better outcome in PH, although this difference has disappeared 2 years later. This finding from earlier studies, was not replicated is some later studies (Creed et al., 1990; Kluiter et al., 1992; Schene et al., 1993), but recently Kallert et al. (2007) did. From their multicentre RCT they concluded that day hospital care was as effective as conventional inpatient care with respect to psychopathological symptoms and quality of life, but more effective on social functioning (at discharge and 3- and 12-month follow-up). Because of its sample size (n = 1117) this study has 'more than doubled the existing evidence base' for the day hospital being a 'viable and clinically effective alternative to inpatient admission for approximately one-fifth of all acute admissions'.

All RCTs together tell us something about contraindications for PH: patients who could harm themselves or others, who fail to care for themselves, who given their symptomatology have no support systems, who are homeless, who also suffer from a severe addiction disorder, patients with organic disorders, and those in need of somatic treatment or nursing care. In all those cases, patients have to be admitted to inpatient services first.

Other outcome measures showed that satisfaction with services is equal or somewhat better in PH (Priebe et al., 2006; Schene et al., 1997). Also family members are more satisfied, while almost all studies have shown no difference in family or care-giver burden. Only Creed et al. (1997) found day hospital patients were less of a burden to their carers at 1 year post-admission. Schene et al. (1993), Wiersma et al. (1995), Sledge et al. (1996a), and Priebe et al. (2006) found no difference in readmissions, while Creed et al. (1990) found more readmissions for those treated in FTH.

Apart from Kris (1965), Herz et al. (1971) and Sledge et al. (1996a) all RCTs found PH to have a longer treatment duration than FTH. This might be related to greater acceptance of PH by patients, more satisfaction, and more compliance with services. However, a relation with the time needed to reach treatment effectiveness as well as Hawthorne effects, are other explanations. Schene et al. (1993) mentioned the interaction of treatment length and treatment intensity as a possible causative factor: PH combines a lower intensity with a longer duration of treatment, while FTH has a higher intensity combined with a shorter duration.

Cost-effectiveness of partial versus full-time hospitalization

Four RCTs have also considered costs. Wiersma et al. (1995) found over a 2-year period direct costs (number of in- and day-patient days and outpatient contacts) for PH and FTH were more or less the same. In this study, costs per day for PH and FTH were the same as well as the number of staff needed to run the service. Because patients' compliance and satisfaction with services both for patient and families was better in PH, they concluded that day treatment can be considered a cost-effective alternative to inpatient treatment.

Sledge et al. (1996b) compared FTH with a day hospital/crisis respite programme. Over a 10-month period the experimental condition was $7100 (20%) cheaper than FTH. In particular the index admission was 43% less expensive due to operating costs which were twice as high in FTH. Personal costs were equal in both conditions as well as effectiveness. Therefore Sledge concluded that in his study PH was less expensive for two reasons: the length of stay during index admission was 7 days less in PH and operating costs were lower.

Creed et al. (1997) assessed costs over 12 months after the date of admission. They found that overall day hospital treatment was £1994 less expensive than FTH for the 30% to 40% of potential admissions that can be treated in this way. Although day hospital patients were less of a burden to their carers the later may bear additional costs.

Priebe et al. (2006) found the costs of the day hospital patients to be higher than the inpatients. Reasons for this were the longer treatment time in the day hospital, the fact that half of the day hospital group also received inpatient care, and the cost per day at the day hospital, which were around 70% of the cost of a day on the inpatient wards, so relatively high.

Acute day hospital care

The percentage of an admissions cohort eligible for PH of course is dependent on other patient, network or support, and service characteristics. If, for instance, patients are well integrated into community support systems this percentage will rise. If the threshold for psychiatric admissions is high, because of a shortage of beds in a certain region, it will be lower because patients will be more severe. Residents and junior staff (Kluiter et al., 1992; Platt et al., 1980; Washburn et al., 1976) also seem to lower this percentage. Acute day hospital care seems to have better opportunities with a well trained and skilled staff with an attitude favouring PH (Herz et al., 1971; Schene 1992). The service has to be closely connected to inpatient services, having available all diagnostic and treatment facilities necessary for acutely ill psychiatric patients.

Practical issues such as transport from home to service and if needed overnight accommodation or a back-up bed (Gudeman et al., 1983) are also important prerequisites. Additional support at home by for instance a community psychiatric nurse, a 24-hour crisis telephone service and the opportunity for outreach to patients in crisis can help to make PH a success for a higher percentage of the admitted patient group.

Partial hospitalization and beds

In a day hospital functioning as an alternative to inpatient hospitalization, Turner and Hoge (1991) studied the use of an overnight hospitalization or backup bed. Twenty per cent of patients admitted to the day hospital used the back-up bed (47% for 1 night, 19% for 2 nights, and 34% for 3 nights). The main reasons were psychotic symptoms (44% of back-up admissions), dangerousness (81%), and extreme agitation (5%). Of all episodes, 73% returned to the day hospital and 27% resulted in FTH. Only 50% of the back-up bed users were able to complete their day hospitalization, the other 50% received a standard FTH.

To really understand the relation between the use of FTH, PH, and outpatient services we first consider for a specific catchment area the total number of days that acutely ill patients should spend in a hospital setting because that setting is more effective or protective than outpatient care. Secondly we consider the percentage of the total amount of days which could be spend just as safely and effectively in an acute day hospital. Of all patients referred for FTH k% will spend their whole admission in FTH, l% will have a combination of x days in FTH and y days in PH (the percentage x/x+y will vary between 1% and 99%) and m% will spend their total time in PH (Schene, 1992).

Effectiveness of partial hospitalization versus outpatient treatment

Comparisons between PHP and outpatient treatment suffers from quite diverse populations and settings and so even more complicated methodologies (Schene 2004). A distinction should be made in: 1) day hospitals or day treatment programmes, emphasizing treatment and run by medical services with the psychotic patient as target group, 2) idem with the non-psychotic patient as target group, and 3) facilities or day care centres run by non-medical services (e.g. social services) and providing long-term care.

Regarding the first category (long-term mostly psychotic patients as target population) only three trials comparing day care medical services with outpatient services were executed in the United States before 1980. Meltzhoff and Blumenthal (1966) found better results for PH for patient with chronic schizophrenia: fewer admissions days, more work, and greater independence. Day treatment changed the deterioration of those patients. Guy et al. (1969) reported that medication and PH for patients with schizoaffective disorder has advantages in terms of reduction of symptoms. Linn et al. (1979) studied 122 male patients with schizophrenia and found a better outcome on symptoms at the end of the 2-year study period and better social functioning during the whole 2-year period. There were no differences in readmissions. Also Weldon et al. (1979) showed better functioning and significant more work or training after 3 months. The quality of these studies was insufficient to show evidence that day hospital care had substantial advantages over outpatient care. Authors of a recently updated Cochrane review (Shek et al., 2009), however, concluded that they had 'the impression' that day hospital does reduce time in inpatient care. Data to support the idea that day hospital or outpatient care helps avoid admission was not strong. Because all trials were undertaken over decades ago, results are difficult to apply in the context of modern outpatient services. It seems that meanwhile this type of PHP has been superseded by case management approaches and vocational rehabilitation programmes.

Regarding the second category of comparison of outpatient and PHP (treatment refractory non-psychotic patients as target population) the Cochrane review of Marshall et al. (2003) could include only four studies, with the following target populations: borderline personality disorders (Bateman and Fonaghy 1999), affective disorders and personality disorders (Piper et al, 1993, 1996), persistent anxiety or depression (Dick et al., 1991), and anxiety or depressive neurosis (Tyrer et al., 1987). Because of the quite different settings and heterogeneous populations definite conclusions could not be drawn. However, considering the total picture the authors concluded tentatively that day treatment might be superior to continued outpatient treatment in terms of improving symptoms and social functioning. Differences in necessary inpatient admissions were not found, patient satisfaction results were equivocal, while participation rates might be lower in day treatment compared to outpatient treatment.

Regarding the third category (facilities or day care centres run by non-medical services) Catty et al. (2007) designed a Cochrane review to determine the effects of non-medical day centre care for people with severe mental illness, but the 12 studies they found were all on medical and not on non-medical day centres. There is a clear need for randomized controlled trials of day centre care compared to other forms of day care.

Therapeutic factors

Hoge et al. (1988) studied therapeutic factors in a day hospital functioning as an alternative to FTH. Patients and staff mentioned the following therapeutic factors in declining frequency: structure, interpersonal contact, medication, altruism, catharsis, learning, mobilization of family support, connection to community, universality, patient autonomy, successful completion, and security. He concluded that it was striking that PH in this setting provides security and structure while simultaneously promoting patient responsibility and autonomy.

Schreer (1988) did a comparable study in a private, non-for-profit, short-term psychiatric partial hospital with more affective and less psychotic disorders than Hoge. She found interpersonal contact just as important, but feedback on behaviour, universality, and learning to be more important, while structure, medication, and security were less important.

Davidson et al. (1996) studied the social environment of a conventional psychiatric inpatient setting with that of a combined day hospital and crisis respite programme. The day hospital programme had higher expectations for patient functioning, a lower tolerance for deviance, more patient choice, and allowing for more continuation of patients' ongoing community involvement. The programme had a more stimulating and attractive physical environment and social milieu. It promoted higher levels of patient functioning and activity, increased help with daily living skills and social and recreational resources and more integration of patients into the community outside the facility.

Discussion and conclusions

PH has become an important, highly differentiated sector of mental health services, representing a spectrum which overlaps with FTH at the one end and outpatient services at the other. There is enough evidence to consider PH to be a good alternative for about one-fifth to one-third of acute patients in need of FTH. Operating costs might be lower, but personal costs are about equal. For this reason integrated admission units which offer FTH and PH in a flexible way seem to be the most practical and need-based way of working. Patients treated on those units start to sleep at home as soon as their clinical condition allows them to do so. The number of nights at home per week can be increased according to their condition. In our own Programme for Mood Disorders all admitted patients are screened for PH at admission. If possible they start PH immediately, if not they start FTH. Some are treated in FTH for the whole length of their admission. For most patients however a combination of FTH and PH is made during their 8- to 16-week stay.

Not only the clinical condition of patients determines the utilization of PH. Staff attitudes and skills, hospital policy, staff-to-patient ratios, structured programming, resources for managing clinical emergencies, distance from home to PH service, attitudes of family members, payment of service, and others certainly also have their influence. Choosing for PH in an early phase and not only when patients' decompensation is so severe that only FTH is still possible makes PH an important function in a comprehensive system of care. For such a short-term PH to be an alternative to FTH, Hoge et al. (1987) described five functions: reduction of acute symptoms (first 2 weeks), decrease of demoralization (week 3 and 4), facilitating community re-entry (weeks 1–4), education and skill building (week 3–4), and connection to community (week 4).

Looking at PH as an extension to outpatient care the conclusions are less clear. For patients with severe psychopathology who do not respond to regular outpatient treatment, PH seems to have some advantages for those with psychosis. For those with personality disorders PH might be an effective alternative for continued outpatient treatment. For both types of patients cost-effectiveness studies are lacking.

Hoge et al. (1992) had the opinion that this type of PH should be changed into assertive community treatment. Rosie et al. (1995) described that this view may be correct for patients with psychotic disorders, but does not hold for patients with personality disorders or severe neurosis. For them a time-limited 4-month programme had good outcome if it had a close relationship to a highly active outpatient clinic. What the future will bring in this field is not clear. Further research with RCTs comparing PH and intensive outpatient treatment with a long-term follow-up is needed.

Finally, the fourth function of PH, rehabilitation or day centre care, is rarely discussed in research terms. It is one of the cornerstones of community support systems, with a strong emphasis on training, support, and continuity of care. However, it lends itself to careful evaluation in the future. Trials comparing day care centres with intermittent day treatment programmes or with intensive forms of outpatient care are certainly lacking.

References

Bateman, A. and Fonaghy, P. (1999). Effectiveness of partial hospitalization in the treatment of borderline personality disorder: a randomized controlled trial. *American Journal of Psychiatry*, **156**, 1563–9.

Bierer, J. (1951). *The day hospital, an experiment in social psychiatry and syntho-analytic psychotherapy*. London: H.K. Lewis and Co.

Bierer, J. (1961). Day hospitals, further developments. *International Journal of Social Psychiatry*, **7**, 148–51.

Block, B.M. and Lefkovitz, P.M. (1991). *Standards and guidelines for partial hospitalization*. Alexandria, VA: American Association for Partial Hospitalization.

Bosch, G. and Veltin, A. (1983). *Die Tagesklinik als teil der psychiatrischen Versorgung*. Köln: Rheinland-Verlag GmbH.

Brocklehurst, J. (1979). The development and present status of day hospitals. *Age and Ageing*, **8**, 76–9.

Bystritsky, A., Muford, P.R., Rosen, R.M., Martin, K.M., Vapnik, T., Borbis, E.E., et al. (1996). A preliminary study of partial hospital management of severe obsessive-compulsive disorder. *Psychiatric Services*, **47**, 170–4.

Cameron, D.E. (1947). The day hospital: an experimental form of hospitalization for psychiatric patients. *Modern Hospital*, **69**, 60–2.

Casarino, J.P., Wilner, M., and Maxey, J.T. (1982). American Association for Partial Hospitalization (AAHP) standards and guideline for partial hospitalization. *International Journal of Partial Hospitalization*, **1**, 15–21.

Catty, J.S., Burns, T., Comas, A. and Poole, Z. (2007). Day centres for severe mental illness. *Cochrane Database of Systematic Reviews*, 1, CD001710.

Creed, F., Black, D., and Anthony, P. (1989a). Day-hospital and community treatment for acute psychiatric illness; a critical appraisal. *British Journal of Psychiatry*, **154**, 300–10.

Creed, F., Anthony, P., Godbert, K., and Huxley, P. (1989b). Treatment of severe psychiatric illness in a day hospital. *British Journal of Psychiatry*, **154**, 341–7.

Creed, F., Black, D., Anthony, P., Osborn, M., Thomas, P., and Tomenson, B. (1990). Randomized controlled trial of day versus inpatient psychiatric treatment. *British Medical Journal*, **300**, 1033–7.

Creed, F., Mbaya, P., Lancashire, S., Tomenson, B., Williams, B., and Holme, S. (1997). Cost-effectiveness of day and inpatient psychiatric treatment. *British Medical Journal*, **314**, 1381–5.

Davidson, L., Kraemer Tebes, J., Rakfeldt, J., and Sledge, W.H. (1996). Differences in social environment between inpatient and day hospital-crisis respite settings. *Psychiatric Services*, **47**, 714–20.

Department of Health and Social Security (1975). *Better Services for the Mentally Ill*. London: HMSO.

De Hert, M., Thys, E., Vercruyssen, V., and Peuskens, J. (1996). Partial hospitalization at night: the Brussels Nighthospital. *Psychiatric Services*, **47**, 527–8.

DiBella, G., Weitz, G.W., Pogntes Bergen, D., and Yurmark, J.L. (eds.) (1982). *Handbook of Partial Hospitalization*. New York: Brunner/Mazel.

Dick, P.H., Ince, A., and Barlow, M. (1985a). Day treatment: suitability and referral procedure. *British Journal of Psychiatry*, **142**, 250–53.

Dick, P.H., Cameron, L., Cohen, D., Barlow, M., and Ince, A. (1985b). Day and full time psychiatric treatment: a controlled comparison. *British Journal of Psychiatry*, **147**, 246–50.

Dick, P.H., Sweeney, M.L., and Crombie, I.K. (1991). Controlled comparison of day-patient and out-patient treatment for persistent anxiety and depression. *British Journal of Psychiatry*, **158**, 24–7.

Dzagharov, M.A. (1937). Experience in organizing a day hospital for mental patients. *Neuropathologi Psikhiatri*, **6**, 137–46.

Farndale, J. (1961). *The day hospital movement in Great Britain*. London: Pergamon Press.

Fink, E.B., Longabaugh, R., and Stout, R. (1978). The paradoxical underutilization of partial hospitalization. *American Journal of Psychiatry*, **135**, 713–16.

Gerlinghoff, M., Backmund, H., and Franzen, U. (1998). Evaluation of a day treatment programme for eating disorders. *European Eating Disorders Review*, **6**, 96–106.

Gudeman, J.E., Shore, M.F., and Dickey B. (1983). Day hospitalization and an inn instead of inpatient care for psychiatric patients. *New England Journal of Medicine*, **308**, 749–53.

Guy, W., Gross, M., Hogarty, G.E., and Dennis, H. (1969). A controlled evaluation of day hospital effectiveness. *Archives of General Psychiatry*, **201**, 329–38.

Herz, M.I., Endicott, J., Spitzer, R.L., and Mesnikoff, A. (1971). Day versus inpatient hospitalization: a controlled study. *American Journal of Psychiatry*, **127**, 1371–81.

Herz, M.I. (1982). Research overview in day treatment. *International Journal of Partial Hospitalization* **1**, 33–45.

Hoge, M.A., Farrell, S.P., Strauss, J.S., and Munchnel Posner, M. (1987). Functions of short-term partial hospitalization in a comprehensive system of care. *International Journal of Partial Hospitalization*, **4**, 177–88.

Hoge, M.A., Farrell, S.P., Munchnel, M.E., and Strauss, J.S. (1988). Therapeutic factors in partial hospitalization. *Psychiatry*, **51**, 199–210.

Hoge, M.A., Davidson, L., Leonard Hill, W., Turner, V.E., and Ameli, R. (1992). The promise of partial hospitalization: a reassessment. *Hospital and Community Psychiatry*, **43**, 345–54.

Holloway, F. (1991). Day care in an inner city I. *Characteristics of the attenders. British Journal of Psychiatry*, **158**, 805–10.

Horvitz-Lennon, M., Normand, S.L., Gaccione, P. and Frank, R.G. (2001). Partial versus full hospitalization for adults in psychiatric distress: a systematic review of the published literature (1957-1997). *American Journal of Psychiatry*, **158**, 676–85.

Kallert, T.W., Glockner, M., Priebe, S., Briscoe, J., Rymaszewska, J., Adamowski, T., et al. (2004). A comparison of psychiatric day hospitals in five European countries: implications of their diversity for day hospital research. *Social Psychiatry & Psychiatric Epidemiology*, **39**, 777–88.

Kallert, T.W., Priebe, S., McCabe, R., Kiejna, A., Rymaszewska, J., Nawka, P., *et al.* (2007). Are day hospitals effective for acutely ill psychiatric patients? A European multicenter randomized controlled trial. *Journal of Clinical Psychiatry*, **68**, 278–87.

Klar, H., Francis, A., and Clarkin, H. (1982). Selection criteria for partial hospitalization. *Hospital and Community Psychiatry*, **33**, 929–33.

Kluiter, H., Giel, R., Nienhuis, F.J., Rüphan, M., and Wiersma, D. (1992). Predicting feasibility of day treatment for unselected patients referred for inpatient psychiatric treatment: results of a randomized trial. *American Journal of Psychiatry*, **149**, 1199–205.

Kris, E.B. (1960). Intensive short-term treatment in a day care facility for the prevention of rehospitalization of patients in the community showing recurrence of psychotic symptoms. *Psychiatric Quarterly*, **34**, 83–8.

Kris, E.B. (1965). Day hospitals. *Current Therapeutic Research*, **7**, 1331–40.

Linn, M.W., Caffey, E.M., Klett, C.J., Hogarty, G.E., and Lamb, H.R. (1979). Day treatment and psychotropic drugs in the aftercare of schizophrenic patients. *Archives of General Psychiatry*, **36**, 1055–66.

Lussier, R.G., Steiner, J., Grey, A., and Hansen, C. (1997). Prevalence of dissociative disorders in an acute care day hospital populaton. *Psychiatric Services*, **48**, 244–6.

Marshall, M., Crowther, R., Almaraz-Serrano, A.M., Creed, F., Sledge, W.H., Kluiter, H, *et al.* (2003). Day hospital versus admission for acute psychiatric disorders. *Cochrane Database of Systematic Reviews*, 1, CD004026.

Mason, J., Louks, J., Burmer, G., and Scher, M. (1982). The efficacy of partial hospitalization: a review of recent literature. *International Journal of Partial Hospitalization*, **1**, 251–69.

Mbaya, P., Creed, F., and Tomenson, B. (1998). The different uses of day hospitals. *Acta Psychiatrica Scandinavica*, **98**, 283–7.

Meltzhoff, J. and Blumenthal, R. (1966). *The day treatment center: principles, application and evaluation*. Springfield Ill.: Charles C. Thomas.

Michaux, M.H., Chelst, M.R., Foster, S.A., Prium, R.J., and Dasinger, E.M. (1972). Day- and full-time treatment, a controlled comparison. *Current Therapeutic Research*, **14**, 279–92.

Parker, S.P. and Knoll III, J.L. (1990). Partial hospitalization: an update. *American Journal of Psychiatry*, **147**, 156–60.

Penk, W.E., Charles, H.L., and Van Hoose, T.A. (1978). Comparative effectiveness of day hospital and inpatient psychiatric treatment. *Journal of Consulting & Clinical Psychology*, **46**, 94–101.

Piper, W.E., Rosie, J.S., Azim, H.F.A. and Joyce, A.S. (1993). A randomized trial of psychiatric day treatment for patients with affective and personality disorders. *Hospital and Community Psychiatry*, **44**, 757–63.

Piper, W.E., Rosie, J.S., Joyce, A.S., and Azim, H.F.A. (1996). *Time-limited day treatment for personality disorders*. Washington, DC: American Psychological Association.

Platt, S.D., Knights, A.C., and Hirsch, S.R. (1980). Caution and conservatism in the use of a psychiatric day hospital; evidence from a research project that failed. *Psychiatric Research*, **3**, 123–32.

Priebe, S., Jones, G., McCabe, R., Briscoe, J., Wright, D., Sleed, M. and Beecham, J. (2006). Effectiveness and costs of acute day hospital treatment compared with conventional in-patient care: Randomised controlled trial. *British Journal of Psychiatry*, **188**, 243–9.

Rosie, J.S. (1987). Partial hospitalization: a review of recent literature. *Hospital and Community Psychiatry*, **38**, 1291–9.

Rosie, J.S., Azim, H.F.A., Piper, W.E., and Joyce, A.S. (1995). Effective psychiatric day treatment: historical lessons. *Psychiatric Services*, **46**, 1019–26.

Schene, A.H. (1985). *Psychiatric partial hospitalization: an overview*. Utrecht: Netherlands Center of Mental Health (in Dutch).

Schene, A.H. (1992). Psychiatric partial and full time hospitalization: a comparative study. Thesis. Utrecht: University of Utrecht.

Schene, A.H. (2004). The effectiveness of psychiatric partial hospitalisation and day care. *Current Opinion in Psychiatry*, **17**, 303–9.

Schene, A.H. and Gersons, B.P.R. (1986). Effectiveness and application of partial hospitalization. *Acta Psychiatrica Scandinavica*, **74**, 335–40.

Schene, A.H., van Lieshout, P., and Mastboom, J. (1986). Development and current status of partial hospitalization in the Netherlands. *International Journal of Partial Hospitalization*, **3**, 237–46.

Schene, A.H., van Lieshout, P., and Mastboom, J. (1988). Different types of partial hospitalization programs: results from a nationwide study. *Acta Psychiatrica Scandinavica*, **75**, 515–20.

Schene, A.H., van Wijngaarden, B., Poelijoe, N.W., and Gersons, B.P.R. (1993). The Utrecht comparative study on psychiatric day treatment and inpatient treatment. *Acta Psychiatrica Scandinavica*, **87**, 427–36.

Schene, A.H., van Wijngaarden, B., and Gersons, B.P.R. (1997). Partial or full-time hospitalization: patients' preferences. In: M. Tansella (ed.) *Making rational mental health services*, pp. 145–54. Roma: Il Pensiero Scientifico Editore.

Schreer, H. (1988). Therapeutic factors in psychiatric day hospital treatment. *International Journal of Partial Hospitalization*, **4**, 307–19.

Shek, E., Stein, A.T., Shansis, F.M., Marshall, M., Crowther, R., and Tyrer, P. (2009). Day hospital versus outpatient care for people with schizophrenia. *Cochrane Database of Systematic Reviews*, **4**, CD003240.

Shepherd, G. (1991). Day treatment and care. In: Bennett, D.H. and Freeman, H.L. (eds.) *Community Psychiatry*. London: Churchill Livingstone.

Sledge, W.H., Tebes, J., Rakfeldt, J., Davidson, L., Lyons, L. and Druss, B. (1996a). Day hospital/crisis respite care versus inpatient care, Part I: clinical outcomes. *American Journal of Psychiatry*, **153**, 1065–73.

Sledge, W.H., Tebes, J., Wolff, N., and Helminiak, T.W. (1996b). Day hospital/crisis respite care versus in-patient care. *Part II. Service utilization and costs. American Journal of Psychiatry*, **153**, 1074–83.

Turner, V.E. and Hoge, M.A. (1991). Overnight hospitalization of acutely ill day hospital patients. *International Journal of Partial Hospitalization*, **7**, 23–36.

Tyrer, P., Remington, M., and Alexander J. (1987). The outcome of neurotic disorders after out-patient and day hospital care. *British Journal of Psychiatry*, **151**, 57–62.

Washburn, S., Vannicelli, R., Longabaugh, R., and Scheff, B.J. (1976). A controlled comparison of psychiatric daytreatment and inpatient hospitalization. *Journal of Consulting & Clinical Psychology*, **44**, 665–75.

Weldon, E., Clarkin, J.E., Hennessy, J.J., and Frances, A. (1979). Day hospital versus outpatient treatment. *A controlled study. Psychiatric Quarterly*, **51**, 144–50.

Wiersma, D., Kluiter, H., Nienhuis, F.J., Ruphan, M., and Giel, R. (1995). Costs and benefits of hospital and day treatment with community care of affective and schizophrenic disorders. *British Journal of Psychiatry*, **27**, 52–9.

Zwerling, I., and Wilder, J.F. (1962). Day hospital treatment for acutely psychotic patients. *Current Psychiatric Therapies*, **2**, 200–10.

Zwerling, I., and Wilder, J.F. (1964). An evaluation of the applicability of the day hospital in treatment for acutely disturbed patients. *Israel Annals of Psychiatry and Related Disciplines*, **2**, 162–85.

CHAPTER 18

Individual placement and support: the evidence-based practice of supported employment

Deborah R. Becker, Gary R. Bond, and Robert E. Drake

Introduction

In most societies, employment is a major avenue to social inclusion (Grove et al., 2005). The benefits of working include increasing one's financial resources, being productive and contributing to society, utilizing one's skills and talents, enhancing self-esteem, improving self-image, meeting other people, and structuring one's time. People with severe mental illness benefit from employment in these same ways. In addition, work enables many to recover from the disabling effects of mental illness.

Expectations for people with severe mental illness have changed drastically in the last two decades. Clients who once were relegated to day treatment 5 days a week are now working competitively. The most successful employment practice to assist people develop a working life is a form of supported employment called individual placement and support (IPS). IPS has been standardized, tested, and implemented in several countries, especially the United States.

Principles and practice of IPS supported employment

Created in the 1980s for people with developmental disabilities, supported employment assists people with disabilities to work competitively alongside others who are not disabled. Modified for people with severe mental illness, IPS supported employment focuses on helping clients find regular part-time or full-time jobs.

The seven guiding principles of IPS supported employment and how they contrast with traditional vocational services are listed in Table 18.1.

First, the only eligibility requirement for services is a desire to work a competitive job. People are not screened for work readiness or other prerequisites.

Second, people are assisted in obtaining comprehensive benefits counselling to learn about work incentive programmes and how work may affect their benefits. Many people with mental illness receive health, disability, welfare, or other benefits (primarily from Social Security, Medicaid, and Medicare in the United States). They are hesitant to return to work because they fear losing these benefits, and accurate information can help them make good decisions.

Third, the goal is competitive employment. People are assisted in finding jobs that pay at least minimum wage and provide the benefits that others receive in the same position. The jobs are not set aside for people with disabilities, such as sheltered work or time-limited positions that are negotiated by a rehabilitation facility or mental health agency.

Fourth, employment specialists assist individuals to seek competitive jobs directly, without requiring lengthy prevocational training or work adjustment activities. While the length of the job search varies, most individuals contact potential employers within 1 month and obtain a desired job within about 3 or 4 months.

Fifth, client preferences determine the type of job, the work environment, decisions about disclosure of disability to the employer, and type of job supports. Employment specialists assist clients to find jobs that are consistent with their job preferences, skills, and previous experiences.

Sixth, support is provided to the client after obtaining employment for as long as he or she wants. Although clients differ in their desire and need for support, the guideline for IPS programmes is to provide regular support for 1 year after a client is working steadily. Afterward, the client transitions off the IPS supported employment caseload, and his/her primary mental health practitioner asks about the job during their regular sessions.

Seventh, IPS supported employment services are team-based. The employment specialist can join one or two multidisciplinary treatment teams and meets at least weekly with each team to review clients, coordinate services, and update plans.

Table 18.1 IPS supported employment compared to traditional approaches

Evidence-based supported employment	Traditional vocational approaches
Integration of mental health, substance abuse and employment services is important. Employment specialists are usually employed by the mental health agency. They attend weekly meetings with clinicians to discuss clients and their goals. State Vocational Rehabilitation also collaborates closely with supported employment programmes	Services are often brokered, meaning that clients receive mental health services, substance abuse services and vocational services at separate agencies
All clients are eligible. Motivation to work is an important predictor of success. Clients are not screened out due to substance abuse, symptoms, hospitalization history, treatment non-adherence, or other factors	It is common for traditional programmes to attempt to assess which clients are 'ready' for employment and to screen out those who appear to have the most significant barriers, including substance abuse, to employment
Clients are encouraged to meet with a person trained in benefits (i.e. Social Security, Medicaid, etc.) to learn how benefits would be affected by part- or full-time employment	Many traditional programmes also offer referrals to benefit specialists
Competitive employment is the goal. These are regular jobs in the community that pay at least minimum wage. They are not jobs that are set aside for people with disabilities	Some programmes focus on competitive jobs, while others focus on sheltered jobs such as sheltered workshops or groups of clients working under the supervision of staff
The job search is rapid. Clients are not asked to participate in vocational evaluation or work adjustment programmes, as these 'pre-vocational, activities' are not related to better employment outcomes	Clients are frequently required to complete vocational testing, vocational adjustment programmes or other pre-vocational groups before searching for a community job
Client preferences are important. Client preferences may refer to type of work, job location, number of hours worked each week, work shift, disclosure of disability to employer, etc.	Some traditional programmes offer only limited choices. This is problematic since, just like anyone else, clients tend to stay employed longer at jobs that meet their preferences
Job supports are offered to working people on a continuous basis. The supported employment team provides long-term supports (typically for at least 1 year). Mental health practitioners sometimes provide supports to people who have been working successfully for more than a year	Follow-along supports are typically offered on a time-limited basis, often for 90 days

Review of the research

IPS supported employment has been designated an evidence-based practice based on several major reviews (Bond, 2004; Bond et al., 2008; Burns et al., 2007; Crowther et al., 2001; Lehman et al., 2004; Twamley et al., 2003) and one large multisite study (Cook et al., 2005). The practice has been well described (Becker and Drake, 2003; Swanson et al., 2008) and a fidelity scale outlines its critical components (Becker et al., 2008; Bond et al., 1997).

Day treatment conversions: quasi-experimental studies

Starting in the late 1980s in the United States, there were several evaluations of day treatment programmes that converted their rehabilitation services to supported employment. Drake and colleagues (1994) compared employment outcomes for people attending day treatment to those people who participated in a former day treatment programme that converted to IPS supported employment. In the conversion site, day treatment counsellor positions were changed to employment specialist positions. Clients continued to receive mental health services (i.e. medication management, case management, etc.) but were encouraged to consider obtaining a competitive job with the support of an employment specialist and the rest of the mental health team.

Employment outcomes significantly increased for those people receiving IPS employment services. Clients, family members, and staff were interviewed 1 year later and reported positively about the changes. The expressed concern about social activities was met by peer support services (Torrey et al., 1995). The finding of increased employment outcomes was replicated in four additional studies (Bailey et al., 1998; Becker et al., 2001a; Drake et al., 1996a; Gold and Marrone, 1998). Clark (1998) demonstrated

that replacing day treatment with IPS supported employment led to cost savings.

Randomized controlled trials

Twelve randomized controlled trials (RCTs) of high-fidelity IPS supported employment demonstrated consistently favourable employment outcomes as compared to traditional stepwise employment services as shown in Fig. 18.1. Across these studies, the competitive employment rate was 62% for people who received IPS supported employment as compared to 23% for people who received traditional vocational services Bond et al., 2008; Davis et al., 2004. The studies conducted in the United States included rural (Gold et al., 2003) and urban (Drake et al., 1999; Lehman et al., 2002; Mueser et al., 2004) communities, diverse populations of African Americans (Bond et al., 2007; Drake et al., 1999, Lehman et al., 2002), Latinos (Mueser, et al., 2004), and older adults (Twamley et al., 2008). These studies compared IPS supported employment to leading vocational approaches of the day, including skills training (Drake et al., 1996b) and psychosocial rehabilitation (Bond et al., 2007). Internationally, RCTs of IPS supported employment have been conducted in Canada (Latimer et al., 2006), a six-country study in Europe (Burns, et al., 2007) and in the Netherlands (van Erp et al., 2007), in Australia with young adults with an initial psychotic episode (Killackey et al., 2008), and in Hong Kong (Wong et al., 2008).

Across these studies Bond et al. (2008) found that about two-thirds of the people who obtained a competitive job worked at least 20 hours. Of the clients who obtained a competitive job, those in IPS supported employment secured their first job about 10 weeks faster than the controls. After the start of the first job, the IPS clients averaged about 24 weeks per year of employment.

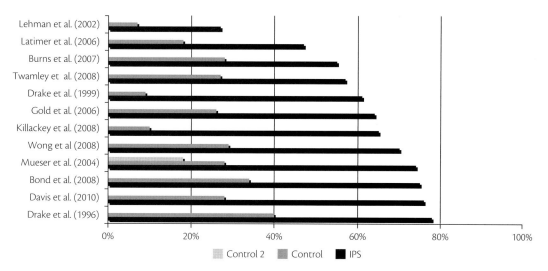

Fig. 18.1 Competitive employment rates in 12 randomized controlled trials of individual placement and support (Bond et al., 2008; Burns et al., 2007; Davis et al., 2010; Drake et al., 1996; Drake et al., 1999; Gold et al., 2008; Killackey et al., 2008; Latimer et al., 2006; Lehman et al., 2008; Mueser et al., 2004; Twamley et al., 2008; Wong et al., 2008).

Most of the studies had a follow-up of 18 or 24 months except for two that had a 12-month follow-up (Latimer et al., 2006; Twamley et al., 2008) and one with a 6-month follow-up (Killackey et al., 2008).

In addition to these 12 high-fidelity IPS studies, four RCTs of supported employment for people with psychiatric disabilities were conducted before the IPS model was first reported in the literature. All four of these early studies also significantly favoured supported employment over usual vocational services (Bond et al., 2008). Two recent RCTs evaluating IPS (Howard et al., 2010) and a vocationally oriented assertive community treatment programme (Macias et al., 2006) have not found an advantage for supported employment over comparison vocational services.

Long-term trajectories

The goal of vocational services is, of course, long-term careers rather than short-term jobs. Findings from two longitudinal, mixed-methods (quantitative and qualitative) studies indicate that many people who receive IPS supported employment continue to work in satisfying jobs that they consider careers over time. Salyers and colleagues (2004) conducted a 10-year follow-up of participants in an IPS supported employment study and found that 47% were working. Becker and colleagues (2007) followed up two groups of clients from the same mental health centre at 8 and 12 years after participating in IPS supported employment studies. At the time of the interview, 71% were currently working and 71% had worked more than half of the follow-up period. Clients reported that medication adjustments, working part time, and continued supports were important factors. Despite consistent employment, neither study found that clients on disability benefits had stopped receiving them completely.

Cost studies

A 2004 study estimated the costs of IPS employment services in seven IPS programmes throughout the United States (Latimer et al., 2004). Although estimates varied according to local salaries and caseload sizes, the cost updated to the present would be approximately $4000 per year for an employment specialist maintaining a caseload of 18 (Drake et al., 2009). Some evidence suggests that supported employment services for clients with psychiatric disabilities are less costly than for clients with other disabilities, possibly because on-site job coaching and training is

less common for people with psychiatric disabilities (Cimera, 2008). Day treatment programmes converting to IPS have resulted in substantial savings (Clark, 1998).

Other studies have suggested a reduction in community mental health treatment costs when clients enrol in supported employment (Bond et al., 1995). A longitudinal outcome study found reduced use of mental health treatment for clients with psychiatric disabilities who became steady workers (Bush et al., 2009). It has also been suggested that substantial cost savings to the federal budget could be realized if IPS were available to young adults experiencing their first psychosis, to reduce the number who begin a lifelong dependence on disability benefits (Drake et al., 2009).

Studies of enhanced supported employment

Several current studies investigate attempts to reach clients who have not expressed interest in employment and those who have been unsuccessful in supported employment.

Motivational counseling

Motivational interviewing is a well-regarded counselling technique pioneered in the treatment of substance use disorders (Miller and Rollnick, 1991). In an application to the vocational rehabilitation field, a single session of motivational interviewing was used to promote participation in vocational rehabilitation; the results were disappointing (Drebing et al., 2009). The results of a second study using motivational interviewing with IPS have not yet been reported (Larson et al., 2007).

Social skills training

Because interpersonal difficulties often precipitate job loss for people with severe mental illness (Becker et al., 1998), social skills training has often been used as a component of vocational services. Research demonstrates that pre-employment skills training as a prerequisite for entry into supported employment is ineffective (Drake et al., 1996). More recently, researchers have examined skills training as an adjunct to supported employment services, either for clients after they have obtained employment or for clients who have not benefited from IPS. Results thus far are mixed (Mueser et al., 2005; Tsang et al., 2009; Wallace and Tauber, 2004).

Cognitive studies

Several researchers are testing approaches to improve problems with memory, concentration, speed, and other cognitive areas in relation to work (McGurk and Mueser, 2004). A restorative approach, for example, includes computerized practice of cognitive functioning. Compensatory approaches may include job-specific coping strategies and job accommodations designed to help clients circumvent cognitive difficulties. Several controlled trials involving supported employment (McGurk et al., 2007) have found higher employment rates for clients receiving a cognitive intervention.

First psychotic episode and work and school

In the past decade, clinical research has emphasized early interventions for people with a first psychotic episode. One strategy involves return to daily life activities like work and school through IPS supported employment. In preliminary findings, Nuechterlein and colleagues (2008) reported that over 90% of the young adults receiving both school and work support through IPS supported employment obtained either a competitive job and/or enrolled in school. Findings are similar in three other studies (Killackey et al., 2008; Major et al., 2010; Rinaldi et al., 2004).

Implementation and fidelity

IPS supported employment has been implemented in routine settings in most states in the United States. Many jurisdictions and local sites utilize the IPS Fidelity Scale (Bond et al., 1997) as a guide to implementation. High-fidelity implementation typically requires initial training, supervision, and fidelity assessment over 6 to 12 months (Becker et al., 2008b). The 15-item IPS Fidelity Scale outlines the critical components of the practice with benchmarks, like a roadmap or a compass. It has been validated and revised based on research and recommendations from expert supported employment trainers (Becker et al., 2007). The updated scale contains 25 items and has an accompanying manual.

Several research studies have demonstrated that supported employment fidelity is significantly positively correlated with employment outcomes (Becker et al., 2001b, 2006; Catty et al., 2008; Henry and Hashemi, 2009; Hepburn and Burns, 2007). In these studies, independent assessors made site visits using the Supported Employment Fidelity Scale and found high-fidelity programmes had superior employment outcomes.

Dissemination

IPS supported employment was developed in the United States, and adoption has occurred more widely in the United States than elsewhere thus far. One large dissemination effort in the United States includes 12 states and the District of Columbia (Becker et al., 2008b; Drake et al., 2006). Over 120 local mental health agencies partner with local vocational rehabilitation providers to implement IPS supported employment. The number of sites continues to increase steadily in this project. Although employment outcomes are clearly affected by the economy and local unemployment (Cook et al., 2006), quarterly employment outcomes in the project have remained above 42% even during the current recession (Becker, 2009).

United States federal reviews advocate IPS supported employment (New Freedom Commission on Mental Health, 2003; U.S. Department of Health and Human Services, 1999), but federal funding mechanisms are not yet aligned with financing IPS supported employment (Lewin Group, 2009).

IPS supported employment is rapidly spreading to other countries as well. RCTs in several other countries (reviewed earlier in this chapter) have spurred this development over the past 5 to 10 years. The increasing numbers of adults on disability due to psychiatric illnesses is stressing democracies with free enterprise systems throughout the world (OECD, 2009). Countries of course vary considerably in terms of economic, workforce, health care, and disability regulations. The degree to which these factors enhance or impede supported employment is termed the 'disability trap' (Burns et al., 2007).

Conclusions

People with severe mental illnesses want to work, not only to improve their economic status but also as part of the process of recovery. Employment enhances one's self-image, self-esteem, relationships, and many other aspects of quality of life. The IPS supported employment model has demonstrated robust success in improving rates of competitive employment in the United States and other countries in which it has been tested. Nevertheless, dissemination progresses slowly in all countries, including the United States, as a result of bureaucratic resistance within the mental health and vocational rehabilitation systems, failures to align funding with evidence-based practices in general, antiquated disability regulations in many countries, and the economic downturn of recent years. Widespread uptake will require attention to all of these factors.

References

Bailey, E., Ricketts, S., Becker, D.R., Xie, H., and Drake, R.E. (1998). Conversion of day treatment to supported employment: One-year outcomes. *Psychiatric Rehabilitation Journal*, **22**, 24–9.

Becker, D.R. (2009). Outcome data from the Johnson & Johnson–Dartmouth Community Mental Health Program. Lebanon, NH: Dartmouth PRC.

Becker, D.R. and Drake, R.E. (2003). *A working life for people with severe mental illness*. New York: Oxford University Press.

Becker, D.R., Drake, R.E., Bond, G.R., Xie, H., Dain, B.J., and Harrison, K. (1998). Job terminations among persons with severe mental illness participating in supported employment. *Community Mental Health Journal*, **34**, 71–82.

Becker, D.R., Bond, G.R., McCarthy, D., Thompson, D., Xie, H., McHugo, G.J., *et al.* (2001a). Converting day treatment centers to supported employment programs in Rhode Island. *Psychiatric Services*, **52**, 351–7.

Becker, D.R., Smith, J., Tanzman, B., Drake, R.E., and Tremblay, T. (2001b). Fidelity of supported employment programs and employment outcomes. *Psychiatric Services*, **52**, 834–6.

Becker, D.R., Xie, H., McHugo, G.J., Halliday, J., and Martinez, R.A. (2006). What predicts supported employment program outcomes? *Community Mental Health Journal*, **42**, 303–13.

Becker, D.R., Whitley, R., Bailey, E.L., and Drake, R.E. (2007a). Long-term employment trajectories among participants with severe mental illness in supported employment. *Psychiatric Services*, **58**, 922–8.

Becker, D.R., Baker, S.R., Carlson, L., Flint, L., Howell, R., Lindsay, S., *et al.* (2007b). Critical strategies for implementing supported employment. *Journal of Vocational Rehabilitation*, **27**, 13–20.

Becker, D.R., Lynde, D., and Swanson, S. (2008b). Strategies for state-wide implementation of supported employment: The Johnson & Johnson-Dartmouth Community Mental Health Program. *Psychiatric Rehabilitation Journal*, **31**, 296–99.

Becker, D.R., Swanson, S.J., Bond, G.R., Carlson, L., Flint, L., Smith, G., et al. (2008a). *Supported employment fidelity scale.* Lebanon, NH: Dartmouth Psychiatric Research Center (http://dms.dartmouth.edu/prc/employment/).

Bond, G.R. (2004). Supported employment: Evidence for an evidence-based practice. *Psychiatric Rehabilitation Journal*, **27**, 345–59.

Bond, G.R., Dietzen, L.L., Vogler, K.M., Katuin, C.H., McGrew, J.H., and Miller, L.D. (1995). Toward a framework for evaluating costs and benefits of psychiatric rehabilitation: Three case examples. *Journal of Vocational Rehabilitation*, **5**, 75–88.

Bond, G.R., Becker, D.R., Drake, R.E., and Vogler, K.M. (1997). A fidelity scale of the Individual Placement and Support model of supported employment. *Rehabilitation Counseling Bulletin*, **40**, 265–84.

Bond, G.R., Salyers, M.P., Dincin, J., Drake, R.E., Becker, D.R., Fraser, V.V., et al. (2007). A randomized controlled trial comparing two vocational models for persons with severe mental illness. *Journal of Consulting and Clinical Psychology*, **75**, 968–82.

Bond, G.R., Drake, R.E., and Becker, D.R. (2008). An update on randomized controlled trials of evidence-based supported employment. *Psychiatric Rehabilitation Journal*, **31**, 280–89.

Burns, T., Catty, J., Becker, T., Drake, R.E., Fioritti, A., Knapp, M, et al. (2007). The effectiveness of supported employment for people with severe mental illness: A randomised controlled trial. *Lancet*, **370**, 1146–52.

Bush, P.W., Drake, R.E., Xie, H., McHugo, G.J., and Haslett, W.R. (2009). The long-term impact of employment on mental health service use and costs. *Psychiatric Services*, **60**, 1024–31.

Catty, J., Lissouba, P., White, S., Becker, T., Drake, R. E., Fioritti, A., et al. (2008). Predictors of employment for people with severe mental illness: results of an international six-centre RCT. *British Journal of Psychiatry*, **192**, 224–31.

Cimera, R.E. (2008). The costs of providing supported employment services to individuals with psychiatric disabilities. *Psychiatric Rehabilitation Journal*, **32**, 110–16.

Clark, R.E. (1998). Supported employment and managed care: Can they co-exist? *Psychiatric Rehabilitation Journal*, **221**, 62–8.

Cook, J.A., Leff, H.S., Blyler, C.R., Gold, P.B., Goldberg, R.W., Mueser, K.T., et al. (2005). Results of a multisite randomized trial of supported employment interventions for individuals with severe mental illness. *Archives of General Psychiatry.* **62**, 505–12.

Cook, J.A., Mulkern, G., Grey, D.D., Burke-Miller, J., Blyler, C.R., Razzano, L.A., et al. (2006). Effects of local unemployment rate on vocational outcomes in a randomized trial of supported employment for individuals with psychiatric disabilities. *Journal of Vocational Rehabilitation*, **25**, 71–84.

Crowther, R.E., Marshall, M., Bond, G.R., and Huxley, P. (2001). Helping people with severe mental illness to obtain work: Systematic review. *British Medical Journal*, **322**, 204–8.

Davis, L.L., Drebing, C., Parker, P.E., Leon, A.C. (2010). *Occupational recovery in persons with PTSD: Results from clinical investigations.* Paper presented at the International Society of Traumatic Stress Studies, Montreal, Quebec.

Drake, R.E., Becker, D.R., Biesanz, J.C., Torrey, W.C., McHugo, G.J., and Wyzik, P.F. (1994). Rehabilitation day treatment vs. supported employment: I. Vocational outcomes. *Community Mental Health Journal*, **30**, 519–32.

Drake, R.E., Becker, D.R., Biesanz, J.C., Wyzik, P.F., and Torrey, W.C. (1996a). Day treatment versus supported employment for persons with severe mental illness: A replication study. *Psychiatric Services*, **47**, 1125–7.

Drake, R.E., McHugo, G.J., Becker, D.R., Anthony, W.A., and Clark, R.E. (1996b). The New Hampshire study of supported employment for people with severe mental illness: Vocational outcomes. *Journal of Consulting and Clinical Psychology*, **64**, 391–99.

Drake, R.E., McHugo, G.J., Bebout, R.R., Becker, D,R., Harris, M., Bond, G.R., et al. (1999). A randomized clinical trial of supported employment for inner-city patients with severe mental illness. *Archives of General Psychiatry*, **56**, 627–33.

Drake, R.E., Becker, D.R., Goldman, H.H., and Martinez, R.A. (2006). Best practices: The Johnson & Johnson Dartmouth Community Mental Health Program: Disseminating evidence-based practice. *Psychiatric Services*, **57**, 302–4.

Drake, R.E., Skinner, J.S., Bond, G.R., and Goldman, H.H. (2009). Social Security and mental illness: Reducing disability with supported employment. *Health Affairs*, **28**, 761–70.

Drebing, C.E., Rosenheck, R.A., Drake, R.E., Penk, W., and Rose, G. (2009). *Pathways to vocational rehabilitation: Enhancing entry and retention.* Bedford, MA: Bedford VHA Hospital.

Gold, M. and Marrone, J. (1998). Mass Bay Employment Services (a service of Bay Cove Human Services, Inc.): A story of leadership, vision and action resulting in employment for people with mental illness, in *Roses and Thorns from the Grassroots.* Boston, MA: Institute for Community Inclusion.

Gold, P.B., Meisler, N., Santos, A.B., Keleher, J., Becker, D.R., Knoedler, W., et al. (2003). The program of assertive community treatment: Implementation and dissemination of an evidence-based model of community-based care for persons with severe and persistent mental illness. *Cognitive and Behavioral Practice*, **10**, 290–303.

Grove, B., Secker, J., and Seebohm, P. (eds.) (2005). *New thinking about mental health and employment.* Abingdon: Radcliffe Publishing.

Henry, A. D. and Hashemi, L. (2009). *Outcomes of supported employment services for adults with serious mental illness in Massachusetts: Findings from the Services for Education and Employment Technical Assistance Project (SEE-TAP).* Paper presented at the Dartmouth Psychiatric Research Center, Lebanon, NH.

Hepburn, B. and Burns, R. (2007). *Extending the welcome mat: Opening DOoRS to employment for individuals with co-occurring mental health and substance use disorders.* Paper presented at the MHA DORS Annual Conference, Baltimore, MD, June 22.

Howard, L.M., Heslin, M., Leese, M., McCrone, P., Rice, C., Jarrett, M., et al. (2010). Supported employment: randomised controlled trial. *British Journal of Psychiatry*, **196**, 404–11.

Killackey, E., Jackson, H.J., and McGorry, P.D. (2008). Vocational intervention in first-episode psychosis: individual placement and support v. treatment as usual. *British Journal of Psychiatry.* **193**, 114–20.

Larson, J.E., Barr, L.K., Kuwabara, S.A., Boyle, M.G., and Glenn, T.L. (2007). Process and outcome analysis of a supported employment program for people with psychiatric disabilities. *American Journal of Psychiatric Rehabilitation*, **10**, 339–53.

Latimer, E.A., Bush, P.W., Becker, D.R., Drake, R.E., and Bond, G.R. (2004). The cost of high-fidelity supported employment programs for people with severe mental illness. *Psychiatric Services*, **55**, 401–6.

Latimer, E.A., Lecomte, T., Becker, D.R., Drake, R.E., Duclos, I., Piat, et al. (2006). Generalisability of the individual placement and support model of supported employment: Results of a Canadian randomised controlled trial. *British Journal of Psychiatry*, **189**, 65–73.

Lehman, A.F., Goldberg, R.W., Dixon, L.B., McNary, S., Postrado, L., Hackman, A., et al. (2002). Improving employment outcomes for persons with severe mental illness. *Archives of General Psychiatry*, **59**, 165–72.

Lehman, A.F., Kreyenbuhl, J., Buchanan, R.W., Dickerson, F.B., Dixon, L.B., Goldberg, R., et al. (2004). The Schizophrenia Patient Outcomes Research Team (PORT): Updated treatment recommendations 2003. *Schizophrenia Bulletin*, **30**, 193–217.

Lewin Group. (2009, May 13). *ASPE Technical Expert Panel on Earlier Intervention for Serious Mental Illness: Summary of Major Themes.* Paper presented at the ASPE Technical Expert Panel, Washington, DC.

Macias, C., Rodican, C. F., Hargreaves, W. A., Jones, D. R., Barreira, P. J., and Wang, Q. (2006). Supported employment outcomes of a randomized controlled trial of ACT and clubhouse models. *Psychiatric Services*, **57**, 1406–15.

Major, B. S., Hinton, M. F., Flint, A., Chalmers-Brown, A., McLoughlin, K., and Johnson, S. (2010). Evidence of the effectiveness of a specialist vocational intervention following first episode psychosis: a naturalistic prospective cohort study. *Social Psychiatry and Psychiatric Epidemiology*, **45**, 1–8.

McGurk, S.R. and Mueser, K.T. (2004). Cognitive functioning, symptoms, and work in supported employment: A review and heuristic model. *Schizophrenia Research*, **70**, 147–73.

McGurk, S.R., Wolfe, R., Pascaris, A., Mueser, K.T., and Feldman, K. (2007). Cognitive training for supported employment: 2-3 year outcomes of a randomized controlled trial. *American Journal of Psychiatry*, **164**, 437–41.

Miller, W. R. and Rollnick, S. (1991). *Motivational interviewing: Preparing people to change addictive behavior*. New York: Guilford Press.

Mueser, K.T., Clark, R.E., Haines, M., Drake, R.E., McHugo, G.J., Bond, G.R., *et al.* (2004). The Hartford study of supported employment for persons with severe mental illness. *Journal of Consulting and Clinical Psychology*, **72**, 479–90.

Mueser, K.T., Aalto, S., Becker, D.R., Ogden, J.S., Wolfe, R.S., Schiavo, D., *et al.* (2005). The effectiveness of skills training for improving outcomes in supported employment. *Psychiatric Services*, **56**, 1254–60.

New Freedom Commission on Mental Health. (2003). *Achieving the promise: Transforming mental health care in America. Final Report.* (DHHS Pub. No. SMA-03-3832.) Rockville, MD: Substance Abuse and Mental Health Services Administration.

Nuechterlein, K.H, Subotnik, K.L., Turner, L.R., Ventura, J., Becker, D.R., and Drake, R.E. (2008). Individual Placement and Support for individuals with recent-onset schizophrenia: Integrating supported education and supported employment. *Psychiatric Rehabilitation Journal.* **31**, 340–9.

OECD (2009). *Sickness, disability and work: Keeping on track in the economic downturn*. Organisation for Economic Co-operation and Development Directorate for Employment, Labour and Social Affairs. Available at: http://www.oecd.org/dataoecd/42/15/42630589.pdf (accessed 4 May 2009).

Rinaldi, M., McNeil, K., Firn, M., Koletsi, M., Perkins, R., and Singh, S.P. (2004). What are the benefits of evidence-based supported employment for patients with first-episode psychosis? *Psychiatric Bulletin*, **28**, 281–4.

Salyers, M.P., Becker, D.R., Drake, R.E., Torrey, W.C., and Wyzik, P.F. (2004). Ten-year follow-up of clients in a supported employment program. *Psychiatric Services*, **55**, 302–8.

Swanson, S.J., Becker, D.R., Drake, R.E., and Merrens, M.R. (2008). *Supported employment: A practical guide for practitioners and s upervisors.* Lebanon, NH: Dartmouth Psychiatric Research Center.

Torrey, W.C., Becker, D.R., and Drake, R.E. (1995). Rehabilitative day treatment versus supported employment: II. Consumer, family and staff reactions to a program change. *Psychosocial Rehabilitation Journal*, **18**, 67–75.

Tsang, H. W., Chan, A., Wong, A., and Liberman, R. P. (2009). Vocational outcomes of an integrated supported employment program for individuals with persistent and severe mental illness. *Journal of Behavior Therapy and Experimental Psychiatry*, **40**, 292–305.

Twamley, E.W., Jeste, D.V., and Lehman, A.F. (2003). Vocational rehabilitation in schizophrenia and other psychotic disorders: A literature review and meta-analysis of randomized controlled trials. *Journal of Nervous and Mental Disease*, **191**, 515–23.

Twamley, E.W., Narvaez, J.M., Becker, D.R., Bartels, S.J., and Jeste, D.V. (2008). Supported employment for middle-aged and older people with schizophrenia. *American Journal of Psychiatric Rehabilitation*, **11**, 76–89.

U.S. Department of Health and Human Services (1999). *Mental Health: A Report of the Surgeon General*. Rockville, MD: U.S. Department of Health and Human Services, Substance Abuse and Mental Health Services Administration, Center for Mental Health Services, National Institutes of Health, National Institute of Mental Health.

van Erp, N.H., Giesen, F.B., van Weeghel, J., Kroon, H., Michon, H.W., Becker, D., *et al.* (2007). A multisite study of implementing supported employment in the Netherlands. *Psychiatric Services*, **58**, 1421–6.

Wallace, C. J., and Tauber, R. (2004). Supplementing supported employment with workplace skills training. *Psychiatric Services*, **55**, 513–15.

Wong, K.K., Chiu, R., Tang, B., Mak, D., Liu, J., and Chiu, S.N. (2008). A randomized controlled trial of a supported employment program for persons with long-term mental illness in Hong Kong. *Psychiatric Services*, **59**, 84–90.

CHAPTER 19

Inpatient treatment

Frank Holloway and Lloyd I. Sederer

Introduction

'Inpatient care is, from the research perspective, the Cinderella of contemporary mental health services' (Szmukler and Holloway, 2001: p. 333). Research on the day-to-day practice of inpatient care remains a step-child of psychiatry and a policy vacuum on the role of inpatient treatment characterizes our field today. In the majority of advanced mental health economies large mental hospitals and institutional care has been vanquished by deinstitutionalization that has produced vast numbers of inpatient bed reductions (see Table 19.1).

Deinstitutionalization was driven by many forces: empirical evidence about the harmful effects of large institutions on patients (Wing and Brown, 1970); a general social movement that emphasized the 'community' as a positive resource for helping people (Hawks, 1975); scandals surrounding institutional care (Martin, 1984); cost containment (Kluiter, 1997); concerns about the importance of patients' liberties and quality of life (Peele and Chodoff, 1999); and improvements in treatment technologies, which included medication, rehabilitation, assertive community treatment, psychological treatments, and crisis care (Ramsay and Holloway, 2007). A consensus developed amongst user groups, government and policy makers, service managers, and practitioners that inpatient treatment represented if not a failure then a barrier to an evolving paradigm of comprehensive community care. However, carers, clinicians in inpatient services, and community mental health staff who recognize the limits of community care however well it is done remain sceptical of such an antihospital proposition.

Table 19.1 Psychiatric inpatient beds in selected high income countries: 2004 data and changes over time

Country	Beds per 100,000 in 2004	% beds in mental hospitals in 2004	Peak year and beds	Ratio of beds maximum or 1965 data: contemporary
United States	77	40%	1955 339/100,000	4.4:1
Canada	193	48%	1965 400/100,000	2.1:1
Australia	39	31%	1965 271/100,000	6.9:1
New Zealand	38	26%	1949 c.500/100,00	13.2:1
Japan	284	73%	Not reached a peak: in 1965 133/100,000	0.46:1
France	120	58%	1974 250/100,000	2.1:1
Germany	75	60%	? 1965 177/100,000	2.4:1
Netherlands	187	65%	1955 260/100,000	1.4:1

(Continued)

Table 19.1 (*Contd.*) Psychiatric inpatient beds in selected high income countries: 2004 data and changes over time

Country	Beds per 100,000 in 2004	% beds in mental hospitals in 2004	Peak year and beds	Ratio of beds maximum or 1965 data: contemporary
Sweden	60	0%	1965–7 >354/100,000	5.9:1
Italy	46	0%	1963 224/100,000	4.9:1
Spain	44	84%	1974 130/1000,000	3.0:1
Ireland	94	79%	1958 500/100,000	5.3:1
United Kingdom	58	Not available	1955 350/100,000	6.0:1
All high-income countries	75	55%		

Given the discourse that has placed community mental health care in opposition to inpatient treatment it might be seen as paradoxical that a textbook of community mental health should contain a chapter on inpatient treatment. There is, in reality, no paradox: despite the advances in community mental health care over the past 50 years, inpatient treatment has not withered away. Inpatient treatment, whether for days or months, forms a necessary, significant, and costly component of any comprehensive mental health system. As an example, after a decade of sustained investment in community mental health services, in England in 2008 (taking account of indirect costs) 45% of the health and social care spending on adult mental health services was on three categories of inpatient care: secure care, acute inpatient care, and continuing care (see Table 19.2). What we stated a decade ago remains true: 'Despite the successful closure of the traditional long-stay mental hospitals, it seems undeniable that, even in the most highly evolved systems of community care, some inpatient beds are required' (Szmukler and Holloway, 2001: p. 333). In the United States the same analysis applies, with inpatient care an essential component of, and asset to, a fully responsive mental health care system.

The past decade has also produced critical information regarding patient experience and quality of care in hospital settings. Increased policy interest in the United Kingdom has produced a significant amount of research activity, though less so in the United States (Markowitz, 2008).

In this chapter we review:

◆ The role and function of inpatient psychiatry

◆ International trends in the provision of inpatient care

◆ Quality of care

◆ The hospital/community interface.

The role and function of inpatient psychiatry

There are many definitions for inpatient care. We define it to be 'treatment and care within a residential setting that is staffed 24 hours a day by nurses with involvement from psychiatrists with overall responsibility for patient care'. These settings admit patients voluntarily who have capacity (or competence); non-dissenting patients who lack capacity; and people who dissent to admission, compulsorily under local mental health legislation. Units vary as to

Table 19.2 Health and social care spending on adult mental health services in England

	2007–8 £1000s	
	Expenditure	% total costs
Secure and High Dependency Provision	859,460.29	16.0
Acute Inpatient Unit/Ward	611,189.53	11.1
Community Mental Health Teams	666,983.54	12.1
Continuing Care	497,800.31	9.0
Housing and Residential Care	429,364.52	8.0
Crisis Resolution/Home Treatment Teams	213,734.78	3.9
Day Services (including NHS)	202,085.51	3.7
Psychological Therapy Services	161,378.39	3.0
Assertive Outreach Teams	124,946.73	2.3
Psychiatric Outpatient Clinics	103,780.19	1.9
Home Support Services	108,587.11	2.0
Specialist mental health services	77,160.47	1.4
Early Intervention in Psychosis Services	69,178.99	1.3
Community Services for Mentally Disordered Offenders	50,368.94	1.0
Carer's Services	23,114.76	0.4
A&E Mental Health Liaison Service	20,065.11	0.4
Personality disorder services	15,642.20	0.3
Mental health promotion	4215.71	0.1
Direct payments	8715.69	0.2
Other direct costs	22,6002.76	4.1
Indirect costs	418,190.68	8.0
Capital charges	165,859.68	3.0
Overheads	440,068.73	8.0
Total	5512,262.49	100.00

Source: The 2007/8 National Survey of Investment in Mental Health Mental Health Strategies (2008)

which populations they will take and there are some crisis and rehabilitation units which do not take involuntary patients but otherwise have the characteristics of an inpatient unit. In addition to the core staffing of nurses and doctors quality inpatient services also have multidisciplinary clinicians, including occupational therapists, clinical pharmacists and psychologists and some have peer counsellors (individuals with a mental disorder who are in process of recovery). The focus of this chapter is on inpatient services for adults of working age (18–64 years), and acute care, though some of the data will cover broader populations and services.

What's inpatient treatment for?

The traditional psychiatric hospital served many functions. As a total institution offering long-term custodial care of patients with continuing disability it provided for the basic needs of its residents for food, shelter, clothing, and a minimal income (Thornicroft and Bebbington, 1989) and offered some opportunities for occupation, leisure, social interaction, and (secretly) sexual expression. It is now clear that for people with persistent, severe mental illness their continuing care needs can largely, although not entirely, be met satisfactorily outside the hospital (Leff and Trieman, 2000; Trieman and Leff, 2002).

The mental hospital served a range of functions that might be termed 'clinical'. These included crisis intervention; assessment or reassessment of diagnosis; the development and institution of a treatment plan; respite (for patient and carer); removal of the patient from a stressful environment; protection of the patient from exploitation; protection of the patient from himself; and protection of the public from dangerous or deviant behaviour (Bachrach, 1976; Talbott and Glick, 1986). Each of these functions can be undertaken without automatic recourse to admission, particularly where intensive support from crisis resolution/home treatment teams and Assertive Community Treatment (ACT) teams is available.

Even enthusiastic proponents of ACT acknowledge that there are limits to community care. Allness and Knoedler (1998), in a manual for ACT teams, set out criteria for short-term inpatient treatment when ACT crisis intervention does not reduce risk:

◆ Suicidal or homicidal ideation or behaviour

◆ Serious self-neglect or risk of physical harm (due to, for example, confusion, disorganized thinking)

◆ Mental illness and acute drug intoxication requiring a brief period of medical care

◆ Adjustment of medication where concern for medical complications, side effects, risk of symptomatic exacerbation requires medical supervision

◆ Serious physical illness comorbidity.

These criteria abide with studies on reasons for acute hospital admission. Abas et al. (2003), in a study of inpatient services in Auckland, New Zealand, identified reasons for admission as: reinstatement of medication (46%); intensive observation (43%); non-compliance with medication (35%); assaultive behaviour (32%); risk of self-neglect (24%); risk of suicide (22%); and misuse of medication/drugs (11%) (often with more than one reason per patient). Similar results appear in other studies (e.g. Preti et al., 2009).

Social and service contexts are also central in determining whether someone is admitted or not. The service context is obvious: if beds become less available or alternatives to admission are in place, thresholds for admission rise. Social issues that affect the decision to admit include relief for, or conflict with, carers, removal from stressful situations, prevention of psychosocial harm, and lack of social supports. Diversion from admission is particularly difficult where people are homeless or lack social supports.

Bowers (2005) identified seven reasons for admission: dangerousness, assessment, medical treatment, severe mental disorder, self-care deficits, respite for carers, and respite for the patient. He concluded that the role of inpatient staff (his interest is in nurses) is in 'providing safety for the patient and others; collecting and communicating information about patients; giving and monitoring treatment; tolerating and managing disturbed behaviour; providing personal care; and managing an environment where patients can comfortably stay'. To this we would add as a key role for staff: planning, with the patient and their carers, for prompt and safe discharge.

One inescapable dimension of inpatient treatment is to manage involuntary patients whose safety and that of the community are in peril. In all jurisdictions people with a mental disorder can be admitted against their will if they meet certain legal criteria, principally evidence of risk to themselves or others. In the United Kingdom, compulsory admission can also take place if treatment is deemed to be in the interests of the individual's health in the absence of overt dangerousness; in the United States many jurisdictions hold to the same criterion, but not all. For some jurisdictions compulsory admission is not necessarily linked to compulsory treatment— which can only occur if the individual is incapacitated (the United Kingdom term) or incompetent (the United States term). It may seem an irony that the authority to admit is not always coupled with the authority to treat; however, court ordered treatment is often needed when involuntary patients refuse treatment. Many jurisdictions now also have provision for compulsory treatment in the community (43 states in the United States have outpatient commitment), almost always after an episode of compulsory inpatient treatment (O'Brien et al., 2009). Reports on its efficacy are variable: some report doubt (Kisley et al., 2005) while others report clear success (Swartz et al., 2004).

Today's answers to the question 'what's inpatient admission for?' reflect a focused, if not limited, role for inpatient psychiatry. There was an earlier era where institutions served as centres for therapeutic activities, and were where 'milieu therapy' and the 'therapeutic community' were developed (see Jones, 2004 for a brief historical account). Some work continues in particular services (Campling et al., 2004) which includes a role for group therapies in inpatient settings (Radcliffe et al., 2010) as well as the systematic use of other therapies for inpatients. As an example, Markowitz (2008) reviewed a successful randomized controlled trial of interpersonal psychotherapy for patients admitted with major depression (Schramm et al., 2007) that was carried out in Germany, which would not be possible in the United States because of the much shorter length of stay for acute patients.

The spectrum of inpatient services

Inpatient services for adults of a working age vary in terms of their location, the level of acuity that they manage, the level of security they provide, and the degree of clinical specialism they offer. Inpatient wards may be free-standing (as a psychiatric hospital) or as a distinct unit within a general hospital. Acuity and security often go together: in the United Kingdom units may be 'open wards' or 'psychiatric intensive care units', the latter providing enhanced staffing and a degree of perimeter security for patients who are behaviourally disturbed or an abscondion risk (Beer et al., 2008); in the United States virtually all units are locked to provide safety since admission is almost invariably based on concerns about danger to self or others. United Kingdom facilities for offender patients can sometimes be 'open' but more typically have a secure perimeter, which may be designated 'low', 'medium', or 'high' depending on the level of risk patients are perceived to present; forensic facilities in the United States are locked and some have perimeter security.

Typically adult acute wards take a wide range of patients. Local mental health services (state mental health authorities in the United States) will, in addition to intensive care facilities, often have dedicated rehabilitation and continuing care wards for a longer-term population, who usually suffer from severe treatment-resistant psychotic illnesses (Killaspy et al., 2005). Tertiary centres in the United Kingdom may contain a large number of specialized inpatient units and can provide specialized care for perinatal psychiatry, eating disorders, neuropsychiatry and brain injury, comorbid mental illness and learning disability, anxiety disorders (including obsessive compulsive disorder), affective disorder, treatment resistant psychosis and self-harm/personality disorder (see, for example, South London and Maudsley NHS Foundation Trust (2010)).

Tertiary care state hospitals in the United States focus especially on people with psychotic illness that is not responsive to acute care, often characterized by danger to self or others; some units are further specialized for violence or personality disorders (especially borderline personality) with self-harm, or individuals with psychosis and significant cognitive impairments. The United States has both a complex pattern of funding health care and a very mixed economy of providers which include state mental hospitals, community hospitals, academic centres, and for-profit hospitals. A few private, not for profit, hospitals are centres for excellence and sites for highly specialized inpatient treatment in the United States, (e.g. McLean Hospital, Cornell-Westchester, Menninger and Shepard-Pratt), although the number of these tertiary centres has declined.

In England, where almost all psychiatric inpatient care is funded by the state, a significant proportion of inpatient beds are provided by the non-state sector (14% in 2008 (Healthcare Commission, 2008)), most of which is run for profit. This sector tends to offer more niche care to complex patient groups with comorbidities, often in small free-standing units.

Who becomes an inpatient?

Cross-sectional data provides a different picture of the inpatient population to prospective data since it will reflect individuals with longer length of stay; in general these are people with psychotic illnesses, who are more likely to be detained in hospital and exhibit comorbid substance misuse. In England in 1999 to 2000 the commonest admission diagnoses for working age adults were depression and anxiety (30%); schizophrenia and related psychoses (26%); substance misuse (19%); and mania (11%) (Thompson et al., 2004). A slightly different pattern is seen in the data from Italy where the commonest admission diagnoses (all ages) were schizophrenia (35%), depression and anxiety (20%), bipolar disorder (18%), and substance misuse (9%) (Preti et al., 2009).

A point-prevalence study of inpatient services in five Middle European countries (all ages) found a rather similar pattern with 33% of patients having a diagnosis of schizophrenia, 35% an affective disorder (subsuming bipolar disorder, depression and anxiety) and 13% substance misuse (Rittmannsberger et al., 2004). In the United States, mood disorders, schizophrenia, and schizoaffective disorders predominate.

Where there is a mixed economy of psychiatric care there are marked differences between patient characteristics in different sectors. In Italy people are significantly more likely to be admitted to the private sector for organic mental disorders and substance misuse and significantly less likely to be admitted for schizophrenia (Preti et al., 2009). In the United States, admissions to the state hospitals serve as the safety net for patients who are uninsured or do not respond to acute care; in recent years, as well, there is increasing presence of patients committed with forensic histories or on court order for restoration of competence or NGRI (not guilty for reason of insanity). (Bloom, 2008). In many states, the public hospitals serve as sites for individuals with serious paraphilias that have led to sex offending and whose sentence has expired but because of continuing risk may require continue containment (and treatment) (Hepburn and Sederer, 2009).

In the United Kingdom, a significant number of admissions are for the primary treatment of substance misuse either to specialist services for planned detoxification or following crisis presentation into acute wards: in the latter situation a key interface will be between the inpatient service and local substance misuse services. In the United States, unlocked residential programmes treat individuals with primary alcohol and drug problems that do not respond to ambulatory care. Comorbid substance misuse is also a very significant and common problem in inpatient services (Department of Health, 2006). Reported prevalence is in the region of 35% to 50%. We know that comorbid cannabis use significantly increases length of stay, possibly because cannabis can exacerbate psychotic symptoms (Isaac et al., 2005). One study has suggested that comorbid alcohol abuse was associated with significantly shorter lengths of stay (Sinclair et al., 2008). Substance misuse (both drugs and alcohol) is a very robust risk factor for violence and other offending behaviour, both in the population as whole and amongst psychiatric patients (Fazel et al., 2009). This reality is relevant to the reasons people get admitted in the first place, to diagnostic considerations, to day-to-day management of inpatients, and to the challenges of discharge planning in a risk-averse culture.

A further characteristic and key issue for people who become inpatients is their limited decision-making capacity or competence. Many inpatients, particularly those who are admitted compulsorily, lack capacity to make treatment decisions, at least in the early part of their admission (Owen et al., 2008). Capacity is decision-specific and we do not have data about inpatients' capacity in other aspects of their lives: however it is clear that care planning and discharge planning in inpatient settings must take account of capacity issues and relevant local legislation surrounding decision-making for incapacitated individuals.

International trends in inpatient provision

The development of inpatient services (in what were then known as asylums) during the 19th century was the basis for an organized system of mental health care, strongly associated with the Industrial

Table 19.3 Psychiatric beds per 100,000 population in each income group[a] of countries

Low	2.4
Lower middle	15.9
Higher middle	77.0
High	75.0

[a] Income groups as defined by the World Bank in 2004

Source: World Health Organization (2005). *Mental Health Atlas*. Geneva: World Health Organization.

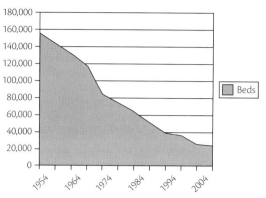

Fig. 19.1 Decline in psychiatric bed numbers in England and Wales 1954–2007. Source: NHS Information Centre

Revolution (Killaspy, 2006; Sederer, 1977). There is a continuing relationship between the numbers of inpatient beds in a country and its per capita income, with wealthier countries having more beds (Table 19.3). However the countries with the highest incomes now have, on average, slightly fewer beds than the next income tier: with the exception of Japan (which has begun the process) the wealthiest countries have gone through a process of deinstitutionalization that has seen the development of a wide range of community mental health care programmes; a critical lesson learned is that unless the funding spent on inpatient services is dedicated to community based care then patients, families, and communities will all suffer the consequences of untreated illness and social burden.

Inpatient provision varies markedly even across high-income countries in ways that cannot plausibly be explained by underlying need. According to the WHO Project Atlas (2005), which documented mental health care across all countries, Japan reports more than seven times as many inpatient beds per capita as New Zealand (see Table 19.1). High-income countries below the mean for inpatient provision include Australia, Italy, Spain, Sweden, and the United Kingdom. Germany and the United States are at the mean whilst Ireland, France, the Netherlands, and Canada are well above the mean. All these countries have advanced health and social welfare systems and researchers from them have contributed significantly to the international literature on community care. Even within a country there can be marked local variations in the pace of change (see, for example, Sealy and Whitehead (2004) and Department of Health and Ageing (2007) in relation to Canada and Australia).

Bed reduction

The outstanding feature of the landscape of mental health services in wealthy countries has been that psychiatric inpatient beds have reduced (see Fig. 19.1 for England and Wales data). It is difficult to obtain reliable dates for when the decline in the numbers of psychiatric beds started but by the 1970s the trend was established for all wealthy countries, with the notable exception of Japan. The extent and rate of change has been markedly different (see Table 19.1). New Zealand and Australia have shown the sharpest declines (New Zealand beginning its process of deinstitutionalization in the late 1940s) to a very low number of beds. Declines in bed numbers have been much less marked in Germany, France, the Netherlands, and Canada.

The process of deinstitutionalization has been associated with a reduction in the proportion of psychiatric beds located within mental hospitals, although again there are differences between countries. Italy and Sweden report no beds within traditional psychiatric institutions whilst in Spain, Ireland and Japan over 70% of psychiatric

beds remain within these settings. In England the majority of the traditional mental hospitals closed (Johnson et al., 2009) whilst in Germany during the deinstitutionalization period few mental hospitals closed but they became much smaller. The Italian experience of deinstitutionalization has been particularly influential in Europe, with a compelling story of idealistic legislation to close all traditional mental hospitals being passed in 1978 and acted upon rapidly. It is also well documented (Burti et al., 2001).

Thresholds for admission

In the early stages of deinstitutionalization the threshold for admission and readmission decreased. Between 1954 and 1968 admissions to mental hospitals in England and Wales went up from 78,586 to 170,527 whilst the inpatient population declined from a peak of 148,100 to 116,400 (Scull, 1977: pp. 64–78). Bed numbers decreased in the United States and the United Kingdom from 1955 while psychiatric admission rates increased for four decades. Mental hospitals (and their alternatives) became more permeable, with patients coming and going rather than becoming long-stay hospital residents. The traditional locked door of the institution became a revolving door. Average lengths of stay decreased and indeed continue to do so. In effect, many patients had more admissions but far fewer bed days per year.

More recently, as community services have improved and acute inpatient beds have become less accessible, admission thresholds have increased. In the United States the criterion for admission and continued stay, administered by for-profit managed care companies, has been the principal means of controlling utilization of inpatient beds in all sectors, except the state hospitals. It is hard to believe that people presenting to emergency rooms with the phenomenology used in Rosenhan's notorious study of mental health care (Rosenhan, 1973)—simple auditory hallucinations—would be admitted today. An obvious practical consequence is that people coming into contemporary inpatient services show ever higher levels of psychiatric and social morbidity: this can have a very significant impact on patient and staff experience (Patrick et al., 1989). These changes have had a particularly strong impact on the state hospital sector in the United States, the safety net and services of last resort (Hepburn and Sederer, 2009).

Alternatives to inpatient care

Advanced mental health systems have sought to develop alternatives to inpatient care. In England, arguably the most highly developed mental health care system in Europe, the decade to 2006 saw an 11% decline in admissions (Keown et al., 2008), which suggests that improving community service can result in decreased demand for inpatient care. This decline in admissions was associated both with continuing bed reductions and a strong policy emphasis on alternatives to inpatient admission, with the development of Assertive Outreach Teams, Early Onset Psychosis Teams, and Crisis Resolution/Home Treatment Teams (Department of Health, 2001). Community Mental Health Teams, the bedrock of mental health care in England, have also been required to deploy evidence-based interventions that should reduce relapse rates for mental illness (e.g. provision of cognitive behaviour therapy for psychosis) (NICE, 2009).

There is a substantial literature on the role of the acute day hospital as an alternative to inpatient admission for informal (voluntary) patients (Kallert et al., 2007; Marshall et al., 2003; Priebe et al., 2006). There has also been a small but significant development of crisis residential facilities as an alternative to acute inpatient care in England (Johnson et al., 2009). Because they are uncommon, crisis residential alternatives to inpatient admission and acute day care (even with their evidence base) cannot have contributed significantly to the reductions in admissions seen in England. There is evidence from routinely collected data that Crisis Resolution/Home Treatment Teams, which now cover the whole of England, have contributed to the decline in admissions; Assertive Outreach Teams do not appear to have had this effect (Glover et al., 2006).

Determinants of demand for inpatient care

How many psychiatric beds do we need? This is no simple question, and may be unanswerable. History tells us that we need fewer beds than we once did. Figures cited in the previous edition of this textbook for the United Kingdom (Szmukler and Holloway, 2001: p. 327) now seem outdated, with estimates of need for general acute beds too high and secure provision too low for contemporary practice.

Supply-side factors are obviously relevant ('if you build it, they will come'). Conversely, decreases in the funding of mental health care may result in rapid disinvestment in psychiatric beds, particularly in sectors that are commercially dependent (Hepburn and Sederer, 2009; Markowitz, 2008). Sociocultural factors are also significant: contemporary bed use between countries cannot plausibly be explained by differences in psychiatric morbidity. The steady decline in inpatient beds seen in England from 1955 on predated by two decades any specific policy initiative in favour of community mental health care: this suggests that changes in professional practice are instrumental in determining the 'need' for beds.

Ideology and policy can determine bed numbers where there are effective policy levers to bring about change. Australia, which has deinstitutionalized aggressively in most states, is a good example of policy into practice (Department of Health and Ageing, 2007). In England, bed numbers, constrained by purchasing reductions of commissioners of services, have continued to decline in the past decade to well below the international average to meet savings goals on baseline budgets (historically relating to inpatient care)—though there was reinvestment into community services. The Netherlands, one of the earlier countries to begin deinstitutionalization, provides an example of investment in community services that has not resulted in matching reduction in beds (Pijl et al.,

2000): in this complex health care system, policy levers seem to have been lacking to achieve the bed reductions seen elsewhere.

We do know that within a particular service system sociodemographic variables also influence the underlying demand for admission: factors include social class, marital status, ethnicity, aspects of domicile such as living alone, in overcrowded circumstances or in a neighbourhood with a large transitory population, and inner urban areas with high population densities and poverty (Croudace et al., 2000; Thornicroft 1991). In rural areas distance from the hospital is a factor (Burgess et al., 1992). At an area level deprivation is associated with prolonged inpatient admissions (Abas et al., 2008): sociodemographic factors impact on discharge after an episode of inpatient treatment with the availability of family support and appropriate housing being particularly salient in maintaining community tenure.

Deinstitutionalization and reinstitutionalization

Although there has been a marked reduction in inpatient beds during this era of community care we also see a countervailing trend towards 'reinsitutionalization'. Three separate strands to this phenomenon have been described: the movement of chronically mentally ill people into alternative, often quite institutionalized, community care; the expansion of secure/forensic hospital care; and the diversion of people with a mental illness into the Criminal Justice System (Priebe et al., 2005).

Analysing data from six European countries Priebe et al. (2005) concluded that 'Most of the data are consistent with the assumption that deinstitutionalisation, the defining process of mental healthcare reforms since the 1950s, has come to an end.'. There is other evidence that we may be nearing the end of the deinstitutionalization era: in Australia, which has one of the lowest bed numbers per capita of wealthy countries, decades of decline recently have been modestly reversed (Department of Health and Ageing, 2007). Certainly current trends in societal attitudes towards risk are powerful drivers towards increasing inpatient provision for people with mental disorders (whether treatable or not) deemed to be potentially risky. As previously noted, this issue has had a significant impact on the state hospital sector in the United States, where an increasing proportion of beds are devoted to management of forensic patients and sex offenders (Bloom, 2008; Hepburn and Sederer, 2009)

Quality of care in inpatient units
Ward atmosphere and environment

Policy concern in England has led to the development of a large contemporary literature on patient experience of psychiatric wards (Quirk and Lelliott, 2004). Patients report being bored, frightened, and not infrequently victims of violence or sexual harassment (Baker, 2000; Sainsbury Centre for Mental Health, 1998). Physical conditions on wards have been described as poor, with reports of a cramped, poorly maintained rather dismal environment. One early study noted, depressingly, that a pass or leave from the ward was the most valued aspect of inpatient stays (McIntyre et al., 1989). That said, patients do consistently report valuing the quality of the nursing care they receive, particularly the empathy, warmth, and respect that they experience. These positives are balanced by negatives when patients experience apparently arbitrary behaviour by nurses, coercion and punishment, and a tendency for staff to congregate in the office to the exclusion of the patients (Quirk and Lelliott, 2004). Too often the inpatient experience is a place to stay whilst receiving drug treatments in a controlled environment during ever-shorter stays (Markowitz, 2008).

Staff also report their concerns, which have striking parallels with the patient perspective. The first *National Audit of Violence* (Royal College of Psychiatrists Research Unit, 2005) identified the main staff concerns as poorly designed and unsafe environments; inadequate levels of staffing with unacceptably high vacancy factors and a reliance on bank and agency staff; overcrowding and inappropriate client mix; high prevalence of substance misuse; lack of access to relevant training for staff; and high levels of boredom for patients.

What do patients and carers want?

Research has identified a range of broad-brush constructs that describe quality of care from a patient perspective: respect for one's dignity; providing a sense of security; participation in care; a focus on recovery; and a quality care environment (Schroder et al., 2006). These are added to by more personal accounts, which underline the importance of adequate information and advice, access to creative therapies and opportunities for occupation and recreation (McCann, 2004). Carers have similar views but also emphasize the importance of maintaining patient safety, accurate diagnosis and open communication between the staff team and the carer (Ruane, 2004).

Violence and its management

Violence is a common feature on inpatient psychiatric wards. Two national audits carried out in England (Royal College of Psychiatrists Centre for Quality Improvement, 2007; Royal College of Psychiatrists Research Unit, 2005) document the problem. From 2003 to 2005, 80% of nursing staff and 36% of patients reported having been attacked, threatened or intimidated during their time on an inpatient unit. In a 2006–7 audit 46% of nursing staff and 18% of patients reported having been physically assaulted. The 2006–7 audit concluded that 'recent national policy and practice drivers that have emphasised the use of prevention and de-escalation, rather than physical interventions, were firmly embedded in ward-based practices in many services. Staff, patients and visitors were clearly aware of this changing culture, and were responding positively to it'.

This important improvement in ward violence has been linked to clinical guidelines for staff management of violence (National Institute for health and Clinical Excellence, 2005; Wing et al., 1998). These emphasize prevention, based on understanding the environmental and clinical factors (including both patient characteristics and staff behaviours) that foster violence (Johnson 2004).

Improving quality of care in inpatient services

Writing in a United Kingdom context, Lelliott et al. (2006) have neatly summarized the problems of acute inpatient psychiatry. These include a policy and practice focus on more 'glamorous' community services; the ill-defined role of inpatient care, which is often seen as a dumping ground; problems with the environment on wards, which are often perceived as chaotic and dangerous; poor leadership; bureaucratic overload; lack of adequately trained staff; and difficulties associated with bed management systems that provide inpatient staff with little control over their work.

How to address these problems? The first step is for professionals and policy-makers to acknowledge there is a problem. England has seen the publication of policy guidance on inpatient and intensive care units (Department of Health 2002 a,b), regulatory oversight from the Health Care Commission (now the Care Quality Commission) (Health Care Commission, 2008) and initiatives to support good practice within inpatient settings, such as the STAR Wards programme (http://starwards.org.uk).

England has also seen the development of a voluntary accreditation system, AIMS (Accreditation for Inpatient Mental Health Services; http://www.rcpsych.ac.uk/clinicalservicestandards/centreforqualityimprovement/aims.aspx). The AIMS acute inpatient standards cover four interlinked domains: General Standards that relate to staffing, policies and procedures; Timely and Purposeful Admission (relating to admission, assessment, care planning, discharge planning, management, skill-mix); Safety; and the Therapeutic Environment (Cresswell et al., 2007). The standards require that wards achieving accreditation through AIMS provide a safe environment and offer effective treatments (not just medication) to their patients. Both AIMS and Star Wards stress the importance of engaging patients in structured activities (often provided in group settings) and the life of the ward, through regular meetings of the ward community, which reflect therapeutic community principles rediscovered and reinterpreted in the light of contemporary practice (Firth, 2004). England has begun to link the funding of mental health services with the routine assessment by service users of the quality of their care: this is having a powerful effect on focusing managers on the service user experience, known as the consumer's perspective in the United States.

The Care Quality Commission, which is the regulator of all health care and adult social care in England, has recently published its accreditation standards (Care Quality Commission, 2010). These are entirely generic other than specific reporting requirements to the CQC in relation to the death of or unauthorized absence of detained patients. The United States has a rigorous accreditation system for inpatient psychiatry (Joint Commission, 2009), focused on evidence of admission screening for violence and substance misuse; use of physical restraint and seclusion; discharge medication; and post-discharge care planning as well as what is called the 'tracer methodology' where individual patients care is traced from admission to discharge to assess processes of care and the patient experience.

It is not clear that accreditation systems lead to a genuine improvement in inpatient services. Improving quality of care is a complex, but not intractable, problem. As an example, seclusion and restraint (including mechanical restraint) have been common to inpatient psychiatry across the world (although in some countries, such as the United Kingdom, mechanical restraint is rarely or never used). There is evidence that concerted efforts to decrease the use of seclusion and restraint can be effective but likely require multiple interventions including regulatory oversight, local monitoring, staff training, review of skill-mix and staffing levels, revised psychopharmacological management and better involvement of patients in their care (Gaskin et al., 2007).

Hospital/community interfaces

Inpatient admission should only ever be an element in the system of care available to someone with a mental illness. Two useful metaphors here are the patient journey (from illness to wellness or recovery) and the care pathway, through which a patient receives the help they need. As mental health services have become more sophisticated they have, in general, become more complex: the patient journey is more varied and the potential care pathways more challenging for patients, staff and carers to negotiate.

The acute care pathway

In England the acute care pathway for hospital admission involves contact with a community mental health team (including specialist teams for Early Intervention in Psychosis and Assertive Outreach) or crisis assessment within an Accident and Emergency Department (Rooney et al., 2008). Screening by the Home Treatment/Crisis Resolution Team (HTT/CRT) then takes place and admission occurs only if the HTT/CRT cannot provide safe treatment outside hospital. (Patients presenting through Criminal Justice System may bypass the gatekeeping function of the HTT/CRT). (See Fig. 19.2 for an example of an acute care pathway developed in one local service.)

Following an episode of inpatient treatment there is a requirement to plan discharge with the patient, their informal carers (family and others) and the community team. The HTT/CRT may, if necessary, provide support in the immediate post-discharge period. As a result of epidemiological data on patient suicide post-discharge, which shows a peak immediately after discharge (Appleby et al., 2001), there is a requirement in England that all inpatients be offered follow-up by mental health services within 7 days of discharge. Some people will need to use step-down accommodation. In the United States, outpatient appointment within 7 days is a quality measure for some systems of care but meeting this standard has yet to be achieved.

Effective inpatient treatment requires close cooperation between inpatient and community teams, with clear expectations at the outset of the outcomes for the episode of inpatient care. Quality

services commence discharge planning early and work with family and other carers and the community mental health services. Barriers to discharge include clinical issues (e.g. continuing symptoms and risk) and social problems. Demands for brief stays often resort to immediate pharmacological treatment of acute disturbance and rapid discharge once safety is restored.

Long-stay patients

Despite decades of deinstitutionalization there are a significant number of long-stay patients (however defined locally; in New York State it is 1 year) even in the most advanced service system. Their heterogeneous characteristics and needs, which will include intractable psychosis, challenging behaviours, and perceived continuing risk of dangerousness, also require robust hospital/community interfaces to return to a life in the community (Holloway, 2004).

Conclusion: inpatient treatment and community mental health

Despite more than five decades of reductions in inpatient beds (New Zealand is now into its sixth) and the impressive developments we have seen in community mental health care, inpatient psychiatry remains vital to an effective mental health service. Utilization of hospital beds depends on a complex interaction between supply (as historically determined) and demand. Demand reflects professional behaviours, societal expectations of care and control of the mentally ill, and acceptance of their return to the community, the local epidemiology of mental illness and the availability of alternative forms of psychiatric provision. The Italian and Australian experience have shown that major systemic change can be successfully introduced: but a change strategy should be incremental, evidence-based and adequately resourced. However, if a publicly funded system does

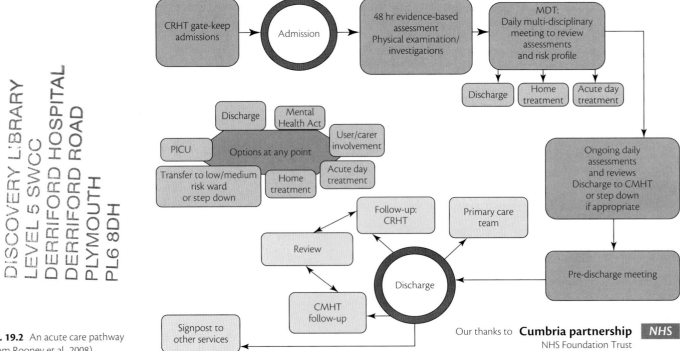

Fig. 19.2 An acute care pathway (from Rooney et al., 2008).

Our thanks to **Cumbria partnership** NHS Foundation Trust

not have adequate bed provision mental health service costs can escalate as can general medical, shelter, welfare, and criminal justice system expenditures.

A particular concern for community mental health care is long-stay individuals, if only because they consume a disproportionate amount of mental health funding (32% of the total in England); these costs could increase as more patients are given long-term mental health disposals by the courts. Effective engagement by community services with the most hard to help patients is vital if funding for community mental health care is to be maintained in a highly risk-averse era.

Quality of inpatient services, access by and their integration with community based care, and a recovery orientation are the essential elements of inpatient care today. There will always be a place for hospital care and it should be held, like all care, to the highest standards for patients and their families.

References

Abas, M., Vanderpyl, J., Le Prou, T., Kydd, R., Emery, B., and Foliaki, S. (2003). Psychiatric hospitalization: reasons for admission and alternatives to admission in South Auckland, New Zealand. *The Australian and New Zealand Journal of Psychiatry*, **37**, 620–5.

Abas, M., Vanderpyl, J., and Robinson, E. (2008). Socio-demographic deprivation and extended hospitalization in severe mental disorder.: A two year follow-up study. *Psychiatric Services*, **59**, 322–25.

Allness, D.J. and Knoedler, W.H. (1998). *The PACT Model of Community-Based Treatment for Persons with Severe and Persistent Mental Illnesses. A Manual for PACT Start-Up.* Arlington, VA: NAMI.

Appleby, L., Shaw, J., Sherratt, J., Amos, T., and Robinson, J. (2001). *Safety First: Five Year Report of the National Confidential Inquiry into Homicides and Suicides by People with a Mental Illness.* London: Department of Health.

Bachrach, L. (1976). *Deinstitutionalization: An Analytical Review and Sociological Perspective.* Rockville, MD: US Department of Health, Education and Welfare, NIMH.

Baker, S. (2000). *Environmentally friendly? Patients' views of conditions on psychiatric wards.* London: MIND.

Beer, M.D., Pereira, S.D., and Paton, C. (2008). *Psychiatric Intensive Care,* 2nd edn. Cambridge: Cambridge University Press.

Bloom, J.D., Krishnan, B., and Lockley, C. (2008). The majority of inpatient psychiatric beds should not be appropriated by the forensic system. *Journal of the American Academy of Psychiatry and the Law*, **36**, 438–42.

Bowers, L. (2005). Reasons for admission and their implications for the nature of acute inpatient psychiatric nursing. *Journal of Psychiatric and Mental Health Nursing*, **12**, 231–6.

Burgess, P.M., Joyce C.M., Pattison P.E., and Finch S.J. (1992). Social indicators and the prediction of psychiatric inpatient service utilisation. *Social Psychiatry Psychiatric Epidemiology*, **27**, 83–94.

Burti, L. (2001). Italian psychiatric reform 20 plus years after. *Acta Psychiatrica Scandinavica*, **104**, 41–6.

Campling, P., Davies, S., and Farquharson, G. (2004). *From Toxic Institutions to Therapeutic Environments: Residential Settings in Mental Health Services.* London: Gaskell.

Care Quality Commission (2010). *Guidance about compliance. Summary of regulations, outcomes and judgement framework.* London: Care Quality Commission. Available at: http://www.cqc.org.uk/aboutcqc/whatwedo/monitoringessentialstandardsofqualityandsafety.cfm

Cresswell, J., Beavon, M., and Hood, C. (2007). *Standards for Acute Inpatient Wards,* 2nd edn. London: Royal College of Psychiatrists' Research and Training Unit.

Croudace, T.J., Kayne, R., Jones, P.B., and Harrison, G.L. (2000). Non-linear relationship between an index of social deprivation,

psychiatric admission prevalence and the incidence of psychosis. *Psychological Medicine*, **30**, 177–85.

Department of Health (2001). *Mental Health Policy Implementation Guide.* London: Department of Health.

Department of Health (2002a). *Acute Inpatient Provision Care Provision: Mental Health Policy Implementation Guide.* London: Department of Health.

Department of Health (2002b). *National Standards for PICU and Low Secure Environments.* London: Department of Health.

Department of Health (2006). *Dual diagnosis in mental health inpatient and day hospital settings.* London: Department of Health

Department of Health and Ageing (2007). *National Mental Health Report 2007: Summary of Twelve Years of Reform in Australia's Mental Health Services under the National Mental Health Strategy 1993-2005.* Canberra: Commonwealth of Australia.

Cresswell, J., Beavon, M., and Hood, C. (2007). *Standards for Acute Inpatient Wards,* 2nd edn. London: Royal College of Psychiatrists' Research and Training Unit.

Fazel, S., Langstrom, N., Hjem, A., et al.(2009). Schizophrenia, substance misuse and violent crime. *Journal of the American Medical Association*, **301**, 2016–23.

Firth, W. (2004). Acute psychiatric wards: an overview. In: Campling, P., Davies, S., and Farquharson, G. (eds.) *From Toxic Institutions to Therapeutic Environments: Residential Settings in Mental Health Services,* pp. 174–87. London: Gaskell.

Gaskin, C.J., Elsom, S.J., and Happell, B. (2007). Interventions for reducing the use of seclusion in psychiatric facilities. Review of the literature. *British Journal of Psychiatry*, **191**, 298–303.

Glover, G., Arts, G., and Babu, K.S (2006). Crisis resolution teams and psychiatric admission rates in England. *British Journal of Psychiatry*, **189**, 441–45.

Hawks, D. (1975). Community Care: an analysis of assumptions. *British Journal of Psychiatry*, **127**, 276–85.

Healthcare Commission (2008). *Count Me In Census 2008.* London: Healthcare Comission.

Hepburn, B. and Sederer, L.I. (2009). The state hospital. In: Sharfstein, S.S., Dickerson, F.B., and Oldham, I.M. (eds.) *Textbook of Hospital Psychiatry,* pp. 207–32. Arlington VA: American Psychiatry Publishing Inc.

Holloway, F. (2004). Reprovision for the long-stay patient. *Psychiatry*, **3**, 5–7.

Isaac, M.B., Isaac, M.T., and Holloway, F. (2005). Is cannabis an anti-antipsychotic? *Human Psychopharmacology*, **20**, 207–10.

Johnson, S., Gilburt, H., Lloyd-Evans, B., Osborn, D.P.J., Boardman, J., Leese, M., et al. (2009). In-patient and residential alternatives to standard acute psychiatric wards in England. *British Journal of Psychiatry* **194**, 456–63.

Johnson, M.E. (2004). Violence on inpatient psychiatric units: state of the science. *Journal of the American Psychiatric Nurses Association*, **10**, 113–21.

Jones, K. (2004). The historical context of therapeutic environments. In: Campling, P., Davies, S., and Farquharson, G. (eds.) *From Toxic Institutions to Therapeutic Environments: Residential Settings in Mental Health Services,* pp. 3–11. London: Gaskell.

Keown, P., Mercer, G., and Scott, J. (2008). Retrospective analysis of hospital episode statistics, involuntary admissions under the Mental Health Act 1983, and number of psychiatric beds in England 1996-2006. *British Medical Journal*, **337**, 1837.

Killaspy, H. (2006). From the asylum to community care: learning from experience. *British Medical Bulletin*, **79-80**, 245–58.

Killaspy, H., Harden, C., Holloway, F. and King, M. (2005). What do mental health rehabilitation services do and what are they for? A national survey in England. *Journal of Mental Health*, **14**, 157–65.

Kisley, S., Smith, M., Preston, N.J., Xiao, J., (2005). A comparison of health service use in two jurisdictions with and without compulsory community treatment. *Psychological Medicine*, **35**, 1–11.

Kluiter, H. (1997). Inpatient treatment and care arrangements to replace or avoid it–searching for an evidence-based balance. *Current Opinion in Psychiatry*, **13**, 333–41.

Joint Commission (2009). *Specification Manual for National Hospital Inpatient Quality Measures–Hospital-Based Inpatient Psychiatric Services Core Measure Set Version 2.2*. Available at: http://www.jointcommission. org/PerformanceMeasurement/PerformanceMeasurement/Hospital+Bas ed+Inpatient+Psychiatric+Services.htm (accessed 26 September 2009).

Kallert, T.W., Priebe, S., McCabe, R., Kiejna, A., Rymaszewska, J., Nawka, P., et al. (2007). Are day hospitals effective for acutely ill psychiatric patients? A European, multicenter randomized controlled trial. *Journal of Clinical Psychiatry* **68**, 278–87.

Leff, L. and Trieman, N. (2000). Long-stay patients discharged from psychiatric hospitals. Social and clinical outcomes after five years in the community. The TAPS Project 46. *British Journal of Psychiatry* **176**, 217–23.

Lelliott, P., Bennett, H., McGeorge, M., and Turner, T. (2006). Accreditation of acute inpatient mental health services. *Psychiatric Bulletin*, **206**, 361–3.

McCann, J. (2004). What users want. In: Campling, P., Davies, S., and Farquharson, G. (eds.) *From Toxic Institutions to Therapeutic Environments: Residential Settings in Mental Health Services*, pp. 159–65. London: Gaskell.

McIntyre, K., Farrell, M., and David, A.S. (1989). What do psychiatric in-patients really want? *British Medical Journal*, **298**, 159–60.

Markowitz, J.C. (2008). A letter from America: rescuing inpatient psychiatry *Evidence Based Mental Health*, **11**, 68–9.

Marshall, M., Crowther, R., Almaraz-Serrano, A., Creed, F., Sledge, W.H., Kluiter, H., et al.(2003). Day hospital *versus* admission for acute psychiatric disorders. *Cochrane Database of Systematic Reviews*, 1, CD004026.

Martin JP (1984). *Hospitals in Trouble*. Oxford, Blackwell.

National Institute for Health and Clinical Excellence (2005). *Violence: The short-term management of disturbed/violent behaviour in psychiatric in-patient settings and emergency departments. Clinical Guideline 25*. London: NICE.

National Institute for Health and Clinical Excellence (2009). *Core Interventions in the Treatment and Management of Schizophrenia in Primary and Secondary Care. Clinical Guideline 82*. London: NICE.

O'Brien, A.J., McKenna, B., and Kydd, R.R. (2009). Compulsory community mental health treatment. Literature review. *International Journal of Nursing Studies* **46**, 1245–55.

Owen, G.S., Richardson, G., David, A., Szmukler, G., and Hotopf, M (2008). Mental capacity to make decisions on treatment in people admitted to psychiatric hospitals: cross-sectional study. *British Medical Journal*, **337**, a448.

Patrick, M., Higgitt, A., Holloway, F., and Silverman, M. (1989). Changes in an inner city psychiatric inpatient service following bed losses: a follow-up of the East Lambeth 1986 Survey. *Health Trends*, **21**, 121–3.

Peele, R., and Chodoff, P. (1999). The ethics of involuntary treatment and deisntitutionalization. In: Bloch, S., Chodoff, P., and Green, S. (eds.) *Psychiatric Ethics*, 3rd edn., pp. 423–40. Oxford: Oxford University Press.

Pijl, Y.J., Kluiter, H., and Wiersma D. (2000). Calculated change in Dutch mental health care. *Social Psychiatry and Psychiatric Epidemiology*, **35**, 548–53.

Preti, A., Rucci, P., Santone, G., Picardi, A., Miglio, R., Bracco R., et al. (2009). Patterns of admission to acute psychiatric in-patient facilities: a national survey in Italy. *Psychological Medicine* **39**, 485–96.

Priebe, S., Badesconyi, A., Fioritti, A., Hansonn, L., Kilian, R., Torres-Gonzales, F., et al. (2005). Reinstitutionalisation in mental health care: comparison of data on service provision from six European countries. *British Medical Journal*, **330**, 123–6.

Priebe, S., Jones, G., McCabe, R., Briscoe, J., Wright, D., Sleed, M., et al. (2006). Effectiveness and costs of acute day hospital treatment compared with conventional in-patient care. Randomised controlled trial. *British Journal of Psychiatry*, **188**, 243–9.

Quirk, A. and Lelliott, P. (2004). Users' experience of in-patient services. In: Campling, P., Davies, S., and Farquharson, G. (eds.) *From Toxic Institutions to Therapeutic Environments: Residential Settings in Mental Health Services*, pp. 45–54. London: Gaskell.

Radcliffe, J., Hajek, K., Carson, J., and Manor, O. (eds.) (2010). *Psychological Groupwork with Acute Psychatric Inpatients*. London: Whiting & Birch.

Ramsay, R. and Holloway, F. (2007). Mental health services. In: Stein, G. and Wilkinson, G. (eds.) *General Psychiatry. College Seminars in Psychiatry*, 2nd edn., pp. 724–46. London: Gaskell.

Rittmannsberger, H., Sartorius, N., and Brad, M (2004). Changing aspects of psychiatric inpatient treatment. A census investigation in five European countries. *European Psychiatry* **19**, 483–8.

Rooney, P., Plumb, J., and Shaw, C (2008). *Laying The Foundations for better Acute Mental Health Care: A Service Redesign and Capital Investment Workbook*. Norwich: The Stationery Office.

Rosenhan, D.L (1973). On being sane in insane places. *Science* **179**, 250–8.

Royal College of Psychiatrists Research Unit (2005). *The Healthcare Commission National Audit of Violence (2003-2005)*. London: Royal College of Psychiatrists Research Unit.

Royal College of Psychiatrists Centre for Quality Improvement (2007). *The Healthcare Commission National Audit of Violence 2006-7 Final Report–Working Age Adult Services*. London: Royal College of Psychiatrists Centre for Quality Improvement.

Ruane, P. (2004). A carer's perception of the value of inpatient settings In: Campling, P., Davies, S., and Farquharson, G. (eds.) *From Toxic Institutions to Therapeutic Environments: Residential Settings in Mental Health Services*, pp. 166–73. London: Gaskell.

Sainsbury Centre for Mental Health (1998). *Acute Problems: A Survey of the Quality of Care in Acute Psychiatric Wards (ACIS)*. London: Sainsbury Centre for Mental Health.

Schramm, E., van Calker, D., Dykierk, P., Lieb, K., Kech, S., Zobel I., et al. (2007). An intensive treatment programme of interpersonal psychotherapy plus pharmacotherapy for depressed inpatients: acute and long-term results. *American Journal of Psychiatry* **164**, 768–77.

Scull, A. (1977). *Decareration. Community Treatment and the Deviant–A Radical View*, 2nd edn. Cambridge: Polity Press.

Sealy, P. and Whitehead, P.C. (2004). Forty years of deinstitutionalization of psychiatric services: An empirical assessment. *Canadian Journal of Psychiatry* **49**, 249–57.

Sederer, L.I. (1977). Moral therapy and the problem of morale. *American Journal of Psychiatry*, **134**, 267–72.

Sinclair, J.M.A., Latifi, A.H., and Latifi, A.W. (2008). Co-morbid substance misuse in psychiatric patients: prevalence and association with length of inpatient stay. *Journal of Psychopharmacology*, **22**, 92–9.

South London and Maudsley NHS Foundation Trust (2010). National Services Directory. A guide to our mental health services for adults. Available at http://www.national.slam.nhs.uk/wp-content/uploads/2010/08/SLaM-NSD-%C2%AD-Adults_singlepp.pdf

Swartz, M,S. and Swanson, J.W. (2004). Involuntary outpatient commitment community treatment orders, and assisted outpatient treatment: What's in the data? *Canadian Journal of Psychiatry*, **49**, 585–91.

Schroder, A., Larsson, B.W., and Ahlstrom, G. (2007). Quality in psychiatric care: an instrument evaluating patients' expectations and experiences. *International Journal of Health Care Quality Assurance* **20**, 141–60.

Szmukler, G. and Holloway, F. (2001). In-patient treatment. In: Thornicroft, G. and Szmukler, G. (eds.) *Textbook of Community Psychiatry*, pp. 321–37. Oxford: Oxford University Press.

Talbott, J. and Glick, I. (1986). The inpatient care of the chronically mentally ill. *Schizophrenia Bulletin*, **12**, 129–40.

Thompson, A., Shaw, M., Harrison, G., Davidson, H., Gunnel, D., and Verne, J. (2004). Patterns of hospital admission for adult psychiatric illness in England: analysis of Hospital Episode Statistics data. *British Journal of Psychiatry*, **185**, 334–41.

Thornicroft, G., and Bebbington, P. (1989). Deinstitutionalisation from hospital closure to service development. *British Journal of Psychiatry,* **155**, 739–53.

Thornicroft, G. (1991). Social deprivation and rates of treated mental disorder. Developing statistical models to predict psychiatric service utilization. *British Journal of Psychiatry,* **158**, 475–84.

Trieman, N. and Leff, J (2002). Long-term outcome of long-stay inpatients considered unsuitable to live in the community. TAPS Project 44. *British Journal of Psychiatry,* **181**, 428–32.

Wing J.K. and Brown G.W. (1970). *Institutionalism and Schizophrenia.* Cambridge: Cambridge University Press.

Wing, J.K., Marriott, S., Palmer, C. and Thomas, V. (1998). *The Management of Imminent Violence: Clinical Practice Guidelines to Support Mental Health Services. Occasional Paper OP41.* London: Royal College of Psychiatrists.

World Health Organization (2005). *Mental Health Atlas 2005.* Available at: http://www.who.int/mental_health/evidence/atlas/en/.

CHAPTER 20

Residential care

Geoff Shepherd and Rob Macpherson

Introduction

We all need somewhere to live where we feel safe and comfortable. Given this simple fact, it is unfortunate that for far too long, housing has been seen as at the periphery of the concerns of most mental health professionals, service providers, and researchers. While the importance of adequate housing may be recognized in principle, little research has been done to identify staffing and management practices associated with high quality care, or to improve outcomes. Meanwhile, people with severe mental health problems continue to live in substandard accommodation and struggle to gain access to decent and affordable housing (Kirby and Keon, 2006). This chapter explores these issues. We will describe the historical and policy background, review current issues, and bring together the available research to make practical, evidence-based suggestions for improving the quality of residential care. The context is the 'mixed economy' of care that now characterizes housing provision for people with mental health problems in the United Kingdom and in most of northern Europe, Australasia, and North America. This has grown up as we have moved away from long-term care in hospital. The 'total institution' has thus disappeared, but we now have many smaller 'institutions', with different management authorities, cultures, and values. How have we arrived at this point?

Historical and policy background

In England, the central theme in the development of residential care for people with mental health problems over the last 50 years has been the move from National Health Service (NHS)-funded hospital care to a multiplicity of independent 'for-profit'—and 'not-for-profit'—community providers. Similar developments have taken place in most other developed countries. Thus, long-stay hospital beds in England and Wales reduced from 155,000 in 1955 to less than 3000 today (O'Brien, 2010). The policy background that drove this dramatic change was signalled in the NHS 'Hospital Plan' almost 50 years ago (Ministry of Health, 1962) which announced an intention to move towards a more community-based system of care. *Care in the Community* (DHSS, 1981) then shifted the responsibility for managing residential care from Regional Health Authorities towards Local Authorities (local

government) and in 1990 the *NHS and Community Care Act* (Department of Health, 1990) enabled agencies other than the NHS and Local Authorities to become involved in providing these facilities. Subsequently *Partnerships in Action* (Department of Health, 1998a) emphasized the importance of joint working between statutory and independent sector agencies and, more recently, *Supporting People* (ODPM, 2002) set out explicitly to co-ordinate all housing support for vulnerable people, including those with mental health problems.

During these changes a tension has emerged between the aims of 'community care' for most people and the needs of a relatively small group of highly disabled patients who require some kind of specialist, 'institutional' provision—albeit resembling community facilities as much as possible. Despite the successes of community care, patients continue to present to services with multiple and complex needs of such severity that care in non-specialist facilities does not seem feasible. Up to now, their needs have also been included in policy. For example, the *National Service Framework for Mental Health* (Department of Health, 1999) recommended a small number of intensive, high dependency places in specialist residential facilities which would provide high quality medical and nursing care for the most disabled. These were called '24-hour nursed care' or 'hospital hostels' (Shepherd, 1995). At the time of writing, a new mental health policy document to replace the NSF has just been published (*New Horizons*; Department of Health, 2009). Its vision is for improved prevention of mental health problems, through early intervention and 'social inclusion' and the successful challenging of inequality and stigma. But, it says little about those with the greatest and most complex needs. There is therefore a danger that the needs of this group will be overlooked as policy moves towards more 'preventative' and 'public health' models (Mountain et al., 2009).

Another important policy theme which has emerged as the hospitals have been run down, has been the most appropriate mechanisms for regulation and quality inspection in a new, multiple provider, environment. In England and Wales a range of monitoring frameworks have been established by different bodies to set standards and attempt to shape practice (e.g. Department of Health, 2003, 2007; ODPM, 2005; Royal College of Psychiatrists, 2010). There has also been a succession of regulatory bodies (in England, three in the last 10 years) to oversee arrangements for the inspection of standards. The latest, the 'Care Quality Commission' (CQC), was set up in 2009 to regulate all adult heath and social care services. It will use a system of registration, together with a familiar combination of standards, self-assessment and emergency inspections (much as its predecessors the Commission for Health Improvement and the Healthcare Commission). The threat to 'deregister' individual providers for conspicuously poor standards of care suggests that it may have more impact than previous regulatory bodies; whether it will be any more effective in raising **general** standards waits to be seen. Previous experience suggests not (Walshe, 2003). Improving the quality of local care is essentially a local matter and this has not changed in the last 200 years.

A new area of policy development that is now beginning to impact across mental health services, including residential care, is that associated with the principles of 'recovery' (Shepherd et al., 2008; Slade, 2009a,b). These aim to make services more supportive of individual's recovery 'journeys', recognizing the centrality of life goals as opposed to symptom management, the importance of a sense of being 'in control' rather than continually directed by others, and of personal hopes and ambitions as opposed to the often reduced expectations of professionals. These ideas now underpin public mental health policy in several countries and we will examine their specific implications for residential care later. Before doing that, let us try to clarify terms.

Defining terms

The range of residential alternatives is notoriously difficult to classify. However, Lelliott et al. (1996) produced a typology some years ago which is still useful. This is shown in Table 20.1.

This classificatory scheme suggests that the different forms of supported accommodation can be arranged on a dimension of staffing levels from acute inpatient wards with constant staffing and relatively high numbers of staff; through high staffed hostels, low staffed hostels; staffed care homes with sleeping night staff; and group homes without staff on the premises, but regular visiting. The problem of this kind of classification for modern residential services is that the changes in the pattern of care over the past 50 years towards a more mixed model of providers have also been associated with a move towards more 'supported housing', where the care is delivered to the person in their home by peripatetic staff teams, rather than by fixed staffing associated with a single facility (hence, these options need to be added). This means that levels of care are much more flexible and the person can live as independently as possible most of the time. It also reflects the consistent research findings that service users generally favour more autonomy and wish to avoid shared housing options that seem too like the institutions they were set up to replace (see 'Quality of care' and 'quality of life' section). At the same time it opens up the possibility of using a much greater range of 'ordinary housing' options in a more cost efficient way and accords with current thinking on the importance of 'social inclusion'.

Estimating needs

One of the major practical reasons for wishing to develop agreed and consistent definitions of sheltered and supported housing is so that these can be used to inform planning for the range of different kinds of accommodation required to meet the needs of a specific, local population. For the reasons given above, this has become increasingly difficult as planning has come to depend more and more on the simple availability of general housing stock. Nevertheless, there are some interesting examples in the literature of attempts to do this and these are summarized in Table 20.2.

Despite these kinds of studies, there is still no generally agreed system of local needs assessment for residential care and no recognized instrument to assess housing need at an individual level (Strathdee and Jenkins, 1996). In practice, the development of local provisions appears to be largely determined by history and factors such as demography, transport, unemployment,

Table 20.1 The spectrum of residential care (modified from Lelliott et al., 1996)

Facility Type	Usual number of places	Night cover	Day cover	Ratio of staff: residents	% staff with care qualification
Forensic unit	>6	Waking	Constant	1.3	62%
Acute ward	>6	Waking	Constant	1.3	63%
Long-stay ward	>6	Waking	Constant	0.9	49%
High-staffed hostel	>6	Waking	Constant	0.7	15%
Mid-staffed hostel	>6	Sleep-in	Constant	0.4	14%
Low-staffed hostel	>6	On call/none	Regular	0.2	15%
Group home	<6	On call/none	Visited	0.2	33%
Staffed care home	>6	Sleep-in	Constant	1.0	7%
Dedicated supported housing schemes	Individual flats/small houses up to 4 places	No	Available in complex	0.5 (average)	Unknown
Outreach support in individual tenancy	Usually individual flats	Rarely	Intermittent	0.5 up to 3	Unknown

Table 20.2 Examples of attempts to estimate local housing needs through survey methods

Authors	Country	Method	Main findings
Shepherd et al. (1997)	United Kingdom	Census of acute bed usage in a nationally representative sample	Highlighted the need for specialist rehabilitation placements or 24-hour, 'nursed care' units
Fitz and Evenson (1999)	United States	Large-scale, systematic assessment of local needs	Community living skills, social skills and problem behaviour were the primary characteristics affecting adjustment to residential settings
Durbin et al. (2001)	Canada	Survey of in-patients	Five levels of care developed, only 10% of current inpatients needed to remain in hospital, 60% could live independently in the community with appropriate support
Bartlett et al. (2001)	United Kingdom	Analysis of 730 acute admissions	Many patients might have benefited from alternative, community-based services. A quarter could have been supported effectively in the community in specialist accommodation if available.
Freeman et al. (2004)	Australia	Survey of all State and non-governmental high support housing services	State and non-government services useful, but significant numbers of unmet social and psychological needs in residents
Commander and Rooprai, (2008)	United Kingdom	Survey of acute in-patients	Almost 20% of acute beds occupied by patients for more than 6 months. 'By far the majority' required 24-hour nursed care, need to improve access to this provision.

ethnic composition, funding priorities, attitudes of primary care, effectiveness of specialist mental health services, etc. Some of these can be partially taken into account by sophisticated quantitative modelling (e.g. Glover, 1996), but at the heart of such algorithms remain guesses—albeit sensible and well-informed guesses—about what numbers of different kinds of provisions a given pattern of local morbidity implies.

The problem of accurately estimating demand is further complicated by the fact that one kind of housing or accommodation can often 'substitute' for another. Thus, high support hostels may substitute for inpatient beds; flexible community teams may substitute for sheltered housing (or hospital beds); family care with intensive professional support may substitute for professional support or specialist housing; and so on. Housing needs assessments therefore cannot be separated from the functioning and dynamics of the total service 'system' and the confidence limits surrounding any estimates of need for different kinds of accommodation remain large (Johnson et al., 1996).

For all these reasons, it is probably more sensible to begin a local planning process by conducting a simple inventory of local housing availability to see who is currently accommodated (i.e. survey of levels of disability and case-mix in existing provision). If one then adds in information on who is currently excluded (e.g. homeless) and these figures are combined with local information about the availability of general housing stock, then this should give a starting point in terms of development priorities. On the basis of national information, shortages in high dependency housing and flexible, intensive community support are likely to be the areas of greatest deficiencies (Audit Commission, 1998; Department of Health, 1998b).

The impact of service developments

In England, the National Service Framework for Mental Health (Department of Health, 1999) prompted the development of a range of new specialist community based teams, focusing on patients with specific needs (crisis and home treatment; assertive outreach; and early intervention). This new pattern of services led, in turn, to a significant reappraisal of traditional concepts of the limits of 'community care'. Thus, it is now clear that many service users who would previously have been in hospital for long periods, or in the 'revolving door' of repeated admissions, can now be successfully supported in the community with well-functioning, specialist teams. However, the success of these specialist teams has resulted in a further reduction in acute beds and this has put pressure on the community teams in terms of their ability to support people with severe and complex problems living in facilities that are run by largely non-statutory providers.

Whether this constitutes a process of 'reinstitutionalization' depends on what you count as an 'institution'. In England, the majority of the residential alternatives that have been developed in the community show few of the common features of institutional care (large size, impersonal routines, lack of contact with the community). Indeed, it is their lack of 'institutionalization' that seems to account for the higher rates of satisfaction reported by patients resettled from the large hospitals (Leff et al., 1994; Thornicroft et al., 1995). Of course, this is not necessarily the same in countries where larger, more 'institutional' units are common.

In all cases, tensions have emerged around the problems of 'partnership working' between mental health services and housing providers in the new system. For example, there is often a perception on the part of clinical teams that housing providers can choose who they will accept and, not surprisingly, tend to choose the apparently 'easier' clients. Conversely, many independent sector providers believe that statutory services simply want to 'dump' difficult problems on to them and then fail to give adequate support and follow-up. Both views reflect stereotypes, but both also contain a degree of truth. These attitudes underline the need for statutory and non-statutory agencies to work closely together (e.g. through joint training). But, given its importance as an everyday, practical problem, the problems of improving joint working has received surprisingly little attention as a research topic.

As indicated above, in England the process of 'de-institutionalization' is now effectively complete and there are only a few remaining long-stay in-patient units, providing mainly medium stay (i.e. 1 to 2 years), 24-hour nursed care for 'new' long-stay patients (Killaspy et al., 2005). A study of changes in services across nine European countries by Priebe et al. (2008) showed a similar picture.

In addition to the increase in placements in sheltered and supported housing, what other changes in services have occurred? There has certainly been a growth in forensic beds and prison places which cannot be explained by changes in prevalence or patterns of morbidity among patients with severe mental illness (Priebe et al., 2008). For example, between 1994 and 2003 the number of NHS secure beds rose from 1080 to 2560 and detained admissions increased from 600 to 1400/year (of which one in five were treated in private or independent sector facilities). Similarly, in England and Wales the number of prison places increased by 32,500 (66%) from 1995 to 2009 (Ministry of Justice, 2009). However, when one considers the case mix of residents in these different facilities it is clear that while there is some overlap between patients in secure and semi-secure beds and those who might have been in 'mainstream' hospitals, the diagnostic profile of those with mental illness in the prison system is quite different—less than 10% with psychosis, high rates of personality disorder, low levels of literacy, and frequent drug and alcohol abuse (Singleton, Meltzer and Gatward, 1998). Thus, while it is possible that there may have been some 'reinstitutionalization' of people with mental health problems from 'open' hospitals to secure and semi-secure provisions, it is unlikely that there has been much 'reinstitutionalization' back to prison.

Perhaps more importantly, there have been changes in public perceptions regarding the risks posed by people with mental illness in the community. These were exacerbated, in the early days of the run-down of the mental hospitals in England, by cases like that of Christopher Clunis, a man with schizophrenia who was well-known to local services, but who had fallen out of follow-up and eventually murdered a member of the public in an Underground station in London (Coid, 1994). Not surprisingly, these kinds of events attracted substantial media attention and, despite the lack of evidence of any actual increase in homicides committed by people with mental illness (Shaw et al., 1999), they contributed to a shift in attitudes—public and professional—towards the need for greater use of secure provisions.

Changes in the pattern of residential provisions have also been driven directly by an increasing emphasis on a 'market philosophy', where private providers are encouraged to try to increase their 'market share' in competition with traditional state provisions. This has also happened across Europe (Priebe et al., 2005) and, as indicated, has been 'successful' in that new providers have been encouraged into the 'market'. However, it has led to concerns regarding the costs and quality of care provided. Secure services are often remote from the geographical area where the patient originated and this makes it difficult to maintain contact with local community services. It can also lead to difficulties in monitoring progress and unnecessarily protracted lengths of stay. The separation of vulnerable patients from their families and friends then makes successful resettlement more difficult (Ryan et al., 2006). Finally, physical and organizational isolation has repeatedly been shown to be a common factor in hospital abuse scandals (Martin, 1984) and these same factors can operate within residential units if they become similarly isolated. It is therefore welcome that the new regulator in England (CQC) will include private and independent sector provisions within its remit.

Staffing and staff training

As indicated above, one of the biggest challenges resulting from the growth of non-statutory providers is that many more staff are now involved who do not have formal mental health training or qualifications (Phelan and Strathdee, 1994). In some ways this is an advantage since they are less likely to have traditional, 'institutional' attitudes but, as we noted earlier, staff untrained to deal with difficult clinical problems are more likely to be reluctant to accept such individuals into their care. In terms of the development and evaluation of training programmes for residential care staff, the evidence is limited and mixed. It is summarized in Table 20.3.

Part of the reason for the failure to develop and evaluate training programmes for residential care staff is that it has not been clear

Table 20.3 Training and quality of care

Authors	Country	Method	Main findings
Sorensen-Snyder et al. (1994)	Sweden	Survey of staff in 15 residential care homes	Association between staff critical comments and resident subjective quality of life. Staff high EE associated with illness severity, suggesting a complex interaction between attitudes and levels of morbidity
Peterson and Barland (1995)	United States	State hospital staff trained workers in community care facilities caring for people with severe mental illness	After a 17-week programme community staff reported high satisfaction and the overall quality of the service was reported to improve, with reduced staff turnover
Shepherd et al. (1996)	United Kingdom	Survey of residential care	Patients with the highest levels of disability tended to receive the least interaction and more negative interactions when they did occur
Senn et al. (1997)	United Kingdom	Survey as part of the TAPS study	Almost a quarter of reprovision schemes offered no training at all, not even in the management of violence or risk
Raskin et al. (1998)	United States	Psychoeducational programme for staff in community residences	Staff liked the networking and mental health component. Service users also became more active and had fewer admissions

exactly what skills they require. The application of 'expressed emotion' (EE) models from the research with family carers (Ball et al., 1992) is one model that seems intuitively plausible. Regarding recruitment and selection of staff, while it is recognized that staff characteristics are important, almost no attention has been given to developing more reliable and valid selection criteria. Again, the 'low EE' model may have applicability as a framework for staff selection (e.g. select staff who are low on blame and criticism) but has not been empirically tested. The involvement of service users (consumers) as part of the selection process also appears to be widely used but, to our knowledge, has not been formally evaluated.

The qualities of effective leaders in residential care teams and how best to develop and support them have also received little specific attention. In other areas of teamwork, successful leaders seem to able to combine good 'task' skills (analysing problems, setting clear goals, agreeing responsibilities) with good 'socioemotional' skills (involving colleagues, recognizing their strengths, inviting collaborative decision-making, etc.), see Alimo-Metcalfe and Alban-Metcalf (2006). There is no reason why this same mix of positive qualities should not apply to leaders in residential staff teams but, again, this has not been investigated within an evaluative framework.

'Quality of care' and 'quality of life'

Before discussing more of the research literature, we should clarify what we mean by the terms '**quality of care**' and '**quality of life**'. 'Quality of care' implies evaluation from an external perspective (e.g. as reflected in positive changes in functioning) whereas 'quality of life' refers to subjective satisfaction by residents with the care delivered and the physical environment.

In terms of quality of care, the most important factor appears to be the effectiveness of individually-centred, targeted programmes of care. The strongest evidence for this comes from studies of 'hospital hostels' where there is 24-hour professional care (Fakhoury et al., 2002). Service users going through these units tend to show positive improvements in functioning—including some reductions in violence—compared with controls and this seems to be associated with the delivery of highly individualized, 'user-centred' programmes (Shepherd et al., 1996; Trieman and Leff, 1996). Such programmes combine structure and support, in the context of frequent, high-quality ('low EE') staff–resident interactions.

Quality of the physical environment may also affect quality of care. For example, Baker and Douglas (1990) studied the effect of the quality of the housing environment on community adjustment over a nine month period in a large sample (n = 729) of clients in community support programmes in upstate New York. Clients who were resident in housing rated 'good' or 'fair' showed significant improvements in functioning and no increases in maladaptive behaviour compared with those in housing rated as 'poor'. In a large-scale systematic review of the quality of institutional care for people with longer-term mental health problems, Taylor et al. (2009) found eight domains of institutional care that were key to recovery: living conditions, interventions for schizophrenia, physical health, restraint and seclusion, staff training and support, therapeutic relationships, autonomy, and service-user involvement. Evidence was strongest for specific interventions for schizophrenia, but this may have been due to the mixed quality of the available research evidence.

Among the most important factors in determining **quality of life** as perceived by the service user are choice (including choice over which setting in which to live) and the absence of unnecessary rules and restrictions (Owen et al., 1996). In relation to choice, as indicated earlier, it is a consistent finding that service users tend to express a preference for more independent living, in ordinary housing, with flexible, domiciliary support, rather than living with staff (Hogberg et al., 2006; Owen et al., 1996; Tanzman, 1993). In addition, if these choices are followed then there is good evidence that satisfaction will increase (Keck, 1990; Nelson et al., 2007; Srebnick et al., 1995).

However, the literature also contains several examples where staff or family perceptions conflict with service users' preferences. Minsky and colleagues (1995) found that the choice of 80 long-term inpatients was overwhelmingly to live alone, with family, or chosen room mate: only 4% preferring options with live-in staff. By contrast, 61% of staff felt this to be the best option. Massey and Wu (1993) surveyed service users in a Florida mental health centre and found similarly that service users prioritized personal choice, location and (interestingly) proximity to mental health services more often than staff. A Canadian study by Piat et al. (2008) found that mental health case managers tended to prefer supported accommodation with structure, i.e. staffing 'built-in' to the accommodation, whereas service users preferred their own apartments. Friedrichs et al. (1999) found that for service users living independently, they and their families reported isolation to be a significant problem and family members tended to prefer housing which provided support and structure. The research therefore suggests that staff—and family members—tend to opt for more 'safe' housing options, with staff on site; while service users value independence and privacy.

Regarding the importance of minimizing 'unnecessary rules and restrictions', in the TAPS study (see 'Outcomes' section) it is striking how much change there was in measures of 'restrictiveness' when patients moved from hospital to community settings (Leff, 1997). These changes were often small (e.g. being able to access the kitchen at 9.00 p.m. and make a cup of tea; having the choice over what to eat and who to eat with) but these small choices made a big difference to the quality of peoples' lives (Borge et al., 1999). The increased satisfaction ('quality of life') consistently associated with the move from hospital to community seems to be largely a direct reflection of the value of these small increments in perceived autonomy (Shepherd et al., 1996).

Stigma

Another important consequence of moving care from hospital to community is that it becomes necessary to deal directly with public attitudes, specifically stigma. In England, public attitudes towards people with mental health problems living in the community have generally softened in recent years. For example, in 2010, 66% agreed with the statement, 'Residents have nothing to fear from people coming into their neighbourhoods to obtain mental health services', this compares with 62% in 2009 (TNS UK, 2010). However, while the public may have become generally less fearful, they are still likely to have specific fears about actual developments in their neighbourhood. Hence, the study by Wolff et al. (1996) is still relevant. They evaluated the effectiveness of a community education programme aimed at preparing a local neighbourhood for a new supported housing scheme. Targeting approximately

150 people, providing information sheets, a video, a public meeting with a 'question-and-answer' session, a barbecue and other social events. Common stereotypes of dangerousness were addressed and the public were reassured that residents would not be simply 'dumped' and left to fend for themselves. The study found a small increase in knowledge concerning mental illness, but a significant reduction in fearful and rejecting attitudes. This confirms several different antistigma programmes and shows that they **can** make a difference providing they are clearly targeted and involve direct contact, in controlled conditions, between those holding the prejudice and those who are the object of it (Thornicroft et al., 2007).

Recovery

As indicated earlier, there is currently considerable interest in the concept of 'recovery' in residential care (e.g. Dinniss et al., 2007). However, there is also still confusion concerning the meaning of 'recovery' and what evidence is available to support the approach (Shepherd et al., 2008; Warner, 2009). In residential care, recovery is mainly about the style and quality of care, in particular the extent to which attempts are made to empower the person to take their own decisions and pursue their own priorities, rather than those of professionals. Hence, it relates closely to the key dimensions of 'choice' and 'control' mentioned above. A new method of improving the quality of recovery-oriented services has recently been proposed by Shepherd et al. (2010) and is to be tested in an empirical study over the next few years.

In England, the move towards a 'recovery-orientation' has been encouraged by attempts to increase the *personalization* of care (Department of Health, 2008). Recently, this has included attempts to provide patients with individual 'budgets', where they are given direct funding and helped to make their own choices about residential (and day care) options. This approach is still controversial and uptake has been slow (SCIE, 2009). The central problem is providing appropriate help and support to individuals who find it difficult to express their views and difficult to manage their own care. There are also obvious dangers of exploitation and abuse. Nevertheless, this approach is becoming more common in relation to residential options for people over 65 and, with increasing pressures on budgets, it is likely to become more widely used for adults of all ages in the future.

Outcomes

Finally, we come to the question of outcomes. Predictably, due to ethical, logistical, and conceptual problems, the evaluation of different forms of residential care is not an area where there are many randomized controlled trials (RCTs). However, there are many other ways of assessing outcomes and we will consider attempts to assess housing initiatives at the whole service level, individual housing schemes, and also narrative approaches, which give rich, qualitative information from an individual perspective.

The research on 'deinstitutionalization' has consistently demonstrated that the functioning of long-stay patients resettled in the community is generally improved and they are more satisfied compared with those remaining in hospital. The TAPS study examined the progress of more than 700 patients leaving Friern and Claybury hospitals in north London over a period of more than 5 years (Leff, 1997). Following resettlement, service users showed reduced negative symptoms, increased social networks and

functioning, and reported higher levels of satisfaction with their living situation compared with the matched controls. There were no differences regarding the severity of positive symptoms or the rates of suicide or crime. Forty per cent of the 72 patients who were initially 'difficult to place' went on to be resettled from hospital over the next 5 years, suggesting that even the most disabled people could manage in less institutional settings, providing appropriate support is available. There were some concerns regarding fragmentation and the possible inadequacy of community services, but overall the results are generally viewed as demonstrating that properly funded, planned resettlement of long-stay patients from asylums results in significant social benefits and increased quality of life without any increased risk of harmful outcomes. If all costs were taken into account, care was slightly less expensive for the community group, but increased with increasing levels of disability (Beecham et al., 1997).

Uncontrolled, prospective follow-up studies of community resettlement in several different countries show a very similar picture. Studies in Australia (Andrews et al., 1990), California (Segal and Kotler, 1993), Northern Ireland (Donnelly et al., 1996), Norway (Borge et al., 1999) and Italy (Barbato et al., 2004) have all generally found improved satisfaction for people moving to the community, stable levels of symptomatology (no increase or decrease) and relatively few subsequent long-term readmissions.

Turning now to specific types of residential care, the one which has probably been most studied is '24-hour nursed care' ('hospital hostels'). The outcome evidence for these kinds of units was reviewed by Macpherson and Jerrom (1999). The data from one random controlled trial and a number of matched controlled trials and uncontrolled follow-up studies suggest that they are effective in improving the functioning of up to 40% of residents sufficiently for them to be resettled into the community after an average of 2 to 3 years. Residents generally made more progress than controls regarding their social functioning; they showed increased contact with the community; and higher levels of satisfaction. Overall, costs were generally less than acute beds.

The outcome evidence for other forms of accommodation is very limited. In their review, Fakhoury et al. (2002) found 28 largely descriptive studies from the United States, Canada, and Europe. They noted that the research was of variable quality and problems of definition, design, and methodology made it difficult to draw firm conclusions regarding the clinical and cost-effectiveness of differing forms of supported accommodation. Similarly, Chilvers et al. (2002) attempted a Cochrane review of studies of supported flats within designated housing schemes (staffed 'core and cluster' facilities) compared with dispersed, 'ordinary housing', outreach support. They found no randomized controlled studies and highlighted the need for more—and better—research. Kyle and Dunn (2008) systematically reviewed 29 studies, using a method to allocate levels of evidence according to the robustness of the research method. They found good evidence that housing interventions impact positively on hospital use in the homeless, but weak evidence for similar effects with people with severe mental illness who were not homeless. There was generally weak, or very weak, evidence of a beneficial effect of supported housing on psychiatric symptoms and, at best, medium evidence of an association between housing and quality of life. These reviews illustrate the wide variety of study methods used and the complex, and at times conflicting, results of studies in this area. A selection of studies that are worth considering in more detail are summarized in Table 20.4.

Table 20.4 Reasonable quality outcome studies

Authors	Country	Method	Main findings
Hodgkins et al. (1990)	Canada	Comparison of 61 inpatients in Montreal placed into designated supported apartments with 51 individuals on the waiting list	No differences in service use after 2 years, but control group showed significantly more thought disorder from 12 months attributed to the stress of living closely with other mentally ill individuals in a poorly supervised setting
Nelson et al. (1998)	Canada	Study of the quality of care provided in a variety of care settings	Number of living companions, housing concerns and having a private room predicted 'community adaptation' (measured by scales rating emotional well-being and personal empowerment).
Seidman et al. (2003)	United States	RCT, followed-up homeless people with severe mental illness for 18 months after random allocation to independent apartments or to group homes	Neuropsychological functioning improved significantly for both groups, but executive functioning decreased significantly for the group living in independent apartments. Authors suggest that living alone may result in a lack of social interaction leading to deleterious effects on cognitive functioning
Tsemberis et al. (2004)	United States	Random allocation of 208 participants with severe mental illness and substance misuse to a housing programme which offered immediate housing without expectation of psychiatric treatment compliance or abstinence from substance use, compared with transitional housing which required compliance and sobriety.	No differences in psychiatric symptoms or substance abuse. Results challenge the common practice of linking access to housing with a requirement to accept treatment and sobriety

Turning now to the qualitative studies, Chesters et al. (2005) reported on the narratives of 15 residents of supported housing programme in Australia. These highlighted the importance of supported housing as an integral part of recovery focused services. The participants reported that people with mental health problems found it difficult to get effective care and treatment (other than education) in the community. The authors concluded that people need the benefits of decent public housing *and* ongoing support. They also warned that not all communities are welcoming and that friendships can be even less easy to secure than housing and support. In a study using interviews with supported housing residents in Ontario, Walker and Seasons (2002) found that four themes emerged: loneliness, poor quality of housing, a desire for greater understanding, and social inclusion. Forchuk et al. (2006), again working in Canada, used a focus group methodology to study the housing experiences of people with severe mental illness living in the community. They likened the devastating impact of loss through mental illness to the effects of a tornado, with periods of losing ground, struggling to survive, and then eventually gaining stability. From a professional perspective, Hogberg and colleagues (2006) carried out a qualitative analysis of interviews with nine nurses in Sweden. They noted a central theme of respect for the service user's self-determination, but also saw a key role for the professional in providing a link between the service user and their local neighbourhood.

These qualitative studies give insights into the lives of people living with serious mental illness in the community. However, they are most useful when it is possible to relate peoples' subjective experience to quantitative data regarding 'quality of care'—staffing levels, quality of interaction, leadership, management regimes, etc. Thus, it is not just the case that 'more research' would be useful, but more 'mixed method' research is most likely to help us improve the quality of resident's experience.

Summary and conclusions

1 In terms of **planning and estimating needs**, any definitions of residential alternatives must be multidimensional and should include a consideration of the whole system of supported accommodation, including all the available private, charitable, and statutory services. They should also reflect the established value and attraction to service users, of flexible, 'supported housing' models, rather than traditional group homes and hostels with fixed staffing. Local planning should be built on locally collected information about *who* the housing network is serving (and who it is not). It should not rely on 'norms'. Any planning process must not neglect the needs of those requiring the highest levels of support and a range of models of specialist residential provision, including '24-hour nursed care' should be available in each locality.

2 In terms of **housing developments**, new projects are increasingly likely to be managed by independent sector providers. To improve 'partnership working' between statutory and non-statutory agencies there needs to be a mutual respect and understanding regarding their respective roles and responsibilities. Support for providers through education and joint working with community mental health teams is necessary and should be seen as an integral part of the work of both agencies.

3 In terms of **user preferences**, new housing developments should try to take into account, as far as possible, the expressed preferences of service users regarding their living arrangements, even if these are different from professionals and family carers. Apart from expressed preferences, there is little evidence to assist in the judgement as to which service users will fare well in which different kinds of accommodation. Resident satisfaction should also be regularly assessed as it may show significant changes over time. Loneliness and isolation may be problems for some people,

but so can stress caused by close proximity to others who show disturbed and distressing behaviour. Staff in housing services should consider carefully whether there is any justification for excluding service users with a history of substance abuse or 'challenging behaviour'. Every attempt should be made to manage these kinds of problems as part of the ongoing support provided.

4 In terms of **staffing and interventions**, more attention needs to be given to the development and evaluation of joint training initiatives, aimed at improving the knowledge and skills of residential care workers. Attention should also be given to staff selection processes in order to identify those who will be most effective in their interactions with residents. Particularly careful consideration should be given to the desirable attributes of project leaders and to mechanisms for supporting and helping them develop their leadership skills. Housing regimes which maximize choice and independence are likely to be most highly valued by residents.

5 The adoption of a **'recovery orientation'** in mental health services will challenge those working in residential care to provide good quality accommodation of the type service users want and maintain a focus on the individual and the importance of choice and control. This may conflict with aspects of a 'business' model where there is an emphasis on 'throughput' and cost efficiency.

6 In terms of **outcomes**, in general those resettled from long-stay hospitals show few advantages in terms of clinical symptoms but function better socially, are happier, and cost less than their counterparts remaining in hospital. The evidence in favour of transitional 24-hour nursed care for the 'new' long stay is generally positive, however it may be unattractive to some service users. Other 'high-support' options may therefore need to be developed. Regarding the differential effectiveness of other types of provision, the evidence is limited and, once again, user preferences should probably predominate as these are most reliably associated with good outcomes.

7 There is a need for better quality, carefully designed, **quantitative research** which investigates the relationship between 'quality of care' variables and objective improvements in clinical and/or social functioning. There is also a need for better quality, carefully designed, **qualitative research** which explores the experience of service users and staff in residential care settings and investigates the relationship between 'quality of care' variables and 'quality of life' (satisfaction). Both methods should be combined for maximum effect.

Conclusions

Housing should be at the centre of community psychiatry. In order to achieve meaningful improvements in housing provision, we need to adopt a whole-systems, multiagency, collaborative approach. Services have evolved rapidly since the closure of the psychiatric institutions and further changes in response to various ideological and policy developments are inevitable. The challenges for professionals working with people who need supported accommodation are as much to do with promoting social inclusion and challenging stigma, as they are about providing the right clinical support and treatment. Residential care is certainly an area where 'more research is needed', but we would also be able to make considerable progress **now** if we were simply to implement what we already know.

References

Alimo-Metcalf, B. and Alban-Metcalf, J. (2006). More good leaders for the public sector. *International Journal of Public Sector Management*, **19**, 293–315.

Andrews, G., Teesson, M., Stewart, G., and Hoult, J. (1990). Follow-up of community placement of the chronic mentally ill in New South Wales. *Hospital and Community Psychiatry*, **41**, 184–8.

Audit Commission (1998). *Home Alone*. London: Audit Commission.

Baker, F. and Douglas, C. (1990). Housing environments and community adjustments of severely mentally ill patients. *Community Mental Health Journal*, **26**, 497–505.

Ball, R.A., Moore, E., and Kuipers, L. (1992). Expressed emotion in community care staff. A comparison of patient outcomes in a nine month follow-up of two hostels. *Social Psychiatry and Psychiatric Epidemiology*, **27**, 35–9.

Barbato, A., D'Avanzo, B., Rocca, G., Amatulli, A., and Lampugnani, D. (2004). A study of long-stay patients resettled in the community after closure of a psychiatric hospital in Italy. *Psychiatric Services*, **55**, 67–70.

Bartlett, C., Holloway, J., Evans, M., Owens, J., and Harrison, G. (2001). Alternatives to psychiatric in-patient care: a case-by-case survey of clinician judgements. *Journal of Mental Health*, **10**, 535–46.

Beecham, J., Hallam, A., Knapp, M., Baines, B., Fenyo, A. and Asbury, M. (1997). Costing care in hospital and in the community. In: Leff, J. (ed.) *Care in the community: Illusion or reality?* pp. 93–108. Chichester: John Wiley & Sons.

Borge, L., Martinsen, E.W., Ruud, T., Watne, O., and Friis, S. (1999). Quality of life, loneliness and social contact among long-term psychiatric patients. *Psychiatric Services*, **50**, 81–4.

Chesters, J., Fletcher, M., and Jones, R. (2005). Mental illness, recovery and place. *Australian e-journal for the advancement of mental health*, **4**, 89–97.

Chilvers, R., MacDonald, G.M. and Hayes, A.A. (2002). Supported housing for people with severe mental disorders. *Cochrane Database of Systematic Reviews, Issue 3*. Oxford: Oxford Update Software.

Coid, J. (1994). The Christopher Clunis Enquiry. *Psychiatric Bulletin*, **18**, 449–52.

Commander, M. and Rooprai, D (2008). Survey of long-stay patients on acute psychiatric wards. *The Psychiatrist*, **32**, 380–3.

DHSS (1981). *Care in the Community*. London: HMSO.

Department of Health (1990). *NHS and Community Care Act*. London: HMSO.

Department of Health (1996). *The Spectrum of Care: Local services for People with Mental Health problems*. London: HMSO.

Department of Health (1998a). *Partnerships in Action–New Opportunities for Joint Working between Health and Social Services: A discussion document*. London: HMSO.

Department of Health (1998b). *Modernising Mental Health Services–safe, sound and supportive*. London: HMSO.

Department of Health (1999). *National Service Framework for Mental Health: Modern standards and service models*. London: Department of Health.

Department of Health (2003). *Care homes for adults (18-65) and supplementary standards for care homes accommodating young people aged 16 and 17: national minimum standards*. London: TSO.

Department of Health (2007). *Essence of Care–Benchmarks for the Care Environment*. Available at: http://www.dh.gov.uk/publications.

Department of Health (2008). *An introduction to personalisation*. Available at: http://www.dh.gov.uk/en/SocialCare/Socialcarereform/Personalisation/.

Department of Health (2009). *New Horizons: A shared vision for mental health*. London: Mental Health Division, Department of Health. Available at: http://www.dh.gov.uk/publications

Dinniss, S., Roberts, G., Hubbard, C., Hounsell, J., and Webb, R. (2007). User-led assessment of a recovery service using DREEM. *Psychiatric Bulletin*, **31**, 124–7.

Donnelly, M., McGilloway, S., Mays, N., Knapp, M., Kavanagh, S., Beecham, J., and Fenyo, A. (1996). Leaving hospital: one and two-year outcomes of long-stay psychiatric patients discharged to the community. *Journal of Mental Health*, **5**, 245–55.

Durbin, J., Cochrane, J., Goering, P., and Macfarlane, D. (2001). Needs-based planning: evaluation of a level of care planning model. *Journal of Behavioural Health Services and Research*, **28**, 67–80.

Elbogen, E.B. and Johnson, S.C. (2009). The intricate link between violence and mental disorder. Results from the National Epidemiologic Survey on Alcohol and Related Conditions. *Archives of General Psychiatry*, **66**, 152–61.

Fitz, D. and Evenson, R.C. (1999). Recommending client residence: a comparison of the St Louis Inventory of Community Living Skills and global assessment. *Psychiatric Rehabilitation Journal*, **23**, 107–12.

Fakhoury, W.K.H., Murray, A., Shepherd, G., and Priebe, S. (2002). Research in supported housing. *Social Psychiatry and Psychiatric Epidemiology*, **37**, 301–15.

Fakhoury, W.K.H., Priebe, S., and Quraishi, M. (2005). Goals of new long stay patients in supported housing a UK study. *International Journal of Social Psychiatry*, **51**, 45–54.

Forchuk, C., Ward-Griffin, C., Csiernik, R., and Turner, C. (2006). Surviving the tornado of mental illness: Psychiatric survivors' experiences of getting, losing and keeping housing. *Psychiatric Services*, **57**, 558–62.

Freeman, A., Malone, J., and Hunt, G.E. (2004). A statewide survey of high support services for people with chronic mental illness: assessment of needs for care, level of functioning and satisfaction. *Australian and New Zealand Journal of Psychiatry*, **38**, 811–19.

Friedrich, R., Hollingsworth, B., Hradeck, E., and Culp, K.R. (1999). Family and client perspectives on alternative residential settings for persons with severe mental illness. *Psychiatric Services*, **50**, 509–14.

Glover, G. (1996). The Mental Illness Needs Index (MINI). In: Thornicroft, G. and Strathdee, G. (eds.) *Commissioning Mental Health Services*. London: HMSO.

Hodgkins, S., Cyr, M., and Gaston, L. (1990). Impact of supervised apartments on the functioning of mentally disordered adults. *Community Mental Health Journal*, **26**, 507–15.

Hogberg, T, Magnusson, H. T. and Lutzen, K. (2006). Living by themselves? Psychiatric nurses' views on supported housing for persons with severe and persistent mental illness. *Journal of Psychiatric and Mental Health Nursing*, **13**, 735–41.

Johnson, S., Thornicroft, G., and Strathdee, G. (1996). Population-based assessment of needs for services. In: Thornicroft, G. and Strathdee, G. (eds.) *Commissioning Mental Health Services*. London: HMSO.

Keck, J. (1990). Responding to consumer housing preferences: the Toledo experience. *Psychosocial Rehabilitation Journal*, **13**, 51–8.

Killaspy, H., Harden, C., Holloway, F., and King, M. (2005). *What do mental health rehabilitation services do and what are they for? A national survey in England. Journal of Mental Health*, **14**, 157–65.

Kirby, M. and Keon, W.J. (2006). Voices of people living with mental illness. In: *Out of the Shadows at Last: Transforming Mental Health, Mental Illness and Addiction Services in Canada*. Ottawa: Standing Senate Committee on Social Affairs, Science and Technology. Available at: http://www.parl.gc.ca

Kyle, T. and Dunn, J.R. (2008). Effects of housing circumstances on health, quality of life and healthcare use for people with severe mental illness: a review. *Health and Social Care in the Community*, **16**, 1–15.

Leff, J., Thornicroft, G., Coxhead, N., and Crawford, C. (1994). A five year follow up of long stay patients discharged to the community. *British Journal of Psychiatry*, **165**(Suppl. 25), 13–17.

Leff, J. (1997). *Care in the community: Illusion or reality?* London: Wiley.

Lelliott, P., Audini, B., Knapp, M., and Chisholm, D. (1996). The mental health residential care study: classification of facilities and descriptions of residents. *British Journal of Psychiatry*, **169**, 39–47.

Macpherson, R. and Jerrom, W. (1999). Review of twenty-four hour nursed care. *Advances in Psychiatric Treatment*, **5**, 146–53.

Martin, J. P. (1984). *Hospitals in Trouble*. Oxford: Basil Blackwell.

Massey, O.T. and Wu, L. (1993). Important characteristics of independent housing for people with severe mental illness: perspectives of case managers and consumers. *Psychosocial Rehabilitation Journal*, **17**, 81–92.

Minsky, S., Riesser, G.G., and Duffy, M. (1995). The eye of the beholder: housing preferences of inpatients and treatment teams. *Psychiatric Services*, **46**, 173–6.

Ministry of Health (1962). *The Hospital Plan for England and Wales (Cmnd, 1604)*. London: HMSO.

Ministry of Justice (2009). *Story of the prison population 1995–2009 England and Wales. Ministry of Justice, Statistics bulletin*. London: Ministry of Justice.

Mountain, D., Killaspy, H., and Holloway, F. (2009). Mental health rehabilitation services in the UK in 2007. *The Psychiatrist*, **33**, 215–18.

Nelson, G., Brent Hall, G., and Walsh-Bowers, R. (1998). The relationship between housing characteristics, emotional well-being and the personal empowerment of psychiatric consumer/survivors. *Community Mental Health Journal*, **34**, 57–69.

Nelson, G., Sylvestre, J., and Aubry, T. (2007). Housing Choice and Control, Housing Quality, and Control over Professional Support as Contributors to the Subjective Quality of Life and Community Adaptation of People with Severe Mental Illness. *Administration and Policy in Mental Health and Mental Health Services Research*, **34**, 89–100.

O'Brien, M. (2010). *Written answer*, 5 February 2010. Available at: http://www.theyworkforyou.com/wrans/?id=2010-02-05a.315539.h&s=O%27Brien+Mike#g315539.r0

ODPM (2002). *The NHS and the supporting people strategy: building the links*. London: Office of the Deputy Prime Minister.

ODPM (2005). *Using the Quality Assessment Framework*. London: Office of the Deputy Prime Minister.

Owen, C., Rutherford, V., Jones, M., Wright, C., Tennant, C., and Smallman, A. (1996). Housing accommodation preferences of people with psychiatric disabilities. *Psychiatric Services*, **47**, 628–32.

Peterson, P. and Borland, A. (1995). Use of state hospital staff to provide training for staff of community residential facilities. *Psychiatric services*, **46**, 506–8.

Phelan, M. and Strathdee, G. (1994). Living in the community: Training house officers in mental health. *Journal of Mental Health*, **3**, 229–33.

Piat, M., Lesage, A., Boyer, R., Dorvil, H., Couture, A., Grenier, G., et al. (2008). Housing for persons with serious mental illness: consumer and service provider preferences. *Psychiatric Services*, **59**, 1011–17.

Priebe, S., Badesconyi, A., Fioritti, A., Hansson, L., Kilian, R., Torres-Gonzales, F., et al. (2005). Reinstitutionalisation in mental health care: comparison of data on service provision from six European countries. *British Medical Journal*, **330**, 123–6.

Priebe, S., Frottier, P., Gaddini, A., Killian, R., Lauber, C., Martinez-Leal, R., et al. (2008). Mental Health care institutions in nine European Countries, 2002 to 2006. *Psychiatric Services*, **59**, 570–3.

Prosser, D., Johnson, S., Kuipers, E., Szmukler, G., Bebbington, P., and Thornicroft, G. (1997). Perceived sources of work stress and satisfaction among hospital and community mental health staff, and their relation to mental health, burnout and job satisfaction. *Journal of Psychosomatic Research*, **43**, 51–9.

Raskin, A., Mghir, R., Peszke, M., and York, D. (1998). A psychoeducational program for caregivers of the chronic mentally ill residing in community residences. *Community Mental Health Journal*, **34**, 393–402.

Ridgeway, P.A. and Press, A. (2004). *Assessing the recovery commitment of your mental health services: A users's guide for the Developing Recovery Enhancing Environments Measure (DREEM)–UK version 1 December, 2004* (Allott, P. and Higginson, P., eds.). Mentalhealthrecovery@blueyonder.co.uk

Royal College of Psychiatrists (2010). *Accreditation for Inpatient Mental Health Services (AIMS)* Available at: http://www.rcpsych.ac.uk/pdf/Standards%20for%20Inpatient%20Wards%20-%20Working%20Age%20Adults%20-%20Fourth%20Edition.pdf

Ryan, T., Pearsall, A., Hatfield, B. and Poole, R. (2006). Long term care for serious mental illness outside the NHS. A study of out of area placements. *Journal of Mental Health*, **13**, 425–9.

SCIE (2009). Research briefing 20: The implementation of individual budget schemes in adult social care. Available at: http://www.scie.org.uk/publications/briefings/briefing20/index.asp.

Segal, S.P. and Kotler. P.L. (1993). Sheltered care residence: ten-year personal outcomes. *American Journal of Orthopsychiatry*, **63**, 80–83.

Seidman, L.J., Schutt, R.K., Caplan, B.C., Tolomiczenko, G.S., Turner, W.M., and Goldfinger, S.M. (2003). The effect of housing interventions on neuropsychological functioning among homeless people with mental illness. *Psychiatric Services*, **54**, 905–8.

Senn, V., Kendal, R., and Trieman, N. (1997). The TAPS project 38: level of training and its availability to carers within group homes in a London district. *Social Psychiatry & Psychiatric Epidemiology*, **32**, 317–22.

Shaw, J., Appleby, L., Amos, T., McDonnell, R., Harris, C., McCann, K., et al. (1999). Homicide, mental disorder and clinical care in people convicted of homicide: national clinical survey. *British Medical Journal*, **318**, 1240–4.

Shepherd, G. (1995). The ward in a house: residential care for the severely disabled. *Journal of Mental Health*, **31**, 53–69.

Shepherd, G., Muijen, M., Dean, R., and Cooney, M. (1996). Residential care in hospital and in the community–Quality of care and quality of life. *British Journal of Psychiatry*, **168**, 448–56.

Shepherd, G., Beadsmoore, A., Moore, C., Hardy, P., and Muijen, M. (1997). Relation between bed use, social deprivation, and overall bed availability in acute psychiatric units and alternative residential options: a cross sectional survey, one day census data and staff interviews. *British Medical Journal*, **314**, 262–6.

Shepherd, G., Boardman, J., and Slade, M. (2008). *Implementing Recovery–A methodology for organisational change. Policy Paper*. London: Sainsbury Centre for Mental Health.

Shepherd, G., Boardman, J., and Burns, M. (2010). *Making recovery a reality. Briefing Paper*. London: Sainsbury Centre for Mental Health.

Singleton, N., Meltzer, H., and Gatward, R. (1998). *Psychiatric morbidity among prisoners in England and Wales*. London: Office for National Statistics.

Slade, M. (2009a). *Personal Recovery and Mental Illness: A Guide for Mental Health Professionals*. Cambridge: Cambridge University Press.

Slade, M. (2009b). *100 Ways to Support Recovery*. London: Rethink. Available at: www.mentalhealthshop.org/rethink_publications

Sorensen-Snyder, K., Wallace, C., Moe, K., and Liberman, R. (1994). Expressed emotion by residential care operators and residents' symptoms and quality of life. *Hospital and Community Psychiatry*, **45**, 1141–3.

Srebnik, D, Livingstone, J, Gordon, L. and King, D. (1995). Housing choice and community success for individuaks with serious and persistent mantal illness. *Community Mental Health Journal*, **31**, 139–52.

Strathdee, G. and Jenkins, R. (1996). Purchasing mental health care for primary care. In Thornicroft, G & Strathdee, G. (eds.) *Commissioning Mental Health Services*, pp. 71–83. London: HMSO.

Tanzman, B. (1993). An overview of surveys of mental health consumers' preferences for housing and support services. *Hospital & Community Psychiatry*, **44**, 450–5.

Taylor, T.L., Killaspy, H., Wright, C., Turton, P., White, S., Kallert, T.W., et al. (2009). A systematic review of the international published literature relating to quality of institutional care for people with longer term mental health problems. *BMC Psychiatry*, **9**, 55–73.

Tempier, R., Mercier, C., Leouffre, P., and Caron, J. (1997). Quality of life and social integration of severely mentally ill patients: a longitudinal study. *Journal of Psychiatry & Neuroscience*, **22**, 249–55.

Thornicroft, G., Bebbington, P., and Leff, J. (2005). Outcomes for long-term patients one year after discharge from a psychiatric hospital. *Psychiatric Services*, **56**, 1416–22.

Thornicroft, G., Diana, R., Kassam, A., and Sartorius, N. (2007). Stigma: ignorance, prejudice or discrimination? *British Journal of Psychiatry*, **190**, 192–3.

TNS UK (2010). *Attitudes to Mental Illness 2010 Research Report*. Available at: http://www.dh.gov.uk/en/Publicationsandstatistics/Publications/PublicationsStatistics/DH_114795

Trieman, N. and Leff, J. (1996). The TAPS Project. 36: the most difficult to place long-stay psychiatric in-patients outcome one year after relocation. *British Journal of Psychiatry*, **169**, 289–92.

Tsemberis, S., Gulcur, L., and Nakae, M. (2004). Housing first, consumer choice and harm reduction for homeless individuals with a dual diagnosis. *Research and Practice*, **94**, 651–6.

Walker, R. and Seasons, M. (2002). Supported Housing for People with Serious Mental Illness: Resident Perspectives on Housing. *Canadian Journal of Community Mental Health*, **21**, 137–51.

Walshe, K. (2003). *Regulating Healthcare*. Maidenhead: Open University Press.

Warner, R. (2009). Recovery from schizophrenia and the recovery model. *Current Opinion in Psychiatry*, **22**, 374–80.

Wolff, G., Pathare, S., Craig T. and Leff, J. (1996). Public education for community care: a new approach. *British Journal of Psychiatry*, **168**, 441–7.

CHAPTER 21

Programmes to support family members and caregivers

Amy L. Drapalski and Lisa B. Dixon

Introduction

Most individuals with schizophrenia or other serious mental illnesses have regular contact with family members and these family members often provide substantial support and assistance to their ill relative (Chien et al., 2006; Hackman and Dixon, 2008; Resnick et al., 2005). Although providing support to a relative with mental illness is often rewarding on many levels, caring for a relative with a mental illness can also be extremely demanding and can lead to feeling of being overwhelmed, frustrated, worried, and depressed. Oftentimes, limited knowledge of mental illness, mental health treatments, and the mental health service system coupled with the increased demands associated with taking on a caregiver role can contribute to significant family stress, distress, and burden. In turn, this increased burden may impede a family's ability to continue to provide the support and assistance that their ill relative may need to help effectively manage an illness and achieve recovery goals. Several programmes have been developed in an effort to address the varying needs and preferences of family members and caregivers of individuals with serious mental illness. This chapter aims to discuss the potential impact of mental illness on the family and its relationship to family needs, to highlight the basic tenets or principles of effective family programmes, and to describe several prominent family interventions and outline the evidence for their effectiveness.

The impact of mental illness on the family

Many aspects of providing support for an individual with a serious mental illness can be rewarding. However, observing mental illness in a family member and experiencing its effects can be traumatic for families and the time and effort required to provide this support in these situations can create additional burden for family members. Family members are often the first to notice emerging signs or symptoms of an illness. However, due to limited prior experience with mental illness these behaviours are rarely recognized as such and even when they are can be distressing and disturbing for family members. Consequently, families may alternate between

periods of denial or avoidance of emerging issues or problems and feeling overwhelmed or overcome by the illness and its effect on the family functioning (Lucksted et al., 2008). These changes may lead family members to experience additional burden—often described in terms of objective and subjective burden. Objective burden typically refer to clear, observable disruptions in the family unit or family roles that stem from the added responsibilities associated with caring for a relative with an illness (Hackman and Dixon, 2008). These can include financial strain or hardship created by the need to financially support a relative who may be unable to support him- or herself, loss of social support or social disengagement due to active efforts to avoid others in an effort to minimize rejection or limited time to engage in social activities as a result of the time constraints created by additional caregiver responsibilities, and disruption in daily routines and family relationships and roles. Subjective burden refers to the psychological impact of the illness on the family, often manifested in the form of psychological distress, particularly depression, anxiety, and anger (Lefley, 1989). Family members often worry about the health and welfare of their ill relative, the potential for future relapses and hospitalization, and their ability to help their family member successfully cope with an illness (Drapalski et al., 2009). Depression is also common and may result from feelings of grief and loss as family members attempt to come to terms with the potential need to change their own expectations concerning their relative's future functioning and goals. Moreover, depression, frustration and anger may also occur in reaction to the added responsibility associated with supporting a relative, the challenges family members may face in their attempts to support their relative, and the potential changes family members may need to make in their own lives or in terms of their own future plans as a result of their relative's illness (Drapalski et al., 2009).

Not surprisingly, greater objective and subjective burden may produce a family environment that is stressful for both the family and the individual with the illness. However, providing family members with information to help them better understanding a relative's illness and ways to help them cope with their illness, assistance with developing more effective communication and problem-solving skills, and support in helping family members better manage the difficulties and struggles than may come with supporting a relative with an illness, can all serve to minimize family burden (Dixon et al., 2001b; Falloon and Pederson, 1985; Hazel et al., 2004). Results of several studies assessing the perceived needs of family members of individuals with serious mental illness echo this sentiment, with family members expressing the need for information on mental illness and its treatment, coping strategies and problem-solving skills, the structure and function of the mental health system and the different roles of mental health treatment providers, community resources (e.g. housing, employment, social/recreational programmes) and future planning (Drapalski et al, 2008; Hatfield, 1978; Lefley, 1989; Smith, 2003; Winefield and Harvey, 1994).

Basic principles and goals of family programmes

Over the past 30 years, a number of family programmes have been developed in an attempt to meet the needs of individuals with serious mental illness and their families. It should be noted that with regards to these programmes, family is defined somewhat broadly to include any individual who is serves as a support to the individual with the illness. As such, 'family' may include parents, siblings, spouses or significant others, or children; extended family such as cousins, aunts, or uncles; or persons outside the family such as close friends or peers. Although these programmes can differ in terms of their content, structure, and format, effective, evidence-based family treatments all tend to adhere to several core principles and incorporate several critical features (Dixon et al., 2001b). These core elements, outlined by a panel of international experts convened by the World Schizophrenia Fellowship (1998), are viewed central in helping providers to work collaboratively with individuals with serious mental illness and their families to best promote positive outcomes for both the individual with the illness and their family (Dixon et al., 2001b). These features include:

- Establishing and maintaining a collaborative and supportive relationship with the consumer and family

- Attention to the needs of the consumer and the family

- Treat family as equal partners in treatment planning and delivery

- Exploration and clarification of the consumer and families treatment expectations

- Assessment and evaluation of family strengths and weaknesses as they pertain to their ability to support their ill relative

- Address feelings of loss

- Sensitivity to the family distress and conflict

- Provision of relevant information/education when needed

- Development of crisis management and response plan

- Communication and problem-solving skill development

- Assisting families in the expansion of social support networks (e.g. National Alliance for Mental Illness—NAMI)

- Awareness of potential differences in the needs of families and be flexible in meeting those needs

- Connecting the family with other professionals once the family work has been completed.

Programmes to support family members and caregivers

As noted previously, a number of family programmes have been developed in an effort to address the need of individuals with serious mental illness and their families. Although these programmes vary substantially in terms of their structure, content, and focus, all share several common features including developing a supportive, collaborative relationship with the consumer and family member, providing education and information on mental illness and its treatment, and helping families develop more effective skills for coping with some of the effects of the illness (often including communication and problem-solving skills) (Murray-Swank et al., 2007; Pfammatter et al., 2006). Moreover, each programme has demonstrated a number of benefits for both consumers and family members. Thus, the availability of a variety of programmes allows providers to work with consumers and family members to decide which programme best meets their individual needs and preferences concerning involvement.

Family psychoeducation

Family Psychoeducation (FPE) programmes were initially developed with the goal of improving consumer outcomes by reducing or minimizing the level of expressed emotion exhibited by family members of individuals with schizophrenia and other serious mental illnesses. Expressed emotion refers to the extent of criticism or emotional over-involvement directed towards an individual with mental illness by another individual (typically a family member) (Bebbington and Kuipers, 1994). High levels of expressed emotion among family members has been associated with greater relapse rates in individuals with both schizophrenia (Bebbington and Kuipers, 1994) and bipolar disorder (Miklowitz et al., 1988). For example, in a study of individuals with schizophrenia, Bebbington and Kuipers (1994) found that individuals with high expressed-emotion families evidenced more than double the relapse rate (50%) compared to low expressed-emotion families (21%). Despite its initial focus, research on family psychoeducation over the past several decades suggests that there are a number of benefits to participation in FPE programmes and that these benefits extend to all families, regardless of the level of expressed emotion (Bebbington and Kuipers, 1994; Murray-Swank and Dixon, 2005).

Although specific FPE programmes may vary somewhat in terms of content, structure, and format, most FPE programmes include several core features: 1) provision of psychoeducation, 2) skill building (particularly communication and problem solving), and 3) increased opportunities for receiving support (Murray-Swank et al., 2007). However, as noted earlier, the way in which these components are delivered can vary depending on the specific programme. For example, some FPE programmes are designed to be conducted with an individual family (Anderson et al., 1986; Falloon et al., 1984; Mueser and Glynn, 1999), while others are conducted in a group setting with several families participating at one time (McFarlane, 2002). Some programmes, such as those developed by Leff and colleagues allows families to attend biweekly family groups without their ill relative in addition to regular joint meetings with the ill relative in the home (Murray-Swank and Dixon, 2005).

While many programmes have been developed primarily with families of individuals with schizophrenia in mind, in the Family-Focused Treatment (FFT) programme the content and focus of the sessions has been modified to better address the specific needs of families of individuals with bipolar disorder (Miklowitz and Goldstein, 1997). Finally, some programmes such as Behavioural Family Treatment (BFT; Falloon et al., 1984; Mueser and Glynn, 1999) and Multifamily Group Therapy (MFGT; McFarlane, 2002) include both the family and the individual with mental illness in sessions, others involve only the family.

Regardless of the differences in the content, structure, and format of the programme, the effectiveness of FPE for individuals with serious mental illness has been clearly established. Results from several meta-analyses of FPE programmes have demonstrated the effectiveness of FPE for individuals with schizophrenia, particularly with regards to relapse and rehospitalization rates (Baucom et al., 1998; Pfammater, et al., 2006; Pitschel-Walz et al., 2001). In an analysis of 25 studies, Pitschel-Walz and colleagues (2001) found that there was a 20% reduction in relapse rates (defined as a significant increase in symptoms or rehospitalization) for individuals with schizophrenia when a family member participated in FPE and that better outcomes were associated with length in treatment with greater benefits evidenced in those that participated in programmes for more than 3 months. Results from other meta-analyses are even more pronounced. Baucom and colleagues (1998) found that participation in an FPE programme lasting at least 9 months can reduce relapse and rehospitalization rates by approximately 50%. Other studies have found that participation in FPE was associated with a number of positive outcomes including better rates of employment (McFarlane et al., 1996, 2000), social functioning (Montero et al., 2001), life satisfaction (Resnick et al., 2004), and reduced negative symptoms (Dyck et al., 2000).

While a majority of studies on FPE has been conducted with families of individuals with schizophrenia, recent studies examining the effects for families of individuals with other diagnosis such as bipolar disorder and major depression have suggested similar positive effects. Modelled after BFT programmes for schizophrenia (Falloon et al., 1984), FFT is a psychoeducation programme that includes the same core components found in FPE programmes for individuals with schizophrenia (e.g. illness education, communication skills development, and problem-solving training); however, if FFT these elements are modified or tailored to address the specific needs of individuals with bipolar disorder and their families (Miklowitz and Goldstein, 1997). In a randomized clinical trial comparing FFT to usual care, Miklowitz and colleagues (2003) found that participation in FFT was associated with significantly lower relapse rates (34% vs. 54%), more extended periods of time between periods of symptom exacerbation (53.2 days vs. 73.2 days), better medication adherence, and less depression 2 years after completing the programme (Miklowitz et al., 2003). Similarly, Rea and colleagues (2003) compared the effects of using FFT as an adjunct to medication management to individual treatment and medication management (Rea et al., 2003). Results were even more pronounced with individuals receiving FFT being less likely to relapse (28% vs. 60%) or be rehospitalized (12% vs. 60%) 1 year after hospital discharge than those who received individual therapy as an adjunct to medication. Other studies have suggested benefits of participation in psychoeducational programmes for couples for individuals with depression (Emanuels-Zuurveen and Emmelkamp, 1997; Leff et al., 2000). Although these findings

suggest that FPE may be equally beneficial for individuals with other serious mental illnesses and their families, particularly when programmes are tailored to meet the specific needs and experiences of those individuals and families, additional studies are needed.

Of importance is the fact that the benefits associated with participation in FPE programmes appear to be sustained well after the completion of the programme. Pitschel-Walz and colleagues (2007) examined relapse rates and days of hospitalization over a 7-year period following discharge. They found that individuals with schizophrenia whose families participated in FPE during the index hospitalization were significantly less likely to relapse (54%) during the 7 years post-hospitalization than those who did not (88%). In addition, individuals who families received FPE spent significantly fewer days in the hospital (75 days) than those whose families did not receive FPE (225 days); thus, suggesting that the benefits of FPE programmes may be maintained and possibly enhanced over time (Pitschel-Walz et al., 2006). Additional studies are needed to determine the long-term impact of FPE on consumer outcomes including relapse and rehospitalization rates as well as family outcomes.

Participation in FPE can also impact family outcomes. A meta-analysis reviewing outcomes of FPE across numerous settings found that participation was associated with a significant decrease in the objective and subjective burden, negative feelings towards the family member with the illness, and family conflict experienced by family members (Cuijpers, 1999). Other studies have found that participation in FPE was associated with improved well-being (Falloon et al., 1985) and better overall family functioning (Cuipers, 1999). Thus, given the overwhelming evidence of the positive effects of FPE, particularly in terms of relapse and rehospitalization rates, it is not surprising that numerous groups such as the American Psychiatric Association, the Schizophrenia Patient Outcomes Research Team (PORT), and others have recommended that family psychoeducation programmes be offered to the families of individuals with serious mental illness. In fact, in the most recent iteration of the PORT recommendations suggested that all individuals with schizophrenia be offered family psychoeducation that includes illness education, coping and crisis management skills training, and support that lasts at least 6 months (Dixon et al., 2010).

Brief education and family consultation

Similar to FPE, briefer educational programmes and family consultation were developed with the goals of increasing knowledge, reducing burden, and minimizing distress in families of individuals with serious mental illness. However, differences in the structure and focus of these programmes may allow them to serve as alternative or in many some complementary programmes to FPE, particularly in cases where participation in FPE may not be feasible, practical, or perceived as needed (Cohen et al., 2008). In these cases, shorter, more targeted programmes or services, such as brief family education or family consultation may be beneficial.

Brief family education

Brief education programmes are time-limited and focused, often lasting anywhere from 6 to 12 weeks or more. Sessions are usually led by a mental health professional and often focus on specific educational and/or skills training goals such as providing families with education on mental illness, its aetiology, and its treatment; helping families develop effective communication and problem-solving skills; and improving self-care and coping skills; crisis management and relapse prevention; and increasing the opportunity for mutual support. For example, Posner and colleagues (1992) had family members attend eight, 90-minute sessions that focus on educating family members concerning schizophrenia, its aetiology, and illness treatment; the effects of mental illness on the family; and available community resources. Another programme developed and evaluated by Magliano and colleagues (2006) had families participating in educational sessions for 6 months that proceeded in stages starting with an assessment of family needs, then informational/educational sessions, communication skills training and finally problem-solving.

Although the benefits of briefer family intervention programmes may be somewhat diminished in comparison to longer programmes, participation in these programmes has been shown to lead to a number of positive outcomes for individuals with schizophrenia. These benefits appear to differ from study to study and have included fewer symptoms (Merinder et al., 1999), better self-care (Magliano et al., 2006; Xiong et al., 1994), and better treatment adherence (Pitschel-Walz et al., 2006; Xiong et al., 1994) in individuals with illness and greater knowledge of the illness (Posner et al., 1992) and less perceived burden and distress among family members (Cuijpers, 1999). However, the impact on relapse and rehospitalization rates is less clear. While results from some studies have suggested that participation in brief educational programmes may be associated with longer periods of time between relapses (Merinder et al., 1999), fewer hospitalizations (Chien and Lee, 2010) and shorter hospitalizations (Chien and Lee, 2010), other have not (Posner et al., 1992). Despite the variability in outcomes found, the apparent benefits of brief family education programme has led to the recently updated schizophrenia PORT recommendation that individuals with schizophrenia and their families be offered brief educational programmes in cases where participation in longer FPE programmes are not possible or not of interest to family members (Dixon et al., 2010). Few studies have examined the use of brief psychoeducational programmes for families of individuals with other serious mental illnesses.

Family consultation

Family consultation offers another alternative to working with families of individuals with mental illness. Similar to the psychoeducational programmes previously mentioned, family consultation involves providing families with information and educational on mental illness and its treatment and helps families to develop better coping skills. However, in contrast, family consultation typically involves a provider meeting with an individual family (rather than several families at a time), is specifically designed to target the individual needs of the family, and can vary in length depending on the needs and goals of the family. Thus, family consultation may be particularly useful in situations where the family can identify a specific problem or needs that can be addressed in a relatively short period of time. In addition, since family consultation can be conducted in the absence of with the illness, it can be useful in situations where the individual with the illness is unwilling or unable to participate.

Most family consultations begin with an assessment with the client and/or the family to determine the focus or primary goal of the consultation effort. After identifying a particular problem or goal to be addressed, potential options for addressing the problem are discussed and a joint decision concerning how best to address

that goal is reached. This may include providing families with additional education on relevant topics, helping families identify and access community resources, working with families to help them develop more effective communication, problem-solving, and other coping skills, or engaging the family in problem-solving around a particular issue (Family Institute for Education, Practice, and Research, and New York State Office of Mental Health, 2007). As such, the consultation length is often dependent on both the problem and the method by which the family has chosen to attempt to address the problem.

Only a few studies have systematically evaluated the effectiveness of family consultation; however, these studies suggest potential benefits to participation in these programmes. In one such study, Solomon and colleagues (1997) compared a brief psychoeducational programme to a family consultation programme. Participants included individuals with schizophrenia spectrum disorders, bipolar disorder or major depression. The brief educational programme included 10, 2-hour sessions that involved both education on mental illness and its treatment and assistance in developing coping skills. In contrast, family consultation involved the family engaging in individual consultation with a mental health provider. Consultation sessions were conducted either in person or over the telephone and were provided as needed basis up to a maximum of 15 hours of consultation over a 3-month period of time. They found that participation in both brief family education and family consultation led to improved self-efficacy concerning the family's ability to successfully manage and cope with their relative's mental illness (Solomon et al., 1996, 1997). Participation did not however lead to greater family contact with the mental health services system, suggesting that specific attention be paid to helping family members connect with the relative's treatment providers (Solomon et al., 1998). Spiegel and Wissler (1987) evaluated a family consultation programme in which a consultation team came to the family's home for 4 to 6 weeks following discharge from an inpatient setting to provide them with education, problem-solving, and crisis intervention skills development. Although conducted with only a small number of families, results show that those whose family received the consultation had fewer days in the hospital, greater use of outpatient services, and better self-reported adjustment than those who did not receive consultation. Although additional research on the impact of family consultation is clearly needed, these studies suggest that family consultation could be useful for some families, particularly in situations where an identified a problem or goal can be addressed in a short period of time.

Peer-led programmes

In addition to family programmes offered by mental health providers, several peer-lead, community based programmes have also been developed to address the needs of families. Based on theories of stress, coping, and adaptation, the primary goal of these programmes are to improve family outcomes, and, as such, differ in several ways from the family programmes mentioned earlier (Dixon et al., 2001a). The central feature of peer-lead family education programmes, such as the NAMI Family-to-Family Education Programme and Journey of Hope, is that they are led by trained family members of individuals with mental illness who have previously completed the programme. These programmes tend to be shorter in length (8 and 12 weeks, respectively), attended by several families at one time, held in the community (rather than a treatment facility) and are aimed at providing family members with education on mental illness, mental health treatments, and the mental health services system, helping them the family to develop skills to both help their relative better cope with their illness and to help the family better cope with stressors that may be associated with their caregiver role, and allowing opportunities for mutual support.

A number of studies have been recently conducted aimed at evaluating the effectiveness of these community-based, peer-lead programmes. Participants in these studies have typically included family members of individuals with a range of serious mental illnesses, such as schizophrenia spectrum disorders, bipolar disorder, and major depression. Participation in peer-lead family education programmes has been associated with a number of positive client and family outcomes. Benefits to the family have included greater sense of empowerment (Dixon et al., 2001a; Dixon et al., 2004), less displeasure or worry associated with their relative (Dixon et al., 2000a; Dixon et al., 2004), reduced depression (Pickett-Schenk et al., 2006a), more knowledge of mental illness and the mental health care system (Dixon et al., 2004; Pickett-Schenk et al., 2006a, 2008), improved self-care (Dixon et al., 2004), and greater caregiver satisfaction (Pickett-Schenck et al., 2006b). Some suggest that the impact of these programmes may be due in part to the fact that the information and support is provided by an individual with similar lived experiences (Solomon 2004). Thus, through that shared experience, group leaders may be able to offer families a different and more 'real' perspective on the family relationship and caregiver role and provide examples of effective strategies for helping their relative better manage their illness, which may be received more positively by participants and lead to increased confidence in the participants' own ability to successfully cope with a relative's illness (Pickett-Schenk et al., 2006a, 2008; Solomon 2004). In addition, many mental health education and advocacy organizations such as National Alliance for the Mentally Ill (NAMI; United States), Depression and Related Affective Disorders (DRADA; United States), the National Schizophrenia Fellowship (United Kingdom), sponsor or provide information on support groups available to family members. Family support groups often afford family members the opportunity to obtain mutual support and understanding from others that share common experiences. Thus, these groups may be useful for family members that may need additional emotional support.

Informal family involvement

Although, as discussed earlier, the benefits for family members and caregivers of individuals with serious mental illness appear to be more pronounced when family members participate in formal programmes, containing certain critical elements, over an extended period of time (more than 6 months), even minimal, more informal contact with family members may help to address some of the families needs. As little as 8% to 15% of families participate in formal family programmes (Dixon et al., 1999; Magliano et al., 2006; Resnick et al., 2005). There are a number of system/provider, consumer, and family-related barriers may prevent family members from participation in these programmes and make participation in these programmes impractical or impossible. Thus, both in the absence of and in conjunction with family programmes family members attempting to involve family members in the ongoing clinical care an individual with serious mental illness could prove beneficial.

Although research on the impact of more informal family involvement is limited, more informal family-provider contact may allow for the needs to the family to be addressed in similar, albeit somewhat diminished or diluted, way to more structured programmes. This involvement may include intermittent telephone contacts with family members, a family member's attendance for part of an individual's treatment session, participation in treatment planning, period family meeting with a provider, or written information or handouts sent or brought home for family members (Drapalski et al., 2009). More informal contact with family members may create opportunities for educating family members on mental illness, its aetiology and its treatment, correcting any misconceptions family members may have regarding the illness, and working collaboratively with family members to identify strategies and develop skills for helping the ill relative cope with the illness, all of which may serve to improve the family relationship and reduce family burden.

Conclusion

Families often require considerable information, education, and support to minimize the additional burden that may come with caring for an individual with serious mental illness and help them in supporting their relative in their mental illness recovery. Several programmes aimed at providing family members and caregivers of individuals with serious mental illness with the information and education, skills, and support they need to support an ill relative have been developed. While research suggests that longer family psychoeducational programmes may produce the best outcomes, briefer programmes such as brief family education and family consultation as well as family involvement in ongoing care or treatment have also proven beneficial and, in some cases, may be preferable for some families. By helping consumers and family members to consider ways to involve family in treatment and explore options concerning family programmes, mental health providers can better determine which of these programmes would best address the needs and potentially produce the most positive outcomes for each family.

References

Anderson, C.M., Reiss, D.J., and Hogarty, G.E. (1986). *Schizophrenia and the Family*. New York: Guilford Press.

Baucom, D.H., Shoham, V., Mueser, K.T., Daiuto, A.D., and Stickle, T.R. (1998). Empirically supported couple and family interventions for marital distress and adult mental health problems. *Journal of Consulting and Clinical Psychology*, **66**, 53–8.

Bebbington, P. and Kuipers, L. (1994). The clinical utility of expressed emotion in schizophrenia. *Acta Psychiatria Scandanavia*, **382**, 46–53.

Chien, W.T. and Lee, I.Y.L. (2010). The schizophrenia care management program for family caregivers of Chinese patient with schizophrenia. *Psychiatric Services*, **61**, 317–20.

Chien, W.T., Chan, S.W.C., Thompson, D.R. (2006). Effects of a mutual support group for families of Chinese people with schizophrenia: 18 month follow-up. *British Journal of Psychiatry*, **189**, 41–9.

Cohen, A.N., Glynn, S.M., Murray-Swank, A., Barrio, C., Fischer, E.P. McCutcheon, S.I., *et al.* (2008). The family forum: directions for the implementation of family psychoeducation for severe mental illness. *Community Mental Health Journal*, **42**, 213–19.

Cuijpers, P. (1999). The effects of family intervention on relatives' burden: A meta-analysis. *Journal of Mental Health*, **8**, 275–85.

Dixon, L., Lyles, A., Scott, J., Lehman, A., Postrado, L., Goldman, H., et al. (1999). Services to families of adults with schizophrenia: from treatment recommendations to dissemination. *Psychiatric Services*, **50**, 233–8.

Dixon, L., Stewart, B., Burland, J., Delahanty, J., Lucksted, A., and Hoffman, M. (2001a). Pilot study of the effectiveness of the family-to-family education program. *Psychiatric Services*, **52**, 965–7.

Dixon, L., McFarlane, W.R., Lefley, H., Lucksted, A., Cohen, M., Falloon, I., et al. (2001b). Evidence-based practices for services to families of people with psychiatric disabilities. *Psychiatric Services*, **52**, 903–10.

Dixon, L., Lucksted, A., Stewart, B., Burland,.J, Brown, C.H., Postrado, L., McGuire, C., Hoffman, M. (2004). Outcomes of the peer-taught 12-week family-to-family education program for severe mental illness. *Acta Psychiatrica Scandinavica*, **109**, 207–15.

Dixon, L.B., Dickerson, F., Bellack, A.S., Bennett, M., Dickinson, D., Goldberg, R.W., et al. (2010). The 2009 Schizophrenia PORT psychosocial treatment recommendations and summary statements. *Schizophrenia Bulletin*, **36**, 48–70.

Drapalski, A.L., Marshall, T., Seybolt, D., Medoff, D., Peer, J., Leith, J., et al. (2008). The unmet needs of families of adults with mental illness and preferences regarding family services. *Psychiatric Services*, **59**, 655–62.

Drapalski, A.L., Leith, J., and Dixon, L. (2009). Involving families in the care of persons with schizophrenia and other serious mental illnesses: history, evidence, and recommendations. *Clinical Schizophrenia and Related Psychosis*, **3**, 39–49.

Dyck, D., Short, R., Hendryx, M., Norell, D., Myers, M., Patterson, T., et al. (2000). Management of negative symptoms among patients with schizophrenia attending multiple-family groups. *Psychiatric Services*, **51**, 513–19.

Emanuaels-Zuurveen, L. and Emmelkamp, P.M.G. (1997). Spouse-aided therapy with depressed patients. *Behavior Modification*, **21**, 62–77.

Falloon, I.R. and Pederson, J. (1985). Family management in the prevention of morbidity of schizophrenia: the adjustment of the family unit. *British Journal of Psychiatry*, **147**, 156–63.

Fallon, I.R.H., Boyd, J., and McGill, C. (1984). *Family Care of Schizophrenia*. New York: Guilford Press.

Falloon, I.R., Boyd, J.L., McGill, C.W. Williamson, M., Razani, J., Moss, H.B., et al. (1985). Family management in the prevention of morbidity of schizophrenia: clinical outcome of a two-year longitudinal study. *Archives of General Psychiatry*, **42**, 887–96.

Family Institute for Education, Practice and Research, New York State Office of Mental Health. (2007). 'Competency training in Consumer Centered Family Consultation.' Unpublished manuscript, Department of Psychiatry, University of Rochester, Rochester, NY.

Hackman, A. and Dixon, L. (2008). Issues in family services for persons with schizophrenia. *Psychiatric Times*, **25**, 1–2. Available at: http://www.psychiatrictimes.com/showArticle.jhtml? articleID=206900852. (ccessed 1 March 2008).

Hatfield A.B. (1978). Psychological costs of schizophrenia to the family. *Social Work*, **23**, 355–59.

Hazel, N.A., McDonell, M.G., Short, R.A., Berry, C.M. Voss, W.D., Rodgers, M.I., et al. (2004). Impact of multiple-family groups for outpatients with schizophrenia on caregiver's distress and resources. *Psychiatric Services*, **55**, 34–41.

Leff, J., Vearnals, S., Brewin, C.R., Wolff, G., Alexander, B., Asen, E., et al. (2000). Randomized controlled trial of antidepressants v. couple therapy in the treatment and maintenance of people with depression living with a partner: clinical outcome and costs. *British Journal of Psychiatry*, **177**, 95–100.

Lefley H.P. (1989). Family burden and family stigma in major mental illness. *American Psychologist*, **44**(3), 556–60.

Magliano, L., Fiorillo, A., Malangone, C., De Rosa, C., and Maj, M. (2006). Patient functioning and family burden in a controlled, real-world trial of family psychoeducation for schizophrenia. *Psychiatric Services*, **57**, 1784–91.

McFarlane, W.R. (2002). *Multifamily groups in the treatment of severe psychiatric disorders*. New York: The Guilford Press.

McFarlane, W.R., Dushay, R.A., Stastny, P., Deakins, S.M., and Link, B. (1996). A comparison of two levels of family-aided assertive community treatment. *Psychiatric Services*, **47**, 744–50.

McFarlane W.R., Dushay, R.A., Deakins, S.M., Stastny, P., Lukens, E.P., Toran J, et al. (2000). Employment outcomes in Family-aided Assertive Community Treatment. *American Journal of Orthopsychiatry*, **70**, 203–14.

McFarlane, W.R., Dixon, L., Lukens, E., and Lucksted, A. (2003). Family psychoeducation and schizophrenia: a review of the literature. *Journal of Marital Therapy*, **29**, 223–45.

Merinder, L.B., Viuff, A.G., Laugensen, H.D., Clemmensen, K., Misfelt, S., and Espensen, B. (1999). Patient and relative education in community psychiatry: a randomized controlled trial regarding its effectiveness. *Social Psychiatry and Psychiatric Epidemiology*, **34**, 287–94.

Miklowitz, D.J. and Goldstein, M.J. (1997). *A family-focused treatment approach*. New York: Guilford Press.

Miklowitz, D.J., Goldstein, M.J., Nuechterlein, K.H., Snyder, K.S., and Mintz, J. (1988). Family factors and the course of bipolar affective disorder. *Archives of General Psychiatry*, **45**, 225–31.

Miklowitz, D.J., George, E.L., Richards, J.A., Simoneau, T.L., and Suddath, R.L. (2003). A randomized study of family-focused psychoeducation and pharmacotherapy in the outpatient management of bipolar disorder. *Archives of General Psychiatry*, **60**, 904–912.

Montero, I., Asencio, A., Hernandez, I., Masanet, M.S.J., Lacruz, M., Bellver, F., et al. (2001). Two strategies for family intervention in schizophrenia: a randomized trial in a mediterranean environment. *Schizophrenia Bulletin*, **27**, 661–70.

Mueser, K.T. and Glynn, S.M. (1999). *Behavioral family therapy for psychiatric disorders*. 2nd edn. Oakland, CA: New Harbinger Publications.

Murray-Swank, A. and Dixon, L. (2005). Evidence based practices for working with families of individuals with serious mental illness. In: Drake, R., Merrens, M., and Lynde, D. (eds.) *Evidence-based Mental Health Practice: A Textbook,* pp. 424–52. New York: W.W. Norton and Company.

Murray-Swank, A., Glynn, S., Cohen, A.N., Sherman, M., Medoff, D.P. Fang, L.J., et al. (2007). Family contact, experience of family relationships, and views about family involvement in treatment among VA consumers with serious mental illness. *Journal of Rehabilitation Research and Development*, **44**, 801–12.

Pfammatter, M., Junghan, U.M., and Brenner, H.D. (2006). Efficacy of psychological therapy in schizophrenia: conclusions from meta-analyses. *Schizophrenia Bulletin*, **32**(Suppl. 1), S64–S80.

Pickett-Schenk, S.A., Cook, J.A., Steigman, P., Lippencott, R., Bennett, C., and Grey, D.D. (2006a). Psychological well-being and relationship outcomes in a randomized study of family-led education. *Archives of General Psychiatry*, **63**, 1043–50.

Pickett-Schenk, S.A., Bennett, C., Cook, J.A., Steigman, P., Lippincott, R., Villagracia, I., et al. (2006b). Changes in caregiving satisfaction and information needs among relatives of adults with mental illness: Results of a randomized evaluation of a family-led education intervention. *American Journal of Orthopsychiatry*, **76**, 545–53.

Pickett-Schenk, S.A., Lippincott, R.C., Bennett, C., and Steigman, P.J. (2008). Improving knowledge about mental illness through family-led education: The journey of hope. *Psychiatric Services*, **59**, 49–56.

Pitschel-Walz, G., Leucht, S., Bauml, J, Kissling, W., and Engel, R.R. (2001). The effect of family interventions on relapse and rehospitalization in schizophrenia-a meta-analysis. *Schizophrenia Bulletin*, **21**, 73–92.

Pitschel-Walz, G., Bauml, J., Bender, W., Engel, R.R., Wagner, M., and Kissling, W. (2006). Psychoeducation and compliance in the treatment of schizophrenia: results of the Munich Psychosis Information Project Study. *Journal of Clinical Psychiatry*, **67**, 443–52.

Posner, C.M., Wilson, K.G, Kral, M.J., Lander, S., and McIIwraith, R.D. (1992). Family psychoeducational support groups in schizophrenia. *American Journal of Orthopsychiatry*, **62**, 206–218.

Rea, M.M., Tompson, M.C., Miklowitz, D.J., Goldstein, M.J., Hwang, S., and Mintz, J. (2003). Family-focused treatment versus individual treatment for bipolar disorder: results of a randomized clinical trial. *Journal of Consulting and Clinical Psychology*, **71**, 482–92.

Resnick, S.G., Rosenheck, R.A., and Lehman, A.F. (2004). An exploratory analysis of correlates of recovery. *Psychiatric Services*, **55**, 540–7.

Resnick, S.G., Rosenheck, R.A., Dixon, L., and Lehman, A.F. (2005). Correlates of family contact with the mental health system: allocation of a scarce resource. *Mental Health Services Research*, **7**, 113–21.

Smith, G.C. (2003). Patterns and predictors of service use and unmet needs among aging families of adults with severe mental illness. *Psychiatric Services*, **4**(6), 871–7.

Solomon, P. (2004). Peer support/peer provided services underlying processes, benefits, and critical ingredients. *Psychiatric Rehabilitation Journal*, **25**, 281–8.

Solomon, P., Draine, J., Mannion, E., and Meisel, M. (1996). Impact of brief family psychoeducation on self-efficacy. *Schizophrenia Bulletin*, **22**, 41–50.

Solomon, P., Draine, J., Mannion, E., and Meisel, M. (1997). Effectiveness of two models of brief family education: retention of gains by family members of adults with serious mental illness. *American Journal of Orthopsychiatry*, **67**, 177–86.

Solomon, P., Draine, J., Mannion, E., and Meisel, M. (1998). Increased contact with community mental health resources as a potential benefit of family education. *Psychiatric Services*, **49**, 333–9.

Spiegel, D. and Wissler, T. (1987). Using family consultation as psychiatric aftercare for schizophrenic patients. *Hospital and Community Psychiatry*, **38**, 1096–9.

Winefield, H. and Harvey, E. (1994). Needs of family caregivers in chronic schizophrenia. *Schizophrenia Bulletin*, **20**, 557–66.

World Schizophrenia Fellowship (1998). *Families as partners in care: a document developed to launch a strategy for the implementation of family education, training, and support.* Toronto: World Schizophrenia Fellowship.

Xiong, W., Phillips, M.R., Hu, X., Wang, R., Dai, Q., Kleinman, J., and Kleinman, A. (1994) Family-based intervention for schizophrenic patients in China: a randomized controlled trial. *British Journal of Psychiatry*, **165**, 239–47.

CHAPTER 22

Medication treatment for anxiety, depression, schizophrenia, and bipolar disorder in the community setting

Jonathan Shaywitz and Stephen Marder

In the community setting, four of the most common mental health syndromes affecting individuals include anxiety, depression, psychosis, and bipolar disorder. While the disorders can be quite debilitating, fortunately recent advances in both behavioural therapy as well as pharmacotherapy have helped improve the lives of countless individuals. In this chapter we will focus our discussion on pharmacotherapy with an emphasis on providing practical information that will be particularly useful to the community psychiatrist in selecting the most optimal therapeutic agents for his/her patient. Specifically, we first briefly introduce each clinical syndrome, and the classes of medications used in treatment; then we go on to discuss in detail each disorder within the general syndrome with the current pharmacological treatments available for each entity, including both their short-term and long-term efficacy. The potential adverse (side) effects associated with each of these medications will also be discussed. Our goal is for this chapter to serve as a clinical tool box providing the reader with a practical and effective approach to these very common psychiatric disorders.

Anxiolytics in community treatment

Anxiety is a normal reaction to stress. It helps one deal with a tense situation in the office, study harder for an exam, and keep focused on an important speech. In general, it helps one cope. But when anxiety becomes an excessive, irrational dread of everyday situations, it has become a disabling disorder. (National Institute of Mental Health, 2010a.)

Available anxiolytic/antidepressant drugs

In reviewing the most current arsenal of medications that are employed to treat anxiety disorders, they are **in general** the same medications (with the exception of benzodiazepines) that are also utilized in the treatment of depression. Specifically, they fall into four general classes:

Benzodiazepines

This group of medications is perhaps the most widely prescribed medication to treat individuals suffering from anxiety. While often viewed as a homogeneous drug class, they display a heterogeneous pharmacokinetic property profile with regard to their potency, onset, and duration of action, and adverse effect profile (Janicak et al., 2006b). Having an understanding of these differences helps the clinician in his or her selection of a particular benzodiazepine. For instance, benzodiazepines that stay longer in an individual's system (those with longer half-lives) such as chlordiazepoxide and clonazepam will mean less rebound anxiety and more prophylaxis in prevention of future anxiety attacks than shorter acting benzodiazepines, including alprazolam and lorazepam. However, long acting benzodiazepines have more of a potential for accumulation with multiple dosing which is especially a concern in the elderly population.

Adverse events

The most common side effects of benzodiazepines include sedation, cognitive impairment, anterograde amnesia, dizziness, and ataxia (Albers et al., 2008).

Selective serotonergic reuptake inhibitors (SSRIs)

The SSRIs as a class are thought to exert both their anxiolytic and antidepressant effects by blockade of serotonin reuptake in the brain. Commonly prescribed SSRIs for anxiety and depressive disorders include fluoxetine, paroxetine, sertraline, citalopram, escitalopram, and fluvoxamine. Within the SSRI class, fluoxetine is believed to be the most activating and stays in the body the longest. On the opposite spectrum, paroxetine is the most sedating and stays in the system the shortest. Sertraline is thought to be somewhere in the middle with regards to both activation and half-life. Within the SSRI drug class, citalopram is unique in that it has the fewest drug–drug interactions.

Adverse events

While generally better tolerated than the tricyclic antidepressants, the SSRIs do have adverse effects. They include nausea, vomiting, headaches, jitteriness, insomnia, dizziness, diarrhoea, reduced libido, and delayed orgasm.

Tricyclic antidepressants (TCAs)

TCAs are believed to work in alleviating anxiety and depression through their effects on blockade of monoamine neurotransmitters including serotonin, norepinephrine, and dopamine. The TCAs are comprised of tertiary amine antidepressants (amitriptyline, clomipramine, imipramine, and doxepin) and secondary amine antidepressants (nortriptyline and desipramine).

Adverse events

Unlike the SSRIs which, as their name implies, are 'selective' in their serotonin reuptake, the TCAs interact with multiple neurotransmitters, which explains their increased side-effect profile. Specifically (Albers et al., 2008):

- Anticholinergic interaction: blurred vision, dry mouth, constipation, urinary retention, heat intolerance, and reflex tachycardia.

- Alpha-adrenergic interaction: dizziness, tachycardia, and orthostatic hypotension.

- Histaminergic effects: potential weight gain and sedation.

Additionally, the TCAs can lead to potential cardiac conduction problems as well as require a fairly long duration (as much as 8 weeks) for a therapeutic response.

Miscellaneous agents

Selective norepinephrine dopamine reuptake inhibitors (SNDRIs)

SNDRIs are medications, such as bupropion, that are postulated to exert their antidepressant and anxiolytic effects through blockade of norepinephrine and dopaminergic reuptake (Albers et al., 2008). Bupropion is considered to be an activating medication and thus, should be started at initial low doses with those individuals with primarily anxiety symptoms.

Adverse events   Unlike the TCAs and SSRIs, bupropion causes less sexual side effects, less weight gain, and is not thought to interfere with cardiac conduction. However, bupropion can cause insomnia, tremors, and headaches. It is also contraindicated in individuals with a history of seizures and should be avoided in individuals with anorexia or bulimia.

Selective norepinephrine reuptake inhibitors (SNRIs)

SNRIs are medications, such as venlafaxine, that exert their effects through selective reuptake of serotonin and norepinephrine. Venlafaxine is also considered to be an activating medication and should be initiated at low doses. However, unlike SSRIs which seem to have a flat dose response curve with respect to depression, it has been demonstrated that venlafaxine possesses greater overall effectiveness at higher doses. Other advantages include more rapid onset of antidepressant action (Janicak et al., 2006c) and less interactions relating to CYP (cytochrome P450) isoenzymes.

Adverse events   The major side effects of venlafaxine include potential increase in blood pressure, nausea, nervousness, headaches, and sexual dysfunction.

Mirtazapine

Mirtazapine is a medication that exerts its antidepressant and anxiolytic effects through blockade of serotonin and central alpha 2 adrenergic receptors. The indirect blockade of the alpha 2 receptors, in turn, increases the release of norepinephrine. Unlike the SNRIs, mirtazapine does not cause an increase in blood pressure and unlike the TCAs has minimal anticholinergic activity. It is also quite sedating which is particularly useful for the depressed patient with comorbid anxiety. Mirtazapine is also a particularly effective choice for those individuals who are having a difficult time gaining weight due to their depression or anxiety.

Adverse events   The major side effects of mirtazapine include sedation, weight gain, and rare cases of transient and severe neutropenia.

Buspirone

Buspirone is a medication that exerts its anxiolytic and antidepressant effects through its action on a specific subtype of serotonin receptor (5H1A agonist) (Albers et al., 2008). This medication's side effect profile is minimal—there are no anticholinergic or cardiotoxic effects—and it is generally well tolerated by all age groups with minimal abuse potential.

Adverse events   The major side effects of buspirone include potential for headaches, dizziness and fatigue.

Trazadone

Trazadone is a medication that is postulated to work through inhibition of both presynaptic and postsynaptic serotonin reuptake (Albers et al., 2008). Trazadone is quite sedating and in addition to its efficacy in treating anxiety and depression can also be utilized (in low doses) for insomnia as well.

Adverse events   The major side effects of trazadone are its sedating properties and potential for orthostatic hypotension. There is also a small risk (1/6000) for male patients for priapism.

Generalized anxiety disorder

Of all the anxiety disorders, generalized anxiety disorder (GAD) is perhaps the most difficult to define as evidenced by the many changes its definition has undergone within the last two decades. First introduced into the DSM III in 1980, GAD became more of an exclusionary disorder of what it was not—panic and social anxiety. The definition has evolved throughout the years and most currently is defined as a condition that involves 'continual excessive worry that is hard to control which is accompanied by at least three of the following symptoms (restlessness, fatigue, difficulty concentrating, irritability, muscle tension, sleep disturbance)' (American Psychiatric Association, 2000). The prevalence of GAD is approximately 5%, with women more commonly affected than men. Moreover, as with many of the anxiety disorders, GAD is highly comorbid with other psychiatric disorders. The benzodiazepines are effective for non-specific anxiety symptoms and have the advantage of having a relatively rapid onset of action. However, their potential for sedation, abuse, and accumulation (especially in the elderly) prevent benzodiazepines from being the first choice for treatment. Instead, buspirone is generally the first choice for treating GAD. Studies have shown that buspirone is also effective in the treatment of GAD with comorbid conditions—specifically GAD with comorbid depression as well as GAD with comorbid alcohol use (Laakmann et al., 1998; Sramek et al., 1997). Furthermore, buspirone has been shown to provide decreased relapse rates after treatment discontinuation. However, buspirone does have some disadvantages. It has a relatively short half-life requiring multiple dosing (often three times a day) and, unlike the benzodiazepines, has no immediate effect and often takes a minimum of 2 to 3 weeks to take effect. Several of the SSRIs and miscellaneous agents have demonstrated positive efficacy in treating GAD in both short- and long-term trials. Specifically, both escitalopram and paroxetine have demonstrated effectiveness in short term trials of GAD (Baldwin et al., 2006; Davidson et al., 2004; Goodman et al., 2005; Rickels et al., 2003; Rocca et al., 1997). Regarding miscellaneous agents, and their use in treating GAD, a small study of affected patients showed bupropion XR to be superior compared to escitalopram (Bystritsky, 2005). Additionally short-term studies of venlafaxine XR and duloxetine have also demonstrated their effectiveness in decreasing anxiety in GAD patients (Endicott et al., 2007; Nimatoudies et al., 2004). Regarding long-term treatment studies, venlafaxine XR showed particularly greater reductions in anxiety up to 8 months, while escitalopram was also found to be effective in a 6-month study (Davidson et al., 2004; Gelenberg et al., 2000). Anticonvulsants have been shown to be especially effective in the treatment of GAD. Specifically pregabalin—a lipophilic GABA analogue—has been demonstrated to effectively decrease anxiety symptoms in GAD patients (Shaywitz and Liebowitz, 2003). The most common adverse events included somnolence and dizziness.

Panic disorder (PD)

PD, also classified as an anxiety disorder, affects approximately 3.5% of the population and more commonly affects women than men. It is characterized by random occurrence of unprovoked attacks of intense fear (American Psychiatric Association, 2000). These panic attacks are characterized by discrete periods of intense terror and fear of impending doom. The SSRIs are generally the first line of treatment for individuals suffering from this disorder (Bandelow et al., 2004; Michelson et al., 2001; Wade et al., 1997). It is important to again note that many of the SSRIs can initially be quite activating and cause restlessness, jitteriness, and insomnia in addition to sexual dysfunction. Thus, it is helpful to obey the mantra 'start low and go slow' with respect to this class of medications in treating PD. For example, it is often necessary to begin with either 25 mg of sertraline or 10 mg of fluoxetine and very gradually increase to a treatment dose of 100 to 200 mg and 20 to 40 mg respectively. The tricyclic antidepressants are considered the second-line treatment for patients with PD (Bystritsky et al., 1994). Studies have shown no difference in efficacy between the SSRIs and TCAs for the treatment of PD, although the SSRIs are generally better tolerated. Also, it should be noted that no differences have been found between the SSRIs, themselves, regarding efficacy in treating PD (Bandelow and Baldwin, 2010). Similar to the SSRIs, the TCAs have a latency of up to 4 to 6 weeks before improvement of anxiety symptoms. Benzodiazepines are also employed (Rosenbaum et al., 1997) in treating PD and are specifically effective in their rapid onset. While the potential of abuse, cognitive impairment, and sedation continue to be disadvantages, a clinician will often concomitantly administer a low-dose, long-acting benzodiazepine such as klonopin with an SSRI at the beginning of treatment to both counter any initial jitteriness from the SSRI as well as prophylactically serving to prevent future panic attacks.

Post-traumatic stress disorder (PTSD)

PTSD is a highly debilitating anxiety disorder that affects about 7% of the population and occurs more often in women than men.

Similar to GAD, PTSD has also evolved over the years in terms of its definition. Currently, the core definition involves an individual having witnessed or experienced a life-threatening event and then re-experiencing this event through recurrent dreams, thoughts, or images. In addition, the affected individual exhibits persistent avoidance of stimuli that he/she associates with this event. These symptoms are required to last longer than 1 month and to cause significant impairment in occupational and social functioning (American Psychiatric Association, 2000). Unfortunately, perhaps due to the complexity involving the number of different core symptoms involved in PTSD, the data for the pharmacotherapy of PTSD have been somewhat disappointing. The SSRIs, specifically sertraline, which is Food and Drug Administration (FDA) approved for PTSD, are the first line of treatment with the most promising data (Brady et al., 2000; Ursano et al., 2004). Other medications have shown more mixed results. The TCAs have shown some (amitriptyline) or no (desipramine) effect. (Davidson et al., 1990; Reist et al., 1989) Moreover, bupropion and the benzodiazepines have not demonstrated any benefit over placebo in addressing the core symptoms of PTSD (Becker et al., 2007; Braun et al., 1990; Hertzberg et al., 2001). Other medications have shown effect only for specific symptoms, such as trazodone for sleep and prazosin in reducing nightmares. However, there have been data demonstrating that augmentation with low dose antipsychotics have some benefit, while the anticonvulsant lamotrigine has also demonstrated some efficacy in treating several of the core symptoms (Hertzberg et al., 1999).

Obsessive–compulsive disorder (OCD)

OCD, affecting approximately 2% of the population, is characterized by recurrent intrusive thoughts, ideas, or images (obsessions) and repetitive ritualistic behaviours (compulsions) (American Psychiatric Association, 2000). The tricyclic antidepressant clomipramine as well as the SSRIs are two of the first-line pharmacotherapy treatments for the symptoms of this disorder (Fineberg and Craig, 2006; Goodman et al., 1990; Insel et al., 1985; Leonard et al., 1988). Unlike other TCAs, clomipramine has a particularly potent serotonergic blockade and studies have shown its efficacy within 1 to 2 weeks of initiating treatment with a flexible dose of up to 300 mg (Devaugh-Geiss et al., 1992). Moreover, clomipramine has also shown effectiveness in treating OCD with comorbid depression. The SSRIs, too, have shown efficacy in OCD; however, currently there is not substantial evidence supporting clinical superiority within the SSRI class (Fineberg and Craig, 2006). Moreover, studies comparing the clinical effectiveness between the SSRIs and clomipramine, have failed to show superior efficacy of one over the other (Fineberg and Craig, 2006). However, considering their adverse effect profile, the SSRIs generally have fewer adverse events and are better tolerated. Overall, studies of OCD have shown a dose–response relationship with higher dosing being equated with a better treatment response. The general consensus regarding switching antidepressants is to delay a switch in medications until an adequate treatment trial consisting of two or, even, three months has been completed (Fineberg and Craig, 2006). If, after switching to another medication an adequate trial again fails, options that have shown some promise include augmentation with a typical or atypical antipsychotic. Unfortunately, other alternatives including augmentation with buspirone, clonazepam, lithium, and pindolol have not demonstrated efficacy in treating refractory OCD (Crockett et al., 2004; Dannon et al., 2000; Grady et al., 1993; McDougle et al., 1995).

Social anxiety disorder (SAD)

SAD is the third most common psychiatric disorder and affects approximately 10% of the population. The onset of SAD is usually in childhood or adolescence and the disorder occurs more often in women than men. Individuals suffering from SAD are extremely fearful and avoidant of social situations (American Psychiatric Association, 2000). This fear is caused primarily by feelings that they will be humiliated or embarrassed and can be quite debilitating. Similar to other anxiety disorders, the first-line pharmacotherapy includes the SSRIs with paroxetine, sertraline, and fluvoxamine CR each FDA approved for the treatment of SAD (Blanco et al., 2003, 2009; Stein et al., 1996). The SNRIs (specifically venlafaxine) have also been demonstrated to be quite effective in treating individuals with this disorder (Algulander et al., 2004: Stein et al., 2005, Rickels et al., 2004). It is important to understand that there have been no robust studies that have established superiority within the SSRI class or between the SSRIs and SNRIs in treating SAD (Blanco et al., 2003). Benzodiazepines are considered a second-line treatment for SAD with longer-acting agents such as klonopin being preferred over shorter-acting medications such as alprazolam (Davidson et al., 1993; Gelertner et al., 1991; Munjack et al., 1990). Unlike in panic disorder, the TCAs have demonstrated little efficacy in treating individuals with SAD (Simpson et al., 1998). Other agents such as bupropion and mirtazapine have shown some promise in early open label studies, but more large controlled studies are needed to evaluate their effectiveness for treating SAD (Emmanuel et al., 2000). For those individuals diagnosed with non-generalized social anxiety (performance anxiety), beta blockers (such as propranolol) have been demonstrated to be quite effective in alleviating some of the symptoms (Gorman et al., 1985).

Depression

> Everyone occasionally feels blue or sad, but these feelings are usually fleeting and pass within a couple of days. When a person has a depressive disorder, it interferes with daily life, normal functioning, and causes pain for both the person with the disorder and those who care about him or her). (National Institute of Mental Health, 2010b.)

Depression is one of the most common mental health disorders and affects up to 12% of the population. It is almost twice as common in women than in men with a mean age of onset occurring in the mid to late twenties. The most common subtypes of depression include major depressive disorder and psychotic depression. As mentioned earlier, with the exception of the benzodiazepines, all the medications discussed above for anxiety are also used in treating individuals with depression.

Major depressive disorder (MDD)

Individuals with MDD can either present with classical depression (melancholia) or atypical depression. Classical depression typically has an onset in the early forties with symptoms that include depressed mood, insomnia, weight loss, and psychomotor retardation. Individuals with atypical depression, on the other hand, often have an earlier onset of presentation, endorse symptoms of irritability, have psychomotor agitation, and complain of hypersomnia as well as hyperphagia (Janicak et al., 2006a). The SSRIs are the first-line treatment for classical major depression while TCAs have demonstrated superiority in the treatment of atypical depression. Citalopram, escitalopram, fluoxetine, fluvoxamine, paroxetine, and sertraline are SSRIs with FDA approval for treating MDD. While numerous studies have demonstrated the efficacy of SSRIs in treating this disorder (Bowden et al., 1993; Mendels et al., 1999; Reimherr et al., 1988), there is also strong data demonstrating no difference in efficacy within the SSRI class as well as when compared to different classes of medications (Bielski et al., 2004; Ginestet, 1989). The data is more mixed when focusing on depressed individuals in an **inpatient setting**. Several studies have shown TCAs (specifically clomipramine) to be superior to SSRIs (Danish University Antidepressant Group, 1986, 1990). Other studies focusing on depressed hospitalized patients have also shown venlafaxine and mirtazapine to be more effective than fluoxetine (Clerc et al., 1994). Regarding pharmokinetic differences between the SSRIs and other agents in treating MDD, there is evidence that the SSRIs show a flat dose response curve whereas the SNRIs demonstrate an 'ascending dose response curve'. Clinically this translates to mean that higher doses, compared to lower doses, of SNRIs can have more beneficial effects for depressed patients (Janicak et al., 2006c). Moreover, the SNRIs as well as the SNDRIs have been noted to have an earlier onset of efficacy compared to the SSRIs. Miscellaneous agents such as mirtazapine and trazodone have also been shown to be effective for the treatment of MDD (Janicak et al., 2006c).

Psychotic depression

Individuals with psychotic depression endorse psychotic symptoms along with suffering from severe depression. The prevalence of psychotic depression is estimated to comprise 15% of major depression in the United States (Johnson et al., 1991). The first-line treatment for psychotic depression includes both ECT (electroconvulsive therapy) (Flint and Rifat, 1998) as well as second-generation antipsychotics (SGAs) such as risperidone and olanzapine. There have been several studies, with mostly positive results, documenting the efficacy of SGAs as monotherapy for psychotic depression. It should be noted, however, that many of these studies had a rather small sample size (Bastlet et al., 2002; Hillert et al., 1992; Nelson et al., 2001). The adverse events of SGAs include potential weight gain, hyperlipidaemia, and a risk for developing diabetes.

Antipsychotics in community treatment

Effectiveness of antipsychotic medications

Antipsychotic medications are among the commonest medications prescribed for seriously ill mentally ill patients living in the community. Antipsychotics are prescribed for nearly every patient with schizophrenia or schizoaffective illness; a substantial proportion of patients with bipolar illness; patients with major depression with psychotic features; and other disorders that are commonly associated with psychotic symptoms. For these illnesses, these medications are effective for psychotic symptoms and to a lesser extent for agitation.

It is important to note that these drugs are frequently prescribed for disorders that are not approved by the FDA in the United States. For example, quetiapine is commonly prescribed as a hypnotic since it is rather sedating. These drugs are also used to control aggressive behaviours in a variety of conditions including pervasive developmental disorder, PTSD, and dementia.

Available antipsychotic drugs

A large number of antipsychotic medications have been approved in the United States and throughout the world. The first antipsychotic—chlorpromazine—was developed in France in the 1950s and was followed by the introduction of a number of other drugs that demonstrated similar effectiveness. A number of methods for classifying antipsychotics have been proposed, and the following is currently accepted.

- **First-generation antipsychotics (FGAs)** This group includes antipsychotics that were approved between the 1950s and 1990. Commonly prescribed FGAs include haloperidol (Haldol), fluphenazine (Prolixin), perphenazine (Trilafon), chlorpromazine (Thorazine), thioridazine (Mellaril), molindone (Moban), and loxipine (Loxitane). These drugs differ in their potency and in their side-effect profiles, but all are antagonists at dopamine D_2 receptors. All of the FGAs are associated with neurologic side effects including acute extrapyramidal side effects (EPS)—described below—and a risk of tardive dyskinesia.

- **Second-generation antipsychotics (SGAs)** This group of antipsychotics includes risperidone, olanzapine, quetiapine, ziprasidone, aripiprazole, paliperidone, and iloperidone. These agents show similar effectiveness to FGAs, but are associated with less EPS.

- **Clozapine** Although clozapine is commonly characterized as an SGA, it is more effective than any of the FGAs or SGAs. Because of its side-effect profile, clozapine is usually reserved for patients who respond inadequately to other antipsychotics.

Antipsychotics are available in a number of formulations including tablets, capsules, rapid dissolve formulations, short-acting injectables, and long-acting injectables. Short-acting injectables are reserved for individuals who are acutely disturbed. Their advantage is that patients reach an effective plasma concentration sooner than other forms.

Approved uses of antipsychotic medications

Schizophrenia

Antipsychotic medications are effective for treating psychotic symptoms in schizophrenia (Buchanan et al., 2010). Patients who are experiencing hallucinations, delusional thinking, conceptual disorganization, and suspiciousness will usually experience substantial improvement in these symptoms if they receive an adequate dose of a drug. Although patients vary in their responsiveness to antipsychotics—with some showing only a minimal reduction of symptoms and others showing complete control of symptoms—they are indicated for nearly every acute episode of schizophrenia.

Antipsychotic medications are relatively ineffective for treating the negative symptoms (including restricted affect, apathy, and anhedonia) and cognitive impairments (which include impairments in memory, attention, and executive functions) in schizophrenia. As a result, antipsychotics are not antischizophrenic. This limitation of antipsychotics is important since there is strong evidence that the ability of people with schizophrenia to function in work, school, and social relationships is strongly related to the severity of negative symptoms (Fenton and McGlashan, 1991) and cognitive impairment (Green, 1996).

In addition to reducing psychotic symptoms, there is also evidence that treating patients can have long-term effects on the course of schizophrenia. This evidence comes from studies that compared individuals who had delayed treatment with antipsychotics for months and individuals who had started on medications shortly after the onset of their illness. Those who delayed treatment tended to have a worse long-term outcome (Barnes et al., 2008; Wyatt, 1991). Other studies have found that there is often a substantial interval between the time that patients with schizophrenia demonstrate psychotic symptoms and the time they receive treatment. A recent study from Norway found that community education about the effects of delaying the treatment of psychosis was effective in reducing the severity of negative symptoms at 1 year (Larsen et al., 2006). This finding suggests that clinicians in mental health and primary care settings should be encouraged to detect early evidence of psychosis and to consider treatment at an early stage.

Antipsychotic medications are also effective for reducing the risk of psychotic relapse in stabilized patients with schizophrenia (Buchanan et al., 2010). This effect has been demonstrated by randomly assigning stabilized patients on an antipsychotic to either stay on their medication or change to a placebo. Patients who remain on their medication have lower rates of relapse than those on placebo. This has led to the recommendation that patients who have multiepisode schizophrenia continue on their medication even after they have recovered from an episode. The issue is less clear with individuals who have recovered from a first episode of schizophrenia. These patients are often resistant to continuing on antipsychotics after they have recovered from their psychosis. However, these individuals remain vulnerable to relapse, particularly if they stop their antipsychotic medications (Robinson et al., 1999).

Large studies have recently compared the effectiveness of antipsychotics. Overall, FGAs and SGAs showed similar effectiveness (Jones et al., 2006; Lieberman et al., 2005). The only exception was clozapine, which was more effective than other antipsychotics in patients who showed a poor response in a previous trial (McEvoy et al., 2006). Clinicians and patients in community practice are often reluctant to treat patients with clozapine because of its side-effect profile. However, patients living in the community with a significant burden of symptoms such as hallucinations and delusions should not be considered treatment resistant until they have had a clozapine trial.

Schizoaffective disorder

There is sufficient evidence to recommend antipsychotic medications for patients with schizoaffective disorder (Levinson et al., 1999b). However, very few antipsychotics have been evaluated in studies that only included schizoaffective individuals. As a result, most of these agents are not approved by FDA for schizoaffective patients. Conceivably, the companies that sponsor drugs have concluded that there is not a need to see FDA approval by designing studies that included only schizoaffective patients.

Bipolar mania

Antipsychotics are effective for treating bipolar mania and mixed states Levinson et al., 1999a; McEvoy et al., 2006). They are also effective when combined with drugs such as valproate, carbamazepine, lamotrigine, and lithium that are commonly used to treat mania. Although studies have been carried out that compare an antipsychotic to lithium or valproate, there is no indication that any of these agents are superior for reducing manic symptoms (Smith et al., 2007a). There are some properties of these agents that can help clinicians decide which medication to choose. Some data suggests that haloperidol has a more rapid onset than other agents although its usefulness is limited by a substantial risk of EPS. Other agents—particularly olanzapine and quetiapine—are limited by their metabolic side effects.

Bipolar depression

The role of antipsychotics in treating bipolar depression is a bit confusing. Most available trials were industry sponsored and focused on a single agent or combination. For example, the combination of olanzapine and fluoxetine and monotherapy with quetiapine are approved for bipolar mania. However, there is no evidence that these specific antipsychotics have effects that other antipsychotics do not. A National Institute of Health (NIMH) study compared lamotrigine, inositol, and risperidone as adjuncts in patients with treatment-resistant bipolar depression and found suggestions that lamotrigine had advantages compared to the other agents. This literature does not point to a definitive recommendation, but suggests that patients should be treated with a mood stabilizing agent and that other drugs—including antipsychotics—may be helpful as adjunctive agents (Azorin and Kaladjian, 2009; Smith et al., 2007a).

Bipolar maintenance

The early enthusiasm about the effects of SGAs led some clinicians and researchers to observe that these drugs were effective as monotherapy for relapse prevention in bipolar patients. Studies have found that olanzapine and aripiprazole are effective for preventing mania; however, these studies selected patients who had responded to these drugs during a manic episode (Azorin and Kaladjian, 2009; Beynon et al., 2009). A Cochrane review found that olanzapine appeared to be effective for this indication, but found stronger evidence for the effectiveness of lithium (Cipriani et al., 2009). Moreover, there is no data indicating that olanzapine or aripiprazole are superior to other antipsychotics for bipolar maintenance. Taken together, these studies suggest that antipsychotics may be an alternative for long-term maintenance—although clinicians who weigh the side effects of antipsychotics may choose a medication such as lithium or valproate where there is a stronger evidence base.

Adjunctive treatment in major depressive disorder

Antipsychotics may also be helpful when patients with MDD fail to demonstrate an adequate response to antidepressants. A recent meta-analysis (Nelson and Papakostas, 2009) found that antipsychotics are effective as adjunctive treatments for patients who were somewhat resistant to treatment with an antidepressant. At this time, aripiprazole and quetiapine are approved for this indication. However, there is no indication that other antipsychotics are less effective for this indication.

Irritability associated with autistic disorder

Antipsychotic medications are effective for treating symptoms such as irritability, tantrums, and self-injurious behaviours that are common in autistic disorder and pervasive developmental disorder (Jesner et al., 2007; McCracken et al., 2002; McDougle et al., 2008). There is no indication that antipsychotics are helpful for the social and communication deficits that define these disorders. At the present time, risperidone is the only agent approved for this indication (in children and adolescents aged 5–16 years) although there is no evidence that other agents are less effective.

Adverse effects

Antipsychotic medications can produce a range of adverse effects. Since all of the antipsychotics—with the exception of clozapine— have similar efficacy, drug selection is often driven by the adverse effects that the patient and clinician are most interested in avoiding.

Neurological side effects

The most common neurological side effects are acute extrapyramidal symptoms (EPS). These symptoms can include parkinsonism characterized by stiffness, tremor, shuffling gait; akathisia which include restless movements and a subjective experience of restlessness; and dystonia which includes muscle spasms usually affecting the head and neck. These side effects tend to occur more often and with greater severity in FGAs particularly high potency FGAs. They are clearly dose related and can be managed by decreasing the antipsychotic dose or changing to an antipsychotic that is less likely to cause EPS. If these strategies are not possible or ineffective, anticholinergic medication such as benztropine can be added for parkinsonism or beta blockers for akathisia.

Tardive dyskinesia (TD) is a late appearing neurological side effect of antipsychotics that usually appears after months or years of antipsychotic treatment. It is characterized by abnormal involuntary movements, typically involving the orofacial region, limbs, and trunk. TD movements are usually slower than the movements of acute EPS. Although most TD movements are mild, severe cases can be disfiguring and disabling. Patients who had previously developed acute EPS are more likely to develop TD.

The management of TD usually includes changing to an antipsychotic with a lower liability for EPS such as quetiapine or clozapine. Unfortunately, there are no specific drug treatments for TD.

Metabolic effects

Antipsychotics are associated with a number of serious metabolic effects including weight gain, hyperlipidaemia, and Type II diabetes mellitus. As with EPS, there is considerable variation among drugs with some—for example, olanzapine and clozapine—being associated with substantial metabolic effects and others—including ziprasidone, aripiprazole, and molindone—having little or no effect on metabolic parameters. Since obesity, elevated lipids, and diabetes are all modifiable risk factors for cardiovascular disease and premature death, it is important that clinicians consider these side effects in monitoring drug effects and in drug selection.

There are a number of approaches to managing metabolic side effects. Changes in diet and exercise can be helpful although many patients find it difficult to make these lifestyle changes. A number of studies indicate that changing patients from an antipsychotic associated with weight gain to one that is not, can lead to weight loss and improvements in metabolic parameters (Stroup et al., 2006).

Endocrine effects

Antipsychotics can elevate serum prolactin. This elevation can cause galactorrhoea, amenorrhoea, gynaecomastia, erectile dysfunction, and anorgasmia. As with other side effects, there are large differences among agents. FGAs, risperidone, and paliperidone cause the greatest prolactin elevation, most of the SGAs cause little or no elevation, and aripiprazole can actually lower prolactin. These side effects can be extremely disturbing when they occur.

Other common side effects

Other common side effects of antipsychotics include sedation, orthostatic hypotension, and insomnia. Clozapine can also cause agranulocytosis, a haematological side effect that can be fatal. Because of this risk, patients who are treated with clozapine are required to have regular blood tests.

Mood stabilizing medications

A number of agents are either approved or commonly prescribed to stabilize mood in bipolar disorder and other psychiatric disorders. These include lithium carbonate, valproate, carbamazepine, and lamotrigine. Although other medications including oxycarbamazepine, gabapentin and topiramate are also prescribed, this section will focus on the medications with the strongest evidence base.

Bipolar mania

Lithium, valproate, and carbamazepine are effective for treating the symptoms of bipolar mania including pressured speech, motor hyperactivity, insomnia, flight of ideas, grandiosity, elation, poor judgment, aggressiveness and possibly hostility. Each of these drugs is effective as monotherapy. Adding an antipsychotic to a mood stabilizer may lead to a more rapid response. The evidence is strongest for lithium and valproate (Sachs et al., 2000) and lamotrigine is not effective for treating acute mania. Carbamazepine is usually considered to be a second line mood stabilizer. Lithium is most effective for patients with euphoric mania whereas valproate is effective for both euphoric and dysphoric manias.

Bipolar depression

Bipolar patients are likely to spend more time in a depressed rather than a manic state. Unfortunately, the best strategy for managing bipolar depression is unclear. Lithium and valproate are reasonable choices. Although lamotrigine is only approved for maintenance in bipolar illness, there is evidence that it is effective for bipolar depression (Geddes et al., 2009). There is evidence that adding an antidepressant to a mood stabilizer does not add to effectiveness (Sachs et al., 2007). However, if patients fail to improve on a mood stabilizer alone, adding lamotrigine or an antidepressant may be helpful (van der Loos et al., 2009).

Bipolar maintenance treatment

Lithium, lamotrigine, and valproate are effective for preventing relapse in bipolar patients (Smith et al., 2007b). The evidence is less robust for carbamazepine. Lamotrigine is probably a more effective agent for preventing depressive rather than manic episodes. Lithium also may have the advantage of being more effective than other mood stabilizers in preventing suicidal behaviours in bipolar patients (Tondo and Baldessarini, 2009).

Other uses

Lithium and valproate are frequently added to an antipsychotic for patients with schizoaffective disorder and schizophrenia with mood symptoms. Although anticonvulsant mood stabilizers are not indicated for major depressive disorder, there is evidence that carbamazepine, valproate, and lamotrigine may be helpful when added to an antidepressant, particularly when there is irritability or anxiety (Vigo and Baldessarini, 2009).

Adverse effects

Lithium

Lithium is probably the most difficult mood stabilizer to prescribe. Finding the correct dose should be guided by regular monitoring of the regular serum lithium level. The most serious concern is lithium toxicity which may appear as ataxia, impaired speech, prominent tremor, and confusion. If not managed promptly—usually by stopping lithium and observing the patient—it can progress to seizures, coma, and even death. Although toxicity usually occurs at high lithium serum levels, it may occur at levels that are therapeutic. Patients should also be monitored for renal damage and renal insufficiency. Common and less serious side effects include a fine tremor, hypothyroidism, weight gain, gastrointestinal discomfort (including nausea and diarrhoea).

Carbamazepine

Carbamazepine can cause a number of relatively mild side effects including ataxia, double vision, and fatigue. Patients may develop a benign skin rash which can progress to a more severe rash. There is a risk of aplastic anaemia and agranulocytosis although both are uncommon.

Carbamazepine can have serious pharmacokinetic interactions with other drugs. Carbamazepine will lead to substantial increases in the metabolism of a number of drugs including antidepressants, mood stabilizers, and antipsychotics, lowering their blood levels. When carbamazepine is discontinued, blood levels of these other drugs will increase.

Valproate

Valproate is associated with relatively rare cases of liver toxicity and pancreatitis. As a result, patients should have baseline liver function tests before starting valproate. Common side effects include gastrointestinal discomfort, sedation, tremor, weight gain, and hair loss.

Lamotrigine

Patients treated with lamotrigine should be warned of the risk of a serious rash including Stevens–Johnson syndrome. The occurrence of even a mild rash should be evaluated and discontinuing lamotrigine may be considered. Common side effects of lamotrigine include nausea, drowsiness, and insomnia.

Conclusion

It is important to understand that while the emphasis of this chapter has been devoted to the psychopharmacological management of anxiety and psychotic disorders, the psychosocial management and therapeutic alliance are equally important for the well-being of the psychotic or anxious patient. While there has been a classic study (May et al., 1976) that has demonstrated that psychotherapy, by itself, has little effect in the treatment of psychotic disorders, other studies have demonstrated a beneficial effect of psychosocial treatment in conjunction with medication, on the relapse rates of individuals suffering from psychotic disorders (Hogarty et al., 1991; Tarrier et al., 1988). Furthermore, the most updated Schizophrenia Patient Outcomes Research Team (PORT) review has recommended evidenced-based psychosocial management in combination with psychopharmacotherapy for effective clinical treatment of psychotic individuals (Lehman et al., 2003). Several of their specific psychosocial recommendations include continual family intervention, including education, as well as supported employment for individuals with schizophrenia. The integration of psychotherapy with medication management is equally important for individuals suffering from anxiety disorders. In general, psychotherapy for most of the anxiety disorders involves a three-pronged approach—the first being psycho-education, the second being cognitive restructuring, and the third behavioural modification. The effectiveness of the combination of psychotherapy in addition to medication management for anxiety disorders has also been supported by multiple clinical studies (Bakker et al., 1999; Bradley et al., 2005; Wardle, 1990).

References

Albers, L., Hahn, R., and Reist, C. (2008). *Handbook of Psychiatric Disorders*. Laguna Hills, CA: Current Clinical Strategies Publishing.

Algulander, C., Mangano, R., and Zhang, J. (2004). Efficacy of venlafaxine ER in patients with social anxiety disorder: a double-blind placebo controlled parallel-group comparison with paroxetine. *Human Psychopharmacology*, 19, 387–96.

American Psychiatric Association (2000). *Diagnostic and Statistical Manual of Mental Disorders, 4th Edition, Text Revision*. Washington, DC: APA.

Azorin, J. and Kaladjian, A. (2009). An update on the treatment of bipolar depression. *Expert Opinion on Pharmacotherapy*, 10, 161–72.

Bakker, A., van Dyck, R., Spinhovenn, P., and van Balkom, A. (1999). Paroxetine, clomipramine and cognitive therapy in the treatment of panic disorder. *Journal of Clinical Psychiatry*, 60, 831–8.

Baldwin, D., Hussom, A., and Maehlum, E. (2006). Escitalopram and paroxetine in the treatment of generalized anxiety disorder: randomised, placebo controlled, double-blind study. *British Journal of Psychiatry*, 189, 264–72.

Bandelow, B. and Baldwin, D. (2010). Pharmacotherapy for panic disorder. In: Stein, D., Hollander, E., and Rothbaum, B. (eds) *Textbook of Anxiety Disorders* 399–414. American Psychiatric Publishing.

Bandelow, B., Behnke, K., and Lenoir, S. (2004). Sertraline vs paroxetine in the treatment of panic disorder: an acute, double-blind noninferiority comparison. *Journal of Clinical Psychiatry*, 65, 405–13.

Barnes, T.R., Leeson, V.C., Mutsatsa, S.H., Watt, H.C., Hutton, S.B., and Joyce, E.M. (2008). Duration of untreated psychosis and social function: 1-year follow-up study of first-episode schizophrenia. *British Journal of Psychiatry*, 193, 203–9.

Bastlet, G., Nour, H., and Janiack, P. (2002). The role of second generation antipsychotics in the treatment of mood disorders. *Contemporary Psychiatry*, 2, 1–8.

Becker, M., Hertzberg, M., and Moore, S. (2007). A placebo-controlled trial of bupropion SR in the treatment of chronic posttraumatic stress disorder. *Journal of Clinical Psychopharmacology*, 27, 193–7.

Beynon, S., Soares-Weiser, K., Woolacott, N., Duffy, S., and Geddes, J. (2009). Pharmacological interventions for the prevention of relapse in bipolar disorder: A systematic review of controlled trials. *Journal of Psychopharmacology*, 23, 574–91.

Bielski, R., Ventura, D., and Chang, C. (2004). A double blind comparison of escitalopram and venlafaxine extended release in the treatment of major depressive disorder. *Journal of Clinical Psychiatry*, 65, 1190–6.

Blanco, C., Schneier, F., and Schmidt, A. (2003). Pharmacological treatment of social anxiety disorder: a meta-analysis. *Depression and Anxiety*, 18, 29–40.

Blanco, C., Schneier, F., Vesga-Lopez, O., and Liebowitz, M. (2009). Pharmacotherapy for social anxiety disorder. In: Stein, D., Hollander, E., and Rothbaum, B. (eds.) *Textbook of Anxiety Disorders*, pp. 471–495. Arlington, VA: American Psychiatric Publishing.

Bowden, C., Schatzberg, A., and Rosenbaum, A. (1993). Fluoxetine and desipramine in major depressive disorder. *Journal of Clinical Psychopharmacology*, 13, 305–11.

Bradley, R., Greene, J., Russ, E., Dutra, L., and Westen, D. (2005). A multidimensional meta-analysis of psychotherapy for PTSD. *American Journal of Psychiatry*, 162, 214–27.

Brady, K., Pearlstein, T., and Asnis, G. (2000). Efficacy and safety of sertraline treatment of posttraumatic stress disorder: a randomized controlled trial. *Journal of the American Medical Association*, 283, 1837–44.

Braun, P., Greenberg, D., and Dasberg, H. (1990). Core symptoms of posttraumatic stress disorder unimproved by alprazolam treatment. *Journal of Clinical Psychiatry*, 51, 236–8.

Buchanan, R.W., Kreyenbuhl, J., Kelly, D.L., Noel, J.M., Boggs, D.L., Fischer, B.A., *et al.* (2010). The 2009 Schizophrenia PORT Psychopharmacological Treatment Recommendations and Summary Statements. *Schizophrenia Bulletin*, 36, 71–93.

Bystritsky, A. (2005). A pilot controlled trial of bupropion vs escitalopram in generalized anxiety disorder. *Neuropsychopharmacology*, 30, s101.

Bystritsky, A., Rosen, R., and Murphy, K. 1994. Double-blind pilot trials of desipramine versus fluoxetine in panic patients. *Anxiety*, 1, 287–90.

Cipriani, A., Rendell, J., and Geddes, J. (2009). Olanzapine in long-term treatment for bipolar disorder. *Cochrane Database of Systematic Reviews*, 1, CD004367.

Clerc, G., Ruimy, P., and Verdeau-Pailles 1994. Double-blind comparison of venlafaxine and fluoxetine in patients hospitalized for major depression and melancholia. *International Clinical Psychopharmacology*, 9, 139–43.

Crockett, B., Churchill, E., and Davidson, J. (2004). A double-blind combination study of clonazepam with sertaline in obsessive-compulsive disorder. *Annals of Clinical Psychiatry*, 16, 127–32.

Danish University Antidepressant Group (1986). Citalopram: clinical effect profile in comparison with clomipramine: a controlled multicenter trial. *Psychopharmacology*, 90, 131–8.

Danish University Antidepressant Group (1990). Paroxetine: a selective serotonin reuptake inhibitor showing better tolerance, but weaker antidepressant effect than clomipramine in a controlled multicenter study. *Journal of Affective Disorders*, 18, 289–99.

Dannon, P., Sasson, Y., and Hirschmann, S. (2000). Pindolol augmentation in treatment resistant obsessive compulsive disorder: a double blind placebo-conrolled trial. *European Neuropsychopharmacology*, 10, 165–9.

Davidson, J., Bose, A., and Korotzer, A. (2004). Escitalopram in the treatment of generalized anxiety disorder: double blind, placebo controlled, flexible-dose study. *Depression and Anxiety*, 60, 528–35.

Davidson, J., Kudler, H., and Smith, R. (1990). Treatment of posttraumatic stress disorder with amitripyline and placebo. *Archives of General Psychiatry*, 47, 259–66.

Davidson, J., Potts, N., and Richichi, E. (1993). Treatment of social phobia with clonazepam and placebo. *Journal of Clinical Psychopharmacology*, 13, 423–8.

Devaugh-Geiss, J., Moroz, G., and Biederman, J. (1992). Clomipramine hydrochloride in childhood and adolescent obsessive-compulsive disorder: a multicenter trial. *Journal of the American Academy of Child and Adolescent Psychiatry*, 31, 45–9.

Emmanuel, N., Brawman-Mintzer, O., and Morton, W. (2000). Bupropion-SR in treatment of social phobia. *Depression and Anxiety*, 12, 111–13.

Endicott, J., Russell, J., and Raskin, J. (2007). Duloxetine treatment for role functioning improvement in generalized anxiety disorders: three independent studies. *Journal of Clinical Psychiatry*, 68, 518–24.

Fenton, W. S. and Mcglashan, T. H. 1991. Natural history of schizophrenia subtypes. II. Positive and negative symptoms and long-term course. *Archives of General Psychiatry*, 48, 978–86.

Fineberg, N. and Craig, K. (2006). Pharmacotherapy for obsessive-compulsive disorder. In: *Textbook of Anxiety Disorders*, pp. 311–31. Washington, DC: American Psychiatric Publishing.

Flint, A. and Rifat, S. (1998). The treatment of psychotic depression in late later life: a comparison of pharmacotherapy and ECT. *International Journal of Geriatric Psychiatry*, 13, 23–8.

Geddes, J.R., Calabrese, J.R., and Goodwin, G.M. (2009). Lamotrigine for treatment of bipolar depression: independent meta-analysis and meta-regression of individual patient data from five randomised trials. *British Journal of Psychiatry*, **194**, 4–9.

Gelenberg, A., Lydiard, B., and Rudolph, R. (2000). Efficacy of venlafaxine extended-release capsules in nondepressed outpatients with generalized anxiety disorder. *Journal of the American Medical Association*, **283**, 3082–8.

Gelertner, C., Uhde, T., and Cimbolic, P. (1991). Cognitive-behavioral and pharmacological treatments of social phobia: a controlled study. *Archives of General Psychiatry*, **48**, 938–45.

Ginestet, D. (1989). Fluoxetine in endogenous depression and melancholia versus clomipramine. *International Clinical Psychopharmacology*, **4**, 37–40.

Goodman, W., Bose, A., and Wang, Q. (2005). Treatment of generalized anxiety disorder with escitalopram: pooled results from double-blind placebo controlled trials. *Journal of Affective Disorders*, **87**, 161–7.

Goodman, W., Price, L., and Delgado, P. (1990). Specificity of serotonin reuptake inhibitors in the treatment of obsessive-compulsive disorder: a comparison of fluvoxamine and desipramine. *Archives of General Psychiatry*, **47**, 577–85.

Gorman, J., Liebowitz, M., and Fryer, A. 1985. Treatment of social phobia with atenolol. *Journal of Clinical Psychopharmacology*, **5**, 298–301.

Grady, T., Pigott, T., and L'heureux (1993). Double-blind study of adjuvant buspirone for fluoxetine-treated patients with obsessive-compulsive disorder. *American Journal of Psychiatry*, **150**, 819–21.

Green, M. F. (1996). What are the functional consequences of neurocognitive deficits in schizophrenia? *American Journal of Psychiatry*, **153**, 321–30.

Hertzberg, M., Butterfield, M., and Feldman, M. 1999. A preliminary study of lamotrigine for the treatment of posttraumatic stress disorder. *Biological Psychiatry*, **45**, 1226–9.

Hertzberg, M., Moore, S., and Feldman, M. (2001). A preliminary study of bupropion sustained release for smoking cessation in patients with chronic post-traumatic stress disorder. *Journal of Clinical Psychopharmacology*, **21**, 94–8.

Hillert, A., Maier, W., and Wetzel, H. (1992). Risperidone in the treatment of disorders with a combined psychotic and depressive syndrome: A functional approach. *Pharmacopsychiatry*, **25**, 213–17.

Hogarty, G., Anderson, C., Reiss, D., Kornblith, S., Greenwald, D., Ulrich, R., et al. 1991. Family psychoeducation, social skills training and maintenance chemotherapy in the aftercare treatment of schizophrenia. Two year effects of a controlled study on relapse and adjustment. *Archives of General Psychiatry*, **48**, 340–7.

Insel, T., Mueller, E., and Alterman, I. (1985). Obsessive-compulsive disorder and serotonin: is there a connection? *Biological Psychiatry*, **20**, 1174–88.

Janicak, P., Davis, J., Preskorn, S., Ayd, F., Jr, Marder, S., and Pavuluri, M. (2006a). Indications for antidepressants. In: *Principles and Practice of Psychopharmacology*, pp. 75–150. Lippincott Williams and Wilkins.

Janicak, P., Davis, J., Preskorn, S., Ayd, F., Jr, Marder, S., and Pavuluri, M. (2006b). *Principles and Practice of Psychopharmacology*. Lippincott Williams and Wilkins.

Janicak, P., Davis, J., Preskorn, S., Ayd, F., Jr, Marder, S., and Pavuluri, M. (2006c). Treatment with antidepressants. In: *Principles and Practice of Psychopharmacology*, pp. 00–00. Lippincott Williams and Wilkins.

Jesner, O.S., Aref-Adib, M., and Coren, E. (2007). Risperidone for autism spectrum disorder. *Cochrane Database Systematic of Reviews*, **1**, CD005040.

Johnson, J., Horwath, E., and Wiesmann, M. (1991). The validity of major depression with psychotic features based on a community study. *Archives of General Psychiatry*, **48**, 1075–81.

Jones, P.B., Barnes, T.R., Davies, L., Dunn, G., Lloyd, H., Hayhurst, K.P., et al. (2006). Randomized controlled trial of the effect on quality of life of second- vs first-generation antipsychotic drugs in schizophrenia: Cost Utility of the Latest Antipsychotic Drugs in Schizophrenia Study (CUtLASS 1). *Archives of General Psychiatry*, **63**, 1079–87.

Laakmann, G., Schule, C., and Lorkowski, G. (1998). Buspirone and lorazepam in the treatment of generalized anxiety disorder in outpatients. *Psychopharmacology*, **136**, 357–66.

Larsen, T.K., Melle, I., Auestad, B., Friis, S., Haahr, U., Johannessen, J.O., et al. (2006). Early detection of first-episode psychosis: the effect on 1-year outcome. *Schizophrenia Bulletin*, **32**, 758–64.

Lehman, A., Kreyenbuhl, J., Buchanan, R., Dickerson, F., Dixon, L., Goldberg, R., et al. (2003). The Schizophrenia Patient Outcome Research Team (PORT): Updated treatment recommendations. *Schizophrenia Bulletin*, **30**, 193–217.

Leonard, H., Swedo, S., and Rapoport, J. (1988). Treatment of childhood obsessive compulsive disorder with clomipramine and desmethylimipramine: a double blind crossover comparison. *Psychopharmacology Bulletin*, **24**, 93–5.

Levinson, D., Umapathy, C., and Musthaq, M. (1999a). Treatment of schizoaffective disorder and schizophrenia with mood symptoms. *American Journal of Psychiatry*, **156**, 1138–48.

Levinson, D.F., Umapathy, C., and Musthaq, M. (1999b). Treatment of schizoaffective disorder and schizophrenia with mood symptoms. *American Journal of Psychiatry*, **156**, 1138–48.

Lieberman, J.A., Stroup, T.S., McEvoy, J.P., Swartz, M.S., Rosenheck, R.A., Perkins, D.O., et al. (2005). Effectiveness of antipsychotic drugs in patients with chronic schizophrenia. *New England Journal of Medicine*, **353**, 1209–23.

May, P., Tuma, A., Yale, C., Potepan, P., and Dixon, W. (1976). Schizophrenia - a follow-up study of results of treatment. *Archives of General Psychiatry*, **33**, 481–6.

McCracken, J.T., McGough, J., Shah, B., Cronin, P., Hong, D., Aman, M.G., et al. (2002). Risperidone in children with autism and serious behavioral problems. *New England Journal of Medicine*, **347**, 314–21.

McDougle, C., Barr, L., and Goodman, W. (1995). Lack of efficacy of clozapine monotherapy in refractory obsessive-compulsive disorder. *American Journal of Psychiatry*, **152**, 1812–14.

McDougle, C.J., Stigler, K.A., Erickson, C.A., and Posey, D.J. (2008). Atypical antipsychotics in children and adolescents with autistic and other pervasive developmental disorders. *Journal of Clinical Psychiatry*, **69**(Suppl. 4), 15–20.

McEvoy, J., Lieberman, J., Stroup, T., Davis, S., Meltzer, H., Rosenheck, R., et al. (2006). Effectiveness of clozapine versus olanzapine, quetiapine, and risperidone in patients with chronic schizophrenia who did not respond to prior atypical antipsychotic treatment. *American Journal of Psychiatry*, **163**, 600–10.

Mendels, J., Kiev, A., and Fabre, L. (1999). Double-blind comparisons of citalopram and placebo in depressed outpatients with melancholia. *Depression and Anxiety*, **9**, 54–60.

Michelson, D., Allgunlander, C., and Dantendorfer, K. (2001). Efficacy of usual antidepressant dosing regimens of fluoxetine in panic disorder: randomized, placebo-controlled trials. *British Journal of Psychiatry*, **179**, 514–18.

Munjack, D., Baltazar, P., and Bohn, P. (1990). Clonazepam in the treatment of social phobia: a pilot study. *Journal of Clinical Psychiatry*, **51**, 35–40.

Nelson, E., Rielage, F., and Welge, J. (2001). An open trial of olanzapine in the treatment of patients with psychotic depression. *Annals of Clinical Psychiatry*, **13**, 147–51.

Nelson, J.C. and Papakostas, G.I. (2009). Atypical antipsychotic augmentation in major depressive disorder: a meta-analysis of placebo-controlled randomized trials. *American Journal of Psychiatry*, **166**, 980–91.

Nimatoudies, I., Zissis, N., and Kogeorgos, J. (2004). Remission rates with venlafaxine extended release in Greek outpatients with generalized anxiety disorder: a double-blind, randomized, placebo controlled study. *International Clinical Psychopharmacology*, **19**, 331–6.

National Institute of Mental Health (2010a). *What is anxiety?* Available at: http://www.nimh.nih.gov/health/topics/anxiety-disorders/index.shtml

National Institute of Mental Health (2010b). *What is depression?* Available at: http://www.nimh.nih.gov/health/topics/depression/index.shtml

Reimherr, F., Byerley, W., and Ward, M. (1988). Sertraline, a selective inhibitor of serotonin uptake for the treatment of outpatients with major depressive disorder. *Psychopharmacology Bulletin*, **24**, 200–5.

Reist, C., Kaufmann, C., and Haier, R. (1989). A controlled trail of desipramine in 18 men with posttraumatic stress disorder. *American Journal of Psychiatry*, **146**, 513–16.

Rickels, K., Zaninelli, R., and Mccafferty, J. (2003). Paroxetine treatment of generalized anxiety disorder: a double blind placebo contolled study. *American Journal of Psychiatry*, **160**, 749–56.

Rickels, K., Mangano, R., and Kahn, A. (2004). A double-blind placebo controlled study of a flexible dose of venlafaxine ER in adult outpatients with generalized social anxiety disorder. *Journal of Clinical Psychopharmacology*, **24**, 488–96.

Robinson, D., Woerner, M.G., Alvir, J.M., Bilder, R., Goldman, R., Geisler, S., *et al.* 1999. Predictors of relapse following response from a first episode of schizophrenia or schizoaffective disorder. *Archives of General Psychiatry*, **56**, 241–7.

Rocca, P., Fonzo, V., and Scotta, M. 1997. Paroxetine efficacy in the treatment of generalized anxiety disorder. *Acta Psychiatrica Scandinavica*, **95**, 444–50.

Rosenbaum, J., Moroz, G., and Bowden, C. (1997). Clonazepam in the treatment of panic disorder with or without agoraphobia: a dose-response study of efficacy, safety and discontinuance. *Journal of Clinical Psychopharmacology*, **17**, 390–400.

Sachs, G.S., Printz, D.J., Kahn, D.A., Carpenter, D., and Docherty, J.P. (2000). The Expert Consensus Guideline Series: Medication Treatment of Bipolar Disorder 2000. *Postgraduate Medicine*, Spec No, 1–104.

Sachs, G.S., Nierenberg, A.A., Calabrese, J.R., Marangell, L.B., Wisniewski, S.R., Gyulai, L., *et al.* (2007). Effectiveness of adjunctive antidepressant treatment for bipolar depression. *New England Journal of Medicine*, **356**, 1711–22.

Shaywitz, J. and Liebowitz, M. (2003). Antiepileptic treatment of anxiety disorders. *Primary Psychiatry*, **10**, 51–6.

Simpson, H., Schneier, F., and Campeas, R. (1998). Imiprammine in the treatment of social phobia. *Journal of Clinical Psychopharmacology*, **18**, 132–5.

Smith, L., Cornelius, V., Warnock, A., Tacchi, M., and Taylor, D. (2007a). Acute bipolar mania: A systematic review and meta-analysis of co-therapy vs. monotherapy. *Acta Psychiatrica Scandinavica*, **115**, 12–20.

Smith, L. A., Cornelius, V., Warnock, A., BELL, A., and Young, A. H. (2007b). Effectiveness of mood stabilizers and antipsychotics in the maintenance phase of bipolar disorder: a systematic review of randomized controlled trials. *Bipolar Disorders*, **9**, 394–412.

Sramek, J., Fackiewicz, E., and Cutler, N. (1997). Efficacy and safety of two dosing regimens of buspirone in the treatment of outpatients with persistent anxiety. *Clinical Therapeutics*, **19**, 498–506.

Stein, M., Chartier, M., and Hazen, A., Kroft, C.D.L., Charle, R., and Walker, J.R. (1996). Paroxetine treatment of generalized social phobia: open-label treatment and double-blind placebo controlled discontinuation. *Journal of Clincal Psychopharmacology*, **16**, 218–22.

Stein, M., Pollack, M., and Bystritsky, A. (2005). Efficacy of low and higher dose extended-release venlafaxine in generalized social anxiety disorder: a 6 month randomized controlled trial. *Psychopharmacology*, **177**, 280–8.

Stroup, T.S., Lieberman, J.A., Mcevoy, J.P., Swartz, M.S., Davis, S.M., Rosenheck, R.A., *et al.* (2006). Effectiveness of olanzapine, quetiapine, risperidone, and ziprasidone in patients with chronic schizophrenia following discontinuation of a previous atypical antipsychotic. *American Journal of Psychiatry*, **163**, 611–22.

Tarrier, N., Barrowclough, C., Vaughn, C., Bamrah, J., Porceddu, K., Watts, S., et al. (1988). The community management of schizophrenia. A controlled trial of a behavioural intervention with families to reduce relapse. *British Journal of Psychiatry*, **153**, 532–42.

Tohen, M. and Vieta, E. (2009). Antipsychotic agents in the treatment of bipolar mania. *Bipolar Disord*, **11**(Suppl. 2), 45–54.

Tondo, L. and Baldessarini, R.J. (2009). Long-term lithium treatment in the prevention of suicidal behavior in bipolar disorder patients. *Epidemiologica e Psichiatria Sociale*, **18**, 179–83.

Ursano, R., Bell, C., and Eth, S. (2004). Practice guideline for the treatment of patients with acute stress disorder and post-traumatic stress disorder. *American Journal of Psychiatry*, **161**, 3–31.

Van Der Loos, M.L., Mulder, P.G., Hartong, E.G., Blom, MB., Vergouwen, A.C., de Keyzer, H. J., *et al.* (2009). Efficacy and safety of lamotrigine as add-on treatment to lithium in bipolar depression: a multicenter, double-blind, placebo-controlled trial. *Journal of Clinical Psychiatry*, **70**, 223–31.

Vigo, D.V. and Baldessarini, R. J. (2009). Anticonvulsants in the treatment of major depressive disorder: an overview. *Harvard Review of Psychiatry*, **17**, 231–41.

Wade, A., Lepola, U., and Koponen, H. 1997. The effect of citalopram in panic disorder. *British Journal of Psychiatry*, **170**, 549–53.

Wardle, J. (1990). Behavioral therapy and benzodiazepines: Allies or antagonists? *British Journal of Psychiatry*, **156**, 163–8.

Wyatt, R.J. (1991). Neuroleptics and thc natural course of schizophrenia. *Schizophrenia Bulletin*, **17**, 325–51.

CHAPTER 23

Managing co-occurring physical disorders in mental health care

Delia Cimpean and Bob Drake

Individuals with serious mental illness (SMI) have increased rates of medical comorbidity. The most common serious medical conditions in this population include cardiovascular disease, cardiovascular risk conditions (obesity, hyperlipidaemia, type 2 diabetes), and blood-borne viral infections. The cluster of cardiovascular risk factors that includes high body-mass index (BMI), high blood pressure, high blood sugar and cholesterol, sometimes called metabolic syndrome, is found in 35% to 63% of people with schizophrenia and is associated with a fivefold increase in risk of diabetes and twofold increased cardiovascular risk (Table 23.1).

As consequences of high rates of medical comorbidity, people with SMI have greatly reduced physical functioning, are vulnerable to early institutionalization in nursing homes, experience worse mental health outcomes, and ultimately, high levels of early mortality, especially cardiovascular mortality. Indeed, on average, people with SMI have 30-year shorter lifespans compared to people of the same age without mental illness (Dickey et al., 2002; Miller et al., 2006).

Morbidity, disability, and early mortality observed in people with SMI are outcomes that resemble that of people 20 years older in the general population. In other populations with premature aging or 'weathering', chronic pervasive socioeconomic stress was associated with increased allostatic load, measured by several cardiovascular, metabolic, and inflammatory biomarkers (Bird et al., 2010; Geronimus et al., 2006). Similarly, people with SMI are subjected to pervasive stress, such as poverty, unemployment, homelessness, and overt or subtle chronic stigma and discrimination. Over the course of a lifetime, psychological and physiological response to pervasive stress and the high effort required for coping, produce premature aging of people with SMI. This underlines the importance of coupling socioeconomic measures to the health improvement programmes to address the high medical burden and early mortality of people with SMI.

Reasons for medical morbidity and early mortality

Poor medical health and early mortality among individuals with SMI are due to several factors, summarized in Table 23.2 and described in detail below.

Table 23.1 Comparison of metabolic syndrome and individual criterion prevalence in fasting CATIE (Clinical Antipsychotic Trials of Intervention Effectiveness) subjects and matched NHANES III (National Health and Nutrition Examination Survey) subjects (Lieberman et al., 2005; Meyer et al., 2005a; Zahran et al., 2005).

	Men (n=509)		p	Women (n=180)		p
	CATIE %	NHANES III %		CATIE %	NHANES III %	
Metabolic syndrome prevalence	36.0	19.7	0.0001	51.6	25.1	0.0001
Waist circumference criterion	35.5	24.8	0.0001	76.3	57.0	0.0001
Triglyceride criterion	50.7	32.1	0.0001	42.3	19.6	0.0001
HDL criterion	48.9	31.9	0.0001	63.3	36.3	0.0001
BP criterion	47.2	31.1	0.0001	49.6	26.8	0.0001
Glucose criterion	14.1	14.2	0.9635	21.7	11.2	0.0075

Table 23.2 Causes of medical morbidity and early mortality

1. Poor health care behaviours	◆ Poor diet ◆ Inactivity ◆ Toxic effects of nicotine, alcohol, and other drugs
2. Medication side effects	◆ Endocrine and metabolic (obesity, diabetes mellitus, hyperlipidaemia, hyperprolactinaemia) ◆ Cardiovascular (coronary artery disease, strokes, sudden death) ◆ Neurological (tardive dyskinesia)
3. Inadequate medical care	◆ Inattention to physical health ◆ Poor access to health care ◆ Poor quality of health care
4. Violent premature death	◆ Suicide ◆ Accidents, violence, overdoses
5. Other factors	◆ Genetic or illness-related vulnerabilities

Poor health care behaviours

People with SMI tend to have sedentary lifestyles and unhealthy diets, which are risk factors for obesity, hyperlipidaemia, diabetes mellitus, and cardiovascular disease. Unemployment and poor social skills undoubtedly contribute to inactivity and dietary problems. Features of the mental illness itself, the treatment, and effects of stigma and discrimination contribute through decreased focus and function, social isolation, and poverty to unhealthy lifestyles as well. The elevated rates of addictions, including high rates of nicotine, alcohol, and other drug abuse/dependence represent other critical behavioural risks. As a direct result of their alcohol/drug use, people with SMI are also prone to engage in dangerous behaviours, which increase the risk of HIV and other blood-borne viral infections.

Medication side effects

Psychiatric medications contribute substantially to excess medical morbidity and mortality.

There is a hierarchy of the risk of weight gain with most antipsychotics, the highest risk occurring with clozapine and olanzapine (Fig. 23.1).

Hypercholesterolaemia, hypertriglyceridaemia, and diabetes have been observed with certain second-generation antipsychotics. Factors that were associated with the magnitude of these effects induced by antipsychotics include younger age, pre-treatment BMI, length of treatment, concomitant treatment with lithium, valproate, or depot progesterone.

Occasionally, the acute onset of marked increases in lipids and/or blood sugar after the start of an antipsychotic, has led to life-threatening complications such as acute pancreatitis due to severe hypertriglyceridaemia or diabetic ketoacidosis (Jin et al., 2002; Koller et al., 2003; Wilson et al., 2003).

In addition to producing metabolic conditions, and thus vastly increasing the risk for occurrence of coronary artery disease and cardiovascular events, the antipsychotics were implicated in an increase in cardiac sudden death. In a large data base analysis in the United States, users of typical and atypical antipsychotics had higher risk of sudden death, without significant difference between the groups (typical antipsychotics: incidence rate ratio (IRR) 1.99, 95% confidence interval (CI) 1.68–2.34; atypical antipsychotics: IRR 2.26, 95% CI 1.88–2.72) (Ray et al., 2009).

Inadequate medical care

Although 50% of psychiatric clients have known medical problems, and another 35% suffer from previously unidentified medical problems, people with SMI tend to receive inadequate medical care. Regardless of the quality of access to care, people with SMI have a decreased likelihood of receiving preventive care, tend not to be treated for the conditions they have, and tend to receive less specialized medical procedures, such as cardiac interventions following a heart attack. In the United States, the CATIE trials identified rates of non-treatment of 30% for diabetes, 60% for hypertension, and almost 90.0% for dyslipidaemia in people with schizophrenia (Nasrallah, et al., 2006). In the United Kingdom, although the rates of non-treatment are far lower than in the United States, there is still evidence that some usual general medical checks are much less common in people with SMI (Roberts et al., 2007). Obstacles to obtaining adequate medical care are likely related to the disease, providers, patients, and the health care system. See Table 23.3.

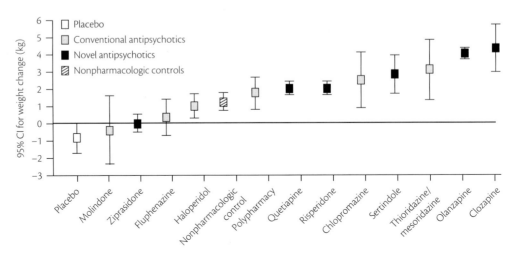

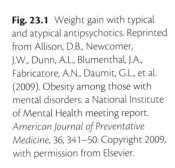

Fig. 23.1 Weight gain with typical and atypical antipsychotics. Reprinted from Allison, D.B., Newcomer, J.W., Dunn, A.L., Blumenthal, J.A., Fabricatore, A.N., Daumit, G.L., et al. (2009). Obesity among those with mental disorders: a National Institute of Mental Health meeting report. *American Journal of Preventative Medicine*, 36, 341–50. Copyright 2009, with permission from Elsevier.

Table 23.3 Reasons for inadequate medical care

Disease-related	◆ Medical problems and psychiatric problems overlap and are difficult to differentiate ◆ Neglect of self-care due to symptoms of mental illnesses (e.g. social withdrawal, paranoia)
Patient-related	◆ Reluctant to seek medical attention: fears of being treated rudely, lack of financial resources ◆ Poor historians, limited ability to describe their symptoms ◆ Impairments in basic self-care skills ◆ Poor medication and health care follow-up adherence
Health-care system related	◆ Poor access to health care ◆ Poor coordination between mental health and general medicine ◆ Poverty and unemployment
Provider related	◆ Biased perceptions of people with mental illnesses ◆ Lack of consensus between psychiatrists and medical providers for assuming responsibility for metabolic screening ◆ Limited knowledge about health risks associated with mental illness ◆ Difficult to differentiate between somatic manifestations of psychiatric illness and general medical problems

Table 23.4 Recommendations to improve physical health and longevity

1. Consumer-centered interventions	Education regarding side effects and polypharmacy
	Shared decision-making
	Health improvement interventions to focus on diet and exercise
	Smoking cessation programmes[a]
	Integrated dual diagnosis interventions[a]
2. Provider-centered interventions	Provider education
	Routine medical screening for side effects
	Treating known medical conditions according to standards of care in the general population
	Changing antipsychotics
3. System-centered interventions	Insure access to prevention, primary care, and specialty care
	Connect medical care and mental health care

[a] These interventions are addressed in other chapters in this textbook

Violent premature death

Intentional suicides, accidents, violence, and overdoses related to substance abuse are discussed in elsewhere in this textbook.

Genetic

Studies of first psychotic episode in schizophrenia show that people have a higher likelihood of having diabetes mellitus and metabolic abnormalities at the time of their first presentation (De Hert et al., 2006; Verma et al., 2009). These facts suggest the possibility of genetic predisposition of people with schizophrenia to these conditions.

Intervention approaches

In this section, we review attempts to help people with mental illness to improve their physical health and decrease their risk of early mortality (Table 23.4).

Consumer-centered interventions

One goal that is receiving increasing attention in the professional literature is helping people become more knowledgeable about their own medications and more active in choosing and monitoring their own medications (Deegan and Drake, 2006). Despite consumer-directed campaigns and internet misinformation, the facts remain that psychiatric medications in general only partially ameliorate the symptoms of psychiatric illnesses for many people, and that the differences in therapeutic effects between antipsychotics are small, while the differences in side effects are often major. Decisions to use specific medications should therefore almost always respond to informed preferences, and people with mental illness should be centrally involved in the process of shared

decision-making. The initial research in mental health shows that shared decision-making increases the quality of decisions (knowledge, participation, and congruence with values) (Beebe et al., 2005; Drake and Deegan 2009; Malm et al., 2003; Priebe et al., 2007).

Improving health care behaviors

Because inactivity, diet, and obesity are such common problems for persons with SMI, many experts recommend exercise and dietary counselling. Reviews of evidence indicate that all behavioural interventions (e.g. individual or group cognitive behavioural counselling or rewards for diet and/or exercise) report weight maintenance or weight reductions (Alvarez-Jimenez et al., 2008; Faulkner and Cohn, 2006; Faulkner et al., 2007; Loh et al., 2006).

Pharmacological interventions for weight management in people on antipsychotics provide modest effects (Table 23.5) (Faulkner et al., 2007; Wu et al., 2008a,b).

Provider-centered interventions

Multiple organizations have issued guidelines for routine monitoring of metabolic, endocrinological, and cardiac side effects (American Diabetes Association 2004; Cohn and Sernyak 2006; Cordes et al., 2008 ; Marder et al., 2002) Some of the recommendations are illustrated in Table 23.6. Most measures are recommended at baseline, and then repeated at variable intervals: from 4 to 12 weeks after initiation or change in antipsychotic treatment to at least once a year in different guidelines, often with the provision of increasing frequency of monitoring if patients are at higher risk (Table 23.6).

Changing antipsychotics is a strategy that has been used to alleviate metabolic risk. Switching from a high-metabolic risk to a low-metabolic risk antipsychotic was associated with improved prevalence of metabolic syndrome, weight maintenance or loss, and cardiovascular risk decrease of 13% to 33% (Meyer, 2002, 2005b; Ried et al., 2003, 2006; Rosenheck et al., 2009). Recently,

Table 23.5 Pharmacological interventions for weight management in people on antipsychotics

Drug	Weight change	Comments
Amantadine	−2.30 kg; CI −4.2 to −0.4	
Metformin	BMI change: of −1.8 (CI −1.3 to −2.3), placebo gained weight	
Nizatidine	−6.80 kg; CI −7.9 to −5.7; and −2.20 kg CI −3.0 to −1.5	
Topiramate	−1.36 kg; CI −2.5 to −0.3	High dose: 200 mg/day

switching from long-acting haloperidol to long-acting risperidone was associated with significant weight gain, and a non-significant decrease in risk for extrapyramidal symptoms (Covell, 2009). Switching from polypharmacy (at least two antipsychotics) to monotherapy resulted in weight loss, and maintained control of symptoms (Essock, 2009). The American Diabetes Association recommends switching antipsychotics when weight gain exceeds 5% during the first few months of starting a medication.

Improving the system of care

Like others in society, people with mental illness need routine primary medical care and specialized care for serious or chronic conditions.

The literature on medical care for people with SMI assumes that greater coordination or integration of medical and mental health care would improve each of these areas. In the United States, there is no consensus regarding a specific approach to connecting mental health care and medical care for people with SMI in order to improve their medical health. Different approaches have been

suggested: dually trained physicians, increasing the role of the psychiatrist in providing primary care, introducing public health nurses in community mental health centres, using case managers or nurses as care coordinators to help link people with SMI with their medical providers, enhancing primary care by establishing specialized medical clinics focused entirely on health of people with SMI, or colocating the medical care team and the mental health team in the same setting. In the United Kingdom, integrated care has been stimulated with increased involvement of the general practitioners, using primary care case registers and incentives, as well as elaborating guidelines for cooperation between primary and secondary care (England and Lester, 2005; National Collaborating Centre for Mental Health, 2009).

Information technology could enhance all approaches to integrating psychiatric and medical care. Computerized reminders, effective in primary medical clinics, might be used to improve the rates of adherence with guidelines for basic medical services in mental health as well. Computerized clinical decision support systems were associated with improvement in outcomes if they had the ability to exchange data with an electronic medical record, generate reports of measures, and provide feedback and computerized prompts to providers (Dorr et al., 2007).

Summary and conclusions

Physical health and threats to normal longevity are ubiquitous issues for people with SMI. People with severe mental illness are particularly vulnerable to poor medical health, considerable morbidity, and early mortality. To reduce the medical comorbidity and mortality, the following issues need to be addressed: 1) improving health care behaviours, such as diet, exercise, and smoking cessation, adherence, and follow-up; 2) enhancing the

Table 23.6 Guidelines for monitoring metabolic parameters

	"Mount Sinai"	Australia	US ADA–APA	Belgium	United Kingdom	Canada (CDA)	France	European Psychiatric Association
FPG	x	x	x	x	x	x	x	x
Random glucose		x			x			
HgbA1C	If FPG not feasible			No	In addition to FPG or RG			
OGTT				x		Tof/up IFG		
Lipids	x	x	x	x	x	x	x	x
Weight	x	x	x	x	x	x	x	x
Waist circ.	x	x	x	x	x	x	x	x
Height	x	x	x	x		x	x	x
Blood pressure		x	x	x		x	x	x
Family history	x	x	x	x		x	x	x
Medical history	x	x	x	x		x	x	x
Ethnicity	x	x		x			x	
Tobacco		x		x	x	x	x	x
Diet-activity	x		x	x	x	x	x	x
ECG							x	x

ADA, American Diabetes Association.; APA, American Psychiatric Association; CDA, Canadian Diabetes Association; ECG, electrocardiogram; FPG, fasting plasma glucose. f/up, follow-up; IFG, impaired fasting glucose; OTGG, oral glucose tolerance test; RG, random glucose.

monitoring and management of side effects related to psychiatric medications; 3) ensuring preventive health care, routine medical care, and specialty referrals.

Physical health is inextricably linked with mental health, functional performance, institutionalization, and quality of life. Real psychiatric rehabilitation cannot occur without holistic, integrated care, which is almost always more accessible and more effective than fragmented care.

References

Allison, D.B., Newcomer, J.W., Dunn, A.L., Blumenthal, J.A., Fabricatore, A.N., Daumit, G.L., et al. (2009). Obesity among those with mental disorders: a National Institute of Mental Health meeting report. *American Journal of Preventative Medicine, 36*, 341–50.

Alvarez-Jimenez, M., Hetrick, S.E., Gonzalez-Blanch, C., Gleeson, J.F., and McGorr, P.D. (2008). Non-pharmacological management of antipsychotic-induced weight gain: systematic review and meta-analysis of randomised controlled trials. *British Journal of Psychiatry, 193*, 101–7.

American Diabetes Association, American Psychiatric Association, American Association of Clinical Endocrinologists, and North American Association for the Study of Obesity (2004). Consensus development conference on antipsychotic drugs and obesity and diabetes. *Diabetes Care, 27*, 596–601.

Beebe, L.H., Tian, L., Morris, N., Goodw, A., Allen, S.S., and Kulda, J. (2005). Effects of exercise on mental and physical health parameters of persons with schizophrenia. *Issues in Mental Health Nursing, 26*, 661–76.

Bird, C.E., TSeeman, .E., Escarce, J.J., Basurto-Dávila, R., Finch, B.K., Dubowitz, T., et al. (2010). Neighborhood socioeconomic status and biological 'wear & tear' in a nationally representative sample of U.S. adults. *Journal of Epidemiology and Community Health, 64*, 860–5.

Cohn, T.A., and Sernyak, M.J. (2006). Metabolic monitoring for patients treated with antipsychotic medications. *Canadian Journal of Psychiatry. Revue Canadienne de Psychiatrie, 51*, 492–501.

Cordes, J., Sinha-Roder, A., Kahl, K.G., Malevani, J., Thuenker, J., Lange-Asschenfeldt, C., et al. (2008). Therapeutic options for weight management in schizophrenic patients treated with atypical antipsychotics. *Fortschritte der Neurologie-Psychiatrie, 76*, 703–14.

Covell, N.H., Schooler, N.R., Stroup, T.S., McEvoy, J.P., and Essock, S.M. (2009). Effectiveness of switching from long-acting first generation antipsychotics to long-acting risperidone. Paper read at Proceedings of the 49th annual meeting of the New Clinical Drug Evaluation Unit of the National Institute of Mental Health, at Hollywood, FL.

De Hert, M., van Winkel, R., Van Eyck, D., Hanssens, L., Wampers, M., Scheenet, A., al. (2006). Prevalence of diabetes, metabolic syndrome and metabolic abnormalities in schizophrenia over the course of the illness: a cross-sectional study. *Clinical Practice and Epidemiology in Mental Health, 2*, 14.

Deegan, P.E., and Drake, R.E. (2006). Shared decision making and medication management in the recovery process. *Psychiatric Services, 57*, 1636–9.

Dickey, B., Normand, S.L., Weiss, R.D., Drake, R.E., and Azeni, H. (2002). Medical morbidity, mental illness, and substance use disorders. *Psychiatric Services, 53*, 861–7.

Dorr, D., Bonner, L.M., Cohen, A.N., Shoai, R.S., Perrin, R., Chaney, E., et al. (2007). Informatics systems to promote improved care for chronic illness: a literature review. *Journal of the American Medical Informatics Association, 14*, 156–63.

Drake, R.E., and Deegan, P.E. (2009). Shared decision making is an ethical imperative. *Psychiatric Services, 60*, 1007.

England, E., and Lester, H. (2005). Integrated mental health services in England: a policy paradox. *International Journal of Integrated Care, 5*, e24.

Essock, S.M., Covell, N.H., Schooler, N.R., Stroup, T.S., and McEvoy, J.P. (2009). Effectiveness of switching from antipsychotic polypharmacy to monotherapy. Paper read at Proceedings of the 49th annual meeting of the New Clinical Drug Evaluation Unit of the National Institute of Mental Health, at Hollywood, FL.

Faulkner, G., and Cohn, T.A. (2006). Pharmacologic and nonpharmacologic strategies for weight gain and metabolic disturbance in patients treated with antipsychotic medications. *Canadian Journal of Psychiatry. Revue Canadienne de Psychiatrie, 51*, 502–11.

Faulkner, G., Cohn, T., and Remington, G. (2007). Interventions to reduce weight gain in schizophrenia. *Cochrane Database of Systematic Reviews, 1*, CD005148.

Geronimus, A.T., Hicken, M., Keene, D., and Bound, J. (2006). 'Weathering' and age patterns of allostatic load scores among blacks and whites in the United States. *American Journal of Public Health, 96*, 826–33.

Jin, H., Meyer, J.M., and Jeste, D.V. (2002). Phenomenology of and risk factors for new-onset diabetes mellitus and diabetic ketoacidosis associated with atypical antipsychotics: an analysis of 45 published cases. *Annals of Clinical Psychiatry, 14*, 59–64.

Koller, E.A., Cross, J.T., Doraiswamy, P.M, and Malozowski, S.N. (2003). Pancreatitis associated with atypical antipsychotics: from the Food and Drug Administration's MedWatch surveillance system and published reports. *Pharmacotherapy, 23*, 1123–30.

Lieberman, J.A., Stroup, T.S., McEvoy, J.P., Swartz, M.S., Rosenheck, R.A., Perkins, D.O. et al. Effectiveness of antipsychotic drugs in patients with chronic schizophrenia, *New England Journal of Medicine 353*(12), 1209–23.

Loh, C., Meyer, J.M., and Leckband, S.G. (2006). A comprehensive review of behavioral interventions for weight management in schizophrenia. *Annals of Clinical Psychiatry, 18*, 23–31.

Malm, U., Ivarsson, B., Allebeck, P., and Falloon, I.R. (2003). Integrated care in schizophrenia: a 2-year randomized controlled study of two community-based treatment programs. *Acta Psychiatrica Scandinavica, 107*, 415–23.

Marder, S.R., Essock, S.M., Miller, A.L., Buchanan, R.W., Davis, J.M., Kane, J.M., et al. (2002). The Mount Sinai conference on the pharmacotherapy of schizophrenia. *Schizophrenia Bulletin, 28*, 5–16.

Meyer, J.M. (2002). A retrospective comparison of weight, lipid, and glucose changes between risperidone- and olanzapine-treated inpatients: metabolic outcomes after 1 year. *Journal of Clinical Psychiatry, 63*, 425–33.

Meyer, J.M., Nasrallah, H.A., McEvoy, J.P., Goff, D.C., Davis, S.M., Chakos, M., et al. (2005a). The Clinical Antipsychotic Trials of Intervention Effectiveness (CATIE) Schizophrenia Trial: clinical comparison of subgroups with and without the metabolic syndrome. *Schizophrenia Research, 80*, 9–18.

Meyer, J.M., Pandina, G., Bossie, C.A., Turkoz, I., and Greenspan, A. (2005b). Effects of switching from olanzapine to risperidone on the prevalence of the metabolic syndrome in overweight or obese patients with schizophrenia or schizoaffective disorder: analysis of a multicenter, rater-blinded, open-label study. *Clinical Therapeutics, 27*, 1930–41.

Miller, B. J., Paschall, 3rd, C.B., and Svendsen, D.P. (2006). Mortality and medical comorbidity among patients with serious mental illness. *Psychiatric Services, 57*, 1482–7.

Nasrallah, H.A. (2006). Metabolic findings from the CATIE trial and their relation to tolerability. *CNS Spectrums, 11*(7 Suppl 7), 32–9.

National Collaborating Centre for Mental Health (2009). Core interventions in the treatment and management of schizophrenia in primary and secondary care (update). In *National Clinical Practice Guideline Number 82*. London: National Institute for Health and Clinical Excellence.

Priebe, S., McCabe, R., Bullenkamp, J., Hansson, L., Lauber, C., Martinez-Leal, R., et al. (2007). Structured patient-clinician communication and 1-year outcome in community mental healthcare: cluster randomised controlled trial. *British Journal of Psychiatry, 191*, 420–6.

Ray, W.A., Chung, C.P., Murray, K.T., Hall, K., and Stein, C.M. (2009). Atypical antipsychotic drugs and the risk of sudden cardiac death. *New England Journal of Medicine,* **360**, 25–35.

Ried, L.D., Renner, B.T., Bengtson, M.A., Wilcox, B.M., and Acholonu, Jr., W.W. (2003). Weight change after an atypical antipsychotic switch. *Annals of Pharmacotherapy,* **37**,1381–6.

Ried, L.D., Renner, B.T., McConkey, J.R., Bengtson, M.A., and Lopez, L.M. (2006). Increased cardiovascular risk with second-generation antipsychotic agent switches. *Journal of the American Pharmacists Association,* **46**, 491–8; quiz 99–501.

Roberts, L., Roalfe, A., Wilson, S., and Lester, H. (2007). Physical health care of patients with schizophrenia in primary care: a comparative study. *Family Practice,* **24**, 34–40.

Rosenheck, R.A., Davis, S., Covell, N., Essock, S., Swartz, M., Stroup, S., *et al.* (2009). Does switching to a new antipsychotic improve outcomes? Data from the CATIE Trial. *Schizophrenia Research,* **107**, 22–9.

Verma, S.K., Subramaniam, M., Liew, A., and Poon, L.Y. (2009). Metabolic risk factors in drug-naive patients with first-episode psychosis. *Journal of Clinical Psychiatry,* **70**, 997–1000.

Wilson, D.R., D'Souza, L., Sarkar, N., Newton, M., and Hammond, C. (2003). New-onset diabetes and ketoacidosis with atypical antipsychotics. *Schizophrenia Research,* **59**, 1–6.

Wu, R.R., Zhao, J.P., Guo, X.F., He, Y.Q., Fang, M.S., Guo, W.B., *et al.* (2008a). Metformin addition attenuates olanzapine-induced weight gain in drug-naive first-episode schizophrenia patients: a double-blind, placebo-controlled study. *American Journal of Psychiatry,* **165**, 352–8.

Wu, R.R., Zhao, J.P. Jin, H. Shao, P. Fang, M.S. Guo, X.F. *et al.* (2008b). Lifestyle intervention and metformin for treatment of antipsychotic-induced weight gain: a randomized controlled trial. *Journal of the American Medical Association,* **299**, 185–93.

Zahran, H.S., Kobau, F., Moriarty, D.G., Zack, M.M., Holt, J., Donehoo, R. Health-related quality of life surveillance-United States, 1993–2002. *MMWR Surveillance summaries: morbidity and mortality weekly report. Surveillance summaries/CDC,* **54**(4), 1–35.

CHAPTER 24

Illness self-management programmes

Kim T. Mueser and Susan Gingerich

In recent years there has been a growth in programmes aimed at teaching illness self-management skills to individuals with a major mental illness. This trend reflects a broader trend in modern medicine towards adopting a more collaborative approach that includes the patient and family members in the management of chronic medical disorders. Education about psychiatric disorders and teaching of illness self-management strategies is now a common practice in the mental health field, and a growing number of programmes have been developed with standard curriculum and teaching methods designed to achieve this. While the goal of these programmes is to improve illness self-management through better adherence to treatment recommendations and improved skills for coping with persistent symptoms and impairments, the management of psychiatric disorders in these programmes is generally viewed as a collaborative process that involves the client, treatment team, and family members or friends.

We begin this chapter with a review of factors that led to the development and growth of illness self-management programmes. We then discuss the goals of illness self-management programmes, followed by a review of different approaches to teaching illness self-management. We then address research supporting illness self-management, and briefly describe several programmes. We conclude with a brief summary of illness self-management for people with serious psychiatric disorders.

Historical factors in the development of self-management programmes for mental illness

The notion that people with a serious psychiatric disorder are capable of helping themselves is not a new one. Over 150 years ago the Alleged Lunatics' Friend Society was founded in England for the purposes of helping people with a serious psychiatric disorder cope with their illness (Frese and Davis, 1997). In the 1940s, former state hospital patients began to meet together to provide support for one another in New York City, which eventually gave rise to Fountain House, and the development of psychosocial clubhouses designed for individuals with a serious mental illness to support one another in moving forward in their lives (Beard et al., 1982). Over the past several decades, a confluence of factors has led to the development of illness self-management programmes for psychiatric disorders. Two important factors merit particular attention, including the rise of the consumer and recovery movement, and the shift toward shared decision-making in general medicine. These factors are briefly described below.

The consumer and recovery movement

The consumer and recovery movement evolved over the past four decades, spurred on by changes in attitudes and beliefs about serious mental illness and its treatment, and research on the long-term course of these disorders. In the wake of deinstitutionalization, and following changes in laws that prohibited people from being hospitalized in the absence of evidence that they presented a grave danger to themselves or others, increasing numbers of people with serious psychiatric disorders began to express dissatisfaction with their treatment in the mental health system, and were afforded the opportunity of meeting and supporting each other in voicing their objections (Chamberlin, 1978). These individuals often objected to the word 'patient' as suggesting a passive role in treatment, with those in the United States opting for the term **consumer** (of mental health services), and those in Great Britain opting for the term **service user**.

Consumers expressed their dissatisfaction with several different aspects of the mental health system. First, they objected to the presumed chronicity of serious mental illnesses such as schizophrenia, and to mental health professionals who sought to explain to them that their psychiatric disorders were lifelong and they should accept this and either modify their hopes and dreams accordingly, or give up on them altogether (Deegan, 1990). Bolstered by a growing body of research demonstrating that the long-term outcome of schizophrenia was in fact much better than previously thought, and that significant numbers of persons demonstrated improvement and even remission of their disorder over the long-term (Harding et al., 1987b; Harrison et al., 2001), consumers argued for a broader definition of recovery that was based not on remission of psychopathology, but rather on the personally meaningful process that involves living and growing beyond or in spite of having a mental illness (Anthony, 1993; Davidson, 2003; Deegan, 1988; Roe and Chopra, 2003). Although the concept of recovery continues to generate debate (Bellack, 2006), and many different definitions have been offered (Ralph and Corrigan, 2005), the shift away from defining recovery in medical terms and towards defining it in more personal terms drew attention to the importance of engaging individuals in identifying their own treatment goals, rather than narrowly focusing on the reduction of symptoms and impairments.

Second, consumers objected to the traditional, hierarchical and often coercive decision-making process that dominated psychiatric treatment (Blaska, 1990; Campbell, 1997; Carling, 1995). They complained that their concerns were frequently ignored by treatment providers, and that rather than providing them with the help and care they needed, they were often further traumatized by the very system that was supposed to serve them (Fisher, 1992; Jennings, 1994). Consumers argued that they needed to be the ones to set the goals of treatment, and demanded respect and collaboration from treatment providers (Segal et al., 1993).

Third, as part of the rise of the self-help movement in the 1970s (Gartner and Riessman, 1977; Kurtz, 1988), consumers began to look to their peers as critical to their own empowerment and recovery. A growing body of writings by consumers testified to the importance of illness self-management strategies to helping individuals get on with their lives (Copeland, 1994; Leete, 1989). As the desire for illness self-management strategies grew, so did curriculum, groups, and settings that responded to this need.

Shared decision-making

Parallel to the rise of the consumer and recovery movement, the modern practice of medicine was undergoing a similar radical shift. While traditional medical practice was hierarchical in nature, with the doctor instructing the patient on what needed to be done to treat the disorder, two trends emerged that led to a reappraisal and change of this practice. First, the problem of poor adherence to doctors' treatment recommendations became increasingly clear. Although effective treatments for many diseases existed, patients often failed to follow their doctor's recommendations, leading to worse than expected outcomes (Blackwell, 1976). Second, as the variety of treatment options for different diseases grew, so did the risks and benefits, and the task of medical decision-making became more complex. The best or optimal treatment for a given disease was often less clear. Patient preferences in treatment decisions became an important consideration, as patients naturally differed in the outcomes they most valued and the side effects they least wanted, resulting in different treatment decisions for the same disease.

Shared decision-making was developed in order to engage and invest patients in making decisions about the treatment and management of an illness, based on the outcomes they desired (Wennberg, 1988). Shared decision-making involves teaching the person about the nature of his or her disease, discussing the advantages and disadvantages of different treatment options, and then involving the person in making treatment decisions based on a consideration of the likely outcomes (Charles et al., 1997, 1999). As shared decision-making required that individuals be educated about the nature of their diseases and the different treatment options, teaching them this information became standard medical practice, which extended to psychiatry (Deegan et al., 2008; Fenton, 2003).

The goals of illness self-management programmes

Psychiatric illness self-management programmes are aimed at teaching clients how to manage their psychiatric disorders in collaboration with others. Although a range of different programmes have been developed, most share a common set of goals, including:

- Instil hope for a better quality of life and a more favourable course of illness by improving illness self-management skills
- Foster the development of a collaborative approach between clients and treatment providers in establishing treatment goals and choosing treatment options
- Provide information about the nature of the individual's psychiatric illness and options for treating it
- Teach strategies for monitoring the course of the illness and for preventing or minimizing symptom relapses and hospitalizations
- Improve social support for illness self-management
- Teach effective strategies for coping with persistent symptoms and illness-related impairments
- Teach strategies for reducing the negative effects of stress
- Assist clients in making lifestyle changes in order to facilitate the management of the psychiatric illness.

Methods for improving illness self-management

A wide range of methods have been developed to achieve the goals of illness self-management. Some of these methods are nearly universal across different programmes, such as psychoeducation, whereas others vary from one programme to another, such as peer support and skills training. In addition to the methods used across programmes, they also differ with respect to the teaching modality (e.g. individual or group) and the provider (e.g. peer, professional). Eight different strategies for teaching illness self-management are briefly described below: psychoeducation, medication adherence strategies, relapse prevention training, coping strategies for persistent symptoms, stress management, social skills training, peer support, and family psychoeducation.

Psychoeducation

Psychoeducation refers to teaching information about a psychiatric disorder in an interactive fashion that engages the clients' interest in the information and its perceived relevance to their lives and goals (Ascher-Svanum and Krause, 1991; Swezey and Swezey, 1976). Psychoeducation includes a combination of didactic teaching strategies with frequent questions and prompts to help individuals relate the information to their own personal experiences and circumstances. A variety of materials may be used to teach information about a psychiatric disorder, including handouts, DVDs, posters, and other media. A summary of the topic areas frequently addressed in psychoeducation programmes for serious mental disorders is provided in Table 24.1.

Table 24.1 Outline of curriculum for psychoeducation about psychiatric disorders

---

◆ Name of psychiatric disorder and how a diagnosis is established

◆ Prevalence, onset, and possible courses of the disorder

◆ Characteristic symptoms and related problems

◆ Theories about the aetiology of the disorder and factors affecting its course (e.g. stress-vulnerability model)

◆ Pharmacological treatment:

- Names and types of medication

- Clinical effects

- Side effects

◆ Psychosocial treatment:

- Psychotherapy and counselling (e.g. cognitive behavioural therapy)

- Illness self-management programmes

- Family psychoeducation

- Psychiatric rehabilitation (e.g. social skills training, cognitive remediation, supported employment)

◆ Family and other social supports

◆ Self help/peer support

Medication adherence strategies

Non-adherence to prescribed medications is an important predictor of relapses and hospitalizations for persons whose psychiatric disorders have been previously stabilized with medication (Miner et al., 1997). There are many different reasons why people do not take their prescribed medications (Roe et al., 2009; Weiden et al., 1995), as described below.

Some clients do not take their medication regularly because they do not fully understand the purpose of the medication, or may have misconceptions about the effects of medication. For example, many clients believe that if they are not experiencing symptoms they do not need to keep taking their medication; they do not know that medication also prevents symptom relapses. Some people do not take medication because they believe it is addictive, or they are afraid of interactions between the medication and alcohol and/or street drugs. Another common reason for non-adherence is that people simply forget to take their medication at the appropriate times. Medication side effects, such as weight gain, sexual difficulties, restlessness, or sedation are other factors that can precipitate medication discontinuation. Lack of accurate information about the effects of medications and their side effects may also lead to medication discontinuation when clients do not feel confident, comfortable, and socially skilled at discussing their concerns with their prescriber. Last, individuals may not take their medication because they do not see how it can improve their lives or help them achieve their goals. Individuals with serious psychiatric disorders vary in their insight into their symptoms, and even those who are aware of their symptoms may not place a high priority on reducing symptoms or reducing symptom relapses.

A wide range of interventions have been developed to increase adherence to prescribed medication. Programmes that target medication adherence typically teach a number of different strategies,

tailored to the individual needs of the client. Commonly used strategies for increasing medication adherence are summarized in Table 24.2.

Relapse prevention training

For many individuals, serious psychiatric disorders are episodic, with the severity of symptoms fluctuating over time, occasionally requiring psychiatric hospitalization when the person poses a threat to self or others. A relapse is defined as either the re-emergence of symptoms (in a client whose symptoms were previously in remission) or the worsening of symptoms (in a client with persistent symptoms), accompanied by a deterioration in functioning, such as increased problems at work or school, social difficulties, or reduction in self-care. Relapses tend to occur gradually, over several weeks, and are often preceded by subtle changes or *early warning signs* that are unique to the individual, such as a mild increase in depression, social withdrawal, or difficulties with concentration. Whether or not early warning signs precede the re-emergence or worsening of psychiatric symptoms, there is usually a window of opportunity for rapid intervention during the early stages of a relapse that can prevent a deterioration in functioning and full-blown relapse from occurring (Herz, 1984). The most common type of rapid intervention that can stave off a relapse if detected early enough is an increase in the individual's medication (Herz et al., 2000).

Relapse prevention training involves teaching the client about the nature of relapse, helping the individual identify his or her early warning signs or first symptoms of relapse, developing a

Table 24.2 Strategies for helping clients increase their adherence to prescribed medications

Strategy	Description
Psychoeducation	Provide information about medications, their effects and side effects
Behavioural tailoring	Help client incorporate taking medication into his or her daily routine
Pill boxes or organizers	Facilitate client taking medication by using pill boxes or organizers
Alarms and other prompts	Teach client how to use alarms and other electronic prompts to take medication
Simplify medication regimen	In collaboration with prescriber, reduce number of different medications and number of times per day medication is taken
Motivational interviewing	Explore with client how taking medication can help him or her achieve personal goals
Social skills training	Teach client skills for interacting with and expressing concerns to medication prescriber
Depot medications	Explore with client potential benefits of taking depot antipsychotic medications over oral medication
Enlisting assistance of family members or other supporters	Explore with client how family members or other supporters could help him or her set up a system for taking medications and/or provide prompts for taking them

plan for monitoring signs and symptoms, and taking rapid action at the first indication of a possible relapse. Relapse prevention plans should be regarded as a 'living document' that can be changed and improved over time to make it more effective. The steps of developing a relapse prevention plan are summarized in Table 24.3.

Coping strategies for persistent symptoms

Many individuals with serious mental disorders experience persistent symptoms, even when they are adherent to their prescribed medications. For example, hallucinations, paranoia, delusions of reference, depression, anxiety, sleep problems, or cognitive difficulties may persist and lead to distress and interference with everyday functioning and the enjoyment of life. Phenomenological studies and personal accounts of individuals with serious mental disorders have shown that many people develop coping strategies for reducing the distress and interference caused by persistent symptoms (Breier and Strauss, 1983; Leete, 1989).

While many individuals with serious mental disorders spontaneously develop strategies for coping with persistent symptoms, many others do not. However, effective coping strategies can be systematically taught using cognitive behavioural teaching principles (Tarrier, 1992). Coping skills can be taught using the following steps:

1 Focus on symptoms that either cause distress or interfere with an area of functioning that the client wants to improve.

2 Explore with the client the situations in which the symptom is most and least problematic.

3 Identify coping strategies that the client currently uses to deal with the target symptom and the effectiveness of those strategies.

4 If the client reports using effective strategies to cope with the symptom, but these strategies are infrequently utilized, make a plan with the client to increase his or her use of those skills on a regular basis.

5 After increasing the utilization of coping skills that the client already uses, review and describe other possible strategies for coping with the symptom.

6 Help the client select another coping strategy to learn.

7 Model (demonstrate) the new coping skill in a role-play for the client.

8 Engage the client in practicing the new coping strategy in a role-play.

9 Praise the client for trying the new strategy, make adaptations to the strategy if necessary, and engage the client in additional role-plays to practice it as needed.

10 Develop a plan with the client to practice the new coping strategy outside of the session, focusing first on easier and more manageable situations.

11 Follow-up on the plan and make modifications to the coping strategy and practice it as needed.

12 Help the client develop at least two or three coping strategies for each symptom, as coping self-efficacy is related to the number of strategies people report using.

A wide range of different coping strategies has been developed to help individuals manage persistent symptoms and impairments more effectively. Table 24.4 summarizes some coping strategies for the most common symptoms.

Table 24.4 Examples of coping strategies for persistent symptoms

Depression	Anxiety
◆ Schedule pleasant events ◆ Use positive self-talk ◆ Challenge negative, self-defeating thoughts ◆ Increase activity level	◆ Learn relaxation strategies ◆ Gradually expose oneself to feared but safe situations ◆ Use positive self-talk ◆ Challenge negative, self-defeating thoughts
Hallucinations	**Cognitive difficulties**
◆ Shift attention (e.g. listen to music) ◆ Use positive self-talk ◆ Accept that voices will not go away but need not be a major focus of your attention ◆ Increase contact with others	◆ Remove distractions to improve attention ◆ Over-practise to improve psychomotor speed ◆ Use memory aids (e.g. pocket calendar) to reduce forgetting ◆ Learn step-by-step problem solving to address problems
Sleep problems	**Negative symptoms**
◆ Choose a standard time to go to bed and get up each day ◆ Avoid napping even if you don't get enough sleep the previous night ◆ Avoid caffeine after 5 p.m. ◆ Develop a relaxing bedtime routine ◆ If you have trouble sleeping for 30 minutes, get out of bed for 10–15 minutes and then return to bed	◆ Break down big goals into smaller goals and steps ◆ Schedule regular pleasant activities to engage in ◆ Focus on the future not the past ◆ Praise yourself for your efforts and accomplishing small steps

Table 24.3 Steps of developing a relapse prevention plan

1.	If possible, try to involve a family member or friend who is close to the client in developing the relapse prevention plan
2.	Identify triggers of previous relapses, such as specific stressful situations
3.	Identify two or three specific early warning signs of relapse based on a discussion of the past one or two relapses
4.	Develop a system for monitoring the early warning signs of relapse
5.	Determine an action plan for responding to early warning signs of relapse, including who should be contacted
6.	Write down the plan, including the specific early warning signs that are being monitored and the telephone numbers of any important contact people
7.	Rehearse the plan in a role play, post the plan in a prominent location, and give copies to anyone with an assigned role in the plan
8.	If a relapse occurs, after the client is safe and the situation has been stabilized, convene a meeting with the client and others who are involved in the plan, praise everyone for implementing those parts of the plan that went well, and then modify the plan to make it more effective

Stress management

Stress is a well-established precipitant of symptom exacerbations (Zubin and Spring, 1977). While the minimization of unnecessary stress can be a valuable illness management strategy, stress is an inherent part of life, and many of the goals that clients have involve stress, such as working in an interesting job, pursuing an educational degree, having a loving relationship, or being a parent. Therefore, teaching stress management skills is another common component of illness self-management programmes.

Illness self-management programmes use a variety of different strategies to improve coping with stress, with most strategies drawn from or adapted from stress management techniques developed for the general population (Davis et al., 2008; Woolfolk et al., 2008). Commonly used stress management techniques include relaxed breathing, using positive imagery, and muscular relaxation (Gingerich and Mueser, 2010).

Social skills training

Social support and social contact are strong predictors of the course of serious mental disorders, including relapses and re-hospitalizations (Erickson et al., 1989; Strauss and Carpenter, 1977). Therefore, improving social support and the quality of social relationships has the potential to facilitate the management and outcome of these disorders. Social skills training, which involves systematically teaching more effective interpersonal skills by breaking complex skills into their constituent elements and then teaching these elements through a combination of modelling, role play rehearsal, positive and corrective feedback, and home assignments to practice skills, is a widely used approach to improving the quality of social relationships for people with serious mental disorders (Bellack et al., 2004). Examples of commonly taught social skills include starting conversations, expressing positive feelings, making a request, and finding common interests.

Peer support

Individuals with a serious mental disorder who are coping effectively and moving ahead with their lives can serve as important peer supports and role models for others who are struggling with their disorder (Clay et al., 2005; Davidson et al., 2006). People who are successfully managing their psychiatric disorder, and who have rewarding lives in areas such as work, school, social relationships, leisure time, and living situation, can provide credible and realistic hope to others who may be discouraged about their lives and their future. Instilling hope for a better life can provide the impetus for learning illness self-management (Deegan, 1996).

Family psychoeducation

Family stress does not cause serious mental disorders, but can be a precipitant of relapse in some individuals (Butzlaff and Hooley, 1998). Family stress may be due in part to the significant challenges of helping a relative deal with a severe mental disorder (Hatfield and Lefley, 1993), but can also be due to a lack of understanding about the nature of the disorder and its treatment (Barrowclough and Hooley, 2003). Many families have not been given information about their relative's psychiatric disorder and its treatment, making it difficult for them to support their relative's adherence to treatment recommendations and work towards personal goals. Families may also not have a working relationship with their relative's treatment team, preventing them from getting timely help when their relative's illness worsens. These families often have significant amounts of contact with their relative, and are in an ideal position to work collaboratively with the treatment team if they are provided with the information and skills they need to help their relative learn how to better manage his or her disorder.

Family psychoeducation programmes have been developed in order to reduce stress in the family, increase the knowledge of family members (including the client) about the mental disorder and its treatment, to improve family support for the client's adherence to the recommended treatments, to monitor the course of the psychiatric disorder, and to work with the client to achieve his or her personal recovery goals. A variety of family programmes have been developed for people with a mental disorder using either single-family or multiple-family group treatment modalities, which include the client in family sessions (Lefley, 2009). Many of the strategies for improving illness self-management previously described are incorporated into family programmes, such as psychoeducation, developing a relapse prevention plan, implementing strategies for reducing stress in the family, and training in communication and problem solving skills to reduce stress and improve social support (Anderson et al., 1986; Barrowclough and Tarrier, 1992; Falloon et al., 1984; Kuipers et al., 2002; Mueser and Glynn, 1999). Multi-family group formats incorporate these strategies and also provide peer support to clients and their relatives (McFarlane, 2002).

Research on illness self-management

Numerous studies have been conducted to evaluate the effectiveness of different approaches to teaching illness self-management to people with serious mental disorders. In a review of 40 randomized controlled trials evaluating different approaches to illness self-management training, Mueser et al. (2002) concluded that there is evidence supporting four major methods for teaching illness self-management: psychoeducation, medication adherence strategies, relapse prevention training, and coping skills training. Several other reviews of research on illness self-management reached similar conclusions (Lincoln et al., 2007; Zygmunt et al., 2002).

Programmes that provided psychoeducation alone were found to lead to significant improvements and knowledge about mental illness and its treatment, but appeared to have no effect on symptoms or relapses. Mueser et al. (2002) suggested that psychoeducation was a necessary part of illness self-management programmes in order to facilitate client involvement in shared decision-making about treatment, but that it alone was not sufficient to equip clients with the skills they need to manage their psychiatric disorder effectively. However, a more recent meta-analysis of research on psychoeducation concluded that it does in fact improve the course of psychiatric illness (Lincoln et al., 2007).

Although Mueser et al. (2002) reviewed research on a wide range of different strategies for improving medication adherence, they found that only one strategy enjoyed consistent support in controlled trials: behavioural tailoring. **Behavioural tailoring** involves helping the client incorporate the taking of medication into his or her daily routine so that the person is reminded to take medication at the appropriate times (e.g. having the client place his medication next to his toothbrush so that he is reminded to take his medication when he brushes his teeth in the morning and evening).

Strong support was also found for the effectiveness of training in the prevention of relapses and hospitalizations (Mueser et al., 2002). Similarly, controlled studies of teaching coping strategies for persistent symptoms also demonstrated significant reductions in symptom severity and distress related to symptoms. Teaching coping strategies is routinely incorporated into cognitive behavioural therapy for psychosis, which has been found to reduce the severity of psychotic and negative symptoms in schizophrenia (Wykes et al., 2008).

The research literature on social skills training has steadily accumulated over the past three decades, with growing evidence supporting its effectiveness. A recent meta-analysis of controlled research on social skills training for schizophrenia reported moderate effect sizes for the impact of skills training on improving both social functioning and role play tests of social competence, a slightly lower effect size on improving negative symptoms, and a small but significant effect size on reducing other symptoms or preventing relapses (Kurtz and Mueser, 2008). An independent meta-analysis research on social skills training reported similar findings (Pfammatter et al., 2006). Thus, social skills training has support for improving illness self-management skills in persons with serious psychiatric disorders.

There is also a strong evidence base supporting the effectiveness of professionally led family psychoeducation programmes for serious psychiatric disorders (Miklowitz et al., 2003; Pitschel-Walz et al., 2006). The most effective family programmes are those that are relatively long-term (minimum 9 months), develop a collaborative relationship between the treatment team and family members, involve educating the family about mental illness and its treatment, help the family develop a relapse prevention plan, and reduce family burden and stress (Glynn et al., 2007). Both single and multi-family group formats have been found to be effective at improving the management of serious psychiatric disorders.

Only a limited amount of research has evaluated the benefits of peer support programmes for improving illness self-management (Barber et al., 2008; Davidson et al., 1999; Davidson et al., 2006). The results of the research conducted thus far is inconclusive, although the study of peer support programmes involves methodological challenges for researchers since those programmes are often embedded within larger self-help programmes that are difficult to randomly assign individuals to. More research is needed on this important approach to illness self-management.

Standardized illness self-management programmes

A number of illness self-management programmes have been standardized and are widely available to people with a serious mental disorder. We briefly describe several of those programmes below.

Illness Management and Recovery programme

The Illness Management and Recovery (IMR) is a programme in which clients set personal recovery goals at the beginning of the programme, break those goals down into smaller goals and steps which they work towards over the course of the programme, and then learn illness self-management information and skills in order to help them achieve their personal goals (Gingerich and Mueser, 2005, 2010). The curriculum is divided into 10 topic areas or modules, each requiring three to seven sessions to complete. It takes an average of 5 to 10 months of either twice-weekly or weekly sessions to complete the overall programme, although persons with more severe symptoms may take longer. The module topics include:

1 Recovery strategies

2 Practical facts about schizophrenia/bipolar disorder/depression

3 Stress-vulnerability model and strategies for treatment

4 Building social support

5 Using medications effectively

6 Drug and alcohol abuse

7 Reducing relapses

8 Coping with stress

9 Coping with problems and persistent symptoms

10 Getting your needs met in the mental health system.

Each module includes a handout for the client and teaching guidelines for the clinician. The guidelines for each module provide recommendations for using psychoeducational, cognitive behavioural, and motivational enhancement teaching strategies. Home assignments are collaboratively developed at the end of each session, and clients are encouraged to involve family members and other supporters in helping them practice their illness management skills and work on their personal goals. The IMR programme can be implemented in either an individual or group modality.

The IMR programme was developed following a comprehensive review of research on illness self-management (Mueser et al., 2002), and was designed to include the core effective elements described in the previous section on research (psychoeducation, behavioural tailoring for medication adherence, relapse prevention training, coping skills training, and social skills training). Controlled research studies on the overall IMR programme have recently been completed and published, including two randomized controlled trials, one in Israel (Hasson-Ohayon et al., 2007) and one in New York (Levitt et al., 2009), with both studies reporting beneficial effects of IMR on illness self-management when compared to usual services.

In addition, one study evaluated whether the IMR programme could be implemented with high fidelity to the treatment model in routine treatment settings serving people with serious mental illness in the United States (McHugo, et al., 2007). Based on a standardized training and consultation model, the IMR programme was implemented at 12 community mental health centres throughout the United States, with fidelity assessments conducted at baseline and every 6 months for 2 years. The results indicated that good levels of fidelity could be achieved 6 months after the initial training, with modest improvements at 1 year that were maintained at the 2-year fidelity assessment. This study supported the feasibility of implementing the IMR programme in routine treatment settings serving people with serious psychiatric disorders.

Social and Independent Living Skills programme

The Medication Management and Symptom Management modules are two of eight different skills training modules that form the Social and Independent Living Skills (SILS) programme (Kopelowicz and Liberman, 1994). These modules were developed for persons with schizophrenia-spectrum disorders with the aim of providing them with information about pharmacological and psychosocial treatments, developing a relapse prevention plan, and teaching strategies for coping with persistent symptoms. Other modules in the SILS programme include Basic Conversational Skills, Recreation for Leisure, Community Reentry (for inpatients anticipating discharge into the community), Substance Abuse Management, Workplace Fundamentals, and Friendship and Intimacy.

All of the modules in this programme are taught using the principles of social skills training, based on video demonstrations of topic areas and skills. Modules are designed to be taught in a group format, although they can also be taught individually. Each module includes a core set of materials, including an instructor's manual, participants' workbooks, a demonstration video, and fidelity and outcome measures. For the Medication Management module, teaching is organized around four topic areas: the benefits of medication, self-administration and self-monitoring of medication effects, coping with side effects, and negotiating medication issues with health providers. The Symptom Management module is organized around four skill areas: identifying early warning signs of relapse and seeking early intervention, devising a relapse prevention plan, coping with persistent symptoms, and avoiding substance abuse. The duration of time needed to complete each module depends on the frequency of sessions and level of functioning of participants, with 3 to 6 months of twice-weekly sessions required to teach a module to outpatients.

A significant amount of research has been conducted on the Medication Management and Symptom Management modules, which are often provided in the context of skills training in other areas (Liberman, 2007). Controlled research shows that clients participating in these modules acquire and retain targeted information and skills over 1 year, as compared with other non-skills training interventions (Eckman et al., 1992; Wirshing et al., 1992). Research on the dissemination of modules in the SILS programme indicates that clinicians can implement the module with high fidelity to the programme (Wallace et al., 1992).

Wellness Recovery Action Plan

The Wellness Recovery Action Plan (WRAP) was developed as a general, standardized programme for helping individuals with recurring health and emotional problems to develop healthier and more rewarding lives (Copeland, 1997; Copeland and Mead, 2004). WRAP is a structured programme in which an individual or group of persons is guided through developing a written plan for managing or reducing distressing symptoms and making other desired changes in their lives. WRAP is aimed at helping people with a variety of mental health problems regain control and balance in their life, and it therefore does not provide information about specific disorders or treatments. The WRAP programme is divided into seven different components, each one including written plans that the client maintains in a workbook:

1 Creating a daily maintenance plan

2 Identifying triggers, early warning signs, and signs of potential crisis

3 Developing a crisis plan

4 Establishing a nurturing lifestyle (e.g. more healthy living)

5 Setting up a support system and self-advocating

6 Increasing self-esteem

7 Relieving tension and stress.

Teaching is typically done through a combination of lecture and discussion, with time taken to complete the plan and receive advice and support. WRAP is usually provided by trained consumers, who use their own experiences to inspire others to realize that they can recover their wellness.

Dialectical behaviour therapy

Dialectical behaviour therapy (DBT) is a comprehensive psychotherapeutic approach that was originally developed with a primary focus on reducing self-injurious and suicidal behaviour, but now is more broadly applied to persons with borderline personality disorder (Linehan, 1993a, b). **Dialectic** or **dialectics** refers to the process of resolving conflict between two apparently contradictory ideas or forces through a synthesis of the two or establishing truths on both sides, rather than attempting to prove one right and the other wrong. In DBT, dialectics are employed at the level of the therapeutic relationship by the clinician's combined use of validation and acceptance of the client as he or she is, with the strategies aimed at changing behaviour and achieving a better balance in the client's functioning. Dialectics are also used to help clients strike a balance between the **reasonable mind** and the **emotional mind** in striving to develop a **wise mind** that combines the two and an integrated fashion.

In practice, DBT involves a wide array of cognitive-behavioural techniques to improve interpersonal skills (e.g. social skills training), self-management of negative emotions (e.g. cognitive restructuring), and practical problem solving. These are combined with mindfulness-based approaches (e.g. focusing on the present, taking a non-judgemental stance) aimed at promoting acceptance and tolerance of the person as he or she is, including any unpleasant feelings and thoughts. DBT is usually provided using a combination of weekly individual psychotherapy and group skills training sessions, with the clinicians providing DBT also participating in weekly case consultation meetings among themselves. Specific guidelines are provided for establishing a clear treatment contract between the client and clinician before the beginning of the programme, and to specify in advance the nature of additional contacts and rules concerning these contacts (e.g. telephone calls regarding thoughts of self-injury).

Following the development of DBT, a body of controlled research has gradually emerged supporting the effectiveness of the approach (Bohus et al., 2004; Linehan et al., 1991, 2006; Verheul et al., 2003). Research on DBT has reported several positive effects, including significant reductions in suicidal behaviour and improvement in common emotional problems such as depression, hopelessness, and anger. Furthermore, there is evidence that providing DBT to persons with borderline personality disorder and substance use disorders can reduce the severity of the substance use disorder when compared to clients receiving the usual services.

Summary and conclusions

It is now widely accepted that people with serious psychiatric disorders are highly capable of being active partners with professionals, family members, and other supporters in the treatment of their disorder and that the provision of optimal mental health treatment requires this kind of partnership. Illness self-management programmes are aimed at developing a collaborative relationship between clients and treatment providers, engaging clients in establishing treatment goals, educating them about the nature of their disorder so that they can make informed decisions about their treatment, teaching them strategies for monitoring their disorder and preventing relapses, teaching them strategies for coping with persistent symptoms or disorder-related impairments, instilling hope for a better future, and increasing social support for improved illness self-management and making progress towards goals. A number of standardized programmes have been developed to teach clients illness self-management information and skills.

Research on approaches to illness self-management provides empirical support for both comprehensive illness self-management programmes as well as specific treatment strategies. Evidence-based illness self-management strategies include: psychoeducation about the disorder and its treatment, behavioural tailoring to help client incorporate taking medication into their daily routines, relapse prevention training, teaching coping skills for persistent symptoms, social skills training to improve social support, and family psychoeducation to develop a collaborative relationship between treatment providers and the family and to teach families (including the client) the principles of illness management. The adoption of more collaboratively-based treatment approaches for serious psychiatric disorders that recognize the importance of involving the client and significant others in decision-making, combined with the growth in empirically supported strategies and programmes for teaching illness self-management, brings the ultimate goal of recovery within reach of many more people with these disorders.

References

Anderson, C.M., Reiss, D.J., and Hogarty, G.E. (1986). *Schizophrenia and the Family*. New York: Guilford Press.

Anthony, W.A. (1993). Recovery from mental illness: The guiding vision of the mental health service system in the 1990s. *Psychosocial Rehabilitation Journal*, **16**, 11–23.

Ascher-Svanum, H. and Krause, A.A. (1991). *Psychoeducational Groups for Patients with Schizophrenia: A Guide for Practitioners*. Gaithersburg, MD: Aspen.

Barber, J., Rosenheck, R., Armstrong, M., and Resnick, S.G. (2008). Monitoring the dissemination of peer support in the VA healthcare system. *Community Mental Health Journal*, **44**, 433–41.

Barrowclough, C. and Hooley, J.M. (2003). Attributions and expressed emotion: A review. *Clinical Psychology Review*, **23**, 849–80.

Barrowclough, C. and Tarrier, N. (1992). *Families of Schizophrenic Patients: Cognitive Behavioural Intervention*. London: Chapman and Hall.

Beard, J.H., Propst, R.N., and Malamud, T.J. (1982). The Fountain House model of rehabilitation. *Psychosocial Rehabilitation Journal*, **5**, 47–53.

Bellack, A.S. (2006). Scientific and consumer models of recovery in schizophrenia: Concordance, contrasts, and implications. *Schizophrenia Bulletin*, **32**, 432–42.

Bellack, A.S., Mueser, K.T., Gingerich, S., and Agresta, J. (2004). *Social Skills Training for Schizophrenia: A Step-by-Step Guide*, 2nd edn. New York: Guilford Press.

Blackwell, B. (1976). Treatment adherence. *British Journal of Psychiatry*, **129**, 513–31.

Blaska, B. (1990). The myriad medication mistakes in psychiatry: A consumer's view. *Hospital and Community Psychiatry*, **41**, 993–97.

Bohus, M., Haaf, B., Simms, T., Limberger, M.F., Schmahl, C., Unckel, C., et al. (2004). Effectiveness of inpatient dialectical behavioral therapy for borderline personality disorder: A controlled trial. *Behaviour Research and Therapy*, **42**, 487–99.

Breier, A.M. and Strauss, J.S. (1983). Self-control of psychotic behavior. *Archives of General Psychiatry*, **40**, 1141–5.

Butzlaff, R.L. and Hooley, J.M. (1998). Expressed emotion and psychiatric relapse. *Archives of General Psychiatry*, **55**, 547–52.

Campbell, J. (1997). How consumers/survivors are evaluating the quality of psychiatric care. *Evaluation Review*, **21**, 357–63.

Carling, P. J. (1995). *Return to Community: Building Support Systems for People with Psychiatric Disabilities*. New York: Guilford Press.

Chamberlin, J. (1978). *On Our Own: Patient-Controlled Alternatives to the Mental Health System*. New York: Hawthorne.

Charles, C., Gafni, A., and Whelan, T. (1997). Shared decision-making in the medical encounter: What does it mean? (or it takes at least two to tango). *Social Science and Medicine*, **44**, 681–92.

Charles, C., Gafni, A., and Whelan, T. (1999). Decision-making in the physician-patient encounter: Revisiting the shared treatment decision-making model. *Social Science and Medicine*, **49**, 651–61.

Clay, S., Schell, B., Corrigan, P., and Ralph, R. (eds.) (2005). *On Our Own, Together: Peer Programs for People with Mental Illness*. Nashville, TN: Vanderbilt University Press.

Copeland, M.E. (1994). *Living Without Depression and Manic Depression*. Oakland, CA: New Harbinger.

Copeland, M.E. (1997). *Wellness Recovery Action Plan*. Brattleboro, VT: Peach Press.

Copeland, M.E., and Mead, S. (2004). *Wellness Recovery Action Plan and Peer Support: Personal, Group and Program Development*. Dummerston, VT: Peach Press.

Davidson, L. (2003). *Living Outside Mental Illness: Qualitative Studies of Recovery in Schizophrenia*. New York: New York University Press.

Davidson, L., Chinman, M., Kloos, B., Weingarten, R., Stayner, D., and Tebes, J.K. (1999). Peer support among individuals with severe mental illness: A review of the evidence. *Clinical Psychology: Science and Practice*, **6**, 165–87.

Davidson, L., Chinman, M., Sells, D., and Rowe, M. (2006). Peer support among adults with serious mental illness: A report from the field. *Schizophrenia Bulletin*, **32**, 443–50.

Davis, M., Eshelman, E.R., McKay, M., and Fanning, P. (2008). *The Relaxation and Stress Reduction Workbook*, 6th edn. Oakland, CA: New Harbinger Publications.

Deegan, P.E. (1988). Recovery: The lived experience of rehabilitation. *Psychosocial Rehabilitation Journal*, **11**, 11–19.

Deegan, P.E. (1990). Spirit breaking: When the helping professionals hurt. *The Humanistic Psychologist*, **18**, 301–313.

Deegan, P.E. (1996). 'Recovery and the Conspiracy of Hope.' Paper presented at the Sixth Annual Mental Health Conference of Australia and New Zealand, Brisbane, Australia, September, 1996.

Deegan, P.E., Rapp, C.A., Holter, M., and Riefer, M. (2008). Best practices: a program to support shared decision making in an outpatient psychiatric medication clinic. *Psychiatric Services*, **59**, 603–605.

Eckman, T.A., Wirshing, W.C., Marder, S.R., Liberman, R.P., Johnston-Cronk, K., Zimmermann, K., et al. (1992). Technique for training schizophrenic patients in illness self-management: A controlled trial. *American Journal of Psychiatry*, **149**, 1549–55.

Erickson, D.H., Beiser, M., Iacono, W.G., Fleming, J.A.E., and Lin, T. (1989). The role of social relationships in the course of first-episode schizophrenia and affective psychosis. *American Journal of Psychiatry*, **146**, 1456–61.

Falloon, I.R.H., Boyd, J.L., and McGill, C.W. (1984). *Family Care of Schizophrenia: A Problem-Solving Approach to the Treatment of Mental Illness*. New York: Guilford Press.

Fenton, W.S. (2003). Shared decision making: A model for the physician-patient relationship in the 21st century? *Acta Psychiatrica Scandinavica*, **107**, 401–2.

Fisher, D.B. (1992). Humanizing the recovery process. *Resources*, **4**, 5–6.

Frese, F.J. and Davis, W.W. (1997). The consumer-survivor movement, recovery, and consumer professionals. *Professional Psychology: Research and Practice*, **28**, 243–5.

Gartner, A. and Riessman, F. (1977). *Self-Help in the Human Services*. San Francisco, CA: Jossey-Bass Publishers.

Gingerich, S. and Mueser, K. T. (2005). Illness management and recovery. In: Drake, R.E., Merrens, M.R. and Lynde, D.W. (eds.) *Evidence-Based Mental Health Practice: A Textbook*, pp. 395–424. New York: Norton.

Gingerich, S. and Mueser, K.T. (2010). *Illness Management and Recovery Implementation Resource Kit* (Revised edn.). Rockville, MD: Center for

Mental Health Services, Substance Abuse and Mental Health Services Administration. Available from: http://mentalhealth.samhsa.gov/cmhs/CommunitySupport/toolkits/illness/

Glynn, S.M., Cohen, A.N., and Niv, N. (2007). New challenges in family interventions for schizophrenia. *Expert Reviews of Neurotherapeutics*, **7**, 33–43.

Harding, C.M., Brooks, G.W., Ashikaga, T., Strauss, J.S., and Breier, A. (1987b). The Vermont longitudinal study of persons with severe mental illness: II. Long-term outcome of subjects who retrospectively met DSM-III criteria for schizophrenia. *American Journal of Psychiatry*, **144**, 727–35.

Harrison, G., Hopper, K., Craig, T., Laska, E., Siegel, C., Wanderling, J., *et al.* (2001). Recovery from psychotic illness: A 15- and 25-year international follow-up study. *British Journal of Psychiatry*, **178**, 506–17.

Hasson-Ohayon, I., Roe, D., and Kravetz, S. (2007). A randomized controlled trial of the effectiveness of the illness management and recovery program. *Psychiatric Services*, **58**, 1461–6.

Hatfield, A.B. and Lefley, H.P. (1993). *Surviving Mental Illness: Stress, Coping, and Adaptation*. New York: Guilford Press.

Herz, M.I. (1984). Recognizing and preventing relapse in patients with schizophrenia. *Hospital and Community Psychiatry*, **35**, 344–9.

Herz, M.I., Lamberti, J.S., Mintz, J., Scott, R., O'Dell, S. P., McCartan, L., *et al.* (2000). A program for relapse prevention in schizophrenia: A controlled study. *Archives of General Psychiatry*, **57**, 277–83.

Jennings, A.F. (1994). On being invisible in the mental health system. *Journal of Mental Health Administration*, **21**, 374–87.

Kopelowicz, A., and Liberman, R.P. (1994). Self-management approaches for seriously mentally ill persons. *Directions in Psychiatry*, **14**, 1–7.

Kuipers, L., Leff, J., and Lam, D. (2002). *Family Work for Schizophrenia: A Practical Guide*, 2nd edn. London: Gaskell.

Kurtz, L. (1988). Mutual aid for affective disorders: The manic depressive and depressive association. *American Journal of Orthopsychiatric Association, Inc.*, **58**, 152–55.

Kurtz, M.M. and Mueser, K.T. (2008). A meta-analysis of controlled research on social skills training for schizophrenia. *Journal of Consulting and Clinical Psychology*, **76**, 491–504.

Leete, E. (1989). How I perceive and manage my illness. *Schizophrenia Bulletin*, **15**, 197–200.

Lefley, H. (2009). *Family Psychoeducation in Serious Mental Illness: Models, Outcomes, Applications*. New York: Oxford University Press.

Levitt, A., Mueser, K.T., DeGenova, J., Lorenzo, J., Bradford-Watt, D., Barbosa, A., *et al.* (2009). A randomized controlled trial of illness management and recovery in multi-unit supported housing. *Psychiatric Services*, **60**, 1629–36.

Liberman, R.P. (2007). Dissemination and adoption of social skills training: Social validation of an evidence-based treatment for the mentally disabled. *Journal of Mental Health*, **16**, 595–623.

Lincoln, T.M., Wilhelma, K., and Nestoriuca, Y. (2007). Effectiveness of psychoeducation for relapse, symptoms, knowledge, adherence and functioning in psychotic disorders: A meta-analysis. *Schizophrenia Research*, **96**, 232–45.

Linehan, M.M. (1993a). *Cognitive-Behavioral Treatment of Borderline Personality Disorder*. New York: Guilford Press.

Linehan, M.M. (1993b). *Skills Training Manual for Treating Borderline Personality Disorder*. New York: Guilford.

Linehan, M.M., Armstrong, H.E., Suarez, A., Allmon, D., and Heard, H.L. (1991). Cognitive behavioral treatment of chronically parasuicidal borderline patients. *Archives of General Psychiatry*, **48**, 1060–4.

Linehan, M.M., Comtois, K.A., Murray, A.M., Brown, M.Z., Gallop, R.J., *et al.* (2006). Two-year randomized controlled trial and follow-up of dialectical behavior therapy vs therapy by experts for suicidal behaviors and borderline personality disorder. *Archives of General Psychiatry*, **63**, 757–66.

McFarlane, W.R. (2002). *Multifamily Groups in the Treatment of Severe Psychiatric Disorders*. New York: Guilford Press.

McHugo, G.J., Drake, R.E., Whitley, R., Bond, G.R., Campbell, K., Rapp, C., et al. (2007). Fidelity outcomes in the national implementing evidence-based project. *Psychiatric Services*, **58**, 1279–84.

Miklowitz, D.J., George, E.L., Richards, J.A., Simoneau, T.L., and Suddath, R.L. (2003). A randomized study of family-focused psychoeducation and pharmacotherapy in the outpatient management of bipolar disorder. *Archives of General Psychiatry*, **60**, 904–12.

Miner, C.R., Rosenthal, R.N., Hellerstein, D.J., and Muenz, L.R. (1997). Prediction of compliance with outpatient referral in patients with schizophrenia and psychoactive substance use disorders. *Archives of General Psychiatry*, **54**, 706–12.

Mueser, K.T. and Glynn, S.M. (1999). *Behavioral Family Therapy for Psychiatric Disorders*, 2nd edn. Oakland, CA: New Harbinger.

Mueser, K.T., Corrigan, P.W., Hilton, D., Tanzman, B., Schaub, A., Gingerich, S., *et al.* (2002). Illness management and recovery for severe mental illness: A review of the research. *Psychiatric Services*, **53**, 1272–84.

Pfammatter, M., Junghan, U.M., and Brenner, H.D. (2006). Efficacy of psychological therapy in schizophrenia: Conclusions from meta-analyses. *Schizophrenia Bulletin*, **32**(Suppl. 1), S64–S68.

Pitschel-Walz, G., Bauml, J., Bender, W., Engel, R.R., Wagner, M., and Kissling, W. (2006). Psychoeducation and compliance in the treatment of schizophrenia: Results of the Munich Psychosis Information Project Study. *Journal of Clinical Psychiatry*, **67**, 443–52.

Ralph, R.O., and Corrigan, P.W. (eds.) (2005). *Recovery in Mental Illness: Broadening Our Understanding of Wellness*. Washington, DC: American Psychological Association.

Roe, D. and Chopra, M. (2003). Beyond coping with mental illness: Toward personal growth. *American Journal of Orthopsychiatry*, **73**, 334–44.

Roe, D., Goldblatt, H., Baloush-Klienman, V., Swarbrick, M., and Davidson, L. (2009). Why and how people decide to stop taking prescribed psychiatric medication: Exploring the subjective process of choice. *Psychiatric Rehabilitation Journal*, **33**, 38–46.

Segal, S.P., Silverman, C., and Temkin, T. (1993). Empowerment and self-help agency practice for people with mental disabilities. *Social Work*, **38**, 705–712.

Strauss, J.S. and Carpenter, W.T. (1977). Prediction of outcome in schizophrenia III. Five-year *outcome and its predictors. Archives of General Psychiatry*, **34**, 159–63.

Swezey, R.L. and Swezey, A.M. (1976). Educational theory as a basis for patient education. *Journal of Chronic Diseases*, **29**, 417–22.

Tarrier, N. (1992). Management and modification of residual positive psychotic symptoms. In: Birchwood, M. and Tarrier, N. (eds.), *Innovations in the Psychological Management of Schizophrenia*, pp. 147–69. Chichester: John Wiley and Sons.

Verheul, R., Van Den Bosch, L.M.C., Koetter, M.W.J., De Ridder, M.A.J., Stijnen, T., and Van Den Brink, W. (2003). Dialectical behaviour therapy for women with borderline personality disorder: 12-month, randomised clinical trial in The Netherlands. *British Journal of Psychiatry*, **182**, 135–40.

Wallace, C.J., Liberman, R.P., MacKain, S.J., Blackwell, G., and Eckman, T. (1992). Effectiveness and replicability of modules for teaching social and instrumental skills to the severely mentally ill. *American Journal of Psychiatry*, **149**, 654–8.

Weiden, P.J., Mott, T., and Curcio, N. (1995). Recognition and management of neuroleptic noncompliance. In: Shriqui, C.L. and Nasrallah, H.A. (eds.), *Contemporary Issues in the Treatment of Schizophrenia*, pp. 411–33. Washington, DC: American Psychiatric Press.

Wennberg, J.E. (1988). Improving the medical decision-making process. *Health Affairs*, **7**, 99–105.

Wirshing, W.C., Marder, S.R., Eckman, T., Liberman, R.P., and Mintz, J. (1992). Acquisition and retention of skills training methods in chronic schizophrenic outpatients. *Psychopharmacology Bulletin*, **28**, 241–5.

Woolfolk, R.L., Sime, W.E., and Barlow, D.H. (2008). *Principles and Practice of Stress Management*, 3rd edn. New York: Guilford Press.

Wykes, T., Steel, C., Everitt, B., and Tarrier, N. (2008). Cognitive behavior therapy (CBTp) for schizophrenia: Effect sizes, clinical models and methodological rigor. *Schizophrenia Bulletin*, **34**, 523–37.

Zubin, J., and Spring, B. (1977). Vulnerability: A new view of schizophrenia. *Journal of Abnormal Psychology*, **86**, 103–26.

Zygmunt, A., Olfson, M., Boyer, C.A., and Mechanic, D. (2002). Interventions to improve medication adherence in schizophrenia. *American Journal of Psychiatry*, **159**, 1653–64.

SECTION 5

Ethical and legal aspects

CHAPTER 25

Ethical framework for community mental health

Abraham Rudnick, Cheryl Forchuk, and George Szmukler

Introduction

Community mental health services have been developing in the last few decades and in the process a number of ethical issues have arisen. Some of these deserve special attention as they are relatively distinct from ethical issues related to hospital mental health services. Application of established ethical approaches in the context of community mental health services may require revision of these approaches or alternatives to them. The aim of this chapter is to review key ethics concepts, to discuss ethical issues in community mental health services, and to provide a basis for an ethical framework for community mental health.

We will present definitions and central theories in ethics, an overview of bioethics, ethical issues related to community mental health services, addressing generic as well as distinctive problems. We will consider conservative and radical approaches (the latter partly based on community psychology research and practice), and challenges arising from an ethics of community mental health services (such as the view that social justice as in 'social inclusion' goes beyond fair resource allocation).

Definitions and central theories in ethics

Ethics addresses moral problems, sometimes termed ethical problems or dilemmas. In health care, ethical problems are commonly viewed as the tension between two or more morally defensible alternative actions, including inaction (Beauchamp and Childress, 2009). Ethical theories suggest various ways of addressing and resolving such ethical problems. The most veteran and well-established ethical theories are 'utilitarianism' (or more generally 'consequentialism'), which considers outcomes; 'deontology', which considers duties; and 'virtue ethics', which considers intentions. More novel ethical theories include 'rights-based theory' and 'care ethics' (Rudnick, 2001), among others.

Consequentialism and deontology are arguably the broadest in scope and the most influential ethical theories in contemporary health care and probably in contemporary life in general—at least in the Western world. For example, the notion of human rights, a mainstay of contemporary attitudes to life in the Western world, can be argued to derive from deontology, since duties to others entail rights of those others and vice versa, and as the notion of duties precedes the notion of rights, at least historically. Both consequentialism and deontology are also considered self-sufficient (unlike most other ethical theories such as virtue ethics). And both may have particular relevance to community mental health, especially in relation to consideration of populations as well as individuals.

Consequentialism is based on the argument that consequences or outcomes of actions (and of inactions) determine whether an action (or an inaction) with ethical implications is moral or immoral. In its simplest form, that of hedonistic-like utilitarianism, consequentialism considers pleasure or happiness and pain or suffering as the outcomes of importance, and determines the morality or immorality of an action (or inaction) based on whether it produces more pleasure or happiness than pain or suffering, either of an individual or counted over a number of individuals if more than one individual is affected by the action (or inaction). Two general types of utilitarianism have been described: act utilitarianism, which maintains that the morality of each action is to be determined in relation to the favourable or unfavourable consequences that emerge from that action; and rule utilitarianism, which maintains that a behavioural code or rule is morally right if the consequences of adopting that rule are more favourable than unfavourable to everyone (Dershowitz, 2004: p. 242). Arguably, rule utilitarianism is conceptually more similar to deontology than act utilitarianism is.

Deontology is based on the argument that moral duties or obligations determine whether an action (or an inaction) is moral or immoral. Deontology was first developed systematically by Kant in the 18th century (MacIntyre, 1998), and since then it has been further developed and diversified. In its simplest form, deontology considers universal obligations as the duties of importance, and determines the morality or immorality of an action (or inaction) based on whether it upholds a universal obligation; famously, Kant argued that there is a universal obligation to tell the truth, even if that means disclosing the location of a potential victim to a person known to plan that victim's murder. More generally, Kant formulated the 'categorical imperative', which is an impartiality—applicable to all people—condition, stating that an action (or inaction) is ethically acceptable if it holds for any person who could hypothetically be involved in the particular circumstances, including the person(s) conducting the action (or inaction) if he were to be at the receiving end of the action (or inaction). A neo-Kantian version of this requirement, developed by John Rawls, is that ethical decision-making should be conducted behind a 'veil of ignorance' (which can be formulated as not knowing whether the person will be the instigator or recipient of the action), which strips the ethical decision-maker of any personal considerations that may disrupt impartiality. A variant of Kant's formulation is that persons should be considered ends in themselves, rather than merely the means for other ends. The question who constitutes a 'person' is still open for discussion, and is particularly relevant in bioethics, e.g. in relation to obligations towards disabled human fetuses and embryos, as mentioned below (Kant claimed that only rational beings are full-fledged persons, hence he declined full-fledged personhood to animals and to human children). Also subject to such considerations are human adults who lack decision-making capacity, such as due to disruptive psychosis (Kant declined full-fledged personhood to such psychotic human adults too).

Overview of bioethics

Health care ethics, or bioethics (as it has been termed since the last few decades), has a history of thousands of years, both in the Western world and elsewhere (Jonsen, 2000). Most well known in relation to ancient health care ethics is the Hippocratic oath. Although partly dated, for example, in its consideration of physician duties to slaves, it has universally applicable components, e.g. its requirements to do no (intentional) harm and to maintain confidentiality (Lloyd, 1983). Admittedly, these Hippocratic requirements are not considered absolute now; sometimes harm may be necessary for benefit (e.g. in relation to chemotherapy for cancer) and sometimes confidentiality may have to be breached (e.g. in order to protect third parties who are at risk due to a patient's illness). However, they are still central considerations in health care ethics. Importantly, self-determination or autonomy, specifically patients' choice in relation to their health care, is not addressed in the Hippocratic oath; it is only since the advent of bioethics, a few decades ago, that it has been widely considered a key component of health care ethics, particularly in the Western world (Jonsen, 1998).

Contemporary bioethics includes various, sometimes conflicting approaches. The most well-known is principlism. Four main moral principles that drive moral action are identified. These may come into conflict with each other (or conflict can occur within one principle), with such conflict resulting in a bioethical problem. These principles are: 1) respect for autonomy or self-determination (sometimes termed respect for persons or their choices), 2) beneficence (i.e. benefiting the person(s) directly involved), 3) non-maleficence (i.e. doing no/least harm, which is sometimes combined with beneficence as a balance of most benefit and least harm), 4) justice (fairness, particularly to third parties or others involved or affected, as in resource allocation) (Beauchamp and Childress, 2009). These principles are considered to ground key tenets of

bioethics, such as confidentiality of personal health information in most circumstances. An example of an alternative approach is care ethics, largely based on virtue ethics and casuistry (context-specific considerations) (Rudnick, 2001). Another example is 'dialogical bioethics', which replaces predetermined principles with reasoned communication, but appears to require the principle of justice as fairness (Rudnick 2002, 2007). Note that contemporary bioethics addresses areas of health care beyond clinical practice, such as health related research, administration, and policy.

Some of the major areas of concern for bioethics to date have addressed end-of-life situations, beginning-of-life situations, and risk/benefit-to-others situations. In these, a bioethical problem is involved, requiring reasoned resolution in order to decide on an acceptable health-related action (or inaction). End-of-life situations address euthanasia (mercy killing), physician-assisted death, withholding or withdrawing life support, and other potential and actual health care procedures that either shorten or do not prolong the life of a person who is terminally ill, irreversibly unconscious, or incurably suffering. Beginning-of-life situations address abortion, artificial insemination, and other potential and actual health care procedures that curtail or alternatively enable the continuation of life of a human fetus, embryo, or newborn.

Risk/benefit-to-others situations address the impact of health, ill health, and health care-related procedures involving one or more individuals on other people. A paradigmatic example of a benefit-to-others situation is that of health-related human research, where persons are invited to participate in health-related research which is not necessarily expected to benefit (and may indeed harm) them, but which is expected to benefit others such as future patients. The need to protect human research participants and to obtain and respect their voluntary informed consent (or refusal) to participate in research was highlighted by the exposure of the Nazi medical experiments in the Doctors' Trial at the Nuremberg Tribunal in 1947, and the resulting 10 principles of human research known as the Nuremberg Code (Jonsen, 2000: pp. 100–2). A paradigmatic psychiatric example of a risk-to-others situation is that of the Tarasoff decisions, whereupon it was determined in the California court system that health care providers are obliged to warn and to protect third parties in relation to identified physical risk posed to these third parties by mentally ill individuals, where the risk is caused by their mental illness (Roberts and Dyer, 2004: p. 104). Such obligations may breach confidentiality of mentally ill individuals, on which see the discussion below.

The context of community psychiatry and related ethical challenges

Community psychiatry involves a change in locus of care (from hospital to community), funding arrangements, and treatment techniques. It establishes a network of services offering crisis intervention, continuing care, accommodation, occupation, and social support which together help people with mental health problems to retain or recover valued social roles (or to promote 'social inclusion'). Usually the focus of services has been on those with severe mental illness. To understand the context of community psychiatry it is important to consider both psychiatric care of **individuals** in the community and psychiatric care in relation to **community**. If the goal of treatment is 'social inclusion' then both aspects require careful consideration.

Mental health care of individuals in the community

To ensure that patients in the community receive the benefits of the range of services that they may require, widespread practice of 'case management' or its variants has been adopted. The aims are to ensure continuity of care, accessibility to often fragmented and independently managed services, accountability, and efficiency. A more intensive model of case management is commonly adopted for people with persistent symptoms who are difficult to engage in treatment—Assertive Community Treatment (ACT). ACT aims to prevent the service user from dropping out of treatment and brings treatment **to** the patient. If he or she defaults from treatment, the community team may actively seek out the patient to re-establish contact.

Patients with severe mental illness have a diverse range of needs that can often only be met by an array of services and agencies. Access to these may require a substantial flow of relevant personal information between care providers concerning the service user. The nature of the therapeutic relationships between staff and service user also change in community-based treatment. The key-worker or other members of the interdisciplinary team provide a broad range of interventions. As well as medication and standard psychological treatments, they may work with the patient in their ordinary community settings to rehabilitate basic living skills. This special relationship may be used to encourage the service user to adhere to treatment.

The role of the community itself is crucial to 'community care'. Public fears that care in the community for persons with mental illness will be a failure are common. Responses to these fears by government, public agencies, and community members may greatly affect practice. 'Risk thinking' leads to attempts at its management, control, or surveillance through classifications of risky persons, registers, databases, regulatory mechanisms, and so on. Risk may become a professional responsibility with new forms of regulation and governance of professional judgement and actions (Rose, 1998). Thus clinical practice in some areas has moved in the direction of greater social control at the expense of autonomy (Holloway, 1996). At the same time, in many places, there has been a move towards more person-centred and recovery-oriented care that encourages the development and use of autonomy, such as in supported (rather than sheltered) programmes (Roberts, et al., 2006).

Key dilemmas in clinical practice in the community

These can be grouped under four headings: privacy, confidentiality, coercion, and conflicts of duty.

1 Privacy

Assertive treatment programmes bring treatment to service users, often in their residence, whether it be home, hostel, or boarding house. Visits may be made by mental health professionals even when uninvited. Indeed, visits may continue even when the patient's explicit desire is that they cease.

Since much treatment occurs in the community, there is also an increased likelihood that it becomes public. The curiosity of neighbours may be aroused, particularly with repeated visits, and especially if attempts to gain entry are rebuffed by the patient. Neighbours may deduce that the person being visited is a service user.

Furthermore, as treatment becomes more visible to the public, new expectations may be generated that a CMHT can be called to deal with a difficult person suspected to be a patient. Even if a public assessment is not carried out, an acknowledgement by the team that they may have a role may reveal to bystanders that the person is a psychiatric patient (if already so) or label them as one (if not).

If the patient assessed as representing a risk defaults from treatment, the team may be expected to make every effort to re-establish contact. The team may inform the police if the person could pose a significant risk to self or others. The nature of the relationship between clinician and service user may shift from care to supervision. In some cases, assertive treatment, instead of ensuring that service users receive the care they need, may lead them to being labelled as 'dangerous' leading to exclusion from community services or amenities, including housing.

2 Confidentiality

In medicine, information obtained from a patient will not be disclosed to others without the patient's consent. In community mental health services, where the patient is commonly treated by an interdisciplinary team, sharing of information is common. Service users may not know that this is to be expected. More complex is the sharing of information between agencies—health, social, voluntary, housing, and so on. Very needy patients' access to benefits and other goods may depend on information about them being revealed to those in a position to supply them. Since information may flow frequently, confidentiality may receive less emphasis. There may develop an attitude that 'the patient has less to lose by certain breaches of confidentiality than other kinds of patients do' (Diamond and Wikler, 1985).

Confidentiality may be breached ostensibly in the interests of the patient as above, or for the protection of others. The latter is considered below, including the interests of family and carers.

3 Treatment pressures and 'coercion'

A range of pressures may be exerted by community mental health teams to gain the patient's cooperation with treatment. These can be placed on a hierarchy—persuasion, interpersonal leverage, inducements (or offers), threats ('coercion' proper), and compulsion. These 'treatment pressures', are described in detail by Szmukler and Appelbaum (2008) and in Chapter 27 in this volume, and will not be further discussed here.

4 Conflict of duty to patient versus others

Risk of harm to others

As previously discussed, the negative climate in which community mental health services may operate often provokes the question of the degree to which a mental health professional has a duty to protect others. If a specific risk to an identified person is established, the clinician's duty to protect that person is usually reasonably clear. When the risk to others is general, judgements are more problematic.

Expectations of the public about what mental health services should do to control disturbed behaviour may change with a growing emphasis on community care. For example, the mental health team may be asked to intervene by neighbours or shopkeepers, when they are disturbed by a service user's behaviour. A further aspect may be the possibility that if the team does not act, prejudice against the service user will increase and his or her community tenure be threatened. The balance between the duty of care to the patient and to the local community may be difficult to strike.

Mental health professionals are expected to be competent in assessing risk to others as well as to patients themselves. This often requires information from a range of informants, particularly concerning previous incidents of violence and risk factors such as substance abuse. On occasion, the mere seeking of information concerning the service user's past behaviour may reveal that the person is being treated by a mental health team. It may even raise unwarranted anxieties in others' minds.

Informal carers

Informal carers, usually family, are often central to effective community care. However, the extent to which carers' own needs should be met is often quite uncertain. Where there is a danger of serious physical harm to the carer, the clinician's responsibility is usually straightforward. Far more common are less grave threats to a carer's well-being which nevertheless have serious effects on well-being. Carers may experience difficulty in coping with burdensome behaviours, lack critical knowledge about their relative's illness, and may not know to whom to turn for support, or what support they might expect or be entitled to. The patient may prohibit any contact with the family. It may be unclear then to what extent the mental health team owes a duty of care to the family (Szmukler and Bloch, 1998).

Approaches to addressing the ethical challenges

Acting in the health interests of the service user

Szmukler and Appelbaum (2008) and in Chapter 27 in this volume discuss two approaches to ethical decision-making based on forms of 'paternalism'. These are a 'capacity-best interests' framework and a 'paternalism' framework. It is argued there that these frameworks can be applied to the full range of ethical dilemmas described above. Note that paternalism may not be fully independent from some principlist considerations, particularly from the consideration of beneficence. The reader is referred to the above-mentioned references for a fuller discussion of these approaches. An alternative approach is that of 'dialogical bioethics', where even incapable service users are engaged in dialogue in order to enhance their participation in ethical decision-making as much as possible and to obtain their input and enrich it (as well as others'), including obtaining their assent (incapable agreement) or dissent (incapable disagreement), as the case may be. Even in situations where grave risk is expected for the person or for others, this approach may be sufficient, considering it involves dialogue and input from all stakeholders involved (although it may not be fully independent from some principlist considerations, particularly from the consideration of justice). For a fuller discussion of this approach, the reader is referred to previous publications by Rudnick (2002; 2007).

Preventing harm to others

Szmukler and Appelbaum elsewhere in this volume discuss the difficulties in deciding when to intervene in a 'coercive' manner for the protection of others. They argue that there is an important conceptual distinction between interventions serving the health interests of service users versus those for the protection of others. The latter may result—through the agency of mental health legislation—in 'preventive detention' or preventive coercive measures that discriminate against people with mental disorders since people not suffering from a mental disorder but who are equally risky cannot be dealt with in such a manner unless they have first committed an offence. Clinical ethical dilemmas in this area are important (see Szmukler and Appelbaum, Chapter 27 in this volume for further discussion of this matter).

Psychiatric care in relation to community: the context

Individual patient goals of social inclusion and community integration imply the need for a receptive community. Considerations include issues of stigma and discrimination, organization of mental health services, and access to social determinants of health. These issues speak to justice, among other moral and ethical considerations.

Oppression, stigma, and discrimination are major issues that impede community integration of individuals with mental illness and perpetuate health disparities (Thornicroft, 2006). People with mental illnesses have been identified to be the most devalued of all people with disabilities (Lyons and Ziviani, 1995). They face negative attitudes and discriminating behaviours, frequently from family members, co-workers, the communities they live in (Schulze and Angermeyer, 2003), and even health care providers (Drake et al., 1999; Geller, 2001). Negative perceptions include beliefs that sufferers are incompetent, unpredictable, violent, hard to talk with, less intelligent, less trustworthy, and less likely to have valuable things to say (Crisp et al., 2000; Overton and Medina, 2008). Fear of this experience is sufficient to prevent some people from seeking help, and is a factor in premature treatment discontinuation (Sirey et al., 2001). Discrimination and stigma play a role in access to social determinants of health such as access to housing (Forchuk et al., 2006a,b), employment (Baldwin and Marcus, 2006; Shied, 2005), and friends (Alexander and Link, 2003).

Other community factors also affect the potential for community integration. Availability and organization of mental health services is important. For example, people in rural areas may relocate to unfamiliar and undesired urban areas solely for accessing mental health services and at times with entire families (Forchuk et al., in press). Unavailability of public transportation can also impede access to services (Forchuk et al., 2006a, in press). These are but a few examples of community level issues that affect the individual.

Discrimination and stigma also play a role in relation to public policy and the priority given (or not given) to people diagnosed with a mental illness. Public policy can have a dramatic effect on the potential for social inclusion. Forchuk, Joplin, and others (2007) described and analysed how the lack of connection between policy changes within the mental health field, housing and income support created a situation which dramatically increased the number of people with mental illnesses who have become homeless. In contrast, using a strategy to explicitly reconnect and partner mental health services with providers of housing and of income support dramatically reduced the number of people discharged from psychiatric wards to homelessness (Forchuk et al., 2008).

When problems with social inclusion occur one cannot assume that the problem is with the individual patient. A conclusion that the underlying problem is either the patient or the community will lead to very different responses and proposed interventions. Thus community level issues have significant ethical implications.

Key dilemmas in community level psychiatry

There is a myriad of potential ethical issues at the community level. Some key dilemmas include: 1) beneficence–doing good for whom?; 2) social justice and basic human rights; 3) the obligation to advocate or to 'whistle-blow', and 4) understanding ethics within legal frameworks.

1 Beneficence–doing good for whom?

When working with individual patients, it is usually clear who the identified 'patient' is. However, with a community focus this is often unclear. There may be multiple vulnerable subgroups and prioritizing the needs of one group will often disadvantage another. For example, the common focus and priority given to people with serious and persistent mental illnesses can mean that people with moderate mental health problems are unable to get services unless they deteriorate sufficiently to 'qualify'. In Ontario, Canada, a priority group for public housing has been people fleeing domestic violence. This group is almost always female and does often include people with mental illness. This seems to be a good policy and practice. However, with the current shortage of public housing, this has made it extremely difficult in many communities for others (such as men with mental illness, or intact families) to get public housing.

2 Social justice and basic human rights

Concerns about 'doing good for whom?' relate to resource allocation within a system with insufficient resources for all. This leads to issues related to social justice and basic human rights. Social justice is based on the ideal of fair distribution (Morris 2002). Essential questions to be addressed include 'which inequalities matter most' (Powers and Faden 2006) and 'is our society just?' (Davison et al., 2006). When people with mental illness are in a community without adequate food and shelter their basic human rights are arguably not being addressed (Forchuk et al., 2006b). Health care providers can contribute to this denial of basic human rights by not looking at the societal context of services. For example, discharging people from psychiatric wards to no fixed addresses has resulted in people, with no previous history of homelessness, being still homeless 6 months later or joining the sex trade to avoid homelessness (Forchuk et al., 2006c).

3 The obligation to advocate or to whistle-blow

If health care professionals witness the denial of basic human rights and other systematic concerns, do obligations follow? In some cases, this will be a part of professional codes of ethics or standards. Some workplaces put restrictions on employees regarding taking information from the workplace to a public forum. To counter this, some jurisdictions have legislation that protects 'whistle-blowers' who bring to light serious problems involving their workplace. Solutions in these situations often involve developing alliances with other groups and individuals to carry forward concerns to the political and public arenas. However, large community issues facing community psychiatric patients, such as homelessness, poverty, and lack of services, will take great efforts and time to overcome.

4 Understanding ethics within legal frameworks

Legal frameworks as well as ethical frameworks require consideration. Legal frameworks underpinning mental health acts, hospital acts, community treatment orders, health professional practices, and privacy can vary considerably, yet they form part of the context of community care. There can be tension between legal and ethical frameworks, which should be identified and addressed as best possible, including implementing legislation changes when possible and appropriate. Many people with mental illness are now entangled with the criminal justice system in myriad ways and are in the community under various conditions of parole, probation, conditional discharge, and so on. The legal system often requests various kinds of reports. Hence coercion, confidentiality and other ethical issues arise. The demands of the legal system should be weighed in relation to the patient's interests. When there is conflict between such demands and such interests, judicial demands may have to take precedence in the short-term, but if deliberation reveals that these judicial demands are ethically unsound, advocacy for legislative and other legal change as well as for related cultural change may be required.

An example of the relation between ethics and law relates to sex offenders, who in many places are now discharged from prison and remanded to mental health care. Mental health care providers may feel unprepared to provide care for these patients, may fear for the safety of community members and may be intimidated by the frequent media accounts of the horrific offences sometimes perpetrated by such patients, while recognizing their fiduciary duty to these patients. To address this set of challenges, mental health care providers and their administrators can champion wide stakeholder collaboration, such as with the police, to try to ensure public safety while keeping confidentiality breaches to the necessary minimum, and with health policy decision-makers and regulators, to try to secure and use adequate specialized resources to provide best care for these patients within legal constraints.

Conclusion

Ethics in relation to community mental health is important and complicated. Such ethics involves knowledge of general ethical approaches, such as the well-established consequentialism, deontology and virtue ethics, as well as more novel approaches, such as care ethics. Skills in bioethics are also required, such as application of principlism, as well as awareness of other bioethical approaches such as dialogical bioethics and—somewhat in contrast—benevolent paternalism. The ethical problems involved in community mental health, in relation to which these approaches can be addressed, range from relatively traditional problems, such as those of coercion, to relatively novel problems, such as those of the community as a unit of ethical analysis. Further discussion and research is required in relation to these and other relevant ethical problems, including some that have not been noted here, in order to address the rapid development of services and policies in relation to community mental health. Community mental health care providers, who may be regularly confronted with ethical problems such as those described here and who may want to seek ethical guidance in relation to these problems, can access written resources, as illustrated in the reference list of this chapter, as well as engage in multidisciplinary team discussions and in consultations by ethicists and ethics committees that are available now in some community mental health settings. Further development of such consultation and capacity building resources in the area of community mental health may be in order.

Table of summary

◆ In health care, ethical problems are commonly viewed as the tension between two or more morally defensible alternative actions, including inaction, and ethical theories such as consequentialism/utilitarianism, deontology and virtue ethics, suggest various ways of addressing and resolving such ethical problems.

◆ Bioethics involves ethics of health related matters, both clinical and other, such as in relation to health policy and research. Principlism, which is a widely used bioethical approach, consists of considerations of autonomy, beneficence, non-maleficence, and justice, in addition to context. Alternatives to principlism, such as dialogical bioethics and–somewhat in contrast–benevolent paternalism, may be helpful in bioethical decision-making, although they may not be fully independent from some principlist considerations (such as justice and beneficence, respectively).

◆ In community mental health, consideration needs to be given to both the individual person/patient as well as to the community as a unit of analysis. Issues of community integration could be related to the person/patient and/or to the broader community as a whole.

◆ Privacy, confidentiality, coercion, and conflicts of duty are key sets of dilemmas in the practice of mental health care in the community.

◆ Community level considerations include: 1) beneficence–doing good for whom?; 2) social justice and basic human rights; 3) the obligation to advocate or to 'whistle-blow', and 4) understanding ethics within legal frameworks.

Further reading

Backlar, P. and Cutler, D.L. (eds). (2002). *Ethics in Community Mental Health Care: Commonplace Concerns*. New York: Kluwer/Plenum.

Blackburn, S. (2001). *Ethics: A Very Short Introduction*. Oxford: Oxford University Press.

References

Alexander, L.A. and Link, B.G. (2003). The impact of contact stigmatizing attitudes toward people with mental illness. *Journal of Mental Health*, **12**, 271–89.

Baldwin, M.L. and Marcus, S.C. (2006). Perceived and measured stigma among workers with serious mental illness. *Psychiatric Services*, **57**, 388–92.

Beauchamp, T.L. and Childress, J.F. (2009). *Principles of Biomedical Ethics*, 6th edn. New York: Oxford University Press.

Crisp, A. H., Gelder, M. G., Rix, S., Meltzer, H., and Rowlands, O. (2000). Stigmatisation of people with mental illnesses. *British Journal of Psychiatry*, **177**, 4–7.

Davison, C., Edwards, N., Robinson, S. (2006). *Social justice: a means to an end, an end in itself*. Ottawa: Canadian Nurses Association. Available at: http://www.cna-nurses.ca/CNA/documents/pdf/publications/Social_Justice_e.pdf (accessed 29 August 2009).

Dershowitz, A. (2004). *Rights from Wrongs: A Secular Theory of the Origins of Rights*. New York: Basic Books.

Diamond, R.J. and Wikler, D. (1985). Ethical problems in the community treatment of the chronically mentally ill. In: Stein, L.I. and Test, M.A. (eds.) *Training in community living model: a decade of experience*, pp. 169–96. San Francisco, CA: Josey-Bass.

Drake, R.E., McHugo, G.J., Bedout, R.R., Becker, D.R., Marris, M., Bond, G.R., *et al*. (1999). A randomized clinical trial of supported employment for inner-city patients with severe mental disorders. *Archives of General Psychiatry*, **56**, 62.

Forchuk, C., Nelson, G., and Hall, G.B. (2006a). It's important to be proud of the place you live in: Housing problems and preferences of psychiatric survivors. *Perspectives in Psychiatric Care*, **42**, 42–52.

Forchuk, C., Ward-Griffin, C., Csiernik, R., and Turner, K. (2006b). Surviving the tornado of mental illness: Psychiatric survivors' experiences of getting, losing, and keeping housing. *Psychiatric Services*, **57**, 558–62.

Forchuk, C., Russell, G., Kingston-Macclure, S., Turner, S., and Dill, S. (2006c). From psychiatric ward to the streets and shelters. *Journal of Psychiatric and Mental Health Nursing*, **13**, 301–8.

Forchuk, C., Joplin, L., Schofield, R., Csiernik, R., Gorlick, C., and Turner, K. (2007). Housing, income support and mental health: Points of disconnection. *Health Research Policy Systems*, **5**, 14.

Forchuk, C., Macclure, S.K., Van Beers, M., Smith, C., Csiernik, R., Hoch, J., *et al*. (2008). Developing and testing an intervention to prevent homelessness among individuals discharged from psychiatric wards to shelters and 'No Fixed Address'. *Journal of Psychiatric and Mental Health Nursing*, **15**, 569–75.

Forchuk, C., Montgomery, P., Berman, H., Ward-Griffin, C., Csiernik, R., Gorlick, C., *et al*. (2010). Gaining Ground, Losing Ground: The Paradoxes of Rural Homelessness. *Canadian Journal of Nursing Research* **42**(2), 138–152.

Geller, J.L. (2001). Taking issue: Ain't no such thing as a schizophrenic. *Psychiatric Services*, **52**, 715.

Holloway, F. (1996). Community psychiatric care: from libertarianism to coercion. Moral panic and mental health policy in Britain. *Health Care Analysis*, **4**, 235–43.

Jonsen, A.R. (1998). *The Birth of Bioethics*. New York: Oxford University Press.

Jonsen, A.R. (2000). *A Short History of Medical Ethics*. New York: Oxford University Press.

Lloyd, G.E.R. (ed). (1983). *Hippocratic Writings*. London: Penguin.

Lyons, M. and Ziviani, J. (1995). Stereotypes, stigma and mental illness: Learning from fieldwork experiences. *American Journal of Occupational Therapy*, **49**, 1002–8.

MacIntyre, A.A. (1998). *Short History of Ethics: A History of Moral Philosophy from the Homeric Age to the Twentieth Century*, 2nd edn. London: Routledge.

Morris, P. (2002). The capabilities perspective. A framework for social justice. *Families in Society*, **83**, 365–73.

Overton, S.L. and Medina, S.L. (2008). The stigma of mental illness. *Journal of Counseling and Development*, **86**, 143–51.

Powers, M. and Faden, R. (2006). *Social justice: the moral foundations of public health and health policy*. New York: Oxford University Press.

Roberts, G., Davenport, S., Holloway, F., and Tattan, T. (eds.) (2006). *Enabling Recovery: The Principles and Practice of Rehabilitation Psychiatry*. London: Gaskell.

Roberts, L.W. and Dyer, A.R. (2004). *Concise Guide to Ethics in Mental Health Care*. Washington, DC: American Psychiatric Publishing.

Rose, N. (1998). Governing risky individuals: the role of psychiatry in new regimes of control. *Psychiatry, Psychology and Law*, **5**, 177–95.

Rudnick, A. (2001). A meta-ethical critique of care ethics. *Theoretical Medicine*, **22**, 505–17.

Rudnick, A. (2002). The ground of dialogical bioethics. *Health Care Analysis*, **10**, 391–402.

Rudnick, A. (2007). Processes and pitfalls of dialogical bioethics. *Health Care Analysis*, **15**, 123–35.

Schulze, B. and Angermeyer, M. (2003). Subjective experiences of stigma: schizophrenic patients, their relatives and mental health professionals. *Social Science & Medicine*, 56, 299–312.

Shied, T. L. (2005). Stigma as a barrier to employment: Mental disability and the Americans with Disabilities Act. *International Journal of Law and Psychiatry*, 28, 670–90.

Sirey, J.A., Bruce, M.L., Alexopoulos, G.S., Perlick, D.A., Raue, P., Friedman, S.J., *et al.* (2001). Perceived stigma as a predictor of treatment discontinuation in young and older outpatients with depression. *American Journal of Psychiatry*, **158**, 479–81.

Szmukler, G. and Appelbaum, P. (2008). Treatment pressures, leverage, coercion and compulsion in mental health care. *Journal of Mental Health*, **17**, 233–44.

Szmukler, G. and Bloch, S. (1998) Family involvement in the care of people with psychoses: an ethical argument. *British Journal of Psychiatry*, **171**, 401–5.

Thornicroft, G. (2006). *Shunned: discrimination against people with mental illness*. New York: Oxford University Press.

CHAPTER 26

International human rights and community mental health

Oliver Lewis and Peter Bartlett

Introduction

This chapter concerns human rights relating to people with mental health problems living in the community. It seeks to explain how international human rights law can work in a variety of ways to foster a person's equal right to live in the community on an equal basis, with choices equal to others.

Each individual country may have legislation and policy to underpin community living. These may include social security payments and personal budgets to help people live independently, housing arrangements, provision of personal assistance and other supports, as well as non-discrimination provisions relating to vocational training and employment, and more widely to the provision of all goods and services. Such legislation and policy are essential in setting and regulating standards of human rights at the domestic level. These arrangements differ widely between countries, and for practical reasons a comparative analysis lies outside the scope of this chapter.

Instead, this chapter concerns the layers of international law and standards that sit above domestic law, directing and influencing domestic law and policy in order to bring about positive changes to the lived experiences of persons with mental health problems living in the community. The second section of the chapter ('International human rights law') is a primer on the treaties, how they are monitored, and how they apply to people with mental health problems living in the community. The third section ('The dawn of a new era?') introduces elements of the United Nations Convention on the Rights of Persons with Disabilities (hereinafter 'CRPD'),[1] and examines its philosophical underpinnings, the obligations on the State to implement it, and sets out its innovative features at the domestic level to coordinate policy action and to monitor implementation. It also outlines the Optional Protocol to

the CRPD and the international mechanism established to monitor State compliance.[2] The fourth section ('Human rights underpinning community mental health') explains some of the CRPD rights which impact upon community mental health, and the next three sections ('Right to health', 'Right to live in the community', and 'Right to legal capacity') provide an analysis of three of these rights in more depth. The conclusion in the final section suggests actions which community mental health practitioners could take in order to ensure that the State respects, protects, and fulfils the rights of people with mental health problems in the community.

International human rights law

International law flows from agreements made between States in intergovernmental organizations such as the Council of Europe[3] and the United Nations (hereinafter 'UN'). International law is, usually, not imposed on a State without its consent. That is to say, States take part in formulating the standards and take part in monitoring the implementation of those standards too. Quite how these various laws and standards work depends on the legal instrument in question. The most important laws are treaties which States (by which we mean the legal entity recognized in international law, usually the national government in federalized countries—thus,

---

1 Convention on the Rights of Persons with Disabilities adopted by the UN General Assembly, New York, 13 December 2006, ref: Doc.A/61/611. A full text of the CRPD may be found at http://www.un.org/disabilities.

2 Optional Protocol to the Convention on the Rights of Persons with Disabilities adopted by the UN General Assembly, New York, 13 December 2006, ref: Doc.A/61/611

3 The Council of Europe (CoE) should not be confused with the European Union (EU). The EU has 27 Member States. While in recent years the EU is becoming more engaged with human rights issues and with health law, it was based in an economic union, and its key features continue to reflect that: EU Member States have open economic borders that preclude favouritism relating to the provision of people, money, goods, and services. The Council of Europe, by comparison, has 47 Member States from across Europe, and includes a wide variety of countries not members of the EU (e.g. Russia, Turkey, the Balkans, the Caucasus). Its remit is to promote and protect democracy, the rule of law, and human rights.

for example, the United Kingdom rather than Scotland or England) have negotiated between themselves. Sometimes civil society organizations have participated in the negotiations. Once these instruments have been adopted, they become open for signature: States may **sign** the treaty, meaning that the State must refrain from acts which would defeat the object and purpose of the treaty.[4] States may also **ratify** the treaty, which means that the treaty will be legally binding in that jurisdiction if it has come into force.[5]

Modifications or additions to human rights treaties may also be adopted and these are usually called 'protocols' or 'optional protocols'. Once ratified, a treaty (and/or its protocols) is binding on the State which that ratifies it, although the mechanism of implementation and enforcement will depend on the treaty. The text of a treaty determines the obligations on States to implement it. This will have knock-on effects for public bodies, private entities, and individual people, since States have duties to respect, protect, and fulfil the rights. Among other things, the State will need to enforce the law (e.g. through its criminal and civil domestic legislation, institutions, and procedures). It is the State that will be held to account under international law, not any particular individual, local authority, or health care service. It is therefore incumbent upon States to ensure that it adopts and amends legislation and policies in line with international human rights standards, and to ensure that these laws and policies are implemented, and that the implementation is independently monitored.

There is a considerable array of international law. People with mental health problems are meant to benefit from these provisions as much—or as little—as anyone else.[6] Thus, for example, a girl does not cease to benefit from the UN Convention on the Rights of the Child because she has a mental health problem. A wide array of international law is relevant to people with mental health problems.

Obvious examples include the International Covenant on Civil and Political Rights (ICCPR),[7] which sets out the right to life, to freedom from torture, to expression and association, freedom from interference with private and family life, and the right to vote. The ICCPR's sister treaty is the International Covenant on Economic, Social and Cultural Rights,[8] which provides, among others, for the right to the enjoyment of the highest attainable standard of physical and mental health,[9] the right to healthy working conditions,[10] social insurance,[11] adequate standard of living and adequacy of housing,[12] education[13] and participation in cultural life.[14] All of these rights are fundamental to enable people with mental health

problems to live in the community. As will be laid out below, they are given further focus in the CRPD.

The treaties covering children,[15] girls and women,[16] people of racial and ethnic minorities,[17] and migrant workers[18] all apply to persons with mental health problems. So too does the treaty dealing with the prohibition of torture, cruel, inhuman and degrading treatment or punishment, whose ambit covers the inappropriate use of psychiatric treatments, restraints and seclusion.[19]

Some of the UN human rights treaties allow individuals, after having exhausted domestic remedies, to take their cases to the relevant treaty body which sits as a quasi-judicial body to adjudicate in individual cases.[20] None of these treaty bodies, however, has developed any significant jurisprudence regarding people with mental health problems.[21] This is unfortunate, as these treaties have considerable potential scope to provide a rights-based approach to support the development of community services and challenge the determinants of mental ill health. That said, the legal technicalities

---

4 See Vienna Convention on the Law of Treaties, 23 May 1969, Art. 18.

5 See Vienna Convention on the Law of Treaties, 23 May 1969, Art. 14.

6 In this chapter, the term 'mental health problems' is taken to include anyone labelled with psychosocial disabilities, mental disorders or mental illness.

7 Adopted by General Assembly resolution 2200A (XXI) on 16 December 1966.

8 International Covenant on Economic, Social and Cultural Rights, adopted by General Assembly resolution 2200A (XXI) on 16 December 1966.

9 Art. 12.

10 Art 7.

11 Art. 9.

12 Art 11.

13 Art 13.

14 Art 15.

15 Convention on the Rights of the Child (Adopted by General Assembly resolution 44/25 on 20 November 1989). See particularly Article 23 which sets out rights specifically for children with physical or mental disabilities and which obliges States to carry out a range of actions to promote the child's self-reliance and facilitate the child's active participation in the community.

16 Convention on the Elimination of All Forms of Discrimination against Women (Adopted by General Assembly resolution 34/180 on 18 December 1979).

17 International Convention on the Elimination of All Forms of Racial Discrimination (Adopted by General Assembly resolution 2106 (XX) on 21 December 1965).

18 International Convention on the Protection of the Rights of All Migrant Workers and Members of Their Families, Adopted by General Assembly resolution 45/158 on 18 December 1990.

19 Convention against Torture and Other Cruel, Inhuman or Degrading Treatment or Punishment, adopted by General Assembly resolution 39/46 on 10 December 1984.

20 In addition to the Optional Protocol to the CRPD, the Human Rights Committee may receive individual communications relating to States parties to the First Optional Protocol to the International Covenant on Civil and Political Rights; the Committee on the Elimination of Discrimination Against Women may receive individual complaints relating to States parties to the Optional Protocol to the Convention on the Elimination of Discrimination Against Women; the Committee against Torture may consider individual communications relating to States parties who have made the necessary declaration under Article 22 of the Convention Against Torture; the Commimttee for the Elimination of Racial Discrimination may consider individual communications relating to States parties who have made the necessary declaration under article 14 of the Convention on the Elimination of Racial Discrimination; and the Convention on Migrant Workers contains provision for allowing individual communications to be considered by the Committee on Migrant Workers and these provisions will become operative when 10 States parties have made the necessary declaration under article 77.

21 Although there have been very few individual complaints brought to the UN treaty monitoring bodies which address concerns of people with mental health problems, it is worth noting that several treaty bodies have issued interpretations of their treaties which address the rights of persons with disabilities. See, for example, Committee on the Elimination of Discrimination against Women, General Recommendation No. 18 (1991) on 'Disabled women'; Committee on Economic, Social and Cultural Rights, General Comment No. 5 (1994) on 'Persons with Disabilities'; and Committee on the Rights of the Child, General Comment No. 9 (2006) on 'The Rights of Children with Disabilities'. Given the interpretation in Article 1 of the UN Convention on the Rights of Persons with Disabilities, references in international law relating to 'disability' can be interpreted as including people with mental health problems also.

of obtaining a remedy can be complex, and the practical barriers to accessing justice can be overwhelming.

Alongside the global UN mechanisms are regional mechanisms to protect human rights. These include the African system, the Inter-American system, and the European system. The European Convention on Human Rights and Fundamental Freedoms (hereinafter 'ECHR'), is particularly important, both because its jurisprudence is more developed than courts in the other regions, and because the ECHR can be invoked and is largely enforceable in domestic courts of the 47 Member States of the Council of Europe. This chapter does not discuss all potentially relevant international law, and readers concerned by specific client groups or human rights issues will need to become acquainted with the international law that relates to their specific concern. The jurisprudence of the ECHR to date has concerned primarily issues relating to detention rather than preventing it, and analyses have been dealt with elsewhere.[22]

Instead, the focus of this chapter is the UN Convention on the Rights of Persons with Disabilities (hereinafter 'CRPD'). Unlike the European Convention on Human Rights which covers human rights broadly, the CRPD focuses specifically on the rights of persons with disabilities. Instead of defining disability, the CRPD defines 'persons with disabilities', to 'include those who have long-term physical, mental, intellectual or sensory impairments which in interaction with various barriers may hinder their full and effective participation in society on an equal basis with others'.[23] It is without doubt that persons with mental health problems fall within the ambit of the CRPD.

One of the reasons that the CRPD came into existence is the global gap between rights rhetoric and lived reality. The CRPD itself points out that international human rights instruments have for many years 'proclaimed and agreed that everyone is entitled to all the rights and freedoms set forth therein, without distinction of any kind',[24] yet the international community is '[c]oncerned that, despite these various instruments and undertakings, persons with disabilities continue to face barriers in their participation as equal members of society and violations of their human rights in all parts of the world'.[25] These statements are likely to resonate with anyone working in mental health systems.

Two reasons for the implementation failure of pre-CRPD human rights treaties are inadequate coordination at the domestic policy level and inadequate independent monitoring of the implementation. The drafters of the CRPD were well aware of these policy failures and ensured that the new treaty binds States to establish implementation mechanisms. These include a governmental coordinating body to facilitate activities relevant to the implementation of the Convention across different ministries and departments, and down into regions and localities.[26] The CRPD also places an obligation on States to establish or designate an independent mechanism (such as an ombudsman or a national human rights institution) to promote and protect the rights of persons with disabilities and

to monitor the domestic implementation of the Convention.[27] States are required to ensure that persons with disabilities and their representative organizations have opportunities to be involved and participate in this monitoring process.[28]

People with mental health problems can play a part in monitoring the CRPD's implementation. The CRPD also makes it a treaty obligation to 'closely consult with and actively involve' people with disabilities (which includes people with mental health problems) '[i]n the development and implementation of legislation and policies to implement the [CRPD], and in other decision-making processes concerning issues relating to persons with disabilities'.[29] This provision echoes a statement in the CRPD's preamble, that 'persons with disabilities should have the opportunity to be actively involved in decision-making processes about policies and programmes, including those directly concerning them'.[30]

At the UN level, the CRPD establishes a treaty monitoring body, the 'Committee on the Rights of Persons with Disabilities',[31] which considers national reports provided by governments and assesses overall compliance by the individual countries.[32] These observations can be influenced other people in those countries—including by organizations of persons with mental health problems or advocacy groups—who may submit their own reports in advance of the Committee's deliberations. The Committee's concluding observations are not legally binding, but are public documents which can be used to advocate politically for laws, policies, and practices to be changed. The Committee also adjudicates on individual complaints submitted to it, from people in States which have ratified the Optional Protocol to the CRPD. In this context, the Committee will behave in a fashion broadly analogous to a court, determining the admissibility and merits of the case before it.

The dawn of a new era?

The CRPD was adopted by the UN General Assembly in December 2006, and it entered into force after 20 ratifications in May 2008. The then UN Secretary General, Kofi Annan, described the adoption of the CRPD as, 'the dawn of a new era—an era in which disabled people will no longer have to endure the discriminatory practices and attitudes that have been permitted to prevail for all too long' (UN Press Release, 2006). The Convention signals an end to a paradigm where people with mental health problems are treated as objects: objects of treatment, management, charity, pity and fear. The new era brings with it a shift in thinking about disability and mental health, one in which people with mental health problems are viewed not as objects, but as subjects: of human rights on an equal basis with others.

Whether the Convention will be meaningful for people remains to be seen. Its success will be largely dependent on whether a variety of stakeholders—including community mental health practitioners—embrace its provisions. Its success will also be dependent on the effectiveness of governmental coordination and on independent monitoring, as noted earlier. Whatever the future

---

22 For an extended discussion of the ECHR jurisprudence relating to people with mental health problems (and people with intellectual disabilities), see Bartlett et al. (2007) (also available on Googlebooks).

23 CRPD, Art. 1.

24 CRPD, perambulatory para (b).

25 CRPD, perambulatory para (k).

26 CRPD, Art. 33(1).

27 CRPD, Art. 33(2).

28 CRPD, Art. 33(3).

29 CRPD, Art. 4(3).

30 CPRD, perambulatory para. (o).

31 CRPD, Art. 34.

32 CRPD, Arts. 35 and 36.

holds in store, the text marks a significant departure from previous human rights instruments for a variety of reasons.

People with disabilities, including global and regional organizations comprising people with mental health problems, were themselves directly involved in the negotiations leading to the Convention.[33] UN Member States were the official negotiators of the CRPD, and they are the duty-bearers to ensure its implementation. That said, persons with disabilities, including people with mental health problems, were key to shaping the text in a way which was unprecedented at the UN. This involvement has resulted in a Convention with great specificity, relevance, and ownership by the disabilities movement. Due to the involvement in and ownership of the process, the CRPD may be more likely than other treaties to be implemented.

The CRPD uses the language and approach of classic human rights expressly and unreservedly in a treaty relating to people with disabilities. Previously, treaties that adopted a clear human rights approach either included people with disabilities by implication, or excluded them specifically (the provision allowing detention of people with mental health problems is an obvious example).[34] There have been other international instruments—of a lower rank than treaties—that have focused on the rights of persons with disabilities. Although these documents used some human rights rhetoric, they pre-supposed that considerably greater control, regulation and substituted decision-making was appropriate for people with mental health problems than for the population as a whole. The UN Mental Illness Principles serve as an example here.[35]

By comparison, the CRPD contains a set of guiding principles, including the 'freedom to make one's own choices' (and by implication the dignity of risk to make one's own mistakes on an equal basis with others),[36] '[r]espect for difference and acceptance of persons with disabilities as part of human diversity and humanity',[37] and the principle that people with disabilities should enjoy '[f]ull and effective participation and inclusion in society'.[38] These philosophical underpinnings come from a human rights model and sit more comfortably with other UN human rights treaties than with the pre-existing specialist instruments which, as noted above, tended to assume that rights needed to be lowered downwards to justify the removal of rights—of autonomy, of liberty, of physical and mental integrity—for people with mental health problems.

In addition to principles, the CRPD articulates a list of general obligations on States in order to ensure compliance with the CRPD's provisions. These obligations include adopting appropriate legislation and taking other measures in order to implement the Convention,[39] and abolishing laws which constitute discrimination.[40] The obligations also include taking 'all appropriate measures to eliminate discrimination on the basis of disability by any person, organization or private enterprise',[41] and 'to take into account the protection and promotion of the human rights of persons with disabilities in all policies and programmes', not only disability policies or mental health policies.[42] Of particular relevance to community mental health practitioners is the general obligation on training on CRPD rights for staff working with people with disabilities, 'so as to better provide the assistance and services guaranteed by those rights'.[43]

One of the top concerns of civil society organizations during the negotiations leading up to the Convention was institutionalization of people with mental health problems and people with other types of disabilities. Removing people from society and placing them in long-term closed institutions is closely connected with other human rights concerns, namely treatment without consent and sometimes by force, as well as the removal of a person's legal capacity rendering them legally unable to make choices about their own lives. The gradual closure of residential institutions and establishing in parallel a variety of community-based services are the focus of this book as a whole, and are of prime importance in the CRPD. In the next sections we will outline how community mental health practitioners can use the CRPD to support independent living.

Human rights underpinning community mental health

This section lays out in general terms the rights contained in the CRPD. The following three sections address provisions which may be of particular relevance for the concerns of community mental health practitioners and their clients.

The CRPD contains a classic array of what have been termed 'civil and political rights' which exist in the ICCPR (see earlier 'International human rights law' section of the chapter), such as the right to liberty (Article 14 of the CRPD) and integrity of the person (Article 17), rights to freedom of expression (Article 21) and privacy (Article 22). The CRPD echoes the ICCPR and the UN Convention against Torture by containing an absolute prohibition on torture, cruel, inhuman, and degrading treatment or punishment. In addition, it outlaws medical and scientific experimentation without consent (Article 15). It sets out rights to equal recognition before the law and to legal capacity (Article 12—a topic which we will address the section 'Right to legal capacity') and access to justice (Article 13). It provides the right to vote and participate in public affairs (Article 29). These are rights that already, at least to a considerable degree, apply to people with mental health problems, through pre-existing international laws. These civil and political rights generally date from 18th-century Western thought, and are generally rights to be free from State intervention. They are potentially significant for persons with mental health problems

---

33 These included the World Network of Users and Survivors of Psychiatry, which, in conjunction with many other non-governmental organizations acted in concert within the International Disability Caucus.

34 See Article 5(1)(e) of the European Convention on Human Rights and Fundamental Freedoms, which suspends the right to liberty for several groups including 'persons of unsound mind'.

35 'Principles for the protection of persons with mental illness and the improvement of mental health care', Adopted by UN General Assembly resolution 46/119 of 17 December 1991.

36 CRPD, Art. 3(a).

37 CRPD, Art. 3(d).

38 CRPD, Art. 3(c).

39 CRPD, Art. 4(1)(a).

---

40 CRPD, Art. 4(1)(b).

41 CRPD, Art. 4(1)(e) (emphasis added).

42 CRPD, Art. 4(1)(c) (emphasis added). This means, for example, that the rights of persons with mental health problems need to be considered not merely in the context of mental health law or legal capacity law, but also in policy areas diverse as housing, travel, insurance, energy, education, transport and international development.

43 CRPD, Art. 4(1)(i).

in the community. A reduction of the power of the State to detain an individual in a psychiatric hospital, for example, is in many ways a pre-requisite for a person with a mental health problem to maintain their life in the community, and Article 14 of the CRPD provides a particularly strong statement framed as a right.

These are sometimes called 'negative rights'—that the State must stop, refrain from doing something, or prevent something from happening. Some people argue that civil and political rights do not cost much money. This assumption is tested by the CRPD. In order to protect people with disabilities against ill-treatment (disability hate crime, for example) a State must actively ensure that there is an adequate criminal law, as well as fund and manage a police force and a justice system including prisons and probation services and the like. The CRPD also places an obligation to provide 'reasonable accommodation'[44] to people with disabilities in order to equalize their rights upwards on an equal basis with others. All of this comes with a price tag. The CRPD further contains a variety of what have traditionally been labelled 'economic, social and cultural rights'. Some of these reflect earlier treaty rights (particularly in the ICESCR, see earlier 'International human rights law' section). These include the right to an adequate standard of living, and the right to health. However, a number of these rights go beyond previously-articulated international law. The right to health and the right to live in the community will be discussed in greater detail in the following sections 'Right to health' and 'Right to live in the community', but it is appropriate also to provide a brief overview of the broader range of rights, as they work in concert with the right to health and the right to community life to provide the legal structure for a new era of community mental health.

The CRPD protects the right to relationships, sexual activity and to family life (Article 23). While other international instruments protect these rights in general, the CRPD provides a detailed articulation of these rights, including the right to decide the number and spacing of one's children, the right to age-appropriate sexual education and information, the right to retain one's fertility, and the right to assistance from the State in the performance of child-rearing duties. While the State retains the right to remove children when it is in the best interests of those children, such removal may not be on the basis of the disability of the parents.

The CRPD also contains the right to education, understood as inclusive education in the general school system, rather than segregated education in facilities only for children with disabilities. It also contains a parallel right to individualized educational support in environments that maximize academic and social development.[45] There are provisions of particular importance for children labelled with mental health problems or behavioural problems, as well as those with intellectual or learning disabilities who are at risk of exclusion from mainstream educational settings.[46]

The CRPD rejects 'special education' where children with disabilities are taught together using different curricula than regular schools and achieving lower educational outcomes. Instead the CRPD calls for an inclusive educational system for all, echoing the preamble to the text which talks about the existing and potential contributions which people with disabilities can make to the well-being and diversity of communities.[47] This is underpinned by one of the principles which must be read into each of the Convention's provisions, namely a '[r]espect for difference and acceptance of persons with disabilities as part of human diversity and humanity'.[48]

In addition to the right to education, the CRPD sets out the right to work and employment. These rights are buttressed by specific requirements that non-discrimination programmes be introduced to cover 'conditions of recruitment, hiring and employment, continuance of employment, career advancement and safe and healthy working conditions',[49] that reasonable accommodation be made of the different needs of employees that flow from their disabilities,[50] and that people with disabilities be employed in the public sector.[51]

The concept of reasonable accommodation is defined in the CRPD as the 'necessary and appropriate modification and adjustments not imposing a disproportionate or undue burden, where needed in a particular case, to ensure to persons with disabilities the enjoyment or exercise on an equal basis with others of all human rights and fundamental freedoms'.[52] The CRPD creates State obligations to equalize upwards so that persons with disabilities can access all rights on an equal basis with others. For example, the right to vote will be meaningful for some people with mental health problems only if the State allows support people into the voting booth, dismantles legal barriers such as deprivation of legal capacity,[53] and removes physical barriers which prevent persons with disabilities from voting: this might mean providing for kerb-side voting so that a person with social anxiety need not leave their car, for example.

The chapter now turns to examine in some detail three clusters of rights of particular relevance to community mental health practitioners: the right to health, the right to live in the community, and the right to legal capacity.

Right to health

The right to health is located in Article 12 of the International Covenant on Economic, Social and Cultural Rights and finds its place in Article 25 of the CRPD. This provision provides that States 'recognize that persons with disabilities have the right to the enjoyment of the highest attainable standard of health without discrimination on the basis of disability', which by definition includes on the basis of a mental health problem. Specifically, States should '[p]rovide persons with disabilities with the same range, quality and standard of free or affordable health care and programmes as

---

44 CRPD, Art. 2.

45 CRPD, Art. 24.

46 For an application of the right to education for children with disabilities, see *Mental Disability Advocacy Center v. Bulgaria*, decided under the European Social Charter by the European Committee on Social Rights, October 2008. For a report which sets out the right for children with disabilities to inclusive education, see Inclusion International, 'Better Education for All When We're Included Too', 2009; and for an overview of how the right to education applies to children with disabilities, see *The right to education of persons with disabilities*, Report to the UN

Human Rights Council of the Special Rapporteur on the Right to Education Vernor Munoz (19 February 2007).

47 CRPD, perambulatory paragraph (m).

48 CRPD, Art. 3(d).

49 Art. 27.(1)(a).

50 Art. 27.(1)(i).

51 Art. 27(1)(g).

52 CRPD, Art. 2.

53 See the European Court of Human Rights judgment in the case of *Alajos Kiss v. Hungary*, Application No. 38832/06, judgment 20 May 2010.

provided to other persons'.[54] This includes sexual and reproductive health and population-based public health programmes. The CRPD also mandates the provision—although not the forcible provision—of 'health services needed by persons with disabilities specifically because of their disabilities, including early identification and intervention as appropriate, and services designed to minimize and prevent further disabilities, including among children and older persons'.[55] Taken together with Article 19 of the Convention which sets out the right to live in the community, it is no stretch to claim that Article 25 requires mental health services to be available in community settings.

Article 25 of the CRPD lays out entitlements to ensure the highest attainable standard of physical and mental health. As Professor Paul Hunt (then UN Special Rapporteur on the Right to Health) stated a year before the CRPD was adopted, such entitlements for persons with mental health problems include obligations on each State to:

> ensure a full package of community-based mental health care and support services conducive to health, dignity, and inclusion, including medication, psychotherapy, ambulatory services, hospital care for acute admissions, residential facilities, rehabilitation for persons with psychiatric disabilities, programmes to maximize the independence and skills of persons with intellectual disabilities, supported housing and employment, income support, inclusive and appropriate education for children with intellectual disabilities, and respite care for families looking after a person with a mental disability 24 hours a day. In this way, unnecessary institutionalization can be avoided.[56]

This language anticipates that of Article 19 of the CRPD (which is examined in the next section of this chapter) in setting out a range of community alternatives which need to be provided so as to avoid institutionalization.

Professor Hunt picks up on a crucial point for community mental health practitioners, namely that 'the right to health includes an entitlement to the underlying determinants of health, including adequate sanitation, safe water and adequate food and shelter. Persons with mental health problems are disproportionately affected by poverty, which is usually characterized by deprivations of these entitlements'.[57] In some countries institutions provide water, food and shelter where such necessities may not be available to a person with mental health problems in the community. That such basic elements to sustain life are provided in institutions but not in the community is no justification for the existence of, and reliance on, institutions. In localities where mental health services are institutional in nature, the language of human rights provides a tool for users of mental health services and those who care for them to advocate for access to the full range of human rights on an equal basis with others in the community. In this sense the right to health goes well beyond access to treatments for mental health problems.

Health services are classically considered to within the 'economic, social or cultural rights' grouping, and as such, the right is subject to 'progressive realization'. This means that States must take demonstrable steps year-on-year to progressively realize the full implementation of the right to health, so that progress can be measured.[58] The right to health includes entitlements, ensuring that people with mental health problems have access to health care services, including services which assist in recovery from mental ill health. As well as entitlements, the right to health also contains freedoms. For people with mental health problems, freedom often means that others should respect a decision to consent to or refuse mental health treatment. Professor Hunt considers forced psychiatric treatment to be 'one of the most important human rights issues relating to mental disability',[59] which is 'intimately connected with a vital element of the right to health: the freedom to control one's health and body'.[60]

The CRPD makes specific reference to the concept of 'consent to treatment' in two places, first by providing that 'no one shall be subjected without his or her free consent to medical or scientific experimentation'.[61] This prohibition sits in the provision setting out the absolute ban on torture and other forms of ill-treatment. Second, consent to treatment is set out in the provision on the right to health, an element of which is that States should '[r]equire health professionals to provide care of the same quality to persons with disabilities as to others, including on the basis of free and informed consent'.[62] This right should be achieved by a variety of activities including human rights awareness-raising,[63] training and standard-setting. In the context of community mental health, it may be helpful to read this provision jointly with the provision prohibiting discrimination on the basis of disability.[64] Given this combination, it is difficult to see that any infringement on the right of any patient to consent would be justified for people with mental health problems, when it would not be so justified for people without such a condition. On this basis, community treatment orders—judicially imposed orders to accept psychiatric treatment in the community—must become suspect, at least when they concern people with capacity to consent to treatment: there is no comparable mechanism for somatic treatments. At least at first glance, it is highly doubtful that psychiatric treatments can be imposed in the community (see Chapter 27, this volume). Any reliance on incapacity as a ground for restricting the right to consent needs to take into account the right to equality before the law, discussed in the following section.

Of direct relevance to community mental health practitioners, the CRPD obliges States to ensure that health services are provided 'as close as possible to people's own communities, including in rural areas'.[65] It is this vision of community living to which the chapter now turns.

54 CRPD, Art. 25(a).

55 CRPD Art. 25(b).

56 Report of the Special Rapporteur on the right of everyone to the enjoyment of the highest attainable standard of physical and mental health, Paul Hunt to the UN Commission on Human Rights (2005), Ref: E/CN.4/2005/51, para. 43.

57 Hunt, para. 45.

58 CRPD, Art. 4(2).

59 Hunt, para. 83.

60 Ibid.

61 CRPD, Art. 15(1).

62 CRPD, Art. 25(d).

63 This wording links with Article 9 of the CRPD which sets out awareness-raising obligations throughout society of the rights of persons with disabilities, including people with mental health problems.

64 CRPD Art. 5.

65 CRPD Art. 25(c).

Right to live in the community

An innovative feature of the CRPD is that unlike other human rights treaties, it is both specific and absolute about inclusion. Article 19 of the CRPD obliges States to 'recognize the equal right of all persons with disabilities to live in the community, with choices equal to others'. The article further specifies that States 'shall take effective and appropriate measures to facilitate full enjoyment by persons with disabilities of this right and their full inclusion and participation in the community,' including ensuring the following three particular things:

a) Persons with disabilities have the opportunity to choose their place of residence and where and with whom they live on an equal basis with others and are not obliged to live in a particular living arrangement;

b) Persons with disabilities have access to a range of in-home, residential and other community support services, including personal assistance necessary to support living and inclusion in the community, and to prevent isolation or segregation from the community;

c) Community services and facilities for the general population are available on an equal basis to persons with disabilities and are responsive to their needs.

Living in the community does not operate in isolation, and other CRPD provisions should be flagged to ensure that people are included into the community rather than stuck at home, as isolated and bored at home as in an institution. The right to personal mobility (Article 20), the right to work and employment (Article 27), the right to participation in cultural life (Article 30), and the right to be free from exploitation and abuse (Article 16) are all relevant. These rights, too, are not new, having been specified in a number of international instruments.[66] But a problematic feature of these pre-CRPD instruments, however, is that the right to live in the community is couched with caveats and qualifications which are have little relevance to people with mental health problems. For example, the UN Mental Illness Principles speak about the 'least restrictive environment', a concept which is meaningless in countries where the only service is institutional: the least restrictive is concurrently the most restrictive.[67] Similarly the 'least restrictive or intrusive treatment' might be the most restrictive where only one treatment is on offer.

These phrases are nowhere to be found in the CRPD, with a corresponding change in tone. While it might be overstating the case to say that the CRPD reads as a clarion call announcing the dignity and social equality of people with mental health problems and pronouncing the end of stigma, it is markedly stronger than any previous international human rights treaty, with a philosophical muscularity absent in previous disability or mental health-specific instruments.

Right to legal capacity

The CRPD provides a new approach to equality before the law, by significantly restricting the scope of traditional decision-making regimes.[68] The preamble to the CRPD itself recognizes the 'importance for persons with disabilities of their individual autonomy and independence, including the freedom to make their own choices'.[69]

Comprehensive and routine deprivations of rights based on blanket findings of 'incapacity' (often, historically and to this day in some parts of the world, based on remarkably flimsy evidence consisting little more than a psychiatric diagnosis) should be a thing of the past. In many jurisdictions, the law allows the relatives of a person with mental health problems, or a local government official, to apply to a court to have that person's legal capacity restricted partially or deprived totally. The person is placed under (what in many countries is called) guardianship of someone else who is empowered to take decisions for and on behalf of the adult with mental health problems. Owing to practical difficulties for people under guardianship to bring cases to court, there are few reported cases highlighting guardianship abuses, but those which do exist make compelling reading.[70]

The CRPD signals a shift away from this approach, towards one in which people who need support in exercising legal capacity are provided with the supports which they need,[71] rather than having their rights taken away.

Legal capacity is crucial for people with mental health problems in the community. Without it there are significant barriers to making decisions in areas of life which others take for granted. These may include the right to take decisions about a one's own finances and property, the right to decide where and with whom to live, the right to work, the right to sign contracts, the right to have relationships, the right to bring up children, the right to vote, to make a will, to join associations and political parties, and the right to access courts and other legal mechanisms.[72] In this sense, legal capacity acts as a gatekeeper of other rights: without providing the right to legal capacity and supports for those who need them, it is likely that full and equal participation in the community will never be achieved.

Community mental health practitioners will perhaps be most cognisant of how legal capacity is connected with the right to consent to or refuse treatment, a topic we outlined in the 'Right to live in the community' section. Any reliance on incapacity as a ground for restricting the right to informed consent needs to take into account the right to legal capacity in Article 12 of the CRPD. This provision requires that safeguards be put in place to ensure that any restrictions on decision-making 'respect the rights, will and preferences of the person, are free of conflict of interest and undue influence, are proportional and tailored to the person's circumstances,

---

66 See, for example Principle 4 of the UN Mental Illness Principles 1991 (op cit) and article 8 of the Council of Europe Recommendation Rec(2004)10 of the Committee of Ministers to member states concerning the protection of the human rights and dignity of persons with mental disorder.

67 'Principles for the protection of persons with mental illness and the improvement of mental health care', Adopted by UN General Assembly resolution 46/119 of 17 December 1991, Principle 9 (treatment).

68 CRPD, Art. 12.

69 CRPD, perambulatory para. (n).

70 See, for example, the European Court of Human Rights judgments *Shtukaturov v. Russia* (Application no. 44009/05, judgment on the merits 27 March 2008 and judgment concerning just satisfaction 4 March 2010) and *Salontaji-Drobnjak v. Serbia* (Application No. 36500/05, judgment 13 October 2009). See also the judgment in the cases *Stanev v. Bulgaria*, *Mitev v. Bulgaria*, and *Kedzior v. Poland*, all which concern legal capacity but which at the time of writing (December 2010) had not yet been decided.

71 CRPD, Art. 12(2).

72 See reports on 'Human Rights and Guardianship in Bulgaria', as well as sister reports covering Czech Republic, Georgia, Hungary, Kyrgyzstan, Russia and Serbia, *Mental Disability Advocacy Center*, 2007. Available at http://www.mdac.info.

apply for the shortest time possible and are subject to regular review by a competent, independent and impartial authority or judicial body'.[73] Simply having a mental health problem is thus not sufficient to remove the right to informed consent, if the individual in fact retains capacity to make the treatment decision in question, and all decisions which need to be taken must have strong regard to the person's will and preferences. A 'best interests' approach—where other people make decisions in isolation from the person with disability—is absent in the CRPD and can no longer be used to 'trump' the views of the individual labelled as incapable. The safeguards must, presumably, include an objective process: it is not obvious at all that decisions to decide whether someone needs supported decision-making, for example, may rest alone with the doctor who is treating the person with mental health problems.

Political motivation is gathering pace internationally now that legal capacity issues have been framed as a matter of law and human rights. In January 2009, the Parliamentary Assembly of the Council of Europe adopted a resolution on participation of people with disabilities.[74] The document's first area of priority action is legal capacity reform which calls on States to ensure that the right of people with disabilities 'to make decisions is not limited or substituted by others, that measures concerning them are individually tailored to their needs and that they may be supported in their decision making by a support person'.[75] The resolution makes clear that 'where they need external assistance so as to exercise those rights, that they are afforded appropriate support, without their wishes or intentions being superseded'.[76] It is likely that many States will embark on legal capacity reforms to provide greater autonomy and self-determination to people with mental health problems and other people with disabilities who have had their decision-making rights removed.

Conclusion

The last section of this chapter speaks directly to community mental health practitioners and sets out ideas about how they can play a part in ensuring that the CRPD is implemented so that their clients benefit from the range of rights set out in the treaty.

At the micro level, practitioners can develop their own understanding by reading about the CRPD in journal articles, on the internet and joining discussion forums. They can distribute copies to their community mental health teams, and professionals with whom they work: social workers, mental health nurses, paramedics, hospital-based colleagues, lawyers, and judges. Practitioners can play an important role in raising awareness about the CRPD at the local level by giving copies of the Convention to clients, as well as their carers and families.[77]

At the mezzo level practitioners could discuss the CRPD with colleagues and see how the local service can make changes to bring the services better in line with the CRPD. Practitioners could engage in a conversation with their clients and ask how they would like the practitioners to change in order that the CRPD is being implemented for them. In this way practitioners breathe life into the CRPD provisions on involvement of persons with disabilities in the implementation of services.[78] Practitioners can encourage their clients to join local advocacy groups in order to be active in improving services and holding their government to account. Practitioners could ensure that people with mental health problems are given the opportunity to serve on decision-making boards which hold services to account. Practitioners could work together with colleagues and people with mental health problems to develop codes of practice for particular CRPD issues which impact on their work.

At the macro level, practitioners are usually more politically powerful than their clients, and it is of prime importance that practitioners do not speak 'for' their clients, but that they support their voices. Practitioners can use their weight to open doors to decision-makers, ombudsman offices, and foreign embassies. Practitioners can speak the language of the CRPD in meetings with decision-makers and call directly for legislative and policy reforms, for the development of services to enable people with disabilities to live in the community, and for adequate resources to be allocated. Practitioners can feed into the changes abroad by asking their government (in countries which are donors) to ensure that all development aid is accessible for people with disabilities, and that there is a specific focus on the rights of people with mental health problems in particular. Practitioners in aid-recipient countries can play a valuable role in supporting their clients and their representative organizations to track development financing and ensuring inclusion of their clients.[79]

This chapter has outlined how the CRPD sets forth a set of guiding principles and lays out specific State obligations for implementation. The Convention rejects the caveats of previous mental illness-specific texts and the hesitancy of previous human rights instruments. It represents the political coming of age of the disability rights movement, of which users, ex-users and survivors of psychiatry are part. The inclusion of the right to health, the right to live in the community and the right to legal capacity, each without discrimination on the basis of disability, is a step change in international law. Community mental health practitioners have a crucial role to play in holding the State accountable for their obligations to respect, protect and fulfil 'the equal right of all persons with disabilities to live in the community, with choices equal to others'.[80] It is a core right for all human beings and it is an invitation for community mental health practitioners to advocate for change.

References

Bartlett, P. Lewis, O., and Thorold, O. (2007). *Mental Disability and the European Convention on Human Rights*. Leiden: Martinus Nijhoff.

UN Press Release (2009). *Secretary General Hails Adoption of Landmark Convention on Rights of People with Disabilities*. UN Press Release, 13 December 2006, Ref SG/SM/10797, HR/4911, L/T/4400.

---

73 CRPD, Art. 12(4).
74 Resolution 1642(2009) of the Parliamentary Assembly of the Council of Europe on 'Access to rights for people with disabilities and their full and active participation in society', 26 January 2009.
75 74 Ibid, para. 7.1.
76 Ibid, para. 7.2.
77 See preambulatory paragraph (x) of the CRPD which states that 'the family is the natural and fundamental group unit of society and is entitled to protection by society and the State, and that persons with disabilities and their family members should receive the necessary protection and assistance to enable families to contribute towards the full and equal enjoyment of the rights of persons with disabilities'.

---

78 See CRPD perambulatory para. (o) as well as Art. 4(3).
79 See CRPD Art on for international cooperation.
80 CRPD, Art. 19.

CHAPTER 27

Treatment pressures, coercion, and compulsion

George Szmukler and Paul S. Appelbaum

Introduction

In the last half of the 20th century and beginning of the 21st century, psychiatrists and other mental health clinicians became increasingly sensitive to the effects and implications of treatment that was not fully consensual. The number of psychiatric inpatients declined by more than two-thirds during that period. Many countries have tightened their procedures and standards for involuntary commitment (Appelbaum, 1997; Dressing and Salize, 2004). Mental health systems have worked harder to protect patients' liberty interests, and to avoid circumstances in which non-consensual treatment occurs.

Nonetheless, the nature of mental illness—with patients frequently manifesting denial of their disorder or of a need for care—and the public's concerns about the propensity of mentally ill persons to injure others or themselves, will probably make it impossible for non-consensual treatment ever to be abandoned completely. Indeed, with the movement to community care, new mechanisms for exerting pressures on patients have developed in services such as Assertive Community Treatment (ACT) (Stein and Santos, 1998). A major focus of ACT—usually targeted at persons with chronic mental illness who are thought likely to drift away from care—is to prevent defaulting from treatment, since loss of contact is likely to lead to relapse and readmission to hospital. Treatment is brought assertively **to** the patient making disengagement difficult. 'Compliance' or 'adherence' with medication is often a central issue. In the background also remains the possibility of compulsory admission to hospital.

This chapter has three aims:

1 To outline a spectrum of treatment pressures in contemporary practice, drawing ethically relevant distinctions between them

2 To consider when the exercise of such treatment pressures can be justified

3 To suggest approaches aimed at reducing the need for treatment pressures in community mental health services.

A range of treatment pressures

The term 'coercion' is often used almost synonymously with pressures exerted by one person (or organization) on another with the intention of making the latter act in accordance with the wishes of the former. We prefer to use the less moralized term 'treatment pressures'; as we shall see, 'coercion' is best applied to specific types of pressure. Within the concept of 'treatment pressures' we cover the whole range of interventions aimed at inducing patients to accept treatment which they have initially declined or seem likely to decline. We seek to identify morally relevant distinctions within the range of treatment pressures.

Here, we attempt to build on our earlier work (Szmukler and Appelbaum, 2008), to outline a hierarchy of pressures for which commensurate justifications must be provided. Our spectrum of pressures is as follows:

◆ Persuasion

◆ Interpersonal leverage

◆ Inducements

◆ Threats

◆ Compulsory treatment (in the community or as an inpatient).

Persuasion

Least problematic is **persuasion**, an appeal to reason. The discussion revolves around an appraisal of the benefits and risks of treatment based on the evidence and the patient's life situation. There is a respect for the patient's arguments. The process does not go beyond a debate.

Interpersonal leverage

Since the clinician (key-worker, case manager), especially in ACT programmes, may have established a relationship with the patient broader in scope and more intimate than a traditional patient–clinician relationship, opportunities for other kinds of pressure arise. Key-workers engage with patients in their ordinary community settings to help with many basic skills, for example, budgeting, shopping, cleaning. The key-worker may act as an advocate in accessing a range of community services. The patient may develop a significant degree of emotional dependency, enabling the exercise of **interpersonal leverage**. The patient may wish to please someone who has proved helpful, or agree to a clinician's proposal in reaction to the clinician's disappointment when a treatment suggestion is rejected.

Inducement and threat

The next level of pressure arises with the introduction of conditional 'if… then' propositions. **If** the patient accepts treatment A, **then** the clinician will do X; or **if** the patient does not accept treatment A, the clinician will do Y. At this point application of the term **coercion** is likely to be considered. A helpful account by Wertheimer (1987) argues that **threats** coerce but **offers** generally do not:

> The crux of the distinction between threats and offers is that A makes a threat when B will be worse off than in some relevant baseline position if B does not accept A's proposal, but that A makes an offer when B will be no worse off than in some relevant baseline position if B does not accept A's proposal.

Therefore the key to what counts as a coercive proposal is to properly fix the **baseline**. Wertheimer favours a '**moral baseline**' and gives an example to clarify this concept: A comes upon B who is drowning. A proposes to rescue B on condition that B pays A a large sum of money. There are no other potential rescuers. Has A made a threat or an offer? The answer depends on where we set the baseline. Under a moral test, the key issue is whether A is **morally required** (ought) to rescue B (or whether B has a **right** to be rescued by A). If A is morally required to rescue B, then B's baseline includes a right to be saved by A. A's proposal is therefore a threat. On the other hand, if A is not morally required to rescue B, then A's proposal is an offer.

A threat thus anticipates making the recipient worse off according to the proposed moral baseline, while an offer—even if declined—typically does not. Threatening to remove something to which the subject is **entitled** (e.g. a housing benefit determined by legal decree; assistance with an application for a disability living allowance) makes the subject worse off if he or she does not accede. An offer of something which is not an entitlement but is in the nature of extra assistance (e.g. the offer of an introduction to a sympathetic second-hand furniture dealer who gives special discounts) made on condition that the patient complies with the treatment would, if rejected, not make the patient worse off compared with the relevant moral baseline—what his or her position would have been if the offer had never been made. Conditional access to monetary benefits (statutory entitlements), as occurs when some patients in the United States have a 'representative payee' under Supplemental Security Income/Social Security Disability Insurance (SSI/SSDI) who only gives the patients their benefits when they comply with treatment is on this account coercive (Elbogen et al., 2003). When it is proposed to a mentally ill person before a Mental Health Court that the usual custodial sentence will be suspended if the person accepts treatment, this is an offer. If rejected by the person, he or she is no worse off than if the offer were never made—a custodial sentence is the standard punishment (Steadman et al., 2001).

Baselines other than 'moral' have been proposed. A 'legal' baseline has been proposed by Bonnie and Monahan (2005). This is more easily defined than a 'moral' baseline, but has the disadvantage of relativity—even in a single country, if it should have different legislatures governing some domains.

A variety of other interventions have been documented in community mental health that may fall along the inducements/threats spectrum. These include access to housing (Robbins et al., 2006), visitation for non-custodial parents or rights to custody (Busch and Redlich, 2007), and release from or avoidance of confinement via probation or parole (Skeem et al., 2006). All may be conditioned on adherence to treatment recommendations, including avoidance of intoxicating substances.

Allied to threats is **deception**. Failing to correct a patient's misconception about the consequences of not accepting treatment may be coercive. Some outpatient commitment orders may depend for their effectiveness on a patient's misapprehension that transgression of the order will result in re-hospitalization or enforced treatment, though it may only permit conveying to a treatment facility or an assessment for compulsory inpatient treatment.

In our hierarchy of pressures, we thus place **offers** (or inducements) before **threats**. Only the latter would count as **coercive**, as would presumably the exercise of compulsion in treatment described below.

Acts which resemble 'coercion': 'exploitation' and 'unwelcome predictions'

A distinction can be made between a coercive threat and exploitation (Rhodes, 2000; Wertheimer, 1987, 1996). Exploitation involves an offer that nevertheless takes unfair advantage of a person in a difficult predicament. Rhodes considers the example of a homeless person in a cold climate who is offered a warm apartment but at a very high rent. The threat is a 'background threat,' and not of the landlord's doing. The key issue is the moral baseline. On Wertheimer's account, exploitation, while often morally questionable, is not 'coercive.' Is it the person's 'right' in this example to be offered a room at a 'fair' rent? Most would say, no. Further, exploitative offers, in some sense, expand possibilities for the recipient; if the offer is not accepted, the person is no worse off than he would have been if the offer had not been made. Both the exploiter and the person exploited can derive advantage from an exploitative offer (a warm room for the former, and a larger income for the latter). The harm lies in taking **unfair advantage** of a person who is at a disadvantage.

If a clinician were to say to a patient that stopping medication will result in involuntary admission to hospital, a distinction can be drawn between this being an **unwelcome prediction**—a statement of fact, over which the clinician has no control—or a threat. Much depends on the factual basis of the prediction; the past history may indicate repeated similar instances that have resulted in a compulsory admission. Whether the clinician will be an instigator of the event is also relevant. A prediction of an unwelcome event, based on sound evidence, would not be considered as 'coercive.' However, a clear line between them may be difficult to draw in practice.

Problematic inducements

Inducements can be problematic. The lure of an offer may be so powerful an inducement that the patient is no longer able to engage in a rational process of weighing the risks and benefits of a decision. An example of a potentially problematic inducement is a proposal to pay non-compliant patients with a psychosis to accept treatment (Claassen, 2007). It has been argued that it is an offer and therefore not 'coercive'. Yet the results of a survey of clinicians in the United Kingdom revealed a widely held intuition that the practice is unethical (Claassen, 2007). There may be a number of explanations for this. First, the transaction involves an exchange of 'goods' involving what might be seen as 'incommensurable values', that is, values that cannot be measured on a single metric, one good being in a higher, and thus separate, domain than the other. Selling a child is a stark example. Such an exchange corrupts or degrades the higher value. In paying patients to take medication, money could be seen as being exchanged for an aspect of respect for the person— that is, there is a failure to respect a patient's considered decision about what is in his or her best interests (assuming the patient has capacity). Second, there may be a possibility of exploitation. It is the patient's vulnerability, psychological or material—often both— which would induce an acceptance of the offer. As noted above, in exploitation one party gains unfairly at the expense of the one who is exploited (even though the exploitee may still derive some gain) (Mayer, 2007). Who gains here? A significant motive for monetary inducements may be to reduce costs to the health service by preventing relapse and rehospitalization. Third, there is an issue concerning the fairness of paying non-treatment adherent patients but not treatment adherent patients. There is also a range of other problems—e.g. ensuring treatment adherence actually occurs, and how possible it would be in practice for payment to be terminated (for a more detailed discussion of the issues see Szmukler, 2009).

Compulsion

Next in our hierarchy of pressures is **compulsion** (backed up by legally authorized force). As the locus of treatment has shifted to the community and concerns about non-adherence to treatment have grown, a number of jurisdictions have introduced **outpatient commitment** orders. Three major types can be discerned:

1 As a substitute for hospital admission: the outpatient commitment order is considered a less restrictive alternative to compulsory inpatient admission, when alternatives to compulsory treatment have been exhausted.

2 To facilitate earlier discharge from hospital (a form of conditional discharge): although the patient may not be well enough for full discharge and requires continued treatment under compulsion, this can be obtained in the community as a less restrictive alternative to the hospital.

3 To prevent relapse: this type of order is applied where there is a proven history of relapse secondary to discontinuation of treatment, usually medication, and relapse is believed to be associated with significant risk to the patient or others.

Outpatient commitment orders carry varying powers (Dawson, 2005). Some allow recall of the patient for compulsory treatment as an inpatient. Others are limited to forced medication 'in the community,' usually achieved by conveying the patient to a clinic where an injection is administered. Still others only permit non-compliant patients to be brought involuntarily to a clinic to be subject to persuasion, leverage or inducements; coercive treatment per se is not authorized. (This is typically the situation in the United States, although there is some variation among the states (Appelbaum, 2001).) Outpatient commitment orders also vary in the range of conditions attached to the order (e.g. specification of clinician, clinic, frequency of reviews, treatments, residence) and their duration (Dawson, 2005).

Finally, there is the option of **compulsory admission to hospital**.

Objective and subjective 'coercion'

An important dimension in thinking about treatment pressures, including coercion, involves the distinction between 'objective' and 'subjective' aspects (Hiday, 1992; Hoge et al., 1997; Lidz et al., 1995). The subjective experience of feeling coerced may not follow an 'objective' schema such as the one outlined above. Indeed, the results of studies of patients' perceived coercion can seem counter-intuitive. Involuntary as opposed to voluntary hospitalization does not necessarily predict subjective coercion, nor does being placed on outpatient commitment compared with receiving voluntary outpatient services (Swartz et al., 2009). Patients' perceptions of how fairly they have been treated and the motives of decision-makers may be more influential in their subjective sense of coercion than actual legal status. From the patient's perspective this may be the most important issue in coercion. Approaches to reducing the need for coercion (discussed below) may also be effective in minimizing subjective coercion.

However, for the clinician seeking to act ethically in pressing a reluctant patient to accept treatment, morally relevant distinctions of an 'objective' kind can be helpful in making justifiable decisions. The hierarchy we have outlined is an attempt to meet this need, but it will require adjustment to take account of a particular patient's preferences and values. Within the domain of **compulsory treatment** there may be variations in restrictions on autonomy or of choice, as well as the subjective experience of constraint.

Justifications for exercising treatment pressures

Two types of justification are usually offered for applying treatment pressures on a patient who declines:

1 Treatment is in the patient's 'best interests' (or 'health or safety'); or

2 Treatment is needed for the protection of others.

If a hierarchy of treatment pressures on reluctant patients is defined as above, then one would ask for a stronger justification the more coercive the pressure to be exerted:

Justification in the best interests of the patient

Before the focus on treatment in the community, the major form of treatment pressure revolved around compulsory treatment in hospital, or its threat. Criteria for involuntary admission embodied in mental health legislation generally rely, at least in part, on evidence of substantial dangers to the patient's health or safety. In the community, however, a wider spectrum of risks or degrees of danger is identified by professionals in closer proximity to the daily lives of their patients. They may suffer from physical disorders that require treatment they are incapable of seeking. A hard-won tenancy may be jeopardized by the patient's failure to take care of an apartment. Significant supportive relationships may be on the verge of breaking down. Criteria of the type set down in mental health legislation governing involuntary hospitalization are simply not sensitive to the broader range of 'risk' encountered in community settings. Nor are they sensitive to 'values' differences in the complex multicultural societies of today, and their role in determining what might be in a person's 'best interests'.

Linking justifications for treatment pressures in the spectrum outlined above to the continuum of risks seen in the community thus requires a broader, more comprehensive ethical framework. It must be able to deal with questions of 'value'.

We outline two 'best interests' frameworks, one deriving from an analysis of 'paternalistic' actions and the other from an analysis of capacity (or mental competence).

A framework based on 'paternalism'

Gert et al. (2006) propose that a person is acting paternalistically towards another if his action benefits the other; his action involves violating a moral rule with regard to the other; and his action does not have the other's past, present, or immediately forthcoming consent. Their approach to 'paternalistic' actions may be helpful. In justifying a paternalistic act, a series of pertinent questions can elicit the 'morally relevant facts':

1 What are the moral rules that would be violated if the clinician were to act against the patient's wishes (e.g. limiting freedom of choice, causing psychological pain)?

2 What are the harms thus perpetrated on the patient and for how long will they last?

3 What is the seriousness of the harms to be avoided through the paternalistic intervention (e.g. death, disability, worsening of the psychiatric disorder), and what is their likelihood?

4 What are the relevant beliefs and desires of the person toward whom a rule is being violated (e.g. religious beliefs)?

5 Are there any alternative actions that would be preferable?

Based on these facts, further questions come into play:

6 How does the clinician rank the two sets of harms compared to the patient?

7 Is the patient's preference when comparing the harms to be avoided with the harms to be incurred, irrational—that is, does the patient have a rational reason to prefer an outcome with apparently greater harms?

8 Can the clinician advocate publicly for his or her ranking of the harms to be perpetrated compared to those to be avoided? Would most rational people agree that this kind of moral violation should in such circumstances be universally allowed?

A decision to exercise a specific treatment pressure in a specific circumstance would depend on a balance informed by the answers to these questions, although no algorithm exists to allow these determinations to be made in a rigorous (or possibly even replicable) way.

A framework based on 'capacity' and 'best interests'

'Mental incapacity' is assuming an increasing emphasis in justifying interventions against a patient's will, in psychiatry as well as in general medicine where it has been long established (Dawson and Szmukler, 2006; Grisso and Appelbaum, 1998). As for physical disorders, it is difficult in psychiatry to argue for treatment against a person's wishes unless that person lacks the capacity (or 'competence,' used by us synonymously) to make treatment decisions for themselves. Definitions of capacity vary, but common elements are the ability to understand and retain information relevant to the decision (including the consequences of deciding one way or the other), and the ability to use that information to make a decision. The latter includes the ability to 'appreciate' that the information applies to the patient's predicament, the ability to reason with that information, and the ability to exercise a choice (Grisso and Appelbaum, 1998; Mental Capacity Act 2005).

Only if the patient lacks capacity, would treatment against a patient's wishes be considered (so-called 'soft paternalism'); but a further test must also be passed—that treatment is in the patient's 'best interests.' Definitions of 'best interests' are difficult, but the United Kingdom Law Commission (1995) has proposed practical guidance for deciding on the matter, now incorporated in the Mental Capacity Act 2005. Regard should be given to the following:

◆ The ascertainable past and present wishes and feelings of the person concerned, and the factors that person would consider if able to do so

◆ The need to permit and encourage the person to participate or improve his or her ability to participate as fully as possible in anything done for and any decision affecting him or her

◆ The views of other persons whom it is appropriate and practical to consult about the person's wishes and feelings and what would be in his or her best interests, and

◆ Whether the purpose for which any action or decision is required can be as effectively achieved in a manner less restrictive of the person's freedom of action.

We insist that if community mental health teams are to exercise their powers to intervene in patients' lives in an ethical manner, an appropriate framework is required. Professionals should be as well versed in using such a framework as they are in assessing 'technical' problems, e.g. the likely benefits of interventions such as medication or psychological treatments.

The application of a framework such as one described above suggests that the degree of pressure to be used should be the minimum necessary, and that the justification should be stronger the more one moves along the spectrum from persuasion to direct force.

These principles should also be considered in relation to involuntary outpatient commitment. As discussed above, blunt criteria similar to those used in mental health legislation are difficult to apply when a wide spectrum of risk is identified by professionals in close and frequent contact with patients in the community. If outpatient commitment is an alternative to admission to hospital or is used to facilitate earlier discharge, criteria for terminating the order are essential. The criteria could be based on one of the frameworks above, e.g. recovery of capacity to make treatment decisions or the compulsory treatment no longer being in the best interests of the patient.

Justification based on protection of others

'Protection of others' is a common criterion for involuntary hospitalization, and generally also for outpatient commitment. However, in a community setting, the definition of risk to others is in danger of expansion; just as there is a spectrum of risk to the well-being of the patient, so is there one for risk to others. In a climate of concern that the safety of the public is threatened, pressures from community members to intervene may intensify. Patients may become subject to treatment pressures under a potentially broad interpretation of the 'protection of others'.

The 'protection of others' is often confused with health interests. However, they are conceptually distinct (Culver and Gert, 1982). When others seek authority to determine what is in a patient's best interests, the legitimacy of their request depends on the patient's lack of capacity to make decisions about the patient's welfare or health. In contrast, the protection of others does not turn on capacity, but on factors such as the risk of harm and its seriousness.

Viewed thus, the fact that 'preventive' detention on the grounds of risk of harm to others is generally restricted only to those with a mental disorder is difficult to defend. The likelihood of serious violence is higher in many non-mentally disordered persons, for example, those who regularly become assaultive when intoxicated or who habitually perpetrate domestic violence. Yet we do not force preventive interventions on such persons before they have been convicted of an offence. It has been argued that separate generic 'dangerousness' legislation is the most appropriate measure for preventing violence if that is deemed a significant societal goal (Campbell and Heginbotham, 1991; Szmukler and Holloway, 1998).

Predicting serious violence is also subject to a major limitation carrying significant ethical implications. Incidents of serious violence are rare. The prediction of rare events inherently lacks accuracy. Even the very best predictive instruments available will have a false positive rate of well over 90% if the rate of serious violence is 1% in the patient population (Szmukler, 2003). If the risk of violence were to lead to coercive interventions, the moral cost of unnecessarily infringing the liberty of a large number of patients to prevent harm by a few is very difficult to justify.

We are left with some thorny issues. Society demands a degree of social control from mental health services. As services move into the community and see at close quarters the lives of their patients and those around them, dilemmas around risk may become especially problematic. The potential for community mental health teams to expand activities directed at social control must be recognized. A dialogue between those advocating on behalf of patients with mental illness and a community often fearful of such persons is essential (and urgent) if abuses are to be avoided.

Reducing the need for treatment pressures

Services can employ a range of measures to reduce the need for exerting pressures on patients to accept treatment. Unfortunately, few of these have been evaluated formally.

Make services as acceptable and attractive to users as possible

Traditionally, mental health service users have had little say in how services ostensibly created to help them are implemented. For services to become more responsive to patients' needs requires an active, not token, involvement of service users in their planning (Pilgrim and Waldron, 1998). Users can make crucial contributions as members of management committees where they ensure that discussion, service developments, and evaluations of quality and outcomes are seen from users', as well as providers' perspective. (Rose et al., 2003).

Enhance patients' involvement in planning their own care

Patients are likely to feel less coerced the more they play an active role in determining their treatment. Recent initiatives employing '**advance statements**' (Henderson et al., 2008a) have provided evidence that their use may reduce the need for 'coercive' interventions.

In the United Kingdom, '**crisis cards**' originated as a service user/voluntary sector initiative to facilitate access to an advocate and to state patients' preferences for care during an emergency when they might be too unwell to express their wishes clearly (Sutherby and Szmukler, 1998). 'Crisis cards' have usually been drawn up by the patient alone, without discussion with the mental health team. They have not proved popular.

The idea of the 'crisis card' has been developed into the '**joint crisis plan**' (JCP) (Sutherby et al., 1999). Here the content of the card, though still ultimately determined by the patient, is negotiated with the treatment team when the patient is able to make competent judgements about what is in his or her best interests. An important aspect of the JCP is the independent 'facilitator' whose role it is to make sure the patient's voice is heard.

Sutherby et al. (1999) reported on the introduction of crisis cards and JCPs in London. Participation was offered to patients with a psychotic illness at high risk of relapse. They chose to include a wide range of information including diagnosis, current treatment, contact information for carers and professionals, first signs of relapse and the preferred treatment, treatment preferences and refusals for established relapses, indications for admission, and practical requests (e.g. who should take care of domestic arrangements in case of admission). A majority of the patients reported feeling empowered in determining details of their care. Subsequently, a randomized controlled trial of JCPs involving patients with a psychosis showed that by 15 months' follow-up, the rate of compulsory admissions was halved in the group completing JCPs (Henderson et al., 2004). Again the effects of drawing up a JCP on patients' attitudes to treatment were, in the main, positive (Henderson et al., 2008b).

Another form of 'advance statement' is a **psychiatric advance directive** (PAD). All states in the United States permit advance directives to be written for health care in general (including psychiatric care), and 25 states now have statutes creating specific provisions for psychiatric advance directives (National Resource Center on Psychiatric Advance Directives, 2009). Advance directives are in principle legally binding, although some PADs statutes stipulate that the patient's wishes may be overridden if they violate 'accepted standards of care.' How this should be interpreted is not clear (Appelbaum, 2004; Swanson et al., 2006). The directives in a PAD may be of three kinds: first, specified treatments that are refused or requested; second, statements about personal values, attitudes, or general preferences that may be used as a guide for those making decisions about treatment; and third, nomination of a person to act a 'substitute' or 'proxy' decision-maker. PAD statutes presume that the patient had decision-making capacity when it was made, in the absence of evidence to the contrary, and their utility is predicated on the assumption that the circumstances in which the PAD is triggered are those that were anticipated.

A variant of the PAD process, termed a **facilitated PAD** (F-PAD), has been introduced following research revealing a low incidence of patients who say they desire a PAD actually completing one. Practical complexities in their execution may act as deterrents to their adoption. In an F-PAD process, a trained facilitator explains what a PAD involves and, if the patient chooses to opt for one, assists with its completion (Swanson et al., 2006b). The service provider may also be asked to become involved.

A randomized controlled study of F-PADs has indeed shown that facilitation results in a highly significant increase in the number of patients who decide to make a PAD (61% vs. 3% of controls). At 1-month follow-up, those with an F-PAD reported a much better working alliance with their clinicians and were more likely to say that they received the services they needed (Swanson et al., 2006b). The number of 'coercive interventions' over the succeeding 2 years for those who made a PAD was considerably fewer compared to patients who did not (Swanson et al., 2008), including for those patients who had suffered a loss of capacity during the crisis.

Thus there is emerging evidence that some forms of 'advance statement' could significantly reduce the number of situations in which clinicians need to act against a patient's competent preferences. Many of the ethical dilemmas discussed above occur precisely at such times of crisis. Independent facilitation, either in a JCP or an F-PAD, may be a critical factor.

Use approaches to reduce levels of perceived coercion

Applying the principles derived from studies such as the MacArthur Foundation coercion project (Hoge et al., 1997; Lidz et al., 1995), though so far untested, may reduce the need for actual coercion as well as reduce patients' 'perceived' coercion. Where situations with the potential for coercive interactions arise, principles of 'procedural justice' can be borne in mind—treating the patient with respect and fairness, giving him or her a 'voice' and taking seriously what is said, and avoiding 'negative pressures' such as threats or force.

Use pressure or coercion only when it is necessary

Using pressures or coercive measures on patients only when justified and to a degree commensurate with the risks to the patient's best interests should minimize their use. The multidisciplinary team is an invaluable resource for ethical decision-making of this kind since the impact of proposed interventions on the values at stake can be tested across a range of team members' perspectives. The views of informal and other formal caregivers should also be considered.

Conclusions

The scope for exerting pressures for treatment on reluctant patients is probably as great in the modern era of community care as it ever was. New forms exist, while ways of thinking about compulsory treatment hallowed by time and convention are not adequate to dealing with the subtle gradations of risk and distinctions among interventions relevant to community psychiatry. We strongly suggest that being adept at using an ethical framework for deciding

when a specific treatment pressure is justified should be a core skill of members of community mental health teams. If community mental health services are to flourish within complex, multicultural and ever-changing societies, they will need to rest on sound ethical foundations. The history of psychiatry, an enterprise in which questions of value are always to the fore, shows that a swing of the moral pendulum is never far away (Appelbaum, 1994).

References

Appelbaum, P.S. (1991). Advance directives for psychiatric treatment. *Hospital and Community Psychiatry*, **42**, 983–4.

Appelbaum, P.S. (1994). *Almost a Revolution: Mental Health Law and the Limits of Change*. New York: Oxford University Press.

Appelbaum, P.S. (1997). Almost a revolution: an international perspective on the law of involuntary commitment. *Journal of American Academy of Psychiatry and the Law*, **25**, 135–48.

Appelbaum, P.S. (2001). Thinking carefully about outpatient commitment. *Psychiatric Services*, **52**, 347–50.

Appelbaum, P.S. (2004). Law and psychiatry: psychiatric advance directives and the treatment of committed patients. *Psychiatric Services*, **55**, 751–2.

Bonnie, R.J. and Monahan, J. (2005). From coercion to contract: reframing the debate on mandated community treatment for people with mental disorders. *Law and Human Behavior*, **29**, 485–503.

Busch, A. and Redlich, A. (2007). Patients' perception of possible child custody or visitation loss if not adherent to psychiatric treatment. *Psychiatric Services*, **58**, 999–1002.

Campbell, T. and Heginbotham, C. (1991). *Mental illness: Prejudice, Discrimination and the Law*. Aldershot: Dartmouth.

Claassen, D. (2007). Financial incentives for antipsychotic depot medication: ethical issues. *Journal of Medical Ethics*, **33**, 189–93.

Claassen, D., Fakhoury, W., Ford, R., and Priebe, S. (2007). Money for medication - financial incentives to improve medication adherence in Assertive Outreach patients. *Psychiatric Bulletin*. **31**, 4–7.

Culver, C.N., and Gert, B. (1982). *Philosophy in Medicine: Conceptual and Ethical Issues in Medicine and Psychiatry*. Oxford: Oxford University Press.

Dawson, J. (2005). *Community Treatment Orders: International Comparisons*. Dunedin: Otago University Press.

Dawson, J. and Szmukler, G. (2006). Fusion of mental health and incapacity legislation. *British Journal of Psychiatry* **188**, 504–9.

Dressing, H. and Salize, H.J. (2004). Compulsory admission of mentally ill patients in European member states. *Social Psychiatry and Psychiatric Epidemiology* **39**, 797–803.

Elbogen, E., Swanson, J., Swartz, M., and Wagner, H. (2003). Characteristics of third-party money management for persons with psychiatric disabilities. *Psychiatric Services*, **54**, 1136–41.

Gert, B, CM Culver, and KD *Clouser* (2006). *Bioethics: a systematic approach*, 2nd edn. New York: Oxford University Press.

Grisso, T. and Appelbaum, PS. (1998). *Assessing competence to consent to treatment: A guide for physicians and other health professionals*. New York: Oxford University Press.

Henderson, C., Flood, C., Leese, M., Thornicroft, G., Sutherby, K., and Szmuckler, G. (2004). Effect of joint crisis plans on use of compulsory treatment in psychiatry: single blind randomised controlled trial. *British Medical Journal*, **329**, 136.

Henderson, C., Swanson, J.W., Szmukler, G., Thornicroft, G., and Zinkler, M. (2008a). A typology of advance statements in mental health care. *Psychiatric Services*, **59**, 63–71.

Henderson, C., Flood, C., Leese, M., Thornicroft, G., Sutherby, K., and Szmukler, G. (2008b). Views of service users and providers on joint crisis plans: Single blind randomized controlled trial. *Social Psychiatry and Psychiatric Epidemiology*, **44**, 369–76.

Hiday, V.A. (1992). Coercion in civil commitment: Process, preferences, and outcome. *International Journal of Law & Psychiatry*, **15**, 359–77.

Hoge, S.K., Lidz, C.W., Eisenberg, Gardner, W., Monahan, J., and Mulvey, E.P., *et al.* (1997). Perceptions of coercion in the admission of voluntary and involuntary psychiatric patients. *International Journal of Law & Psychiatry*, **20**, 167–81.

Law Commission (1995). *Report No. 231. Mental Incapacity.* London: HMSO.

Lidz, C., Hoge, S., Gardner, W., Bennett, N., Monahan, J., Mulvey, E., *et al.* (1995). Perceived coercion in mental hospital admission: Pressures and process. *Archives of General Psychiatry*, **52**, 1034–39.

Mayer, R. (2007). What's wrong with exploitation. *Journal of Applied Philosophy.* **24**, 137–50.

National Resource Centre on Psychiatric Advance Directives (2009). http://www.nrc-pad.org/content/view/41/25/.

Pilgrim, D. and Waldron, L. (1998). User involvement in mental health service development: How far can it go? *Journal of Mental Health*, **7**, 95–104.

Robbins, P., Petrila, J., LeMelle, S., and Monahan, J. (2006). The use of housing as leverage to increase adherence to psychiatric treatment in the community. *Administration and Policy in Mental Health and Mental Health Services Research*, **33**, 226–36.

Rhodes, M. (2000). The nature of coercion. *Journal of Value Inquiry*, **34**, 369–81.

Rose, D., Fleischman, P., Tonkiss, F., Campbell, P., and Wykes, T. (2003). *User and carer involvement in change management in a mental health context: review of the literature.* London: NHS Service Delivery and Organisation R&D Programme.

Skeem, J., Emke-Francis, P., and Eno Louden, J. (2006). Probation, mental health, and mandated treatment: A national survey. *Criminal Justice & Behavior*, **33**, 158–84.

Steadman, H., Davidson, S., and Brown, C. (2001). Mental health courts: Their promise and unanswered questions. *Psychiatric Services*, **52**, 457–58.

Stein, L.I. and Santos, A.B. (1998). *Assertive Community Treatment of Persons with Severe Mental Illness.* New York: Norton.

Sutherby K., Szmukler G.I., Halpern A., Alexander, M., Thornicroft, G., Johnson, C., *et al.* (1999). A study of 'crisis cards' in a community psychiatric service. *Acta Psychiatrica Scandinavica*, **100**, 56–61.

Sutherby, K. & Szmukler, G. (1998). Crisis cards and self-help crisis initiatives. *Psychiatric Bulletin*, **22**, 4–7.

Swanson, J.W., McCrary, S.V., Swartz, M.S., Elbogen, E.B., and Van Dorn, R.A. (2006a). Superseding psychiatric advance directives: ethical and legal considerations. *Journal of the American Academy of Psychiatry and the Law*, **34**, 385–94.

Swanson, J.W., Swartz, M.S., Elbogen, E.B., Van Dorn, R.A., Wagner, H.R., Moser, L.A., *et al.* (2006b). Facilitated psychiatric advance directives: a randomized trial of an intervention to foster advance treatment planning among persons with severe mental illness. *American Journal of Psychiatry*, **163**, 1943–51.

Swanson, J.W., Swartz, M.S., Elbogen, E.B., Van Dorn, R.A., Wagner, H.R., Moser, L.A., *et al.* (2008). Psychiatric advance directives and reduction of coercive crisis interventions. *Journal of Mental Health*, **17**, 255–67.

Swartz, M.D., Swanson, J.W., Steadman, H.J., Robbins, P.C., and Monahan, J. (2009). New York State Assisted Outpatient Treatment Program Evaluation. Duke University School of Medicine, Durham, NC. Available at: http://www.omh.state.ny.us/omhweb/resources/publications/aot_program_evaluation/index.html (accessed 24 August 2009)

Szmukler, G. and Holloway, F. (1998). Mental health legislation is now a harmful anachronism. *Psychiatric Bulletin*, **22**, 662–5.

Szmukler, G. (2003). Risk assessment: 'numbers' and 'values'. *Psychiatric Bulletin*, **27**, 205–7.

Szmukler, G. and Appelbaum, P.S. (2008). Treatment pressures, leverage, coercion, and compulsion in mental health care. *Journal of Mental Health,* **17**, 233–44.

Szmukler, G (2009). Financial incentives for patients in the treatment of psychosis. *Journal of Medical Ethics*, **35**, 224–8.

Wertheimer, A. (1987). *Coercion.* Princeton, NJ: Princeton University Press.

Wertheimer, A. (1996). *Exploitation.* Princeton, NJ: Princeton University Press.

SECTION 6

Stigma and discrimination

CHAPTER 28

Public knowledge and awareness about mental illnesses

Anthony F. Jorm

For major physical health problems, like cancer and cardiovascular disease, members of the public typically have considerable knowledge about what they can do for prevention or early intervention, or have knowledge of treatments and services available. For example, in the area of cardiovascular disease, there is widespread knowledge about modifiable risk factors like smoking and exercise, people know the value of screening and treatment for hypertension and high cholesterol, many people have the first aid skills to apply cardiopulmonary resuscitation in an emergency, and some would know the warning signs of a stroke and the need to call an ambulance immediately.

Knowledge about mental disorders in the community has generally lagged behind that for major physical diseases. This is surprising given the high prevalence of mental disorders. Community surveys in many countries show high rates, with 1-year prevalence rates of 10% to 19% and lifetime prevalence rates of 18% to 36% being typical (Kessler et al., 2009). This high prevalence means that the whole population will either be personally affected by a mental disorder or have close contact with other people who are. Given the high exposure to mental disorders in the population, it can be argued that everyone needs some knowledge and skill to take action to improve community mental health.

The concept of mental health literacy

The term **mental health literacy** has been coined to draw attention to this neglected area. This is defined as 'knowledge and beliefs about mental disorders which aid their recognition, management or prevention' (Jorm et al., 1997). Note that mental health literacy is more than just knowledge about mental disorders; rather it is knowledge that a person can use to guide action to benefit their own mental health or that of others. All of the following are examples of mental health literacy:

◆ Recognition of developing disorders which can guide early help-seeking

◆ Knowledge of the range of professional help and effective treatments available

◆ Knowledge of effective self-help strategies

◆ Knowledge and skills to access quality mental health information

◆ Knowledge and skills to give mental health first aid

◆ Knowledge of risk factors and causes that can be used to guide preventive action.

For people who have a mental disorder, mental health literacy would also involve knowledge and skills for self-management, while for family members it would also involve knowledge and skills of how to be a supportive care-giver. However, this chapter focuses on aspects of mental health literacy that apply to the community as a whole, rather than on those more appropriate to people who have a mental disorder or who provide family support to someone with a mental disorder.

Recognition of developing disorders which can guide early help-seeking

Community surveys of mental disorders show that many people do not get professional help. In developed countries, 36% to 50% of people with a mental disorder have not received treatment in the previous 12 months, while in less-developed countries the rate of non-treatment is 76% to 85% (The WHO World Mental Health Consortium, 2004). Even when professional help is sought, there may be long delays. The length of delay typically varies with the type and severity of the disorder. For example, for anxiety disorders delays of many years are common (Christiana et al., 2000), whereas for psychotic disorders delays of months will be more typical (Marshall et al., 2005).

Delays in recognition are important because early intervention with mental disorders may be associated with a better outcome. With psychotic disorders, many studies have shown that the duration of untreated psychosis is associated with worse outcome (Marshall et al., 2005). There is also some evidence that duration of untreated depression is associated with worse outcomes (Altamura et al., 2008).

Delays in help-seeking are affected by the knowledge a person with a mental disorder has about recognition. For example, a study of people being treated for anxiety or mood disorders found an average delay of 8.2 years (Thompson et al., 2008). Most of this delay was due to a failure to recognize that the symptoms were due to a mental disorder. The average time to recognize the problem as a mental disorder was 6.9 years and it then took an average of 1.3 years between recognition and help-seeking.

Community surveys in a many countries have shown that there are deficiencies in recognition of mental disorders. A typical methodology used in these surveys is to present a case vignette of a person with a mental disorder and ask the respondent what they think is wrong with the person. The results differ from country to country and may depend on local community awareness activities. For example, in Australia, 77% of adults applied the label 'depression' to a vignette of a person who was depressed and suicidal, compared to only 35% of the Japanese public (Jorm et al., 2005a). By contrast, the term 'stress' was applied more in Japan than in Australia. The conceptualization of the problem as a mental disorder versus a life problem can affect help-seeking preferences. For example, people who conceptualize the problem as 'depression' are less likely to think it is helpful to deal with the problem on one's own (Jorm et al., 2006a).

An additional factor contributing to under-recognition is that mental disorders often first develop during adolescence and early adulthood (Kessler et al., 2009). This is a period of life where the knowledge and experience of mental disorders may be less developed and assistance may be needed from family or other supporters to recognize the problem. When a young person recognizes a pattern of symptoms as a mental disorder, they are more likely to choose appropriate help and treatment (Wright et al., 2007). Furthermore, if a young person with a mental disorder attends a general practitioner (GP), the GP is more likely to detect it if the young person conceptualizes their problem as a mental disorder (Haller et al., 2009).

While early recognition of mental disorders may have benefits, caution is needed about unnecessary labelling that may lead to stigma. Sometimes labelling a person as having a 'mental illness' can lead others to avoid or otherwise stigmatize them. Labelling needs to be a positive act that gives a person with a mental disorder earlier treatment and better support, rather than a negative one that leads to avoidance and discrimination.

Knowledge of the range of professional help and effective treatments available

Once a person with a mental disorder recognizes the problem and decides they need help, they need to know about the range of professional help available and what treatments are likely to be helpful.

Surveys have been carried out in many developed countries looking at public beliefs about sources of help and types of treatment (Angermeyer et al., 2005; Croghan et al., 2003; Jorm et al., 2000a, 2005a; Lauber et al., 2001; Magliano et al., 2004; Priest et al., 1996). While many findings are country-specific, there are some that apply across many countries. These include:

- Family and friends are viewed very positively as a source of help, often ahead of health professionals

- Psychiatric medications are seen negatively by many people because of concerns that they do not treat the underlying causes and can cause dependence

- Psychological treatments such as counselling are viewed very positively for a wide range of disorders

- Beliefs about GPs as a source of help for mental disorders are very positive in most countries, but appear to be influenced by the type of healthcare system operating and the perceived appropriateness of GPs for mental health treatment

- A significant minority of the population believes that it is helpful to deal with mental disorders on one's own.

A particular concern is where beliefs about treatments diverge from those of professionals and from what the evidence shows is effective. This is seen most clearly with psychiatric medications. For example, in Germany, only 11% of the public give medication as their first choice of treatment for depression and only 15% as their first choice for schizophrenia (Riedel-Heller et al., 2005). In Australia, around a quarter of the public see antidepressants as likely to be harmful for a person with depression, while in Canada antidepressants are rated at a similar level to non-evidence-based treatments such as vitamins and changes in diet (Wang et al., 2007). Having negative views about medications can have major effects on the benefit received from these treatments. For example, depressed patients who have negative views about antidepressants are less likely to be prescribed these medications, less likely to fill prescriptions and less likely to benefit overall (Pyne et al., 2005). If patients are to get the full benefit of evidence-based health care, community beliefs need to be concordant with the evidence.

Fortunately, community beliefs can be changed. In both Germany and Australia, repeat community surveys show that attitudes towards treatments for mental disorders, including medication, have become more favourable over time (Angermeyer and Matschinger 2005; Jorm, et al., 2006b). Even so, there is considerable room for further improvement.

Knowledge of effective self-help strategies

Self-help strategies are those that a person can use to deal with mental health problems on their own. Sometimes self-help strategies will be used under the guidance of a health professional (e.g. using a book that teaches how to apply cognitive behaviour therapy). However, most self-help is informal and carried out without any professional guidance. Self-help strategies are very commonly used by members of the public to deal with disabling symptoms. For example, in an Australian community sample, the following strategies were commonly used to deal with depression and anxiety symptoms: alcohol to relax, pain relievers, physical activity, help from friends and family, holidays and time off work (Jorm et al., 2000b). Some of these strategies are supported by evidence as likely to be helpful (e.g. physical activity), but others may be counter-productive (e.g. heavy use of alcohol can exacerbate anxiety and depression).

Community surveys show that the public believe in the effectiveness of self-help strategies, often more so than in professional interventions. This preference for self-help extends to more severe mental disorders like schizophrenia, as well as for common ones like depression. Self-help interventions that are endorsed as helpful across a number of countries include: exercise, getting out and about more, taking vitamins, reading self-help books, getting support from family and friends, and consulting a website (Jorm et al., 2005a; Wang et al., 2007).

Self-help strategies are not an effective substitute for professional treatments of mental disorders. However, they can play a very useful role in dealing with anxiety and depressive symptoms that do not reach a diagnostic threshold. Such subthreshold symptoms are very common in the community and cause much disability, but do not justify the use of scarce mental health professional care. It has been proposed that informal self-help strategies that have evidence of effectiveness (such as exercise) should be widely promoted in the community in order to prevent the development of sub-threshold symptoms into clinical disorders (Jorm and Griffiths, 2006). Morgan and Jorm (2009) have produced a list of self-help strategies that could be usefully promoted, based on a review of the available evidence of effectiveness and the consensus of clinicians and consumers. These include physical activity, better sleep practices, scheduling regular activities, seeking support from others, and learning relaxation methods.

Knowledge and skills to give mental health first aid

When a person develops a mental disorder, this will often be recognized by other people in their social network. Whether these others provide appropriate support and encourage appropriate help-seeking may be important to the person's recovery. There is evidence that people with mental disorders are more likely to seek help if someone else suggests it (Cusack et al., 2004; Dew et al., 1991). There is also evidence that receiving good social support is associated with a better outcome for the person with a mental disorder (Keitner et al., 1995). Such findings illustrate the importance of improving the community's knowledge and skills in mental health first aid. **Mental health first aid** is the initial help provided by a person's social network when they are developing a mental health problem or are in a mental health crisis (e.g. are suicidal).

There is only limited evidence from community surveys on mental health first aid knowledge. Australian national surveys have shown that many people see the value of listening to the person and of recommending professional help-seeking, although there are significant minorities who do not (Jorm et al., 2005b). Furthermore, many members of the public do not see it as helpful to ask a person with a mental disorder about suicidal feelings, despite the overwhelming consensus of mental health professionals that this is appropriate (Jorm et al., 2008). A particular concern is evidence from the United States that many young people say that they would not tell a responsible adult if a friend disclosed suicidal intentions (Dunham, 2004).

Knowledge of risk factors and causes that can be used to guide preventive action

Public knowledge of how to prevent mental disorders has received scant research attention. Nevertheless, a German survey on public attitudes to the prevention of depression showed that 75% agreed that prevention of depression is possible and around half of these said that they would take part in prevention programmes (Schomerus et al., 2008). Strategies that were approved of by over 90% of the population included: stable friendships, enjoyable leisure activities, family support, thinking positively, disclosing oneself to a confidant, activities that increases self-confidence, and meaningful activities.

Given these data showing public interest in taking preventive action, it is interesting that there has been so little health promotion activity in this area, in great contrast to the situation with major physical diseases. To some extent, this may be because there is less consensus about modifiable risk factors for mental disorders. However, there is enough known for action to be taken now, as illustrated by the following examples:

◆ **Cannabis and psychosis** There is now fairly consistent evidence that using cannabis increases the risk of psychosis. It has been proposed that the evidence is sufficient to justify warning young people about the risk (Moore et al., 2007).

◆ **Parenting strategies in relation to substance misuse** There is consistent evidence that a number of parenting strategies reduce the risk of alcohol and drug misuse in adolescents. One of these is **parental monitoring**, which refers to parents' knowledge of their child's activities, whereabouts, and friends. Greater parental monitoring reduces risk of both alcohol and cannabis misuse (Hayes et al., 2004; Lae and Crano, 2009).

◆ **Effects of family conflict on children** Longitudinal studies show that conflict between parents increases the risk of a range of mental health problems in their children, including depression and conduct disorder (Kelly, 2000). Parents need to know that their behaviour in settling conflict can potentially have these adverse effects.

Finding quality mental health information

In order to take effective action, the community needs to know how to find quality mental health information. Community surveys show that books, the Internet, and professional experts are all seen as suitable sources by many people (Jorm et al., 2005a). Print media have been a traditional source, but increasingly the internet is becoming a primary source for health information. A United States national survey found that 58% of Internet users reported using it to search for health information for themselves (Atkinson et al., 2009), while a European survey found that it was used by 52% of the population for health purposes (Kummervold et al., 2008). A survey of adults in the United States found that 21% had used the Internet to search for information about depression, anxiety, stress, or mental health issues (Fox and Jones, 2009). As well as being a source of information, the internet can also be a source of mutual support from other consumers and of online therapy.

While there is considerable information available to the public, there has been concern about its quality. A number of evaluations have been carried out on the quality of mental health information on the Internet and have often found it to be poor (e.g. Griffiths and Christensen, 2000; Ipser et al., 2007; Kisely et al., 2003). Similarly, the information given in self-help books for the public is not always of a high standard (Redding et al., 2008). Proposals have been made to improve the quality of internet health information on the internet (Commission of the European Communities, 2002), but these require adherence by website developers. Ultimately the ranking methods used by search engines may be the most practical method of helping consumers get the best information.

Public support for improving services

In many countries, mental health services are not supported by public funds at a level that satisfies the needs of service users, their families, or the clinicians who work in these services. Public knowledge and awareness may be an important factor in persuading policy makers to devote more resources to mental health services.

This is well illustrated by a community survey in Germany where members of the public were asked about what diseases should get a reduction in services if the health care budget had to be cut (Schomerus et al., 2006). In general, mental disorders were more often favoured for cuts than physical diseases, with alcoholism heading the list, followed by depression and schizophrenia. Cancer and myocardial infarction were seldom selected for cuts. The most important determinant of whether an area should be cut was the perceived severity of the disorder. This finding shows the importance of promoting to the public the large contribution that mental disorders make to a country's burden of disease.

Interventions to improve public knowledge and awareness

There have been programmes in many countries to improve public knowledge and awareness. However, many of these have no or limited evaluation. Described here are some programmes that have been evaluated against a control condition of some kind.

Population interventions

beyondblue

beyondblue is an Australian national organization which aims to increase community awareness and reduce stigma around depression and related disorders. It started in 2000 and is primarily funded by the federal and state governments. *beyondblue* has used a variety of means to achieve its community awareness aims, including frequent contacts with the media, advertising campaigns, high-profile supporters, sponsored community activities, and a popular website. A national survey of adults in 2004 to 2005 showed that awareness of *beyondblue* was very high (62%) and that there was a high level of exposure to depression through the media (Highet et al., 2006). However, because some Australian states did not initially provide funding for *beyondblue*, exposure to its work was higher in some parts of the country than in others. A comparison of changes in depression literacy showed that the high-exposure states had greater change than the low-exposure states (Jorm et al., 2005c, 2006c). In particular, there was greater ability to recognize depression, more positive beliefs about the benefits of some treatments, increased belief in the benefits of help-seeking in general, greater awareness of depression in self or others, and greater awareness of discrimination against depressed people.

Nuremberg Alliance Against Depression

In Germany, the Nuremberg Alliance Against Depression involved four components: interventions with GPs, a public campaign (poster, leaflets, events), interventions with community facilitators (e.g. clergy, teachers, police), and interventions with consumers and their relatives (Dietrich et al., 2010). The intervention was run in 2001 to 2002 in Nuremberg, with the city of Wurzburg serving as a comparison. To evaluate the intervention, surveys were carried out before, during and after the campaign in both cities. These showed increased awareness of depression, with the effects being stronger in people directly or indirectly affected by depression. For example, there was an improvement in attitudes to antidepressants and a decline in the belief that depression is due to a lack of self-discipline. The evaluation also showed a reduction in suicidal acts

in Nuremberg compared to Wurzburg. This intervention has now been extended to 17 European countries and called the European Alliance Against Depression.

Treatment and Intervention in Psychosis (TIPS)

TIPS was a programme based in one region of Norway designed to reduce the duration of untreated psychosis in first-episode schizophrenia (Joa et al., 2008). The programme had two components: availability of easy access detection teams and a large-scale information campaign to raise awareness of early recognition of psychosis to the public, schools, and GPs. Before the campaign began, the duration of untreated psychosis was 16 weeks and this reduced to 5 weeks during intervention. However, after the campaign stopped, the duration of untreated psychosis increased back to 15 weeks, despite the continuing availability of the easy access detection teams. These findings show that community awareness is critical to improving early intervention for people with schizophrenia.

Compass Strategy

The Compass Strategy was a community awareness campaign targeting young people aged 12 to 25 in one region of Australia from 2001 to 2003 (Wright et al., 2006). The aim was to encourage earlier detection and treatment of mental disorders during the stage of life when these disorders often have first onset. A variety of methods were used to convey messages, including cinema, radio, newspapers, youth magazines, posters, brochures, postcards, a website, an information line, and training for professionals who might facilitate earlier help-seeking. To evaluate the programme, community surveys of young people were carried out in the intervention region and in an adjacent comparison region. Although the campaign was of relatively short duration and of moderate intensity, a number of aspects of mental health literacy increased more in the intervention region.

Interventions based in educational institutions

Schools have been a popular setting for mental health education. However, very few evaluations have involved control groups. In the United States, one study has evaluated a mental illness awareness week in several high schools (Battaglia et al., 1990). This intervention involved psychiatry residents giving talks to students about topics such as psychiatry, drugs and alcohol, suicide, and depression. Compared to a group of students who did not receive talks, the intervention group was more likely to say that they would seek help from a psychiatrist or counsellor. In another United States evaluation, high school students were giving a lesson teaching them about mental illness and sources of help available (Esters et al., 1998). Compared to a control group, these students' beliefs about mental illness became more like those of health professionals and they developed more favourable attitudes to seeking help.

Higher education has been less popular as a setting for intervention than high school students, despite young adults being a high-risk group. One programme to educate university students about depression has been the subject of a controlled trial (Merritt et al., 2007). The intervention involved posters and postcards about depression and its treatment. Compared to a control group, those who received the intervention were more likely to recognize depressive symptoms and to report that antidepressants are not addictive, but there was no difference in the belief that depression can be treated effectively.

Mental Health First Aid training

A Mental Health First Aid course has been developed in Australia to train members of the public to give early help to people developing a mental disorder and to give assistance in mental health crisis situations (Kitchener and Jorm 2008). Two randomized controlled trials have been carried out to evaluate the effects of the course. These trials showed benefits in knowledge (improved agreement with health professionals about treatment), in behaviour (improved helping behaviour), in intentions (greater confidence in providing help to others), and in attitudes (decreased social distance from people with mental disorders). The Mental Health First Aid course has been widely disseminated in Australia and has spread to many other countries.

Websites

Although websites are now an important source of mental health information, there has been only one controlled trial of their impact. This trial evaluated the BluePages website (http://bluepages. anu.edu.au/) which provides information about depression. To evaluate the website, individuals who had depressive symptoms were randomly assigned to either work through the BluePages website systematically, to work through a website providing cognitive behaviour therapy (MoodGYM), or to an attention placebo control (Christensen et al., 2004). Those who explored BluePages had improved understanding of evidence-based treatments and improved depressive symptoms compared to the control.

How big a difference can interventions make?

While interventions can make a difference, this varies depending on the intensity of the intervention. Population interventions often have small effects on an individual, but can be useful if they can be disseminated cheaply across a whole population. Individual interventions are more likely to have larger effects, but are generally more expensive and difficult to implement. The level of intervention that is appropriate may depend on the degree of knowledge that an individual needs. Population interventions may be appropriate for most members of the community, whereas more intensive interventions will be justified for people in higher risk groups (e.g. young people) and those who having a higher probability of contact with people with mental disorders (e.g. people working in human service occupations).

Conclusions

Across many countries, deficiencies have been found in mental health literacy which limit the ability of the public to take action for prevention, early intervention, uptake of evidence-based treatment, self-help, first aid, and support for better mental health services. While there is some evidence that improvements are possible, this is an area that has not seen the large investment in health education and promotion that has occurred with cancer and heart disease.

References

Altamura, A.C., Dell'osso, B., Vismara, S., and Mundo, E. (2008). May duration of untreated illness influence the long-term course of major depressive disorder? *European Psychiatry*, **23**, 92–6.

Angermeyer, M.C., Breier, P., Dietrich, S., Kenzine, D., and Matschinger, H. (2005). Public attitudes toward psychiatric treatment: An international comparison. *Social Psychiatry and Psychiatric Epidemiology*, **40**, 855–64.

Angermeyer, M.C. and Matschinger, H. (2005). Have there been any changes in the public's attitudes towards psychiatric treatment? Results from representative population surveys in Germany in the years 1990 and 2001. *Acta Psychiatrica Scandinavica*, **111**, 68–73.

Atkinson, N.L., Saperstein, S.L., and Pleis, J. (2009). Using the internet for health related activities: findings from a national probability sample. *Journal of Medical Internet Research*, **11**, e4.

Battaglia, J., Coverdale, J.H., and Bushong, C.P. (1990). Evaluation of a mental illness awareness week program in public schools. *American Journal of Psychiatry*, **147**, 324–9.

Christensen, H., Griffiths, K.M., and Jorm, A.F. (2004). Delivering interventions for depression by using the internet: randomised controlled trial. *British Medical Journal*, **328**, 265.

Christiana, J.M., Gilman, S.E., Guarding, M., Mickelson, K., Morselli,, P.L., Olfson, M., *et al.* (2000). Duration between onset and time of obtaining initial treatment among people with anxiety and mood disorders: an international survey of members of mental health patient advocate groups. *Psychological Medicine*, **30**, 693–703.

Commission of the European Communities, Brussels (2002). eEurope 2002: quality criteria for health related websites. *Journal of Medical Internet Research*, **4**, e15.

Croghan, T.W., Tomlin, M., Pescosolido, B.A., Schnittker, J., Martin, J., Lubell, K. *et al.* (2003). American attitudes toward and willingness to use psychiatric medications. *Journal of Nervous and Mental Disease*, **191**, 166–74.

Cusack, J., Deane, F.P., Wilson, C.J., and Ciarrochi, J. (2004). Who influence men to go to therapy? Reports from men attending psychological services. *International Journal of Advances in Counselling*, **26**, 271–83.

Dew, M.A., Bromet, E.J., Schulberg, H.C., Parkinson, D.K., and Curtis, E.C. (1991). Factors affecting service utilization for depression in a white collar population. *Social Psychiatry and Psychiatric Epidemiology*, **26**, 230–7.

Dietrich, S., Mergl, R., Freudenberg, P., Althaus, D., and Hegerl, U. (2010). Impact of a campaign on the public's attitudes towards depression. *Health Education Research*, **25**, 135–50.

Dunham, K. (2004). Young adults' support strategies when peers disclose suicidal intent. *Suicide and Life-Threatening Behavior*, **34**, 56–65.

Esters, I.G., Cooker, P.G., and Ittenbach, R.F. (1998). Effects of a unit of instruction in mental health on rural adolescents' conceptions of mental illness and attitudes about seeking help. *Adolescence*, **33**, 469–76.

Griffiths, K.M. and Christensen, H. (2000). Quality of web based information on treatment of depression: cross sectional survey. *British Medical Journal*, **321**, 1511–15.

Haller, D.M., Sanci, L.A., Sawyer, S.M., and Patton, G.C. (2009). The identification of young people's emotional distress: a study in primary care. *British Journal of General Practice*, **59**, e61–70.

Hayes, L., Smart, D., Toumbourou, J.W., and Sanson, A. (2004). *Parenting influences on adolescent alcohol use*. Melbourne: Australian Institute of Family Studies.

Highet, N.J., Luscombe, G.M., Davenport, T.A., Burns, J.M., and Hickie, I.B. (2006). Positive relationships between public awareness activity and recognition of the impacts of depression in Australia. *Australian and New Zealand Journal of Psychiatry*, **40**, 55–8.

Ipser, J.C., Dewing, S., and Stein, D.J. (2007). A systematic review of the quality of information on the treatment of anxiety disorders on the internet. *Current Psychiatry Reports* 2007, **9**, 303–9.

Fox, S. and Jones, S. (2009). *The social life of health information.* Washington DC: Pew Internet.

Joa, I., Johannessen, J.O., Auestad, B., Friis, S., McGlashan, T., Melle, I., *et al.* (2008). The key to reducing duration of untreated first psychosis: information campaigns. *Schizophrenia Bulletin*, **34**, 466–72.

Jorm, A.F. and Griffiths, K.M. (2006). Population promotion of informal self-help strategies for early intervention against depression and anxiety. *Psychological Medicine*, **36**, 3–6.

Jorm, A.F., Korten, A.E., Jacomb, P.A., Christensen, H., Rodgers, B., and Pollitt, P (1997). 'Mental health literacy': A survey of the public's ability to recognise mental disorders and their beliefs about the effectiveness of treatment. *Medical Journal of Australia*, **166**, 182–6.

Jorm, A.F., Angermeyer, M.C., and Katschnig, H. (2000a). Public knowledge of and attitudes to mental disorders: A limiting factor in the optimal use of treatment services. In: Andrews, G. and Henderson, S. (eds.) *Unmet Need in Psychiatry: Problems, Resources, Responses*, pp. 399–413 Cambridge: Cambridge University Press.

Jorm, A.F., Medway, J., Christensen, H., Korten, A.E., Jacomb, P.A., and Rodgers, B. (2000b). Public beliefs about the helpfulness of interventions for depression: effects on actions taken when experiencing anxiety and depression symptoms. *Australian and New Zealand Journal of Psychiatry*, **34**, 619–26.

Jorm, A.F., Nakane, Y., Christensen, H., Yoshioka, K., Griffiths, K.M., and Wata, Y (2005a). Public beliefs about treatment and outcome of mental disorders: a comparison of Australia and Japan. *BMC Medicine*, **3**, 12.

Jorm, A.F., Blewitt, K.A., Griffiths, K.M., Kitchener, B.A., and Parslow, R.A. (2005b). Mental health first aid responses of the public: Results from an Australian national survey. *BMC Psychiatry*, **5**, 9.

Jorm, A.F., Christensen, H., and Griffiths, K.M. (2005c). The impact of *beyondblue: the national depression initiative* on the Australian public's recognition of depression and beliefs about treatments. *Australian and New Zealand Journal of Psychiatry*, **39**, 248–54.

Jorm, A.F., Kelly, C.M., Wright, A., Parslow, R.A., Harris, M.G., and McGorry, P.D. (2006a). Belief in dealing with depression alone: Results from community surveys of adolescents and adults. *Journal of Affective Disorders*, **96**, 59–65.

Jorm, A.F., Christensen, H., and Griffiths, K.M. (2006b). The public's ability to recognize mental disorders and their beliefs about treatment: Changes in Australia over 8 years. *Australian and New Zealand Journal of Psychiatry*, **40**, 36–41.

Jorm, A.F., Christensen, H., and Griffiths, K.M. (2006c). Changes in depression awareness and attitudes in Australia: the impact of *beyondblue: the national depression initiative. Australian and New Zealand Journal of Psychiatry*, **40**, 42–6.

Jorm, A.F., Morgan, A.J., and Wright, A. (2008). First aid strategies that are helpful to young people developing a mental disorder: beliefs of health professionals compared to young people and parents. *BMC Psychiatry*, **8**, 42.

Keitner, G.I., Ryan, C.E., Miller, I.W., Kohn, R., Bishop, D.S., and Epstein, N.B. (1995). Role of the family in recovery and major depression. *American Journal of Psychiatry*, **152**, 1002–8.

Kelly, J.B. (2000). Children's adjustment in conflicted marriage and divorce: A decade review of research. *Journal of the American Academy of Child & Adolescent Psychiatry*, **39**, 963–73.

Kessler, R.C., Aguilar-Gaxiola, S., Alonso, J., Chatterji, S., Lee, S., Ormel, J., *et al.* (2009). The global burden of mental disorders: an update from the WHO World Mental Health (WMH) surveys. *Epidemiologia e Psichiatria Sociale*, **18**, 23–33.

Kisely, S., Ong, G., and Takyar, A. (2003). A survey of the quality of web based information on the treatment of schizophrenia and Attention Deficit Hyperactivity Disorder. *Australian and New Zealand Journal of Psychiatry*, 37, 85–91.

Kitchener, B.A. and Jorm, A.F. (2008). Mental health first aid: An international programme for early intervention. *Early Intervention in Psychiatry*, **2**, 55–61.

Kummervold, P.E., Chronaki, C.E., Lausen, B., Prokosch, H.U., Rasmussen, J., Santana, S., *et al.* (2008). eHealth trends in Europe 2005–2007: a population-based survey. *Journal of Medical Internet Research*, **10**, e42.

Lae, A. and Crano, W.D. (2009). Monitoring matters: Meta-analytic review reveals the reliable linkage of parental monitoring with adolescent marijuana use. *Perspectives on Psychological Science*, **4**, 578–86.

Lauber, C., Nordt, C., Falcato, L., and Rössler, W. (2001). Lay recommendations on how to treat mental disorders. *Social Psychiatry and Psychiatric Epidemiology*, **36**, 553–6.

Magliano, L., Fiorillo, A., De Rosa, C., Malangone, C., and Maj, M. (2004). Beliefs about schizophrenia in Italy: A comparative nationwide survey of the general public, mental health professionals, and patients' relatives. *Canadian Journal of Psychiatry*, **49**, 322–30.

Marshall, M., Lewis, S., Lockwood, A., Drake, R., Jones, P., and Croudace, T. (2005). Association between duration of untreated psychosis and outcome in cohorts of first-episode patients: A systematic review. *Archives of General Psychiatry*, **62**, 975–83.

Merritt, R.K., Price, J.R., Mollison, J., and Geddes, J.R. (2007). A cluster randomized controlled trial to assess the effectiveness of an intervention to educate students about depression. *Psychological Medicine*, **37**, 363–72.

Moore, T.H., Zammit, S., Lingford-Hughes, A., Barnes, T.R., Jones, P.B., Burke, M., *et al.* (2007). Cannabis use and risk of psychotic or affective mental health outcomes: a systematic review. *Lancet*, **370**, 319–28.

Morgan, A.J. and Jorm, A.F. (2009). Self-help strategies that are helpful for sub-threshold depression: A Delphi consensus study. *Journal of Affective Disorders*, **115**, 196–200.

Priest, R.G., Vize, C., Roberts, A., Roberts, M., and Tylee, A. (1996). Lay people's attitudes to treatment for depression: Results of opinion poll for Defeat Depression Campaign just before its launch. *British Medical Journal*, **313**, 858–9.

Pyne, J.M., Rost, K.M., Farahati, F., Tripathi, S.P., Smith, J., Willams, D.K., *et al.* (2005). One size fits some: the impact of patient treatment attitudes on the cost-effectiveness of a depression primary-care intervention. *Psychological Medicine*, **35**, 839–54.

Redding, R.E., Herbert, J.D., Forman, E.M., and Gaudiano, B.A. (2008). Popular self-help books for anxiety, depression, and trauma: How scientifically grounded and useful are they? *Professional Psychology: Research and Practice*, **39**, 537–45.

Riedel-Heller, S.G., Matschinger, H., and Angermeyer, M.C. (2005). Mental disorders—who and what might help? Help-seeking and treatment preferences of the lay public. *Social Psychiatry and Psychiatric Epidemiology*, **40**, 167–74.

Schomerus, G., Matschinger, H., and Angermeyer, M.C. (2006). Preferences of the public regarding cutbacks in expenditure for patient care: Are there indications of discrimination against those with mental disorders? *Social Psychiatry and Psychiatric Epidemiology*, **41**, 369–77.

Schomerus, G., Angermeyer, M.C., Matschinger, H., and Riedel-Heller, S.G. (2008). Public attitudes towards prevention of depression. *Journal of Affective Disorders*, **106**, 257–63.

The WHO World Mental Health Consortium (2004). Prevalence, severity, and unmet need for treatment of mental disorders in the World Health Organization World Mental Health Surveys. *Journal of the American Medical Association*, **291**, 1581–90.

Thompson, A., Issakidis, C., and Hunt, C. (2008). Delay to seek treatment for anxiety and mood disorders in an Australian clinical sample. *Behaviour Change*, **25**, 71–84.

Wang, J.L., Adair, C., Fick, G., Lai, D., Evans, B., Perry, B.W., *et al.* (2007). Depression literacy in Alberta: Findings from a general population sample. *Canadian Journal of Psychiatry*, **52**, 442–9.

Wright, A., Jorm, A.F., Harris, M.G., and McGorry, P.D. (2007). What's in a name? Is accurate recognition and labeling of mental disorders by young people associated with better help-seeking and treatment preferences? *Social Psychiatry and Psychiatric Epidemiology*, **42**, 244–50.

Wright, A., McGorry, P.D., Harris, M.G., Jorm, A.F., and Pennell, K. (2006). Development and evaluation of a youth mental health community awareness campaign: The Compass Strategy. *BMC Public Health*, **6**, 215.

CHAPTER 29

Public attitudes towards people with mental illness

Bruce Link, Matthias C. Angermeyer, and Jo Phelan

The increase in research about public knowledge, attitudes, and beliefs concerning mental illnesses is a prominent fact. From just a small number of path-breaking studies in the 1950s and 1960s (Cohen and Struening, 1962; Cumming and Cumming, 1957; Nunnally, 1961; Star, 1955) the field has grown to become an enormous literature that has used multiple measures and multiple methods in studies conducted in a vast array of populations (Link et al., 2004; Thornicroft 2006; Thornicroft et al., 2009). We seek to capture the essence of this body of work by reviewing the core questions it has assessed. We follow this brief review by posing two questions. The first asks why it is important to study knowledge, attitudes, and beliefs (KABs) and turns our attention to KABs as representations of cultural conceptions of mental illness. We argue that KABs are elements of a cultural context that influences how people think about and respond to mental illnesses and that this influence expands beyond the narrow individually-based model that asks whether individual attitudes are good predictors of individual behaviours. To exemplify this point we highlight the importance of cultural conceptions for modified labelling theory and for the creation and sustenance of structural stigma. The second question asks how we can capture changes in KABs towards mental illnesses and leads us to consider the importance of studies that monitor trends in KABs over time.

Knowledge, attitudes, and beliefs: constructs and their meanings

Most of the content found in studies of KABs concerning mental illnesses can be captured in a relatively simple rubric, much of which has been in place since the very earliest studies of these phenomena (e.g. Star, 1955). The reason for this is that studies have sought to achieve the common goal of assessing mental representations of, and emotional responses to, mental illnesses and people who have them. We explicate this multifaceted domain below by briefly describing each component.

What is mental illness?

Each member of the public has his or her own internal (albeit less explicitly formulated) *Diagnostic and Statistical Manual of Mental Disorders* (DSM) or International Classification of Diseases (ICD) that achieves some classification as to what is, and what is not, mental illness. Learning about these lay classification schemes is potentially important for understanding help-seeking—an individual is unlikely to seek mental health treatment for something he/she does not identify as mental illness. On a collective level, societies will not develop mental health treatment options, legal statutes, or insurance policies for conditions few people think of as mental illnesses. Finally the number of people labelled as having a mental illness (for good or ill) will depend on how broad these definitions are in a given context. Studies of KABs have assessed this component by asking open-ended questions such as 'When you hear someone say that a person is "mentally ill" what does that mean to you?' and then coding the open-ended responses (Phelan et al., 2000; Star, 1955). More commonly researchers have constructed vignettes describing individuals with symptoms of mental illness and have asked whether the behaviour constitutes some kind of mental illness or some specific manifestation of mental illness (e.g. major depression, schizophrenia) (Angermeyer and Matschinger, 1994; Link et al., 1999).

What labels are used to describe people with mental illnesses?

Multiple options for labelling mental illnesses are possible. The use of labels can vary from the vernacular (crazy, insane, etc.) to the clinical (obsessive–compulsive disorder (OCD), bipolar, etc.) and from the currently appropriate (user, consumer) to the pejorative (nut job, psycho). Perhaps the most obvious reason for considering this domain to be of importance is the harmful effects that pejorative labelling might have both for individuals who have mental illnesses and people who might develop them. Beyond this, labels (such as OCD, attention deficit hyperactivity disorder, bipolar) help structure experience and influence how people communicate about a problem with doctors and mental health professionals. Given that professionals rely on patient descriptions, this could influence whether a person goes to treatment, where they go, and precisely what kind of treatment they receive when they arrive. This domain can be assessed through direct inquiries in a survey research setting. However, the public has largely learned the 'correct' language for describing mental health problems and is likely to reflect that in their responses. Qualitative research that observes people in contexts in which they are not being 'careful' or content analysis of newspaper headlines or dialogue in television and movies can be quite revealing about variations in the use of labels (Wahl, 1995).

What are people with mental illnesses like?

Stereotypes about mental illnesses can vary considerably in their breadth and strength. One of the most prominent and consequential is the stereotype of dangerousness—the belief that people with mental illness are likely to do something violent towards others (Link et al., 1987, 1999). But other stereotypes such as incompetence, unpredictability, and malevolence are prominent as well. Research can assess whether beliefs about the group—people with mental illnesses or people with schizophrenia—are exaggerated or completely inaccurate. Research can also assess whether the stereotype is applied to individuals within the group whether or not the individual fits the caricature that the stereotype implies. At the individual level, the stereotypes might affect self-stigma as Corrigan and Watson (2002) describe it or the behaviour of others when people apply for jobs, housing, or educational opportunities. At the societal level, coercive policy is more likely if beliefs about dangerousness are prevalent and paternalism is more likely if beliefs about incompetence are strong. Stereotypes have been assessed in many ways including the method of the semantic differential that presents pairs of opposite adjectives focused on a target like a description of a person with mental illness or a history of mental illness (Olmsted and Durham, 1976; Nunnally, 1961). More recently people have begun to develop and deploy Implicit Attitudes Tests in the area of mental illnesses. The value of these tests is that they are less influenced by social desirability bias as they rely on reaction times in making connections between concepts—e.g. 'mental illness' and 'dangerous' as opposed to 'mental illness' and 'harmless.'

What causes mental illnesses?

Public beliefs about causes of mental illnesses vary as to whether genetic and other biological factors, stressful circumstances, social conditions, family factors, individual behaviours, personality, spirit possession or fate play important roles in aetiology. At the individual level beliefs about causes are important in whether and to what extent individuals and families are 'blamed' or 'exculpated'. If personal weakness, reckless behaviours, or poor parenting are emphasized, then so-called attribution theory (Weiner et al., 1988) would lead us to believe that the public would be less likely to help and more likely to blame and punish individuals and families experiencing mental illnesses. If the cause is attributed to factors the individual cannot control such as genes, biochemical processes, or some stressful circumstance, a better public response would be expected. On the other hand, a strong belief in genetic causes could lead members of the public to avoid marrying family members of affected individuals and to see the problem as more serious and intractable (Phelan 2005, 2006). At the societal level beliefs about causes can shape the treatment system we choose to construct for people with mental illnesses. An excellent historical example is Rothman's (1971) account of the discovery of asylums in the early 19th century in America. Rothman argues that the movement to create asylums was powerfully influenced by the reformers'

conviction that the root causes of mental illness lay in the disorder and turmoil caused by the massive industrialization, urbanization, and immigration that was taking place at the time. Imbued with this belief the antidote was obvious, 'asylums'—orderly institutions located in bucolic settings away from the illness-generating turmoil of urban centres. Driven by beliefs about the causes of mental illness, the asylum remained the dominant mode of service delivery for generations, powerfully shaping the lives of people with mental illnesses and their families (Rothman, 1971). Numerous studies have assessed beliefs about cause either by having members of the public respond to individual items in a Likert format or by presenting a vignette followed by questions like 'How likely is it that the condition was caused by "genetic factors", by "stressful circumstances", by a "chemical imbalance in the brain", "the way the person was raised"' and so on.

What is the range of emotional reactions to people with mental illnesses?

The idea that stigmatized individuals experience emotions of guilt, shame, humiliation, and anger is widely acknowledged. At the same time it is also true that emotions of fear, pity, awkwardness, anxiety, and irritation are possible responses to people with mental illnesses among members of the general public. These emotional responses may be a prominent mediator of KABs as when beliefs about dangerousness lead to feelings of fear which then lead to social rejection and exclusion. Emotions can also be 'read' independently of what a person says or the way a person wants to be perceived. For example, someone who feels some combination of pity, awkwardness, and anxiety in the presence of a person with mental illness might modulate their voice and speak in a soft and unnaturally calming tone thereby signalling to the person with mental illness that he/she is being approached from a standpoint of differentness. Assessments of emotional reactions in the literature have generally provided a stimulus—like a vignette describing someone with mental illness— and then asked respondents to indicate whether the stimulus induces any of a number of emotions (e.g. Angermeyer et al., 2010).

What should a person with mental illness do to address their situation?

A consistent concern in studies of KABs has directed attention to professional help seeking and its alternatives. What might the public advise a person with mental illness to do or what might they do themselves if they experienced symptoms—talk to friends, consult a clergyman, see a general practice doctor, go to a mental health professional, wait for the problem to get better on its own, or something else? What the public deems to be appropriate could influence their own and others' help seeking thereby influencing the demand for professional services and the course of symptoms and their consequences.

What policies should be developed for people with mental illnesses?

Another key concern in studies of KABs involves support for broad policies designed to help or manage people with mental illnesses. Questions such as: what level of support do policies favouring community integration of people with mental illnesses enjoy? Does the public support coercive policies and under what circumstances?

Should mental health treatment be covered by insurance or national health plans in the same way as physical illnesses? Should people with a history of mental illness be allowed to adopt children or buy guns? Questions like these have been addressed in studies of KABs by, for example, asking respondents whether they would be willing to have a group home for people with mental illnesses located in their neighbourhood or 'who should be responsible for paying for the treatment of someone with schizophrenia—the government, private insurers, charity, or the person with mental illness and their family?'.

How would I respond to a person with mental illness?

Perhaps the most commonly assessed domain of KABs is so-called social distance. Respondents are queried about their willingness to interact with a person with mental illness across relationships that vary in intimacy from being a mere acquaintance to accepting a person into the family through marriage. Early studies assessed social distance from a person described as a 'mental patient' (Whatley, 1959) whereas more recent studies typically describe a person in a vignette and ask respondents how willing they would be to engage in specific kinds of interaction with the person. Social distance questions can therefore be construed as behavioural intentions with respect to rejecting behaviours.

Summary

KAB studies can be conceptualized as answering a series of questions that capture how people think about mental illness—what is mental illness, what causes it, how do people react to mental illnesses, and what should be done about them. On their face these domains convey some degree of importance, as one can imagine how help-seeking behaviour or policy might be influenced by such beliefs. In the next section we expand our consideration of the importance of KABs by considering them in light of the idea that they assess a critically important contextual factor that shapes many behaviours.

The importance of KABs: cultural conceptions and cultural contexts

One way to think about domains of KABs, and the most common way to do so, is at the individual level that asks about individual differences in each domain, what determines such individual differences, and what consequences such differences might have for individual behaviours. Construed in this way KAB research is sometimes challenged when it either does not assess individual behaviours at all or predicts such behaviours with less than ideal accuracy. The lack of correspondence between attitudes and behaviours is brought to the fore and the utility of research focused on KABs is sharply questioned.

However, another way to reason about KAB domains is to view them at the collective level—as indicators of context. Specifically, if we could obtain an accurate assessment of all of the domains identified above we would have a portrait of the cultural conception of mental illness in a given place and at a particular time. It would tell us how people think and feel about mental illnesses and how such illnesses should be managed. As a context this cultural conception becomes an external reality—something that individuals must take into account when they make decisions and enact behaviours. The idea is that individuals (e.g. people with mental illnesses,

care givers, policy-makers) know about cultural conceptions and shape their behaviours to some significant degree to take account of them no matter what their own knowledge, attitudes, and beliefs happen to be. In this way, cultural conceptions can have an important impact on things that matter for people with mental illnesses through mechanisms that do not involve individual attitudes towards mental illnesses influencing individual behaviours toward people with a mental illness. To the extent that this is true, KABs—as an assessment of cultural conceptions and a cultural context— are critically important factors that need deep and ongoing scrutiny so that they can be better understood and their influence harnessed to achieve desirable ends. Some support for the idea of KABs as an important cultural context can be found in several strands of theory and research including modified labelling theory and the concept of structural stigma.

Modified labelling theory: cultural conceptions and individual outcomes

Constructed in response to a lively debate concerning the labelling theory of mental illness (Gove, 1975; Scheff, 1966), so-called modified labelling theory (Link et al., 1989) identified cultural conceptions as a contextual factor disadvantaging people exposed to mental illness labelling. According to the theory people learn about cultural conceptions of mental illness as part of socialization into the culture they grow up in (Angermeyer and Matschinger, 1996; Scheff 1966; Wahl, 1995). Once in place, people's internalization of cultural conceptions yields a lay theory about what it means to have a mental illness (Angermeyer and Matschinger, 1994; Furnham and Bower, 1992). People know about cultural conceptions and form beliefs about whether people will reject an individual with mental illness as a friend, employee, neighbour, or intimate partner and whether most people will devalue a person with mental illness as less trustworthy, intelligent, and competent. For someone who never develops mental illness and is never exposed to mental illness labelling these beliefs have little personal relevance. But for someone who develops a mental illness and is exposed to mental illness labelling, these beliefs are potentially enormously consequential as they become personally relevant. The person may wonder, 'Will others look down on me, reject me, because I have been identified as having a mental illness?'. Expecting and fearing rejection, a person might feel badly about themselves, act less confidently in social situations, or simply avoid a potentially threatening contact altogether. This can have consequences for strained social interactions (Farina, 1968), constricted social networks (Link et al., 1989; Perlick et al., 2001), a compromised quality of life (Rosenfield, 1997), low self-esteem (Link et al., 2001, 2008), unemployment, and income loss (Link, 1987). To the extent that this theory is apt, KABs attain substantial important because they represent the content of the cultural conception that people internalize. If we can change the cultural conception in beneficial ways we will change the images of mental illness that people internalize and thereby the social psychological situation people face when they develop a mental illness.

Structural stigma refers to accumulated policies and institutional practices that work to the disadvantage of a stigmatized group. For example, insurance coverage for mental illnesses in the United States includes stricter limits on payments and higher cost sharing than physical illnesses (Glied and Frank, 2008). Policies and practices are likely strongly influenced by cultural conceptions for at least four reasons. First, cultural conceptions are the ways we have of thinking about the issue, about what mental illness is, what people who have mental illnesses are like, what people need and how we should manage people who develop mental illnesses. This will influence the kind of policies and practices we conjure to address the problem, putting bounds on what we think makes sense and what we think is possible. As the previously mentioned example of Rothman's (1971) analysis of the asylum makes clear, historical accounts of eras in which very different cultural conceptions than ones we now prefer held sway show how powerful such conceptions can be. The importance of cultural conceptions is also evident when we look across cultures to note how different conceptions of mental illness can lead to different treatment and different outcomes (Yang et al., 2007). Second, to the extent that there is a societal downward placement of mental illness in a hierarchy of importance or worthiness, structural stigma is likely to be a consequence. When studies of the prestige of medical specialties and of specific illnesses have been undertaken, psychiatry and psychiatric illness are rated low (Norredam and Album, 2007). Moreover, coverage of mental illness in high-impact prestigious journals like *The Lancet* is dramatically lower than one would expect given the burden of disease that mental illnesses impose (Griffiths, 2010). Lower prestige and reduced coverage in major journals means less prominence that could lead to lower funding, fewer scientific discoveries, and less money for good patient care. Third, cultural conceptions impose constraints on many policies and practices. For example, as treatment providers and policy makers make decisions about where to locate a new board and care home for people with serious mental illness, they are likely to include in their considerations the expected response of the neighbourhoods they imagine placing the facility in. Processes like these have resulted in a clustering of board and care facilities in neighbourhoods that do not have the clout to exclude such facilities, thereby creating what have been called 'psychiatric ghettos' (Arboleda-Florez, 2006). Fourth and finally, structural stigma is not only induced by cultural conceptions, it is also sustained by such conceptions. Institutional policies and practices that disadvantage people with illnesses that are viewed positively in the culture are likely to be challenged and culled from the existing repertoires of such policies and practices. Imagine for example that, unlike all other illnesses, insurance policies for heart disease (instead of mental illnesses) were capped at lower levels of compensation and included higher co-pays. Despite the fact that a rationale could be conjured for such a policy, given that heart disease is influenced by behaviours people can control, such as sedentarism, fatty diets, and smoking, an insurance policy disadvantaging heart disease is unimaginable at the current time. Similarly, if cultural conceptions deemed some of the disadvantages that people with mental illnesses currently endure as simply outrageous and unthinkable, pressure would be brought to bear to change them and they would not exist.

In sum, because of structural stigma a person who develops a mental illness gets fewer benefits (e.g. knowledge about how to prevent, cure, or treat) and more disadvantages (housing in locations where crime, infectious disease, pollution, and noise are high) than a person who happens to develop heart disease or cancer. Moreover, structural stigma has long-lasting consequences as when people who have schizophrenia are disadvantaged by a history of reduced funding for research or by the general absence of care facilities in safe areas because of policies enacted in earlier eras. Because structural stigma is enabled and sustained by cultural conceptions, it follows that cultural conceptions are broadly important factors in the well-being of people with mental illnesses.

The importance of monitoring KABs and what we have learned from doing so

To the extent that cultural conceptions are important, it becomes critical to understand them and, in our view, understanding them requires multiple assessments over long periods of time. The reason a long-term perspective is required is that cultural conceptions change relatively slowly and it is impossible to observe such change in cross-sectional studies. Cross-sectional (or other studies with a short time frame) direct attention to the variation such studies can capture—individual differences in KABs and their associations with outcomes variables of interest. Important as such studies can be they leave us blind to the impact of changes in levels of KABs over time and to the powerful implications such changes have for the context in which people experience mental illnesses. In keeping with this rationale, we present evidence from several studies that have enacted the same or similar methods over multiple time periods. We begin by considering a study conducted by Phelan et al. (2000) that provided evidence on changes in the stereotype of dangerousness associated with mental illness in the United States.

The dangerousness stereotype in the United States from 1950 to 1996

Over the period from the 1950s to the 1990s two perspectives on public attitudes were in play. On the one hand the 'optimists' (Crocetti and Spiro, 1973) heralded a new era in which the public was more knowledgeable and much more tolerant than it had been in the 1950's. 'Pessimists' took a decidedly different and much more sceptical view attributing any apparent positive trends to surface-level changes in knowledge about the socially desirable response to survey items (Link and Cullen, 1983). There was little if any consideration of the possibility that things might have gotten worse. It was in this context that Phelan undertook a study that could reflect on such changes over long periods of time.

In 1996, teams of investigators at Columbia and Indiana Universities constructed the MacArthur module of the General Social Survey (Pescosolido et al., 2010). Interested in trends over time, the team directed attention to the first nationwide study of public attitudes conducted in 1950 by Shirley Star. Unfortunately, the questions in the original study generally used language that had become 'dated' by 1996. However, the following open-ended question was available and could be repeated, 'Of course, everyone hears a good deal about physical illness and disease, but now, what about the ones we call mental or nervous illness… When you hear someone say that a person is "mentally-ill," what does that mean to you?' In both the Star study and the MacArthur module of the 1996 survey, answers were recorded verbatim. Fortunately, every 10th interview of the original Star survey had been saved by the librarian at the National Opinion Research Center in Chicago where both studies were conduced. This allowed trained coders to reliably rate the 1950 and 1996 responses to this question with respect to whether the respondent spontaneously referred to violent behaviour in describing a person with mental illness. Thereby the study allowed a rare glimpse at trends in one key stereotype in the stigma associated with mental illnesses involving psychosis.

Remarkably, the analysis revealed that despite massive efforts to educate the public about mental illness and enormous advances in treatment, respondents whose descriptions indicated a person with psychosis were nearly two and a half times as likely to mention violent behaviour in 1996 (31.0%) as in 1950 (12.7%) (Phelan et al., 2000). Whatever the reasons for this change, at the very least, it represents a discomforting fact for people with a psychotic illness seeking broader social acceptance.

From the vantage point of our interest in surveillance of KABs over long periods of time, it is important to note that without the 1950 benchmark we would not have known that these beliefs about dangerousness were increasing and that the conventional wisdom, as reflected in the views of both optimists and pessimists, was out of step with this empirical finding. Moreover, once revealed, attention can be directed to factors that might have driven this dramatic change, and since the change is at the population level we are likely to be directed to factors associated with structural stigma. In this regard Phelan and Link (1998, 2004) investigated two possible explanations. In the first, they considered whether the implementation of the policy of deinstitutionalization in the United States might have induced more negative street contact with people with mental illnesses driving beliefs about dangerousness up. In the second they investigated the role of legal criteria for involuntary commitment that focused on widely publicized judgements of 'dangerous to self or others'. Results revealed no support for the deinstitutionalization hypothesis (Phelan and Link, 2004) but some support for the legal dangerousness criterion hypothesis—verbatim descriptions from 1996 were much more likely to use the phrase 'dangerous to self or others' than the 1950 descriptions were (Phelan and Link, 1998). Thus the long-term surveillance of this important KAB revealed a dramatic and unexpected change in its prevalence and directed attention to possible structural stigma sources of these changes that could be evaluated for validity.

Changes in KABs in Germany from 1990 to 2001

Over the last 20 years or so, dramatic efforts have been unleashed aimed at educating the public that mental illnesses are illnesses like other illnesses—that they have a biological basis and are amenable to treatment. The first study that could track changes in KABs over any part of this period was undertaken by Angermeyer and colleagues. In 1990, the first representative survey on KAB was conducted in the 'old' Federal Republic of Germany, involving German citizens aged 18 years and older, living in non-institutional settings. Eleven years later, in 2001, another survey was carried out, using the same sampling procedure and the same personal, fully structured interview which began with the presentation of a vignette depicting an individual suffering from either schizophrenia or major depressive disorder. The main purpose of the study was to examine whether the reforms of German mental health care, which during the 1990s had made considerable progress, were reflected in the public's attitudes towards psychiatric treatment. It was hoped that the change from custodial care provided by large institutions to community-focused services may have reduced the stigma attached to mental illness, resulting in a greater willingness to seek help from mental health professionals and also in less discriminatory attitudes towards people suffering from mental illness.

In fact, the proportion of the public recommending that a person with schizophrenia or major depressive disorder should see a psychiatrist or psychotherapist increased substantially. By contrast, the willingness to recommend other helping sources either remained unchanged (self-help group, taking a cure) or even decreased (general practitioner, priest). As concerns particular treatment modalities, the change was most pronounced for the use of psychotropic medication for schizophrenia. The probability that it was recommended by the public increased by 27%. This was mainly because of a marked decrease of the proportion of those who were opposed to medication. Also the probability of the endorsement of psychotherapy increased while 'alternative' treatment modalities did not show marked changes over time. For the treatment of major depressive disorder, an increase across all treatment modalities could be observed (Angermeyer and Matschinger, 2005a).

Apart from a greater acceptance of psychiatric treatment, there were also changes in the public's beliefs about the causes of the two mental disorders in question. The percentage of those endorsing brain disease and genetic factors as a cause increased substantially, while the attribution to psychosocial stress remained practically unchanged. The readiness to blame the afflicted person for the illness decreased. Thus, there was a tendency towards the public becoming more ready to adopt causal explanations currently favoured by mental health professionals, resulting in the gap between public and professional views becoming narrower (Angermeyer and Matschinger, 2005b).

In sharp contrast to the changes observed with regard to the public's causal beliefs and their help-seeking and treatment preferences was the development of attitudes towards those suffering from mental illnesses. Rather than having become more favourable, the emotional reaction of the public remained unchanged or actually deteriorated over the time period under study. Respondents expressed more fear and anger about an individual with schizophrenia in 2001 than in 1990. There was no change with regard to pro-social reactions. With respect to the depression vignette, there was an increase of pro-social reactions, but also of anger, while fear remained unchanged (Angermeyer et al., 2010). The public's desire for social distance from people with schizophrenia also increased markedly. For instance, while 19% of respondents rejected such an individual as a neighbour in 1990, this number had risen to 35% in 2001. As concerns major depressive disorder, the preference for social distance remained the same (Angermeyer and Matschinger, 2004, 2005b).

These findings could be replicated in another study which was carried out in the eastern part of Germany, covering the time period between 1993 and 2001. Again, the public becoming more 'literate' in terms of their knowledge about mental disorders and showing a greater readiness to recommend treatment provided by mental health professionals was in sharp contrast to emotional reactions remaining unchanged or even deteriorating and the desire for social distance increasing slightly (Angermeyer et al., 2009).

Two conclusions can be drawn from these studies: first, improving mental health services may have a positive effect on the public's attitude towards help-seeking from mental health professionals. However, this may not necessarily translate into an increase of the public's acceptance of those using these services. Second, the promulgation of neurobiological conceptualizations of mental disorders may not help reduce the stigma attached to mental illness, as claimed by biological psychiatrists. It may even have the opposite effect. Again as with the Phelan study, without the benchmark of the earlier period the direction of change from the early 1990s to 2001 could not have been known. Moreover we would not have known that 'improvements' in neurobiological understandings failed to fuel corresponding improvements in emotional or social distancing reactions. This latter finding is critical as such a change was widely touted as an antidote to stigma.

Changes in KABs in the United States from 1996 to 2006

Like the studies conducted by Angermeyer and colleagues in Germany, a 10-year follow-up of KABs in the United States sought to assess whether and to what extent presenting mental illnesses and alcohol dependence as medical diseases increase service use and reduce stigma (Pescosolido et al., 2010). With benchmarks like the 1999 U.S. Surgeon General's report, efforts designed to reduce stigma were often predicated on assumptions that neuroscience offered the most effective tool to lower prejudice and discrimination. For example the National Alliance for the Mentally Ill's (NAMI's) 'Campaign to End Discrimination' sought to improve public understanding of neurobiological bases of mental illnesses and substance abuse, facilitating treatment-seeking and lessening stigma. Over the decade between 1996 and 2006, the American public was taught about the symptoms of mental illnesses, educated about biological theories of aetiology, and informed about the value of treatment to thereby underscore the basic argument that mental illnesses are diseases, no different from others. The National Stigma Study–Replication (NSS-R) which used modules from the 1996 and 2006 General Social Surveys in the United States provides evidence on the consequences of these efforts for KABs.

The NSS-R is a nationally representative study conducted under the umbrella of the General Social Survey that is implemented on an ongoing basis by the National Opinion Research Corporation. Individuals (N = 1956) were interviewed face-to-face and presented with vignettes describing cases meeting DSM-IV criteria for schizophrenia, major depression or alcohol dependence. Approximately half of the respondents were interviewed in 1996, the other half in 2006, and all were randomly assigned to one vignette and then asked about KABs about the described person.

Results show that there were widespread increases in public acceptance of neurobiological theories about the causes of mental illnesses and significant changes in public support for treatment but no reduction in social distance or perceptions of dangerousness to self or others. Further, in both years and across all vignette conditions, holding a neurobiological conception was either unrelated to social distance and perceptions of dangerousness or was actually associated with an increase in these indicators of stigmatizing reactions (Pescosolido et al., 2010).

The striking similarity in the pattern of findings found in the NSS-R and German studies suggests the generality of the changes and provides the reassurance of replication. Again, the changes could not have been revealed without the trend over time, and we could not have known with any precision that the portrait of current KABs is the outcome of changes from an earlier era. Interestingly, the data provide rationales for both optimism and pessimism. On the one hand the data tell us that at least certain aspects of KABs are subject to change—tremendous effort was exerted to realize change and change did in fact occur in some dimensions. The public is much more likely to see mental illnesses as medical conditions and to believe that seeking help from medical and psychiatric sources is appropriate for such conditions. This change in the KAB context has been accompanied by a dramatic increase in the number of people with disorders seeking appropriate help for those disorders (Wang et al., 2005). The rational for pessimism resides in the relatively high and enduring levels of social distance, beliefs in dangerousness and in the Germany study negative emotional reactions. There are three reasons for pessimism associated with this finding. First, a highly touted approach—advancing a neurobiological basis for mental illnesses—that was believed to be a potent factor failed to reduce core aspects of stigma. Second is the possibility that social distance and perceptions of danger are simply more deeply ingrained in history and the human condition and, as a consequence, much more difficult to change. Third is the possibility that social distance and stereotypes are not core concerns of the most powerful groups shaping public opinion—the medical, psychiatric, and psychotherapeutic professions and pharmaceutical companies. The changes that have occurred are consistent with the interests of these groups: to be recognized on a par with other medical conditions for treating a 'real' illness, to underscore the legitimacy of approaches to treatment that these groups deliver and, for the industry, an expansion of the market. Changing stereotypes and social distance are not as essential to the aims of these interest groups. People with mental illnesses who are often deeply harmed by stereotypes and rejection have great interest in these domains but less power to shape messages directed at what matters most to them.

Summary and conclusion

The domains of public knowledge, attitudes, and beliefs that researchers assess can be conceptualized as a reflection of cultural conceptions of mental illnesses. Such conceptions form a cultural context that influences the way we think about mental illnesses and the people who have them. The nature of the cultural context shapes behaviours that range from how individuals respond to the illnesses they develop to the behaviours of policy-makers who set research, treatment, and social-control policies that affect people with mental illnesses. In order to understand cultural contexts, it is critical that we implement studies that allow us to capture variation in these phenomena. Cross-sectional studies are limited in this respect because a one point in time study assesses the cultural context at only one time and does not powerfully reveal variations. Ongoing surveillance, as enacted in the studies we reviewed, serves to overcome this weakness and has helped reveal dramatic changes that have been both surprising and critically important for the evaluation of extant policy. Our conceptualization of KABs and our empirical assessment of changes in them over time convince us of their importance and inspire us to advocate for ongoing research to assess them.

References

Angermeyer, M.C. and Matschinger, H. (1994) Lay beliefs about schizophrenic disorder: The results of a population survey in Germany. *Acta Psychiatrica Scandinavica*, **89**, 39–45.

Angermeyer, M.C. and Matschinger, H. (1996) Public attitude towards psychiatric treatment. *Acta Psychiatrica Scandinavica*, **94**, 326–36.

Angermeyer, M.C. and Matschinger, H. (2004). Public attitudes to people with depression: Have there been any changes over the last decade? *Journal of Affective Disorders*, **83**, 177–82.

Angermeyer, M.C. and Matschinger, H. (2005a) Have there been any changes in the public's attitudes towards psychiatric treatment? Results from representative population surveys in Germany in the years 1990 and 2001. *Acta Psychiatrica Scandinavica*, **111**, 68–73.

Angermeyer, M.C. and Matschinger, H. (2005b). Causal beliefs and attitudes to people with schizophrenia. Trend analysis based on data from two population surveys in Germany. *British Journal of Psychiatry*, **186**, 331–4.

Angermeyer, M.C., Holzinger, A., and Matschinger, H. (2009). Mental health literacy and attitude toward people with mental illness. A trend analysis based on population surveys in the eastern part of Germany. *European Psychiatry*, **24**, 225–32.

Angermeyer, M.C., Holzinger, A., and Matschinger, H. (2010). Emotional reactions to people with mental illness. *Epidemiologia e Psichiatria Sociale*, **19**, 26–32.

Arboleda-Florez, J. (2006). Forensic psychiatry: contemporary scope, challenges and controversies. *World Psychiatry*, **5**, 87–91.

Cohen, J. and Struening, E.L. (1962). Opinions about mental illness in the personnel of two large mentalhospitals. *Journal of Abnormal and Social Psychology*, **64**, 349–60.

Corrigan, P.W. and Watson, A.C. (2002). The paradox of self-stigma and mental illness. *Clinical Psychology: Science and Practice*, **9**, 35–53.

Crocetti, G. and Spiro, H. (1973). *Contemporary attitudes towards mental illness*. Pittsburgh, PA: University of Pittsburgh Press.

Cumming, J. and Cumming, E. (1957). *Closed ranks*. Cambridge, MA: Harvard University Press.

Farina, A., Allen, J.G., and Saul, B. (1968). The role of the stigmatized in affecting social relationships. *Journal of Personality*, **36**, 169–82.

Furnham, A. and Bower, P. (1992). A comparison of academic and lay theories of schizophrenia. *British Journal of Psychiatry*, **161**, 201–10.

Gove, W. R. (1975). *The Labeling of Deviance: Evaluating a Perspective*. New York: Sage.

Glied, S. and Frank, R. (2008). Shuffling toward parity—bringing mental health care under the umbrella. *New England Journal of Medicine*, **359**, 113–15.

Griffiths, K. (2010). Unraveling the Stigma of Depression. Paper presented at the Meetings of the Academy of Eating Disorders, Salzburg, Germany, 10 June 2010.

Link, B.G. (1987). Understanding labeling effects in the area of mental disorders: An assessment of the effects of expectations of rejection. *American Sociological Review*, **52**, 96–112.

Link, B.G., Castille, D., and Stuber, J. (2008). Stigma and coercion in the context of outpatient treatment for people with mental illnesses. *Social Science and Medicine*, **67**, 409–19.

Link, B.G. and Cullen, F.T. (1983). Reconsidering the social rejection of ex-mental patients: Levels of attitudinal response, *American Journal of Community Psychology*, **11**, 261–73.

Link, B.G., Cullen, F.T., Frank, J., and Wozniak, J.F. (1987). The social rejection of former mental patients: understanding why labels matter. *American Journal of Sociology* **92**, 1461–500.

Link, B.G., Cullen, F.T., Struening, E., Shrout, P., and Dohrenwend, B.P. (1989). A modified labeling theory approach in the area of the mental disorders: An empirical assessment. *American Sociological Review* **54**, 400–23.

Link, B.G., Phelan, J.C., Bresnahan, M., Stueve, A., and Pescosolido, B.A. (1999). Public conceptions of mental illness: labels, causes, dangerousness, and social distance. *American Journal of Public Health*, **89**, 1328–33.

Link, B.G., Struening, E.L., Neese-Todd, S., Asmussen, S., and Phelan, J.C. (2001). Stigma as a barrier to recovery: The consequences of stigma for the self-esteem of people with mental illnesses. *Psychiatric Services*, **52**, 1621–6.

Link, B.G., Yang, L., Phelan, J.C., and Collins, P.Y. (2004). Measuring mental illness stigma. *Schizophrenia Bulletin*, **30**, 11–42.

Norredam, M. and Album, D. (2007). Prestige and its significance for medical specialties and diseases. *Scandinavian Journal of Public Health* **35**, 655–61.

Nunnally, J.C. (1961). *Popular conceptions of mental health: Their development and change*. New York: Holt, Rinehart, and Winston.

Olmsted, D.W., and Durham, K. (1976). Stability of mental health attitudes: A semantic differential study. *Journal of Health and Social Behavior*, **17**, 35–44.

Pescosolido, B.A., Martin, J.K., Long, J.S., Medina, T.R., Phelan, J.C., Link, B.G. (2010). A disease like any other? A decade of change in public reactions to schizophrenia, depression and alcohol dependence. *American Journal of Psychiatry*, **167**, 1321–30.

Phelan, J.C. (2005). Geneticization of deviant behavior and consequences for stigma: The case of mental illness. *Journal of Health and Social Behavior*, **46**, 307–22.

Phelan, J.C. and Link, B.G. (1998). The growing belief that people with mental illnesses are violent: the role of the dangerousness criterion for civil commitment. *Social Psychiatry and Psychiatric Epidemiology*, **33**, S7–S12.

Phelan, J.C. and Link, B.G. (2004). Fear of people with mental illnesses: the role of personal and impersonal contact and exposure to threat or harm. *Journal of Health and Social Behavior*, **45**, 68–80.

Phelan, J.C., Link, B.G., Stueve, A., and Pescosolido, B.A. (2000). Public conceptions of mental illness in 1950 and 1996: What is mental illness and is it to be feared? *Journal of Health and Social Behavior* **41**, 188–207.

Phelan, J.C., Yang, L., and Cruz-Rojas, R. (2006). Effects of attributing serious mental illnesses to genetic causes on orientations to treatment. *Psychiatric Services* **57**, 382–7.

Perlick, D.A., Rosenheck, R.A., Clarkin, J.F., *et al.* (2001). Stigma as a barrier to recovery: Adverse effects of perceived stigma on social adaptation of persons diagnosed with bipolar affective disorder. *Psychiatric Services*, **52**, 1627–32.

Rosenfield, S. (1997). Labeling mental illness: the effects of received services and perceived stigma on life satisfaction. *American Sociological Review*, **62**, 660–72.

Rothman, D. (1971). *The Discovery of the Asylum*. Boston: Little Brown & Company.

Scheff, T.J. (1966). *Being Mentally Ill: A Sociological Theory*. Chicago, IL: Aldine.

Star, S. (1995). *The public's ideas about mental illness*. Paper presented at the Annual Meeting of the National Association for Mental Health, Indianapolis, Indiana, 1955.

Thornicroft, G. (2006). *Shunned: Discrimination against People with Mental Illness*. Oxford: Oxford University Press.

Thornicroft, G., Brohan, E., Rose, D., Sartorius, N., and Leese, M. (2009). Global pattern of experienced and anticipated discrimination against people with schizophrenia: A cross-sectional survey. *Lancet*, **373**, 408–15.

Wahl, O.F. (1995). *Media Madness: Public Images of Mental Illness*. New Brunswick, NJ: Rutgers University Press.

Wang, P.S., Lane, M., Olfson, M., Pincus, H.A., Wells, K.B., and Kessler, R.C. (2005). Twelve-Month Use of Mental Health Services in the United States: Results from the National Comorbidity Survey Replication. *Archives of General Psychiatry*, **62**, 629–40.

Whatley, C.D. (1959). Social attitudes toward discharged mental patients. *Social Problems*, **6**, 313–20.

Weiner, B., Perry, R. P., and Magnusson, J. (1988). An attributional analysis of reactions to stigmas. *Journal of Personality and Social Psychology*, **55**, 738–48.

Yang, L.H., Kleinman, A., Link, B.G., Phelan, J.C., Lee, S., and Good, B. (2007) Culture and stigma: adding moral experience to stigma theory. *Social Science and Medicine*, **64**, 1524–35.

CHAPTER 30

Reducing stigma and discrimination

Graham Thornicroft and Nisha Mehta

Defining stigma

The term stigma (plural stigmata) was originally used to refer to an indelible dot left on the skin after stinging with a sharp instrument, sometimes used to identify vagabonds or slaves. The resulting mark led to the metaphorical use of 'stigma' to refer to stained or soiled individuals who were in some way morally diminished. In modern times stigma has come to mean 'any attribute, trait or disorder that marks an individual as being unacceptably different from the "normal" people with whom he or she routinely interacts, and that elicits some form of community sanction' (Goffman, 1963).

Understanding stigma

There is now a voluminous literature on stigma (Corrigan, 2005; Link et al., 1999; Mason, 2001; Sartorius and Schulze, 2005). The stigma of mental illness is the subject of many hundreds of scientific papers (Pickenhagen and Sartorius, 2002). The most complete model of the component processes of stigmatization has four key components (Link and Phelan, 2001): 1) labelling, in which personal characteristics are signalled or noticed as conveying an important difference; 2) stereotyping, which is the linkage of these differences to undesirable characteristics; 3) separating, the categorical distinction between the mainstream/normal group and the labelled group as in some respects fundamentally different; 4) status loss and discrimination: devaluing, rejecting, and excluding the labelled group. Interestingly, more recently the authors of this model have added a revision to include the emotional reactions which may accompany each of these stages (Link et al., 2004).

The three core issues

We shall consider later what needs to be done to allow people with mental illnesses a full opportunity for social participation. First of all we need to have a clear map to know where we are and where we want to go.

Stigma theories have not been enough to understand the feelings and experiences of people with mental illness, nor to know what

practical steps to are needed to reverse social exclusion (Social Exclusion Unit, 2004). Rather stigma can be seen as an overarching term that contains three important elements:

- Problems of knowledge (ignorance)
- Problems of attitudes (prejudice), and
- Problems of behaviour (discrimination).

In terms of social psychology, these are referred to as the cognitive, affective, and behavioural domains (Dovidio et al., 2000), and each will now be discussed.

Ignorance: the problem of knowledge

As we have seen, while some information is available on knowledge about mental illnesses in non-Western nations, the vast majority of information on stigma and discrimination stems from the more economically developed countries. A surprisingly consistent picture emerges: wherever it has been studied it is found that general levels of knowledge about mental illness are remarkably low. One common misunderstanding, for example, is that schizophrenia means 'split-mind', usually misinterpreted to mean a 'split-personality' (as in the 'Dr Jekyll and Mr Hyde' story by Robert Louis Stevenson). Surveys of over 12,000 individuals in several European countries have discovered that such views are common, and are supported by many or people in: Austria (29%), Germany (80%), Greece (81%), Poland (50%), Slovakia 61%), and Turkey (39%) (Gaebel et al., 2002; Sartorius and Schulze, 2005). Commonly older people are less knowledgeable than younger (Stuart and Arboleda-Florez, 2001).

At a time when there is an unprecedented volume of information in the public domain about health problems in general, the level of general knowledge about mental illnesses is universally meagre. In population surveys in England, for example, most people (55%) believe that the statement 'someone who cannot be held responsible for his or her own actions' describes a person who is mentally ill (Department of Health, 2003). Most (63%) thought that fewer that 10% of the population would experience a mental illness at some time in their lives. In Northern Italy it was found that people who had more information about mental illnesses were less fearful and more willing to favour working with people with a history of mental illness (Vezzoli et al., 2001), and exactly the same finding came from a Canadian study (Stuart and Arboleda-Florez, 2001). Most such studies agree with the findings of a Swiss survey that age matters: older people are less well informed about mental illness and less favourable towards people with mental illnesses, although these are relatively small effects (Lauber et al., 2000).

There are also striking knowledge gaps about how to find help. In Scotland most children did not know what to do if they had a mental health problem or what to recommend to a friend with mental health difficulties: only 1% mentioned school counselling, 1% nominated helplines, 4% recommended talking with friends, 10% said that they would turn to a doctor, but over a third (35%) were unsure where to find help (See Me Scotland, 2004).

The public level of knowledge about mental illnesses and their treatments has sometimes been called 'mental health literacy' (Jorm et al., 1997). In Australia over 2000 adults were asked about the features of two mental illnesses and their treatment. Most (72%) could identify the key characteristics of depression, but relatively few (27%) could accurately recognize schizophrenia. Many standard psychiatric treatments (such as antidepressant and antipsychotic medication, or admission to a psychiatric ward) were more often rated as harmful than as helpful, and most people more readily recommended the use of vitamins (Jorm et al., 1997). Similarly, although most people in a nationwide survey in the United States agreed that psychiatric medications are effective, the majority were not willing to take such drugs themselves (Croghan et al., 2003). Also among people with depression, many have strong and often ambivalent feelings about taking antidepressant drugs, although interestingly the rate of acceptance is higher among people who have taken them for a previous episode of depression (Sirey et al., 2001).

Such findings have led may, especially in Australia where much of this work has been pioneered, to conclude that it is necessary to provide far more public information on the nature of conditions, such as depression, and on the treatments options which are available, so that both the general population, and those people who are depressed can make decisions about getting help on a fully informed basis (Jorm et al., 2003). In other words, the best remedy for ignorance is information.

What evidence we do have about trends is contradictory. In Greece, a comparison was made between public views about mental illness in 1980 and 1994 (Madianos et al., 1999). Significant improvements were identified for: social discrimination, restrictiveness, and social integration. For example, more people said that they would accept a mentally ill person as a neighbour or work colleague. By comparison a long-term comparison of popular views about mental illness in Germany has found a hardening of opinion against people with schizophrenia (Angermeyer and Matschinger, 2005a), but no change towards people with depression (Angermeyer and Matschinger, 2004).

There are also some indirect indications that popular views of mental illness have changed, e.g. the fact that increasing numbers of people in many countries do now seek help for mental illnesses (Phelan et al., 2000), although the majority still do not (Kessler et al., 2005). An important study in the United States compared popular views of mental illness in 1950 and 1996. Over this period it found evidence that there was a broadening of what was seen as mental illness, to include non-psychotic disorders, and socially deviant behaviour.

The second focus of the study was on 'frightening characteristics', and the results here were not heartening. There was a significant increase (almost twofold) over the 46-year period in public expectations linking mental illness to violence in terms of: extreme, unstable, excessive, unpredictable, uncontrolled, or irrational behaviour. This link was especially marked for public views of psychotic disorders, whereas dangerousness was less often mentioned as typical of non-psychotic conditions in 1996. In other words depression and anxiety-related disorders had become 'less alien and less extreme', while schizophrenia and similar conditions had grown in their perceived threat (Phelan et al., 2000). The authors examined the hypothesis that closing large psychiatric hospitals had led to this greater disapproval and rejection. In fact they found the opposite: those who reported frequently seeing people in public who seemed to be mentally ill were significantly less likely to perceive them as dangerous (Link et al., 1994). The authors concluded that 'something has occurred in our culture that has increased the connection between psychosis and violence in the public mind'(Phelan et al., 2000).

There have also been changes in public views about mental illness in Germany. A series of surveys between 1990 and 2001 found the German public became more ready to recommend seeking help from psychiatrists or psychotherapists for people with schizophrenia or depression. In particular there was a greater willingness to drug treatment and psychotherapy, especially for schizophrenia. Almost as often residents suggested that mediation or yoga should be recommended (Angermeyer and Matschinger, 2005a). The results suggested that the gap between professional and popular views on treatment was closing (Angermeyer and Matschinger, 2005b).

There is evidence that deliberate interventions to improve public knowledge about depression can be successful. In a campaign in Australia to increase knowledge about depression and its treatment, some states and territories received this coordinated programme, while other did not (Hickie, 2004). In areas which had received this programme respondents more often recognized the features of depression, were more likely to support seeking help for depression, and accepting treatment with counselling and medication (Jorm et al., 2005).

In Great Britain there have been confusing and conflicting findings about trends in attitudes to mental illness. A series of governmental surveys have been carried out from 1993 to 2003 and give a mixed picture (Department of Health, 2000). On one hand there are some clear improvements, for example the proportion thinking that people with mental illness can be easily distinguished from 'normal people' fell from 30% to 20%. On the other hand views became significantly less favourable over this decade, shown by the percentage of those agreeing with the following items:

- It is frightening to think of people with mental problems living in residential neighbourhoods (increased from 33% to 42%)

- Residents have nothing to fear from people coming into their neighbourhood to obtain mental health services (decreased from 70% to 55%)

- People with mental illness are far less of a danger than most people suppose (decreased from 65% to 58%)

- Less emphasis should be placed on protecting the public from people with mental illness (decreased from 38% to 31%).

How is it possible that different studies seem to show that public attitudes seem to becoming both more favourable and more rejecting? One key seems to be diagnosis. Before and after its campaign called 'Changing Minds' the United Kingdom Royal College of Psychiatrists commissioned national opinion polls of nearly 2000 adults, asking about mental illness (Crisp et al., 2004). Unusually, they asked each of the key questions separately for a series of different diagnoses. Significant changes were reported in the following for the percentage of people who agreed with the following items between 1998 and 2003:

◆ 'Danger posed to others': depression (fell from 23% to 19%), schizophrenia (fell from 71% to 66%), but no change for alcoholism or drug addiction

◆ 'Hard to talk to': depression (fell from 62% to 56%), schizophrenia (fell from 58% to 52%), alcoholism (fell from 59% to 55%)

◆ 'Never fully recover': schizophrenia (decrease from 51% to 42%), eating disorders (increase from 11% to 15%), alcoholism (increase from 24% to 29%), and drug addiction (increase from 23% to 26%)

◆ 'Feel different from us': depression (decrease from 43% to 30%), schizophrenia (decrease from 57% to 37%) dementia (decrease from 61% to 42%).

It is clear from these trends that complicated and mixed pictures emerge of both favourable and unfavourable change across a wide spectrum of conditions (Crisp et al., 2005). These marked variations suggest that public opinion surveys, which ask about 'the mentally ill' in general terms, are likely to produce a composite and possibly uninformative response which summarizes these conflicting trends. Overall it seems that popular views about depression in some countries appear to be improving in some Western countries in recent years, in terms of less social rejection, but the evidence about views on people with psychotic disorders is too confused to give a clear picture.

Prejudice: the problem of negative attitudes and emotions

If ignorance is the first great hurdle faced by people with mental illness, prejudice is the second. Although the term prejudice has been used extensively to some groups which undergo particular disadvantage, e.g. minority ethnic groups, it is employed rarely in relation to people with mental illness (Corrigan et al., 2001). Social psychologists have focused for almost a century on thoughts (cognition) rather than feelings (affect) (Bogardus, 1924). In particular they have long been interested in stereotypes (widely held and fixed images about a particular type of person), and degrees of social distance to such stereotypes (Fiske, 1998).

But reactions of rejection usually involve not just negative thoughts but also negative feelings such as anxiety, anger, resentment, hostility, distaste, or disgust (Link et al., 2004). In fact, prejudice may more strongly predict discrimination (negative behaviours to a specific category of people) than do stereotypes (Dovidio et al., 1996). First, so called 'gut level' prejudices (Fiske, 1998) may stem from anticipated group threats, or in other words, how far a member of an 'out-group' is seen to threaten the goals or the interests of the person concerned. Perceiving possible harm may provoke anger (if the person is seen to threaten harm), fear (if the harm is in the certain future), anxiety (if the harm is in the uncertain future),

or sadness (if the harm is in the past) (Fiske, 1998). Some writers have made a distinction between 'hot' prejudices, in which strong emotions are more prominent than negative thoughts, and 'cold' forms of rejection, e.g. in failing to promote a member of staff, when stereotypes are activated in the absence of negative feelings (Fiske, 1993).

Second, emotional reactions may be a consequence of direct contact with the 'target' group. This may be experienced as discomfort, anxiety, ambivalence, or as a rejection of intimacy (Crocker et al., 1998). Such feelings have been shown to be stronger in individuals who have a relatively authoritarian personality, and among people who tend to believe that the world is basically just (and so that people get what they deserve) (Crandall and Eshleman, 2003). Such emotional aspects of rejection have been studied extensively in the fields of HIV/AIDS (Herek et al., 2002), and in those conditions which produce visible marks which contravene aesthetic conventions (Hahn, 1988), such as the use of catheters or colostomies (Wilde, 2003). Interestingly, probably because research on exclusion and mental health has been almost entirely carried out using the concept of stigma rather than prejudice, there is almost nothing published about emotional reactions to mental illness apart from that which describes a fear of violence (Corrigan et al., 2001).

One fascinating exception to this generalization is work carried out in the South Eastern region of the United States, in which students were asked to imagine meeting people some of whom were labelled as having a diagnosis of schizophrenia, while their brow muscle tension, palm skin conductance, and heart rate were monitored. These physiological indicators revealed higher levels of tension during imagery with 'labelled' than 'non-labelled' individuals, and these levels also predicted self-reported attitudes of stigma towards people with schizophrenia. The authors concluded that one reason why individuals avoid those with mental illness is physiological arousal, which is experienced as a negative feeling (Graves et al., 2005).

Discrimination: the problem of rejecting behaviour

Most attention in work on mental illness has concerned attitudes towards mental illness. Much of this work is concerned with asking people, usually members of the general public, about either what they would do in given situations or what they think 'most people' who do, e.g. when faced with a neighbour or work colleague with mental illness. Important lessons have flowed from these findings. At the same time, this work has emphasized what 'normal' people say rather than the accounts of people with mental illness themselves. It also assumes that such statements (usually on knowledge or behavioural intentions) are somehow linked with actual behaviour, rather than assessing such behaviour directly. In short, with some clear exceptions, it has focused on hypothetical rather than real situations (Sayce, 1998), shorn of emotions and feelings (Crocker et al., 1998), divorced from context (Corrigan et al., 2004), indirectly rather than directly experienced, and without clear implications for how to reduce social rejection (Corrigan, 2004). The stigma field has therefore been, to a large extent, beside the point.

Theoretical approaches to mental illness-related stigma

Most of the literature on stigma and discrimination focuses on: theories of psychological processes, attitude scales, opinion surveys, links with violence, and portrayals in the media. Comparative stigma is one of the many areas about which very little has been written (Weiss, 2001).

There have been several studies of social distance (Corrigan et al., 2001). These typically present a vignette or a hypothetical scenario of a person with a particular condition, and ask whether you would want to live next door to that person, let them act as a child-minder to your children, or to allow your son or daughter to marry such a person (Angermeyer et al., 2003). A series of such surveys in Germany found high levels of social distance expressed towards people with schizophrenia, and even higher levels to those with alcohol dependence (Angermeyer and Matschinger, 1997). A United States study asked employers about job offer intentions, and found that ex-convicts were seen to be more acceptable than people with mental illness, and the only group less favoured by employers were those with tuberculosis. Such high levels of concern were also found in a sample of over 1500 members of the general United Kingdom population who were asked about their attitudes to people with five different conditions. Their concern levels were: stress or depression 34%, epilepsy 19%, heart attack 17%, facial disfigurement 9%, or use of a wheelchair 4% (Jacoby et al., 2004).

In a detailed comparison in Kansas, over 100 undergraduate psychology students were asked to compare 66 different medical conditions along 13 dimensions, including social distance. Overall, five of these dimensions predicted rejection: severity of the condition, contagiousness, behavioural causality, availability, and sexual transmission, where the last four were all closely linked to personal control. In other words, how far is the individual directly or indirectly at fault in developing the condition? In an important conclusion the authors stated, 'Severity and behavioural causality account for a significant amount of the **socially shared representation** of what makes an illness stigmatisable' [emphasis added] (Crandall and Moriarty, 1995). Care is needed here. It may not necessarily follow, for example, that emphasizing the biological basis mental illnesses will reduce stigma by reducing blame for a condition over which the person affected is assumed to have little responsibility. Indeed a German survey found the opposite (Dietrich et al., 2004).

Global patterns of stigma and discrimination

Do we know if discrimination varies between countries and cultures? The evidence here is stronger, but still patchy. Although studies on stigma and mental illness have been carried out in many countries, few have been comparisons of two or more places, or have included non-Western nations (Fabrega, 1991a).

In Africa, one study described attitudes to mentally ill people in rural sites in Ethiopia. Among almost 200 relatives of people with diagnoses of schizophrenia or mood disorders, three-quarters said that they had experienced stigma due to the presence of mental illness in the family, and a third (37%) wanted to conceal the fact that a relative was ill. Most family members (65%) said that praying was their preferred of treating the condition (Shibre et al., 2001).

In Ethiopia, 100 members of the general population gave their views about vignettes of people with seven types of disorder. Schizophrenia was judged to be the most severe problem, and talkativeness, aggression, and strange behaviour were rated as the most common symptoms of mental illness (Alem et al., 1999). Traditional treatment methods were preferred to treat symptoms of mental illness, and medications were favoured for physical illnesses.

The authors concluded that it was important to work closely with traditional healers and to reduce 'certain harmful practices' inflicted on people with mental illness in these rural communities.

In South Africa (Stein et al., 1997), a survey was conducted of over 600 members of the public on their knowledge and attitudes towards people with mental illness (Hugo et al., 2003). Different vignettes, portraying depression, schizophrenia, panic disorder, or substance misuse were presented to each person. Most thought that these conditions were either related to stress or to a lack of willpower, rather than seeing them as medical disorders. They therefore preferred to talk the problem over rather than to consult professionals. The results suggest that there is widespread misinformation about mental illness in South Africa. Among one particular group, the Xhosa, the use of traditional remedies and ancestor worship is usual, and it is common for mental distress to be explained as the influence of spirits and therefore to lie in the domain of witchdoctors.

Similar findings, that a lack of will power contributes towards mental illness, have also been observed in other non-Western countries, e.g. in Turkey (Ozmen et al., 2004), Siberia and Mongolia (Dietrich et al., 2004). This suggests that people in such countries may more ready to make the individual responsible for his or her mental illness and less willing to grant the benefits of the sick role.

Most of the published work on stigma is from the United States and Canada (Corrigan, 2005; Link et al., 2004), with a few reports from elsewhere in the Americas and in the Caribbean (Villares and Sartorius, 2003). In a review of studies from Argentina, Brazil, Dominica, Mexico, and Nicaragua, mainly from urban sites, a number of common themes emerged. The conditions most often rated as 'mental illnesses' were psychotic disorders, especially schizophrenia. People with higher levels of education tended to have more favourable attitudes to people with mental illness. Alcoholism was considered to be the most common type of mental disorder. Most people thought that a health professional needs to be consulted by people with mental illnesses (de Toledo Piza and Blay, 2004).

Studies have been conducted in Asian countries and cultures (Leong and Lau, 2001). Within China (Kleinman and Mechanic, 1979), an e-survey was undertaken of over 600 people with a diagnosis of schizophrenia and over 900 family members (Phillips et al., 2002). Over half of the family members said that stigma had had an important effect on them and their family, and levels of stigma were higher in urban areas and for people who were more highly educated. In relation to staff views, another study discovered far more negative views toward people with mental illness among psychiatric nurses than psychiatrists in China (Sevigny et al., 1999). Even so, it seems that both Chinese doctors and nurses may differ from the general population in their views about the causes of mental illness. A survey of almost 400 people with mental illness and their relatives showed that most attributed the cause to social, interpersonal, and psychological problems, whereas staff more often used biomedical explanation for schizophrenia.

Schizophrenia is the primary focus of interest in the field of stigma. It is remarkable that there are almost no studies, for example, on bipolar disorder and stigma. A comparison of attitudes to schizophrenia was undertaken in England and Hong Kong. As predicted, the Chinese respondents expressed more negative attitudes and beliefs about schizophrenia, and preferred a more social model to explain its causation. In both countries most participants, whatever their educational level, showed great ignorance about this condition (Furnham and Chan, 2004). This may well be one reason why most of population in Hong Kong are very concerned about their mental health and hold rather negative views about mentally ill people (Chou et al., 1996). Less favourable attitudes were common in those with less direct personal contact with people with mental illness (as in most Western studies), and by women (the opposite has been found in many Western reports).

Among Chinese people with mental illness, expectations of rejection may be more common than actual experiences. Almost 200 outpatients in Hong Kong, for example, said that most people would agree that someone with a history of mental illness is likely to be untrustworthy, dangerous, looked down upon, and not to be taken seriously. In terms of actual experiences of rejection, the most common was seeing offensive articles in the mass media (49%), being treated as less competent (34%), and being treated differently by friends after they learned about the mental illness (28%). Over a half (56%) concluded that their best course of action was to try to conceal the condition (Chung and Wong, 2004). A similar study in Hong Kong also showed that significantly more people with schizophrenia (40%) than diabetes (15%) experienced stigma from family members, partners, friends, and colleagues (Lee et al., 2005).

To gain some understanding about stigma in India we also need to assemble an overall picture from a few jigsaw pieces of evidence. Among relatives of people with schizophrenia in Chennai (Madras) in Southern India, their main concerns were: effects on marital prospects, fear of rejection by neighbours, and the need to hide the condition from others. Higher levels of stigma were reported by women and by younger people with the condition (Thara and Srinvasan, 2000). Women who have mental illness appear to be at a particular disadvantage in India. If they are divorced, sometimes related to concerns about heredity (Raguram et al., 2004), then they often receive no financial support from their former husbands, and they and their families experience intense distress from the additional stigma of being separated or divorced (Thara et al., 2003).

There are complex relationships in India between depression and somatic disorders. It seems that how these conditions are viewed by others plays a part in framing how psychological distress is experienced and communicated. One study in Bangalore showed higher levels of stigma among psychiatric outpatients who complained of depression than for those who described physical complaints (Raguram et al., 1996). In Kolkata (Calcutta), for example, among outpatients who met Western criteria for major depression, only 5% complained of sadness, while half (48%) described pains and other physical symptoms. This suggests that there is a congruence between the language used by individuals to describe their own suffering, and the forms of distress that are socially allowed (e.g. avoiding stigmatizing rejection) (Chowdhury et al., 2001).

These cultural influences can also shape access to treatment and care. Beliefs that mental illnesses may be caused by religious factors will encourage families to seek help from senior figures in their faith communities in many countries and cultures, and can delay seeking help from health professionals (Conrad and Pacquiao, 2005). In some parts of India and Pakistan mental health service provision has been integrated into the general primary care services, and this is intended to reduce the barriers to accessing care which are related to stigma. Psychiatrists are the least preferred option because of the stigma attached to consultations: The key barrier is the sense of shame, rather than the physical location of doctors and nurses (James et al., 2002)

These themes also emerge from work on stigma in Japan. In particular, mental illnesses are seen to reflect a loss of control, and so are not subject to the force of will power, both of which lead to a sense of shame (Hasui et al., 2000). Although it is tempting to generalize about the degree of stigma in different countries, reality may not allow such simplifications. A comparison of attitudes to mentally ill people in Japan and Bali, for example, showed that views towards people with schizophrenia were less favourable in Japan, but that people with depression and obsessive-compulsive disorder were seen to be less acceptable in Bali (Kurihara et al., 2000).

What different countries do often share is a high level of ignorance and misinformation about mental illnesses. A survey of teachers' opinions in Japan and Taiwan showed that relatively few could describe the main features of schizophrenia with any accuracy. The general profile of knowledge, beliefs, and attitudes was similar to that found in most Western countries, although the degree of social rejection was somewhat greater in Japan (Kurumatani et al., 2004).

In a unique move aimed to reduce social rejection, the name for schizophrenia has been changed in Japan. Following a decade of pressure from family member groups, including Zenkaren, the name for this condition was changed from 'seishi buntetsu byo' (split-mind disorder) to 'togo shiccho sho' (loss of coordination disorder) (Desapriya and Nobutada, 2002). The previous term went against the grain of traditional, culturally-valued concepts of personal autonomy, as a result of which only 20% of people with this condition were told the diagnosis by their doctors (Goto, 2003; Mino et al., 2001). There are indications from service users and family members that the new term is seen as less stigmatizing and is more often discussed openly. This is consistent with work in Germany suggesting that giving the label 'schizophrenia' has a significant and negative effect on public perceptions (Angermeyer and Matschinger, 2005c).

Little is written in the English language literature on stigma in Islamic communities, but despite earlier indications that the intensity of stigma may be relatively low (Fabrega, 1991b), detailed studies indicate that, on balance, it is no less than we have seen described elsewhere (Karim et al., 2004). A study of 100 family members of people with schizophrenia in Morocco found that 76% had no knowledge about the condition, and many considered it chronic (80%), handicapping (48%), incurable (39%), or linked with sorcery (25%). Most said that they had 'hard lives' because of the diagnosis (Kadri et al., 2004). Turning to religious authority figures is reported to be common in some Moslem countries (Al-Krenawi et al., 2004). Some studies have found that direct personal contact was not associated with more favourable attitudes to people with mental illness (Arkar and Eker, 1994), especially where behaviour is seen to threaten the social fabric of the community (Coker, 2005). A large study of public attitudes in Istanbul in Turkey drew similar conclusions noting prominence of social distance and a lack of knowledge about mental illness amongst the 700 respondents (Ozmen et al., 2004).

A recent study used the Discrimination and Stigma Scale (DISC) in a cross-sectional survey in 27 countries using language-equivalent versions of the instrument in face-to-face interviews between research staff and 732 participants with a clinical diagnosis of schizophrenia (Thornicroft et al., 2009). The most frequently occurring areas of negative experienced discrimination were: making or keeping friends (47%), discrimination by family members (43%), keeping a job (29%); finding a job: (29%), and intimate or sexual relationships (29%). Positive experienced discrimination was rare. Anticipated discrimination was common for: applying for work or training or education (64%); looking for a close relationship (55%), and 72% felt the need to conceal the diagnosis. Anticipated discrimination occurred more often than experienced discrimination. This study suggests that rates of experienced discrimination are relatively high and consistent across countries. For two of the most important domains (work and personal relationships) anticipated discrimination occurs in the absence of experienced discrimination in over a third of participants. This has important implications: disability discrimination laws may not be effective without also developing interventions to reduce anticipated discrimination, e.g. by enhancing the self-esteem of people with mental illness, so that they will be more likely to apply for jobs.

What sense can we make of all these fragments of information? Several points are clear. First there is no known country, society, or culture in which people with mental illness are considered to have the same value and to be as acceptable as people who do not have mental illness. Second, the quality of information that we have is relatively poor, with very few comparative studies between countries or over time. Third, there do seem to be clear links between popular understandings of mental illness, people in mental distress seeking help, and whether they feel able to disclose their problems. The core experiences of shame (to oneself) and blame (from others) are common everywhere stigma has been studied, but to differing extents. Where comparisons with other conditions have been made, then mental illnesses are more, or far more, stigmatized (Lee et al., 2005), and have been referred to as the 'ultimate stigma' (Falk, 2001). Finally, rejection and avoidance of people with mental illness appear to be universal phenomena. In this context, the next section considers what actions are needed at the individual, local, and national levels to reduce stigma and discrimination.

Action needed to reduce stigma for individuals in relation to work

For some people with mental illness, allowance needs to be made at work for their personal requirements. In parallel with the modifications made for people with physical disabilities, people with mental illness-related disabilities may need what are called 'reasonable adjustments' in relation to the anti-discrimination laws. In practice this can include the following measures:

- Having a quieter work place with fewer distractions for people with concentration problems, rather than a noisy open plan office, and a rest area for breaks

- Giving more or more frequent supervision than usual to give feedback and guidance on job performance

- Allowing a person to use headphones to block out distracting noise

- Creating flexibility in work hours so that they can attend their healthcare appointments, or work when not impaired by medication

- Funding an external job coach for counselling and support, and to mediate between employee and employer

- Providing a buddy/mentor scheme to provide on-site orientation, and assistance

- Writing clear person specifications, job descriptions, and task assignments to assist people who find ambiguity or uncertainty hard to cope with

- Making contract modifications to specifically allow whatever sickness leave is required by people likely to become unwell for prolonged periods

- Providing a more gradual induction phase, e.g. with more time to complete tasks, for those who return to work after a prolonged absence, or who may have some cognitive impairment

- Improving disability awareness in the workplace to reduce stigma and to underpin all other accommodations

- Reallocating marginal job functions which are disturbing to an individual

- Allowing use of accrued paid and unpaid leave for periods of illness.

Further, community bodies need to act to promote the social inclusion of people with mental illnesses. The following initiatives address discrimination in the workplace, and misinformation about mental health issues (Wheat et al., 2010):

- Employers' federations should inform employers of their legal obligations under existing disability laws towards people with mental illnesses

- Employers in the health and social care sector, when recruiting, should make explicit that a history of mental illness is a valuable attribute for many roles

- Mental health services should work with employers and business confederations to ensure that reasonable accommodations and adjustments in the workplace are made for people with mental illness

- The education, health, and police authorities and commissioners should provide well evaluated interventions to increase integration with, and understanding of, people with mental illness to targeted groups such as schoolchildren, police, and healthcare staff

- Professional training and accreditation organizations should ensure that mental health practitioners are fully aware of the actual recovery rates in mental illness.

Actions needed at the local level

In local communities or health and social care economies the initiatives listed in Table 30.1 are needed to promote the social inclusion of people with mental illness.

Actions needed at the national level

In terms of national policy, a series of changes are necessary which span governmental ministries, the non-governmental and independent sector, along with service user and professional groups. This is a vision of a long-term attack upon individual and systemic/structural discrimination (Corrigan et al., 2004) through a coordinated, multisectoral programme of action to promote the social inclusion of people with mental illness. Further social marketing approaches, the adaptation of advertising methods for a social good rather than for the consumptions of a commodity, are increasingly often being used (Dunion and Gordon, 2005; Sullivan et al., 2005).

In terms of change needed within mental health systems, several elements are necessary. For example, the development of psychological services designed to support people in or seeking

Table 30.1 Initiatives needed to promote the social inclusion of people with mental illness

Action	By
◆ Introduction supported work schemes	◆ Mental health services with specialist independent sector providers
◆ Psychological treatments to improve cognition, self-esteem, and confidence	◆ Mental health and general health services
◆ Health and social care explicitly give credit to applicants with a history of mental illness when hiring staff	◆ Health and social care agencies
◆ Provision of reasonable adjustments/ accommodations at work	◆ Mental health providers engaging with employers and business confederations
◆ Inform employers of their legal obligations under disability laws	◆ Employers' confederations
◆ Deliver and evaluate the widespread implementation of targeted interventions with targeted groups including school children, police, and healthcare staff	◆ Education, police, and health commissioning and providing authorities
◆ Provide accurate data on mental illness recovery rates to mental health practitioners	◆ Professional training and accreditation organizations
◆ Implementation of measures to support care plans negotiated between staff and consumers	◆ Mental health provider organizations and consumer groups

work. Many people with mental illness experience demoralization, reduced self-esteem, loss of confidence, and sometimes depression (Hayward et al., 2002). It is therefore likely that support programmes assisting people with mental illness to gain employment will need to assess whether structured psychological treatment is also needed (Brown et al., 2004). Second, mental health staff may increasingly see the need to widen their remit from direct treatment provision, to also intervening for local populations (Thornicroft et al., 2010). Mental health awareness campaigns towards local programmes which are targeted to specific groups. In the antistigma network of the World Psychiatric Association (called 'Open the Doors'), for example, such interventions have most often been applied to medical staff, journalists, school children, police, employers, and church leaders (Sartorius and Schulze, 2005).

Another key target group is healthcare professionals. Consumers surprisingly often describe that their experiences of general health care and mental health care staff reveal levels of ignorance, prejudice, and discrimination that they find deeply distressing. This has been confirmed in several international studies (White, 2004). Based on the principle 'catch them young', several programmes have given antistigma interventions to medical students (Lethem, 2004). As is usual in the field of stigma and discrimination, there is more research describing stigma than assessing which interventions are effective. In Japan one study found that the traditional medical curriculum led to mixed results: students became more accepting of mentally ill people and mental health services, and more optimistic about the outlook with treatment, but there was no impact on their views about how far people with mental illness should have their

human rights fully observed (Mino et al., 2000). Positive changes in all of these domains were achieved with a 1-hour supplementary educational programme (Mino et al., 2001).

It appears that psychiatrists may not be in the best position to lead such educational programmes. Studies in Switzerland found no overall differences between the general public and psychiatrists in terms of social distance to mentally ill people. Psychiatry itself tries to walk the narrow tightrope between the physical/pharmacological and psychological/social poles (Luhrmann, 2000). Clinicians who keep contact with people who are unwell, and who selectively stop seeing people who have recovered, may therefore develop a pessimistic view of the outlook for people with mental illnesses (Burti and Moshe, 2005). On balance there is mixed evidence about whether psychiatrists can be seen as stigmatizers or destigmatizers (Schlosberg, 1993). Mental health nurses also been found to have more and less favourable views about people with mental illness that the general public (Caldwell and Jorm, 2001). Interestingly, nurses, like the general population, tend to be more favourable if they have a friend who is mentally ill, in other words if there is a perceived similarity and equality with the person affected (Sadow et al., 2002).

In this case what should mental health staff do? Direct involvement in the media is a vital route that professionals can use more often, with proper preparation and training. They also need to set their own house in order by promoting information within their training curricula, continuing professional development (continuing medical education) and relicensing/revalidation procedures which ensures that they have accurate information, for example, on recovery (Crisp, 2004).

Further, in future practitioners need to pay greater attention to what consumers and family members say about their experiences of discrimination, e.g. in relation to work or housing. It is clear that consumer groups increasingly seek to change the terms of engagement between mental health professionals and consumers, and to move from paternalism to negotiation (Chamberlin, 2005). Vehicles to support shared decision-making include: crisis plans (Sutherby et al., 1999) (which seem able to reduce the frequency of compulsory treatment (Henderson et al., 2004)), advance directives (Swanson et al., 2006), shared care agreements (Byng et al., 2004), and consumer-held records (Lester et al., 2003). The key issue is that many consumers want direct participation in their own care plans.

Going into the public advocacy domain, staff in mental health systems may well develop in future a direct campaigning role. A practical approach is for local and national agencies to set aside their differences and to find common cause. In some areas such coordinating groups are called forums, peak bodies, alliances, or consortia. What they have in common is a recognition that what they can achieve together, in political terms, is greater that their individual impact. Core issues able to unite such coalitions are likely to be parity in funding, the use of disability discrimination laws for people with and mental illness related disabilities, and the recognition of international human rights conventions in practice (Thornicroft and Rose, 2005).

Action needed to reduce public stigma at the national level

Public stigma

Three main strategies have been used to reduce public stigma: protest, education, and contact (Corrigan and Penn, 1999). Protest, by stigmatized individuals or members of the public who support them, cxis often applied against stigmatizing public statements, such as media reports and advertisements. Many protest interventions, e.g. against stigmatizing advertisements or soap operas, have successfully suppressed negative public statements and for this purpose they are clearly very useful (Wahl, 1995). However, it has been argued (Corrigan and Penn, 1999) that protest is not effective for improving attitudes toward people with mental illness. Education interventions aim to diminish stigma by replacing myths and negative stereotypes with facts, and have reduced stigmatizing attitudes among members of the public. However, research on educational campaigns suggests that behaviour changes are often not evaluated, and the degree of change achieved is both limited and may fade quickly. The third strategy is personal contact with persons with mental illness. In a number of interventions in secondary schools, education and personal contact have been combined (Pinfold et al., 2003a). Contact appears to be the more efficacious part of the intervention. Factors that create an advantageous environment for interpersonal contact and stigma reduction include equal status among participants, a cooperative interaction, and institutional support for the contact initiative.

For both education and contact, the content of antistigma programmes matters. Biogenetic models of mental illness are often highlighted because viewing mental illness as a biological, mainly inherited problem, may reduce shame and blame associated with it. Evidence supports this optimistic expectation (i.e. that a biogenetic causal model of mental illness will reduce stigma) in terms of reduced blame. However, focusing on biogenetic factors may increase the perception that people with mental illness are fundamentally different, and thus biogenetic interpretations have been associated with increased social distance, perceptions of mental illness as more persistent, serious and dangerous, and with more pessimistic views about treatment outcomes (Phelen et al., 2006). Therefore, a message of mental illness as being 'genetic' or 'neurological' may be overly simplistic and unhelpful for reducing stigma.

Antistigma initiatives can take place nationally as well as locally. National campaigns often adopt a social marketing approach, whereas local initiatives usually focus on target groups. An example of a large multifaceted national campaign is *Time To Change* in England (Henderson and Thornicroft, 2009). It combines mass-media advertising and local initiatives. The latter try to facilitate social contact between members of the general public and mental health service users as well as target specific groups such as medical students and teachers. The programme is evaluated by public surveys assessing knowledge, attitudes, and behaviour, and by measuring the amount of experienced discrimination reported by people with mental illness. Similar initiatives in other countries, e.g. *See Me* in Scotland (Dunion and Gordon, 2005), *Like Minds, Like Mine* in New Zealand (Vaughan and Hansen, 2004), or the World Psychiatric Association antistigma initiative (Sartorius and Schulze, 2005) in, among many other countries, Japan, Brazil, Egypt, have reported positive outcomes.

Action at the international level

What action is necessary at the international level? Such contributions, so far removed from the everyday lives of people, may be hardly noticeable unless they are very sharply focused and coherent. Setting international standards for national polices can be one useful intervention. For example the World Health Organization (WHO) has published standards to guide countries in producing or revising mental health laws (World Health Organization, 2005a). This covers advice on:

◆ Access to care

◆ Confidentiality

◆ Assessments of competence and capacity

◆ Involuntary treatment

◆ Consent

◆ Physical treatments

◆ Seclusion

◆ Restraint

◆ Privacy of communications

◆ Appeals against detention

◆ Review procedures for compulsory detention.

At present, 25% of countries worldwide do not have legislation related to mental health treatment, and for those that do, half of these enacted their law over 15 years ago. Generally lower income countries are more likely to have older legislation.

In the European Union, for example, antidiscrimination laws are now mandatory under the Article 13 Directive (Bartlett et al., 2006). Such laws must make illegal all discrimination in the workplace on grounds that include disability, and also set up institutions to enforce these laws. The time is therefore right to share experience between different countries on how successful such laws have been to reduce discrimination against people with mental illness, and to understand more clearly what is required both for new legislation elsewhere, and for amendments to existing laws that fall short of their original intentions.

International organization, such as the WHO can also contribute towards better care and less discrimination by indicating the need for national mental health policies, and by giving guidance on their content. In 2005, for example, only 62% of countries in the world had a mental health policy (World Health Organization, 2005b). In Europe Health Ministers have signed a Mental Health Declaration and Action Plan which set the following priorities:

◆ foster awareness of mental illness

◆ tackle stigma, discrimination and inequality

◆ provide comprehensive, integrated care systems,

◆ support a competent, effective workforce,

◆ recognize the experience and knowledge of services users and carers (Thornicroft and Rose, 2005; World Health Organization, 2005c)

Conclusion

The strongest evidence at present for active ingredients to reduce stigma refers to direct social contact with people with mental illness which has been shown to be effective, e.g. in relation to police officers, school students, journalists, or the clergy (Pinfold et al., 2003a,b) At the national level, there is emerging evidence that a carefully coordinated approach based using social marketing techniques, namely advertising and promotional methods designed to achieve a social good rather than sales of a commodity, have shown benefit in Australia, New Zealand, and Scotland (Jorm et al., 2005; Vaughan, 2004). The challenge in the coming years will be to identify which interventions (whether directed towards knowledge, attitudes, or behaviour are most cost-effective in reducing the social exclusion of people with mental illness.

If we deliberately shift focus from stigma to discrimination in this way, there are a number of advantages. First attention moves from intentions to actual behaviour, not if an employer **would** hire a person with mental illness, but if he or she **does**. Second, interventions can be tried and tested to change behaviour towards people with mental illness, without **necessarily** changing knowledge or feelings towards such people. Third, people who have a diagnosis of mental illness can expect to benefit from all the relevant antidiscrimination provisions and laws in their country or jurisdiction, or a basis of parity with people with physical disabilities. Fourth a discrimination perspective requires us to change viewpoint from that of the person within the 'in-group' to that of the person in the 'out-group', namely people with mental illness. In sum, this means sharpening our sights upon injustice and human rights as experienced by people with mental illness (Chamberlin, 2005; Estroff, 1981; Rose, 2001).

References

Alem, A., Jacobsson, L., Araya, M., Kebede, D., and Kullgren, G. (1999). How are mental disorders seen and where is help sought in a rural Ethiopian community? A key informant study in Butajira, Ethiopia. *Acta Psychiatrica Scandinavica*, **397**, 40–7.

Al-Krenawi, A., Graham, J.R., Dean, Y.Z., and Eltaiba, N. (2004). Cross-national study of attitudes towards seeking professional help: Jordan, United Arab Emirates (UAE) and Arabs in Israel. *International Journal of Social* Psychiatry, **50**, 102–14.

Angermeyer, M.C. and Matschinger H. (1997). Social distance towards the mentally ill: results of representative surveys in the Federal Republic of Germany. *Psychological Medicine*, **27**, 131–41.

Angermeyer, M.C. and Matschinger H. (2004). Public attitudes to people with depression: have there been any changes over the last decade? *Journal of Affective Disorders*, **83**, 177–82.

Angermeyer, M.C. and Matschinger H. (2005a). Have there been any changes in the public's attitudes towards psychiatric treatment? Results from representative population surveys in Germany in the years 1990 and 2001. *Acta Psychiatrica Scandinavica*, **111**, 68–73.

Angermeyer, M.C. and Matschinger H. (2005b). The stigma of mental illness in Germany: a trend analysis. *International Journal of Social Psychiatry*, **51**, 276–84.

Angermeyer, M.C. and Matschinger H. (2005c). Labeling—stereotype—discrimination. An investigation of the stigma process. *Social Psychiatry and Psychiatric Epidemiology*, **40**, 391–5.

Angermeyer, M.C., Beck, M., Matschinger, H. (2003). Determinants of the public's preference for social distance from people with schizophrenia. *Canadian Journal of Psychiatry*, **48**, 663–8.

Arkar, H. and Eker, D. (1994). Effect of psychiatric labels on attitudes toward mental illness in a Turkish sample. *International Journal of Social Psychiatry*, **40**, 205–13.

Bartlett, P., Lewis, O., Thorold, O. (2006). *Mental Disability and the European Convention on Human Rights*. Leiden: Martinus Nijhoff.

Bogardus, E.S. (1924). Social distance and its origins. *Journal of Applied Sociology*, **9**, 216–26.

Brown, J.S., Elliott, S.A., Boardman, J., Ferns, J., and Morrison, J. (2004). Meeting the unmet need for depression services with psycho-educational self-confidence workshops: preliminary report. *British Journal of Psy*chiatry, **185**, 511–15.

Burti, L. and Mosher, L.R. (2003). Attitudes, values and beliefs of mental health workers. *Epidemiologica e Psichiatria Sociale*, **12**, 227–31.

Byng, R., Jones, R., Leese, M., Hamilton, B., McCrone, P., and Craig, T. (2004). Exploratory cluster randomised controlled trial of shared care development for long-term mental illness. *British Journal of General Practice*, **54**, 259–66.

Caldwell, T.M. and Jorm, A.F. (2001). Mental health nurses' beliefs about likely outcomes for people with schizophrenia or depression: a comparison with the public and other healthcare professionals. *Australian and New Zealand Journal of Mental Health Nursing*, **10**, 42–54.

Chamberlin, J. (2005). User/consumer involvement in mental health service delivery. *Epidemiologica e Psichiatria Sociale*, **14**, 10–14.

Chou, K.L., Mak, K.Y., Chung, P.K., and Ho, K. (1996). Attitudes towards mental patients in Hong Kong. *International Journal of Social Psychiatry*, **42**, 213–19.

Chowdhury, A.N., Sanyal, D., Bhattacharya, A., Dutta, S.K., De R., Banerjee, S., et al. (2001). Prominence of symptoms and level of stigma among depressed patients in Calcutta. *Journal of the Indian Medical Association*, **99**, 20–3.

Chung, K. and Wong, M. (2004). Experiences of stigma among Chinese mental health patients in Hong Kong. *Psychiatric Bulletin*, **28**, 451–4.

Coker, E.M. (2005). Selfhood and social distance: toward a cultural understanding of psychiatric stigma in Egypt. *Social Science & Medicine*, **61**, 920–30.

Conrad, M.M. and Pacquiao, D.F. (2005). Manifestation, attribution, and coping with depression among Asian Indians from the perspectives of health care practitioners. *Journal of Transcultural Nursing*, **16**, 32–40.

Corrigan, P.W. (2004). Target-specific stigma change: a strategy for impacting mental illness stigma. *Psychiatric Rehabilitation Journal*, **28**, 113–21.

Corrigan, P.W. (2005). *On the Stigma of Mental Illness*. Washington, D.C.: American Psychological Association.

Corrigan, P.W. and Penn, D.L. (1999). Lessons from social psychology on discrediting psychiatric stigma. *American Psychologist*, **54**, 765–76.

Corrigan, P.W., Edwards, A.B., Green, A., Diwan, S.L., and Penn, D.L. (2001). Prejudice, social distance, and familiarity with mental illness. *Schizophrenia Bulletin*, **27**, 219–25.

Corrigan, P.W., Markowitz, F.E., and Watson, A.C. (2004). Structural levels of mental illness stigma and discrimination. *Schizophrenia Bulletin*, **30**, 481–91.

Crandall, C.S. and Moriarty, D. (1995). Physical illness stigma and social rejection. *British Journal of Social Psychology*, **34**, 67–83.

Crandall, C.S. and Eshleman, A. (2003). A justification-suppression model of the expression and experience of prejudice. *Psychological Bulletin*, **129**, 414–46.

Crisp, A. (2004). *Every Family in the Land: Understanding Prejudice and Discrimination Against People with Mental Illness*. London: Royal Society of Medicine Press.

Crisp, A.H., Cowan, L., and Hart, D. (2004). The College's anti-stigma campaign 1998-2003. *Psychiatric Bulletin*, **28**, 133–6.

Crisp, A., Gelder, M.G., Goddard, E., and Meltzer, H. (2005). Stigmatization of people with mental illnesses: a follow-up study within the Changing Minds campaign of the Royal College of Psychiatrists. *World Psychiatry*, **4**, 106–13.

Crocker, J., Major, B., and Steele, C. (1998). Social Stigma. In: Gilbert D., Fiske S.T., and Lindzey G. (eds.) *The Handbook of Social Psychology*, 4th edn., pp. 504–33. Boston, MA: McGraw-Hill.

Croghan, T.W., Tomlin, M., Pescosolido, B.A., Schnittker, J., Martin, J., Lubell, K., *et al.* (2003). American attitudes toward and willingness to use psychiatric medications. *Journal of Nervous and Mental Disease*, **191**, 166–74.

de Toledo Piza, P.E. and Blay, S.L. (2004). Community perception of mental disorders - a systematic review of Latin American and Caribbean studies. *Social Psychiatry and Psychiatric Epidemiology*, **39**, 955–61.

Department of Health (2000). *Attitudes to Mental Illness Summary Report 2000*. London: Department of Health.

Department of Health (2003). *Attitudes to Mental Illness 2003 Report*. London: Department of Health.

Desapriya, E.B. and Nobutada, I. (2002). Stigma of mental illness in Japan. *Lancet*, **359**, 1866.

Dietrich, S., Beck, M., Bujantugs, B., Kenzine, D., Matschinger, H., and Angermeyer, M.C. (2004). The relationship between public causal beliefs and social distance toward mentally ill people. *Australian and New Zealand Journal of Psychiatry*, **38**, 348–54.

Dovidio, J., Brigham, J.C., Johnson, B.T., and Gaertner, S.L. (1996). Stereotyping, prejudice and discrimination: another look. In: McCrae, N., Stangor, C., and Hewstone, M. (eds.) *Stereotypes and Stereotyping*, pp. 276–319. New York: Guildford.

Dovidio J, Major B, Crocker J. (2000). Stigma: introduction and overview. In: Heatherton, T.F., Kleck, R.E., Hebl, M.R., and Hull, J.G. (eds) *The Social Psychology of Stigma*, pp. 1–28. New York: Guilford Press.

Dunion, L. and Gordon, L. (2005). Tackling the attitude problem. The achievements to date of Scotland's 'See Me' anti-stigma campaign. *Mental Health Today*, Mar, 22–5.

Estroff, S. (1981). *Making it Crazy: Ethnography of Psychiatric Clients in an American Community*. Berkeley, CA: University of California Press.

Fabrega, H., Jr. (1991b). Psychiatric stigma in non-Western societies. *Comprehensive Psychiatry*, **32**, 534–51.

Fabrega, H., Jr. (1991a). The culture and history of psychiatric stigma in early modern and modern Western societies: a review of recent literature. *Comprehensive Psychiatry*, **32**, 97–119.

Falk, G. (2001). *Stigma: How We Treat Outsiders*. New York: Prometheus Books.

Fiske, S.T. (1993). Social cognition and social perception. *Annual Review of Psychology* 1993; **44**, 155–94.

Fiske, S.T. (1998). Stereotyping, prejudice and discrimination. In: Gilbert, D.T., Fiske, S.T., and Lindzey, G. (eds.) *The Handbook of Social Psychology*, 4th edn., pp. 357–411. Boston, MA: McGraw Hill.

Furnham, A. and Chan, E. (2004). Lay theories of schizophrenia. A cross-cultural comparison of British and Hong Kong Chinese attitudes, attributions and beliefs. *Social Psychiatry and Psychiatric Epidemiology*, **39**, 543–52.

Gaebel, W., Baumann, A., Witte, A.M., and Zaeske, H. (2002). Public attitudes towards people with mental illness in six German cities: results of a public survey under special consideration of schizophrenia. European *Archives of Psychiatry and Clinical Neurosciences*, **252**, 278–87.

Goffman, I. (1963). *Stigma: Notes on the Management of Spoiled Identity*. Harmondsworth, Middlesex: Penguin Books.

Goto, M. (2003). [Family psychoeducation in Japan]. *Seishin Shinkeigaku Zasshi*, **105**, 243–7.

Graves, R.E., Cassisi, J.E., and Penn, D.L. (2005). Psychophysiological evaluation of stigma towards schizophrenia. *Schizophrenia Research*, **76**, 317–27.

Hahn, H. (1988). The politics of physical differences: disability and discrimination. *Journal of Social Issues*, **44**, 39–47.

Hasui, C., Sakamoto, S., Suguira, B., Kitamura, T. (2000). Stigmatization of mental illness in Japan: Images and frequency of encounters with diagnostic categories of mental illness among medical and non-medical university students. *Journal of Psychiatry & Law*, **28**, 253–66.

Hayward, P., Wong, G., Bright, J.A., and Lam, D. (2002). Stigma and self-esteem in manic depression: an exploratory study. *Journal of Affective Disorders*, **69**, 61–7.

Henderson, C. and Thornicroft, G. (2009). Stigma and discrimination in mental illness: Time to Change. *Lancet*, **373**, 1930–2.

Henderson, C., Flood, C., Leese, M., Thornicroft, G., Sutherby, K., and Szmukler, G. (2004). Effect of joint crisis plans on use of compulsory treatment in psychiatry: single blind randomised controlled trial. *British Medical Journal*, **329**, 136–8.

Herek, G.M., Capitanio, J.P., and Widaman, K.F. (2002). HIV-related stigma and knowledge in the United States: prevalence and trends, 1991-1999. *American Journal of Public Health*, **92**, 371–7.

Hickie, I. (2004). Can we reduce the burden of depression? The Australian experience with beyondblue: the national depression initiative. *Australasian Psychiatry*, **12**(Suppl.), S38–46.

Hugo, C.J., Boshoff, D.E., Traut, A., Zungu-Dirwayi, N., and Stein, D.J. (2003). Community attitudes toward and knowledge of mental illness in South Africa. *Social Psychiatry and Psychiatric Epidemiology*, **38**, 715–19.

Jacoby, A., Gorry, J., Gamble, C., and Baker, G.A. (2004). Public knowledge, private grief: a study of public attitudes to epilepsy in the United Kingdom and implications for stigma. *Epilepsia*, **45**, 1405–15.

James, S., Chisholm, D., Murthy, R.S., Kumar, K.K., Sekar, K., Saeed, K., *et al.* (2002). Demand for, access to and use of community mental health care: lessons from a demonstration project in India and Pakistan. *International Journal of Social Psychiatry*, **48**, 163–76.

Jorm, A.F., Korten, A.E., Jacomb, P.A., Christensen, H., Rodgers, B., and Pollitt, P. (1997). 'Mental health literacy': a survey of the public's ability to recognise mental disorders and their beliefs about the effectiveness of treatment. *Medical Journal of Australia*, **166**, 182–6.

Jorm, A.F., Griffiths, K.M., Christensen, H., Korten, A.E., Parslow, R.A., and Rodgers, B. (2003). Providing information about the effectiveness of treatment options to depressed people in the community: a randomized controlled trial of effects on mental health literacy, help-seeking and symptoms. *Psychological Medicine*, **33**, 1071–9.

Jorm, A.F., Christensen, H., and Griffiths, K.M. (2005). The impact of beyondblue: the national depression initiative on the Australian public's recognition of depression and beliefs about treatments. *Australian and New Zealand Journal of Psychiatry*, **39**, 248–54.

Kadri, N., Manoudi, F., Berrada, S., and Moussaoui, D. (2004). Stigma impact on Moroccan families of patients with schizophrenia. *Canadian Journal of Psychiatry*, **49**, 625–9.

Karim, S., Saeed, K., Rana, M.H., Mubbashar, M.H., and Jenkins, R. (2004). Pakistan mental health country profile. *International Review of Psychiatry*, **16**, 83–92.

Kessler, RC., Demler, O., Frank, R.G., Olfson, M., Pincus, H.A., Walters, E.E., *et al.* (2005). Prevalence and treatment of mental disorders, 1990 to 2003. *New England Journal of Medicine*, **352**, 2515–23.

Kleinman, A. and Mechanic, D. (1979). Some observations of mental illness and its treatment in the People's Republic of China. *Journal of Nervous and Mental Disease*, **167**, 267–74.

Kurihara, T., Kato, M., Sakamoto, S., Reverger, R., and Kitamura, T. (2000). Public attitudes towards the mentally ill: a cross-cultural study between Bali and Tokyo. *Psychiatry and Clinical Neurosciences*, **54**, 547–52.

Kurumatani, T., Ukawa, K., Kawaguchi, Y., Miyata, S., Suzuki, M., Ide, H., *et al.* (2004). Teachers' knowledge, beliefs and attitudes concerning schizophrenia- a cross-cultural approach in Japan and Taiwan. *Social Psychiatry and Psychiatric Epidemiology*, **39**, 402–9.

Lauber, C., Nordt, C., Sartorius, N., Falcato, L., and Rossler, W. (2000). Public acceptance of restrictions on mentally ill people. *Acta Psychiatrica Scandinavica*, **102**, 26–32.

Lee, S., Lee, M.T., Chiu, M.Y., and Kleinman, A. (2005). Experience of social stigma by people with schizophrenia in Hong Kong. *British Journal of Psychiatry*, **186**, 153–7.

Leong, F.T. and Lau, A.S. (2001). Barriers to providing effective mental health services to Asian Americans. *Mental Health Services Research*, **3**, 201–14.

Lester, H., Allan, T., Wilson, S., Jowett, S., and Roberts, L. (2003). A cluster randomised controlled trial of patient-held medical records for people with schizophrenia receiving shared care. *British Journal of General Practice*, **53**, 197–203.

Lethem, R. (2004).Mental illness in medical students and doctors: fitness to practice. In: Crisp A. (ed.) *Every Family in the Land*, pp. 356–64. London: Royal Society of Medicine.

Link BG, Phelan JC. (2001). Conceptualizing stigma. Annual Review of Sociology, **27**, 363–85.

Link, B.G., Susser, E., Stueve, A., Phelan, J., Moore, R.E., and Struening, E. (1994). Lifetime and five-year prevalence of homelessness in the United States. *American Journal of Public Health*, **84**, 1907–12.

Link, B.G., Phelan, J.C., Bresnahan, M., Stueve, A., and Pescosolido, B.A. (1999). Public conceptions of mental illness: labels, causes, dangerousness, and social distance. *American Journal of Public Health*, **89**, 1328–33.

Link, B.G., Yang, L.H., Phelan, J.C., and Collins, P.Y. (2004). Measuring mental illness stigma. *Schizophrenia Bulletin*, **30**, 511–41.

Luhrmann, T.M. (2000). *Of Two Minds*. New York: Vintage Books.

Madianos, M.G., Economou, M., Hatjiandreou, M., Papageorgiou, A., and Rogakou, E. (1999). Changes in public attitudes towards mental illness in the Athens area (1979/1980-1994). *Acta Psychiatrica Scandinavica*, **99**, 73–8.

Mason, T. (2001). *Stigma and Social Exclusion in Healthcare*. London: Routledge.

Mino, Y., Yasuda, N., Kanazawa, S., and Inoue, S. (2000). Effects of medical education on attitudes towards mental illness among medical students: a five-year follow-up study. *Acta Medica Okayama*, **54**, 127–32.

Mino, Y., Yasuda, N., Tsuda, T., and Shimodera, S. (2001). Effects of a one-hour educational program on medical students' attitudes to mental illness. *Psychiatry and Clinical Neurosciences*, **55**, 501–7.

Ozmen, E., Ogel, K., Aker, T., Sagduyu, A., Tamar, D., and Boratav, C. (2004). Public attitudes to depression in urban Turkey - the influence of perceptions and causal attributions on social distance towards individuals suffering from depression. *Social Psychiatry and Psychiatric Epidemiology*, **39**, 1010–16.

Phelan, J.C., Link, B.G., Stueve, A., and Pescosolido, B.A. (2000). Public conceptions of mental illness in 1950 and 1996: What is mental illness and it sit to be feared? *Journal of Health and Social Behavior*, **41**, 188–207.

Phelan, J.C., Yang, L.H., and Cruz-Rojas, R. (2006). Effects of attributing serious mental illnesses to genetic causes on orientations to treatment. *Psychiatric Services*, **57**, 382–7.

Phillips, M.R., Pearson, V., Li, F., Xu, M., and Yang, L. (2002). Stigma and expressed emotion: a study of people with schizophrenia and their family members in China. *British Journal of Psychiatry*, **181**, 488–93.

Pickenhagen, A. and Sartorius, N. (2002). *The WPA Global Programme to Reduce Stigma and Discrimination because of Schizophrenia*. Geneva: World Psychiatric Association.

Pinfold, V., Toulmin, H., Thornicroft, G., Huxley, P., Farmer, P., and Graham, T. (2003a). Reducing psychiatric stigma and discrimination: Evaluation of educational interventions in UK secondary schools. *British Journal of Psychiatry*, **182**, 342–6.

Pinfold, V., Huxley, P., Thornicroft, G., Farmer, P., Toulmin, H., and Graham, T. (2003b). Reducing psychiatric stigma and discrimination—evaluating an educational intervention with the police force in England. *Social Psychiatry and Psychiatric Epidemiology*, **38**, 337–44.

Raguram, R., Weiss, M.G., Channabasavanna, S.M., and Devins, G.M. (1996). Stigma, depression, and somatization in South India. *American Journal of Psychiatry*, **153**, 1043–9.

Raguram, R., Raghu, T.M., Vounatsou, P., and Weiss, M.G. (2004). Schizophrenia and the cultural epidemiology of stigma in Bangalore, India. *Journal of Nervous and Mental Disease*, **192**, 734–44.

Rose, D. (2001). *Users' Voices, The perspectives of mental health service users on community and hospital care*. London: The Sainsbury Centre.

Sadow, D., Ryder, M., and Webster, D. (2002). Is education of health professionals encouraging stigma towards the mentally ill? *Journal of Mental Health*, **11**, 657–65.

Sartorius, N. and Schulze, H. (2005). *Reducing the Stigma of Mental Illness: A Report from a Global Association*. Cambridge: Cambridge University Press.

Sayce, L. (1998). Stigma, discrimination and social exclusion: what's in a word? *Journal of Mental Health*, **7**, 331–43.

Schlosberg, A. (1993). Psychiatric stigma and mental health professionals (stigmatizers and destigmatizers). *Medicine and Law*, **12**, 409–16.

See Me Scotland (2004). *The Second National Public Attitudes Survey, 'Well? What do you think?'*. Edinburgh: Scottish Executive.

Sevigny, R., Yang, W., Zhang, P., Marleau, J.D., Yang, Z., Su, L., et al. (1999). Attitudes toward the mentally ill in a sample of professionals working in a psychiatric hospital in Beijing (China). *International Journal of Social Psychiatry*, **45**, 41–55.

Shibre, T., Negash, A., Kullgren, G., Kebede, D., Alem, A., Fekadu, A., et al. (2001). Perception of stigma among family members of individuals with schizophrenia and major affective disorders in rural Ethiopia. *Social Psychiatry and Psychiatric Epidemiology*, **36**, 299–303.

Sirey, J.A., Bruce, M.L., Alexopoulos, G.S., Perlick, D.A., Raue, P., Friedman, S.J., et al. (2001). Perceived stigma as a predictor of treatment discontinuation in young and older outpatients with depression. *American Journal of Psychiatry*, **158**, 479–81.

Social Exclusion Unit (2004). *Mental Health and Social Exclusion*. London: Office of the Deputy Prime Minister.

Stein, D.J., Wessels, C., Van Kradenberg, J., and Emsley, R.A. (1997). The Mental Health Information Centre of South Africa: a report of the first 500 calls. *Central African Journal of Medicine*, **43**, 244–6.

Stuart, H. and Arboleda-Florez, J. (2001). Community attitudes toward people with schizophrenia. *Canadian Journal of Psychiatry*, **46**, 245–52.

Sullivan, M., Hamilton, T., Allen, H. (2005). Changing stigma through the media. In: Corrigan P.W. (ed.) *On the Stigma of Mental Illness. Practical Strategies for Research and Social Change*, pp. 297–312. Washington, DC: American Psychology Association.

Sutherby, K., Szmukler, G.I., Halpern, A., Alexander, M., Thornicroft, G., Johnson, C., et al. (1999). A study of 'crisis cards' in a community psychiatric service. *Acta Psychiatrica Scandinavica*, **100**, 56–61.

Swanson, J., Swartz, M., Ferron, J., Elbogen, E.B., and Van Dom, R. (2006). Psychiatric advance directives among public mental health consumers in five U.S. cities: prevalence, demand, and correlates. *Journal of the American Academy of Psychiatry and the Law*, **34**, 43–57.

Thara, R. and Srinivasan, T.N. (2000). How stigmatising is schizophrenia in India? *International Journal of Social Psychiatry*, **46**, 135–41.

Thara, R., Kamath, S., and Kumar, S. (2003). Women with schizophrenia and broken marriages—doubly disadvantaged? Part II: family perspective. *International Journal of Social Psychiatry*, **49**, 233–40.

Thornicroft, G. and Rose, D. (2005). Mental health in Europe. *British Medical Journal*, 330, 613–14.

Thornicroft, G., Brohan, E., Rose, D., Sartorius, N., and the INDIGO Study Group. (2009). Global pattern of anticipated and experienced discrimination against people with schizophrenia. *Lancet*, **373**, 408–15.

Thornicroft, G., Rose, D.S., Mehta, N. (2010). Discrimination against people with mental illness: what can psychiatrists do? *Advances in Psychiatric Treatment*, **16**, 53–9.

Vaughan, G. and Hansen, C. (2004). 'Like Minds, Like Mine': a New Zealand project to counter the stigma and discrimination associated with mental illness. *Australasian Psychiatry*, **12**, 113–17.

Vezzoli, R., Archiati, L., Buizza, C., Pasqualetti, P., Rossi, G., and Pioli, R. (2001). Attitude towards psychiatric patients: a pilot study in a northern Italian town. *European Psychiatry*, **16**, 451–8.

Villares, C. and Sartorius, N. (2003). Challenging the stigma of schizophrenia. *Revista Brasileira de Psiquiatria*, **25**, 1–2.

Wahl, O.F. (1995). *Media madness: Public images of mental illness*. New Brunswick, NJ: Rutgers University Press.

Weiss, M.G. (2001). Cultural epidemiology. *Anthropology and Medicine*, **8**, 5–29.

Wheat, K., Brohan, E., Henderson, C., and Thornicroft, G. (2010). Mental illness and the workplace: conceal or reveal? *Journal of the Royal Society of Medicine* 2010; **103**, 83–6.

White, R. (2004). Stigmatisation of mentally ill medical students. In: Crisp, A. (ed.) *Every Family in the Land*, pp. 365–6. London: Royal Society of Medicine.

Wilde, M.H. (2003). *Life with an indwelling urinary catheter: the dialectic of stigma and acceptance*. Qualitative Health Research, **13**, 1189–204.

World Health Organization (2005a). *WHO Resource Book on Mental Health, Human Rights and Legislation*. Geneva: World Health Organization.

World Health Organization (2005b). *Mental Health Atlas 2005*. Geneva: World Health Organization.

World Health Organization (2005c). *Mental Health Declaration for Europe*. Copenhagen: World Health Organization.

SECTION 7

Policies and the funding

CHAPTER 31

Shaping national mental health policy

Harvey Whiteford

Introduction

From the perspective of those at the service delivery coalface, national mental health policy often seems a remote activity unrelated to their daily responsibilities. The concept of national policy can be vague and how it is formed opaque. The time taken from the beginnings of policy formulation to adoption and implementation can seem extraordinarily long. When national policy does become relevant it is often because it is driving change that the clinician or service manager finds confronting and difficult. It is therefore easy to be cynical about government policy, but most of us still want and expect explicit national mental health policy, the implementation of which drives improved services for people with mental illness and their families. For the creation of good policy, those working outside of government bureaucracies need to better understand, and be able to exert influence on, the policy-making process.

The aim of this chapter is to describe the policy development cycle and the factors that shape national mental health policy. A good understanding of these should enhance the capacity of service providers and others to influence the content and effectiveness of mental health policy. At the outset it is important to provide a caveat. This chapter is most relevant to countries that operate a democratic system of government. While many of the concepts discussed in the chapter will apply to policy development in any country with an organized system of government, the assumptions that underpin the policy cycle described in the chapter are most applicable in a democratically governed society.

Also at the outset, it is important to clarify the term **policy** which is often used to describe different things, such as government decisions, government programmes, and/or the political process. The following definition would apply to the way the term policy is used in this chapter: 'policy is deciding at any time and place what objectives and substantive measures should be chosen in order to deal with a particular problem, issue or innovation' (Dimock et al., 1983). In this chapter I limit the discussion to government policy. The private for-profit and not-for-profit sectors also make policy

for their own purposes and while many of the principles described here might be relevant, there are also many differences which are beyond the scope of this chapter.

The public policy cycle has been well documented and health policy analysis is becoming an important area for academic research (Walt et al., 2008). Roberts and colleagues (2003) developed a five-part policy cycle (Fig. 31.1) that has been applied to health. Understanding the components of the cycle—problem identification, development of a policy option, policy adoption, policy implementation, and policy evaluation—and the factors that influence and shape them should improve our ability to exert influence on the policy content and outcomes. The description of these five components as a cycle should not be taken to imply that the policy process is uniform and sequential. Policy development and implementation is anything but linear, and flexibility is essential in the policy process. In addition to the impact of the policy environment on the process of policy development it is in fact essential to consider other aspects of the policy process in each phase. For example, it is important for an understanding of implementation to influence policy development and for evaluation to be considered very early in the cycle. This chapter is primarily concerned with **shaping** national policy and will therefore concentrate on the first two of the components of the policy cycle, problem identification and development of a policy option. It is nevertheless important to understand how these two steps relate to the adoption, implementation, and revision of mental health policy.

For economically more developed countries, many improvements in the quality of life for people with mental illness have come from improvements in welfare and health care more generally (Frank and Glied, 2006). Conversely for those countries in economic decline and/or in conflict, the mental health of the population and services for those with mental illness usually suffer (Jacob et al., 2007). The national economic and security situations notwithstanding, it is important to identify what action can be taken, including in low- and middle-income countries, within the mental health sector to improve mental health (Saraceno et al., 2007). Having a national policy on mental health is widely seen as fundamental

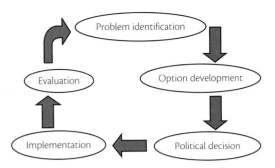

Fig. 31.1 Generic policy cycle as identified by Roberts et al. (2003).

to the promoting mental health in the population and delivering effective mental health services (Jenkins et al., 2002; World Health Organization, 2005a). A review of the health and mental health policy literature identifies the context within which policy development takes place, the factors that influence the process and shape the content of the policy, the factors that impede or facilitate implementation of the policy and the extent to which an evidence base informs policy (Baker, 1996; Lee et al., 2002; Townsend et al., 2004; Walt, 1994; World Health Organization, 2005b).

Problem identification

For an understanding of what shapes mental health policy, it is most important to appreciate what problem or problems the policy is intended to address. Government policy, including mental health policy, is developed in response to real or perceived issues or problems. The identification of any particular problem as needing policy attention occurs within the wider social, economic, historical, and political environment. A problem that those working in mental health services think is deserving of government attention may not necessarily appear the most prominent from a government perspective. For example, the fact that the majority of people with depression in a population do not access treatment might not be a priority for a busy mental health service. However, governments may take a different view about people who do not, or cannot, get treatment and may see improving access to care as a priority needing policy attention.

Among the many demands being made on government, how does one particular issue, in our case mental health, become identified as needing policy attention? These demands, and therefore the factors shaping policy, can arise from inside, or from forces external to, the country. With respect to the latter, international agencies can be influential, particularly in developing countries where international expectations are articulated and development or aid funding is linked to policy attention to a particular area. For example, by highlighting the importance of mental health in *The World Health Report, 2001* (World Health Organization, 2001), the World Health Organization (WHO) made it harder for national governments to ignore this area of health. The potential ranking of country resources allocated to mental health in WHO's mental health atlas (World Health Organization, 2005c) can attract internal and external criticism to those countries with low resource allocation, thereby applying pressure to the government to increase resources.

International aid agencies and development banks, with their focus on social and economic development and poverty

reduction, can greatly influence the content of health policy by the conditions attached to their aid and loans. To the extent that their focus includes mental health and related disability and psychosocial development, national governments will consider mental health more seriously. The relationship between poverty and mental health (Patel and Kleinman, 2003) although controversial according to some researchers (Das et al., 2007) has allowed poverty reduction funding to be linked to improving mental health, through both promotion of psychosocial development at a population level and the improvement of treatment services (Department for International Development, 2009; Flisher et al., 2007). Impaired mental health impacts adversely on many other health conditions and opportunities can be found to improve outcomes in a range of physical health areas by employing strategies to improve mental health (Prince et al., 2007). At a more macro level, when it is possible to link action on mental health to achievement of high level goals, such as the United Nations Millennium Development Goals (Miranda and Patel, 2005), further expectations and opportunities are created for government action.

Some international agencies focus on post-conflict redevelopment and human rights issues and here there have also been opportunities to incorporate a focus on mental health policy and services (Piachaud, 2008; Srinivasa Murthy and Lakshminarayana, 2006). The history of stigma, human rights violations, and social exclusion of people with mental illness (Patel et al., 2006) has led to international efforts to reform mental health legislation and services. For example, major efforts have been made in Eastern Europe to reform mental health legislation encouraged by the European Union and United Nations (Knapp et al., 2007).

New and influential research findings can also provide a base from which policy relevant arguments for attention to mental health can be made. The publication of the Global Burden of Disease Studies in 1996 and 2006 showing the mental disorders to be the leading cause of health related disability in most countries (Lopez et al., 2006; Murray et al., 1996) and the recent *Lancet* series of articles (Horton 2007) outlining the need for increased action in mental health raise the expectation that governments will do more in the area of mental health. International professional organizations such as the World Psychiatric Association (http://www.wpanet.org), non-government organizations (NGOs) such as the World Federation for Mental Health (http://www.wfmh.org), and advocacy movements such as the Global Movement on Mental Health (http://www.globalmentalhealth.org) can and do apply external pressure on governments to address mental health issues. While there are individual examples of government action in response to such external influences (Patel et al., 2008) the extent to which such advocacy has been effective globally has not been quantified.

Complementing these external influences, demand on national governments to address a particular issue arises from inside the country. Most governments feel the need to respond to the demands of their citizens. Information about the needs of individuals within a country can be effective in advocating for mental health resources. For example, the International Consortium in Psychiatric Epidemiology (http://www.hcp.med.harvard.edu/icpe) has undertaken surveys in over 25 countries using the WHO CIDI (Kessler et al., 2007) identifying the prevalence of mental disorders, the disability caused by these disorders and services utilized (or not utilized) by those with the disorders. Dissemination of findings such as these within the country highlights the extent of the health need, and the gap between need and services.

In response to such evidence, WHO has launched a mental health Gap Action Programme aimed at scaling-up care for mental, neurological and substance use disorders (World Health Organization, 2008). The increasing recognition of the economic burden of mental illness, especially in terms of lost productivity, has also been a factor spurring action in some countries (Saxena et al., 2007) especially when there is seen to be a positive economic return on investing in treatment of mental disorders (Wang et al., 2007).

My experience as mental health specialist at the World Bank was that there were four major mental health areas of focus that influenced governments to seek Bank loans that included a mental health component. The first two of these were high-profile public health issues—suicide and substance abuse. Both had received adverse media attention and were emotive topics that the government came to believe were necessary areas for policy attention. The third area was to address the mental health consequences of conflict or natural disasters. Again populations having experienced conflict or a natural disaster were in media focus and were attractive targets for donor countries and organizations with considerable NGO engagements. The fourth area was to facilitate the reorganization of services to move resources from institutional to community care. Here governments were persuaded that reform of services, including a more cost-effective use of existing resources, could lead to better outcomes for more patients with mental illness.

Roberts and colleagues (2003) highlight two mechanisms that determine how these issues can receive selective attention within a country. First, cultural norms and social attitudes in a country provide a set of filters that selectively focus on or divert public and government attention. Attitudes that devalue and minimize the importance of any issue will result in attention being diverted away. A mental health example is the poor living conditions, inadequate quality of care and human rights abuses in psychiatric hospitals during much of the last century. For decades these circumstances were not seen as warranting intervention. A change in societal attitudes saw the extension of the human rights movement to encompass individuals with mental illness, legitimize and later require government action in the form of a major policy shift to either improve conditions in these hospitals and to close wards or even hospitals.

Social norms and attitudes continue to change. The deinstitutionalization that resulted in part from the new policy position is now facing its own backlash. Societal focus has shifted from patient abuse and neglect in institutions to community safety and the 'right' to treatment for mental illness. The right to treatment means often means increased access to inpatient care. A parallel changing of norms and attitudes underpins the fluctuations in the threshold for involuntary detention in our Mental Health Acts. When societal focus is on individual liberty, the threshold for involuntary detention and treatment is higher. When the focus is on 'right to treatment' and public safety, the threshold for involuntary detention and treatment is lower.

The second mechanism identified by Roberts et al (2003) relates to the role of 'issue entrepreneurs'. These individuals or groups are advocates who promote attention to their issue. They highlight and promote the issue as needing attention until it emerges from the societal filters as a problem needing policy attention. These advocates may be political or special interest lobby groups within the

community. Their motives vary. Some groups form on the basis of a conviction about the need to improve a particular area and these individuals or groups often have a stake in that area. In mental health there are professional groupings (e.g. national associations of psychiatrists or psychologists) and consumer and carer groupings. Sometimes these groupings form a coalition and increase their ability to influence government policy. For example, the Australian National Association for Mental Health (a grouping of NGOs, consumers and carers) and the Royal Australian and New Zealand College of Psychiatrists, acted as issue entrepreneurs between 1984 and 1989 to build the momentum for the a National Mental Health Policy to be adopted by the Federal and state governments (Whiteford, 1992).

Advocates target those whom they believe can deliver the decisions they want and these are usually elected or appointed politicians. The motives of these politicians and their staff are usually a mixture of genuine interest and party and/or electoral politics. The balance between these motives is often not clear to the advocacy groups and the willingness of politicians to become involved in particular issues can be influenced by the electoral cycle, with a need to placate activists and minimize adverse publicity in an election year. Advocates need to understand the different roles of politicians, their staff and government officials and public servants in their country. It is generally expected that the departmental officials (a bureaucracy whose members are called public servants in many countries) implement the policies of the government of the day. However, most governments do not come to power with a detailed action plan for how they will deal with mental health. Even when mental health is part of a political party's health policy statement, there is usually little detail about mental health and much room for interpretation. The officials in the ministry of health and related ministries (such as social services, justice, housing, and education) do most of this interpretation. These officials hold the corporate history about government programmes and prepare submissions with options (and often costings of those options) for ministers and governments to consider. They can therefore facilitate or impede problem identification (and policy adoption and implementation). Given they generally hold the keys to making the machinery of government work, it is important for issue entrepreneurs to understand the role they play in having matters considered by the government.

The interaction between the social filters and the efforts of advocates produces fluctuating patterns in the process of problem definition and in this the incentives and behaviour of the media can play an important role (Miller, 2007). The reporting of issues by the media can highlight important problems needing attention or create the perception of a problem where none really exists. This is especially true in countries where there is less government control of the media. While a 'free press' is an important of democratic societies, the media is not unbiased or without its own distorting of facts. The media focus can be captured by scandal and/or personalities, which at its worst is called tabloid journalism. Information is often presented in a way that will sell media products. However, the media can also be an important avenue for disseminating information and improving community knowledge. Nevertheless, there is a herd pattern found among the media. Competitive media outlets can feel compelled to cover a story simply because other outlets are doing so, but the interest in the issue can quickly fade. Mental health advocates have to be patient as their issue cycles in and out of public attention and different perspectives on the issue are presented as problems at different times.

Development of a policy option

Once it has been agreed that a problem exists and needs to be addressed, policy makers have to find a way of doing this. Sometimes the option for fixing the problem is predetermined. This occurs when the government has been elected with a mandate to take certain action. However, this is uncommon in mental health and it is usually after a government has formed that solutions to various problems need to be found. How a solution is chosen among a range of options is policy development.

Governments may try and craft a policy solution in a very generic way. Decision research suggests that decisions about resource allocation by governments are influenced by knowledge of the need and effectiveness of service options, perceptions of resource scarcity, the political ideology of individual decision-makers, and perceptions of responsibility for the recipient's problems that require service (Corrigan et al., 2003).

Solutions to improving service delivery can be sought by considering health as an industry with inputs, processes, outputs, and outcomes and applying industry solutions to problems of quality, equity, and efficiency. Historically mental health services have been measured by counting inputs (numbers of staff or beds) or processes and activities (number of occupied bed days or number of outpatient services provided). In industry, routine outcome measures are considered essential in order to measure efficiency and allow customer feedback and benchmarking. Mental health has historically been disadvantaged by the lack of outcome measures that can be easily collected, clinically relevant to the clinician and consumer and able to be used in cost-effectiveness analyses. However, recent years have seen major advances in these areas with the introduction of routine outcome measures and the development of methodologies for cost effectiveness of mental health interventions (Chisholm, 2005; Thornicroft et al., 2006).

Governments often start by looking at what other jurisdictions or countries have chosen to do in response to similar problems. In mental health policy and service development there is a growing evidence base for what services work and when (Townsend et al., 2004; World Health Organization, 2005a). Whether a policy option is being imported from another jurisdiction or from another industry or is developed generically, it is necessary to arrive at a consensus on the option to be chosen. Achieving this consensus requires the government to consider the possible options and choose from among them. In many countries this choice will be informed by stakeholder consultation. Choosing the stakeholders to consult is important, because excluding any major group from the process will create ill will and potential opposition. It is nearly always better to have all stakeholders involved in the process, even if it is considered that this will result in time-consuming debate and even enmity. Subsequent political support may depend, in large part, on the extent of stakeholder consultation and support for any particular option.

Stakeholder analysis is a recognized methodology used to determine the position of relevant groups and individuals both inside and outside government who are likely to influence the policy choice and the success of its implementation (Sturm, 1999). Stakeholder analysis includes interest group analysis and bureaucratic analysis

and has been refined to the extent that software exists to do the analysis (Reich, 1996).

Mental health reform also requires complementary action in areas outside health. A challenge for national mental health policy is clarifying what policy should be endorsed and action taken in portfolios such as social services, housing, education, police, and justice. The correct policy settings in these areas can greatly improve outcomes for people with mental illness and overcome fragmentation between components of the health, housing and social services (Hogan, 2008) and the government officials and stakeholders from these sectors cannot be excluded from consideration when mental health policy options are being developed.

The opinions of identified stakeholders and views of the general population (often considered to be expressed through the media) sometimes agree. While major policy shifts are often adopted because they fit well with the interests of these major stakeholders, overriding the findings of any stakeholder analysis is the question of whether an option presented as a policy position is politically feasible. The position of experts in the stakeholder community and politics can clash when the two come to irreconcilable conclusions. The debate about needle exchange programmes is an example (Collins and Coates, 2000). The scientific data supported the use of such programmes but in many countries the political view was that they would be unpopular with the electorate. This leads us to consider how the decision is made to adopt a policy, and this decision is political.

Political decision

The environment of political decision-making is complex. Factors such as the relative power of each player (politicians, advisors, government officials, and major stakeholders) in the political landscape, the positions taken by them and the intensity of commitment for or against the policy all come into play. Within the political sphere, these players include not only the health minister, but also his or her staff, other key ministers (especially the minister responsible for finance) and their staff, and the head of the government (the premier or prime minister) and his or her social policy or health policy adviser. Senior bureaucrats and advisory bodies in each of these departments are often exceptionally influential through the advice they give to the minister's office. Successfully negotiating a coalition of support from among these players usually involves bargaining and trade-offs. Throughout the process of negotiation, the content of a policy will be modified, because compromise is usually necessary to achieve consensus.

In trying to arrive at a decision about adopting a policy, the politicians and their advisors will often scan the stakeholder and community landscape to assess the degree of support the policy will have. Determining this is made difficult in health and mental health by levels of complexity. It is necessary to consider the impact of a policy change on other parts of the system because it may be necessary to make multiple changes at the same time in order to achieve the right policy outcome. Failure to do this can undermine the success of good policy decisions in another area. For example, the policy of closing long stay hospital beds was often accompanied by a policy to expand community-based mental health services. However, the lack of community-based accommodation for patients discharged from the hospitals, often the responsibility of the housing department, seriously undermined the mental health policies (Whiteford, 1994).

Another component of this complexity is the concentrated costs, and power, of select groups such as the medical and nursing professions. The potential beneficiaries of a policy, for example consumers, are generally less powerful and less well-organized. The closure of a ward in a psychiatric hospital with the savings going to community-based services is likely to bring a more vigorous response from the staff who are to be affected in the hospital than the potential beneficiaries of the community services.

To create the necessary support for a policy to be adopted, it can be useful to align it with symbols that are seen as ideologically unchallengeable and which would have widespread community support. Community mental health care was aligned with 'least restrictive care'. Concepts such as the 'right' to treatment and 'equity' in access to care were introduced to generate support for the relevant policies.

Sometimes it is also a matter of reframing the explanation around the policy to ensure political adoption. During the revision of mental health legislation in Australia, a debate arose about the policy of the legislation permitting patients to be involuntarily treated in private hospitals. This position was initially seen in Australia as unsupportable because of the perception that the private sector would profit from patients being treated in hospital against their will. With over a third of the population at the time having private health insurance and wanting treatment with the psychiatrist of their choice, the policy position was reframed to argue that a person with mental illness, who had chosen and paid for their private health insurance, should be allowed to remain with the psychiatrist (and hospital) of their choice even when (or especially when) their illness was at its worst. With this reframing of the context, the policy became politically acceptable and was adopted. Perceptions of policy reform are matters of values as well as facts. Political decision-making is about emotion as well as data.

Policy implementation

Many policies are developed and adopted but not implemented. Government options are actually quite limited and in reality they have only five main levers available (Lee et al., 2002; Musgrove, 1996). These are information collection and dissemination; the financing system that determines how resources are collected and who has access to them; the payment system that determines on what terms these resources are made available to individuals and organizations; the organization of the health system in both the distribution of services and how they respond to consumer demands; and the regulatory system, which imposes a set of constraints on services (e.g. how providers are trained and accredited, how any health or pharmaceutical insurance schemes operate and regulations that cover the private sector).

Successful implementation requires an implementation plan and there are many excellent texts on strategic planning (Bryson, 2004; Swayne et al., 2006). A discussion on strategic planning is outside the scope of this chapter but it is important to emphasize that policy implementation is much more likely to be successful if it has the support of those professional and community organizations that came together to ensure that the policy was adopted in the first place. In addition, forging new alliances consolidates support and enhances implementation.

The central government, if it has sufficient financial resources, can tie funding allocations to the implementation of the policy (and the provision of agreed data to allow monitoring of the policy implementation), as can regional or state governments with funding going to districts. The information lever is important as there needs to be agreement to collect data on national progress in implementing the policy. National indicators need to be drawn from data collected around the country at service delivery sites and considerable effort is needed to develop nationally consistent data definitions and collection so comparable data from different parts of the country can be aggregated. National reports on progress should be public documents and benchmarks that can be used as a form of accountability.

Policy implementation requires sustained effort over time. During the implementation stage, which is often over a 5- or 10-year time span, the political party in power when the policy was adopted may well change. However, if the coalition of stakeholders remains largely intact and there is public expectation for change progress should continue. There is however always a risk that new governments, with their need to have policies which distinguish them from the party they replaced will attempt to prematurely change the direction of the implementation. This is just one reason why the implementation of policy virtually never goes as planned. It is also an argument for attempting to gain bipartisan support for the policy when it is developed. Flexibility in responding and adapting to emerging issues, which can create barriers and opportunities, is essential.

There are many examples of the key elements of mental health service programmes (Pirkis et al., 2007; Thornicroft and Tansella, 2004) and WHO's Mental Health Gap Action Programme (mhGAP; World Health Organization, 2008) which provides advice on scaling up services for mental, neurological, and substance use disorders especially with low- and middle-income countries. Each country can adapt the available evidence for their own circumstances. At a local level, implementation of national policy will also tend to be piecemeal in response to specific problems and resources idiosyncratic to the local environment (Garfield, 2009).

Evaluation

The shaping of national mental health policy should be shaped by an evaluation of the successes and failures of implementing existing policy. However, as noted earlier, many polices remain largely unimplemented and even fewer are evaluated in a way that would inform a revised national policy. By the time an evaluation is due to be conducted (at the end of five or ten years), many of the politicians and government officials originally involved in its development will have moved to different areas. During the implementation, organizations that supported the policy may have wilted (or grown), and those who opposed it may be stronger. The environment will be different. For an evaluation to have credibility, it must be as transparent and independent as possible. This means finding people to undertake the evaluation who can demonstrate objectivity. With the availability of higher quality independent data, it has become possible to have the evaluation done by representatives of the key stakeholders.

The results of the evaluation should be used to revise the policy. In revising policy or developing successive implementation plans, it is important to resist the temptation to neglect those areas that have been successful and focus primarily on areas that have been

Table 31.1 Examples of factors influencing the policy cycle

Stage of the cycle	Influencing factors	
Problem identification	Primarily internal influences	*Citizens:* public opinion changes in cultural norms/social attitudes *Media:* focus on high profile areas such as substance use, suicide and conflict *Advocates and stakeholders:* agendas depending on priorities specific to each group *New information:* new research and data informs problem identification *Other factors:* mental health receives focus because of its relationship to physical health priorities (e.g. HIV);mental health issues recognized following conflict or natural disaster
	Primarily external influences	*International agencies:* government responds to leadership of an agency (e.g. WHO); aid/loans linked to health policy and/or outcomes;government responds to criticism, e.g. of inadequate spending or human rights issues
Option development		*Policy mandate and ideology:* public government commitments including in election platform; governments accept responsibility for a solution *Political feasibility and sustainability:* governments seek re-election *Cost:* governments seek cost effective solutions to problems; resources are available *Experience of other jurisdictions* *Available knowledge and evidence* *Stakeholder opinion* *Implementation design* *project scope, process, performance measurement, impact on rest of health system and other sectors*
Decision-making		*Assessment of electoral acceptance* *Intensity of political commitment* *Relative power of advocates in government, bureaucracy and community* *Harnessing stakeholders for long-term sustainability*
Implementation		*Information collection and dissemination:* funding tied to data collection and reporting requirements *Financing system* (how resources are collected) *Payment system* (how resources are distributed) *Organization of the broader health system* *Impact of the broader health regulatory system* *Development of implementation plan:* stakeholders involved in implementation design; include performance monitoring and reporting for transparency
Evaluation		*Designed at the time of policy development and/or implementation* *Conducted independent of those implementing policy utilizing a transparent process* *Use to inform future and revised policy*

less well addressed. There will always be criticism that areas were neglected and the temptation to expand the policy implementation agenda once the policy is revised is enormous. While the policy can and should be broad, it is important to ensure that in policy implementation scarce resources remain focused on key areas where the best outcomes can be achieved. If the effort is diffuse and resources spread too widely, effectiveness will be diluted, with a loss of credibility for the policy.

Conclusion

Policy development, adoption, implementation, and evaluation are often seen as political and bureaucratic exercises out of the reach of clinicians, consumers, and others in the mental health sector. Some of the factors influencing the five stages are summarized in Table 31.1. It is important that the perspectives of clinicians and those who use services and their carers be brought to the policy process so decisions are made more on the basis of relevance and less on the basis of political expediency and ideology. In doing this, it is necessary for information from those intimately engaged in research and service delivery to be communicated in a way that can be assimilated by individuals in government who are unfamiliar with the technical detail. It is often necessary to reframe the information or reduce it to what may seem overly simplistic or inexact.

Mental health professionals should have an advantage in the policy arena because they are trained in systems thinking. Many government policies outside of health can impact on the mental health of populations or the delivery of mental health services and mental health professionals should understand the context within which policy is framed, as well as the resources needed, the inter-related components of provision, and the outcomes that need to be achieved. However, they must be prepared to enter an arena where their opinions are not automatically accepted and which is not only unfamiliar but operates at times in a way that they may find disturbingly irrational.

References

Baker, C. (1996). *The Health Care Policy Process*. London: Sage Publications.

Bryson, J.M. (2004). *Strategic planning for public and nonprofit organizations: A guide to strengthening and sustaining organizational achievement*, 3rd edn. San Francisco, CA: Jossey-Bass Publishers.

Chisholm, D. (2005). Choosing cost-effective interventions in psychiatry: results from the CHOICE programme of the World Health Organization. *World Psychiatry*, **4**, 37–44.

Collins, C. and Coates, T. (2000). Science and health policy: can they cohabit or should they divorce? *American Journal of Public Health*, **90**, 1389–90.

Corrigan, P.W. and Watson, A.C. (2003). Factors that explain how policy makers distribute resources to mental health services. *Psychiatric Services*, **54**, 501–7.

Das, J., Do, Q.-T., Friedman, J., McKenzie, D., and Scott, K. (2007). Mental health and poverty in developing countries: Revisiting the relationship. *Social Science & Medicine*, **65**, 467–80.

Department for International Development, Mental Health and Poverty Project: Mental health policy development and implementation in four African countries. Available at: http://www.research4development.info/SearchResearchDatabase.asp?ProjectID=50165 (accessed 21 December 2009).

Dimock, M.E., Dimock, M.O., and Fox, G.M. (1983.) *Public Administration*. New York: Holt, Rinehart and Winston.

Flisher, A.J., Lund, C., Funk, M., Banda, M., Bhana, A., Doku, V., *et al.* (2007) Mental health policy development and implementation in four African countries. *Journal of Health Psychology*, **12**, 505–16.

Frank, R.G. and Glied, S.A. (2006). *Better but not well: mental health policy in the United States since 1950*. Baltimore, MD: Johns Hopkins University Press.

Garfield, R. (2009). Mental health policy development in the States: The piecemeal nature of transformational change. *Psychiatric Services*, **60**, 1329–35.

Hogan, M.F. (2008). Transforming mental health care: realities, priorities and prospects. *Psychiatric Clinics of North America*, **31**, 1–9.

Horton, R. (2007). Launching a new movement for mental health. *Lancet*, **370**, 806.

International Consortium in Psychiatric Epidemiology. Available at: http://www.hcp.med.harvard.edu/icpe/ (accessed 21 December 2009).

Jacob, K.S., Sharan, P., Mirza, I., Zarrido-Cumbrera, M., Seedat, S., Mari, J.J., *et al.* (2007). Mental health systems in countries: where are we now? *Lancet*, **370**, 1061–77.

Jenkins, R., McCulloch, A., Friedli, L., and Parker, L. (2002). *Developing a national mental health policy. Maudsley Monograph 43*. East Sussex: Psychology Press.

Kessler, R., Angermeyer, M., Anthony, J.C. de Graaf, R., Demyttenaere, K., Gasquet, I., *et al.* (2007). Lifetime prevalence and age-of-onset distributions of mental disorders in the World Health Organization's World Mental Health Survey Initiative. *World Psychiatry*, **6**, 168–76.

Knapp, M., McDaid, D., Mossialos, E., and Thornicroft, G. (2007). *Mental Health Policy and Practice across Europe*. Milton Keynes: Open University Press.

Lopez, A., Mathers, C., Ezzati, M., Jamison, D., and Murray, C. (2006). *Global burden of disease and risk factors*. Washington, DC: Oxford University Press and the World Bank.

Lee, K., Buse, K., and Fustukian, S. (2002). *Health Policy in a Globalising World*. Cambridge: Cambridge University Press.

Miller, G. (2007). Mental health and the mass media: room for improvement. *Lancet*, **370**, 1015–16.

Miranda, J.J. and Patel, V. (2005). Achieving the Millennium Development Goals: Does mental health play a role? *PLoS Med* **2**, e291.

Movement for Global Mental Health. Available at: http://www.globalmentalhealth.org/ (accessed 21 December 2009).

Murray, C.J.L. and Lopez, A.D. (eds.) (1996). *The global burden of disease and injury series, volume 1: a comprehensive assessment of mortality and disability from diseases, injuries, and risk factors in 1990 and projected to 2020*. Cambridge, MA: Harvard University Press.

Musgrove, P. (1996). *Public and Private Roles in Health: Theory and Financing Patterns*. Washington, DC: World Bank.

Patel, V. and Kleinman, A. (2003). Poverty and common mental disorders in developing countries. *Bulletin of the World Health Organization*, **81**, 609–15.

Patel, V., Saraceno, B., and Kleinman, A. (2006). Beyond evidence: The moral case of international mental health. *American Journal of Psychiatry*, **163**, 1312–15.

Patel, V., Garrison, P., de Jesus Mari, J., Minas, H., Prince, M., and Saxena, S. (2008). *The Lancet* Series on Global Mental Health: 1 year on. *Lancet*, **372**, 1354–7.

Piachaud, J. (2008). Globalization, conflict and mental health. *Global Social Policy*, **8**, 315–34.

Pirkis, J., Harris, M., Buckingham, B., Whiteford, H.A., and Townsend-White, C. (2007). International planning directions for provision of mental health services. *Administration and Policy in Mental Health and Mental Health Services Research*, **34**, 377–87.

Prince, M., Patel, V., Saxena, S., Maj, M., Maselko, J., Phillips, M., *et al.* (2007). No health without mental health–a slogan with substance. *Lancet*, **370**, 859–77.

Reich, M.R. (1996). Applied political analysis for health policy reform. *Current Issues in Public Health*, **2**, 186–91.

Roberts, M., Hsiao, W., Berman, P., and Reich, M. (2003). *Getting Health Reform Right: a Guide to Improving Performance and Equity*. Oxford: Oxford University Press.

Saraceno, B., van Ommeren, M., Batniji, R., Cohen, A., Gureje, O., Mahoney, J., *et al.* (2007). Barriers to improvement of mental health services in low-income and middle-income countries. *Lancet*, **370**, 1164–74.

Saxena, S., Thornicroft, G., Knapp, M., and Whiteford, H.A. (2007). Resources for mental health: scarcity, inequity, and inefficiency. *Lancet*, **370**, 878–89.

Srinivasa Murthy, R. and Lakshminarayana, R. (2006). Mental health consequences of war: A brief review of research findings. *World Psychiatry*, **5**, 25–30.

Sturm, R. (1999). What type of information is needed to inform mental health policy. *Journal of Mental Health Policy and Economics*, **2**, 141–4.

Swayne, L.E., Duncan, W.J., and Ginter, P.M. (2006). *Strategic Management of Health Care Organizations*, 5th edn. Oxford: Blackwell publishers.

Thornicroft, G. and Tansella, M. (2004). Components of a modern mental health service: a pragmatic balance of community and hospital care: overview of systematic evidence. *British Journal of Psychiatry*, **185**, 283–90.

Thornicroft, G., Becker, T., Knapp, M., Knudsen, H.C., Schene, A.H., Tansella, M., *et al.* (2006). *International Outcome Measures in Mental Health: Quality of Life, Needs, Service Satisfaction, Costs and Impact on Carers*. London: Gaskell, Royal College of Psychiatrists.

Townsend, C., Whiteford, H., and Baingana, F., Gulbinat, W., Jenkins, R., Baba, A., *et al.* (2004). A mental health policy template. Domains and elements for mental health policy formulation. *International Review of Psychiatry*, **16**, 18–23.

Walt, G. (1994). *Health Policy: an Introduction to Process and Power*. Johannesburg: Witwatersrand University Press.

Walt, G., Shiffman, J., Schneider, H., Murray, S.F., Brugha, R., and Gilson, L. (2008). 'Doing' health policy analysis: methodological and conceptual reflections and challenges. *Health Policy and Planning*, **23**, 308–17.

Wang, P.W., Simon, G.E., Avorn, J., Azocar, F., Ludman, E.J., McCulloch, J., *et al.* (2007). Telephone screening, outreach, and care management for depressed workers and impact on clinical and work productivity outcomes: A randomized controlled trial. *Journal of the American Medical Association*, **298**, 1401–11.

Whiteford, H. (1992). A National Mental Health Policy for Australia. *Medical Journal of Australia*, **157**, 510–11.

Whiteford, H.A. (1994). Intersectoral policy reform is critical to the National Mental Health Strategy. *Australian Journal of Public Health*, **18**, 342–4.

World Federation for Mental Health. Available at: http://www.wfmh.org/ (accessed 21 December 2009).

World Health Organization (2001). *The World Health Report 2001: Mental Health: new understanding, new hope.* Available at: http://www.who.int/whr/2001/en (accessed 21 December 2009).

World Health Organization (2005a). *Mental Health Declaration for Europe: facing the challenges, building solutions.* Copenhagen: World Health Organization.

World Health Organization (2005b). *Mental health policy, plans and programmes (updated version 2).* Geneva: World Health Organization (Mental Health Policy and Service Guidance Package).

World Health Organization (2005c). *Mental Health Atlas.* Available at: http://www.who.int/mental_health/evidence/atlas (accessed 21 December 2009).

World Health Organization (2008). *Mental Health Gap Action Programme – Scaling Up Care for Mental, Neurological, and Substance Use Disorders.* Geneva: World Health Organization. Available at: http://www.who.int/mental_health/mhgap/, (accessed 4 January 2010).

World Psychiatric Association. Available at: http://www.wpanet.org/ (accessed 21 December 2009).

CHAPTER 32

Using information and evidence to improve mental health policy

Michelle Funk, Jodi Morris, and Shekhar Saxena

Background

A mental health policy is the official statement of a government about what they will do to improve the mental health situation in that country. Together with a mental health plan, which details concrete actions to implement the policy, they represent essential tools to improve the way mental health problems are addressed in countries. When well formulated, they can coordinate, through a common vision and plan, all programmes, services, and actions related to mental health. Without this type of organization, mental health problems are likely to be dealt with in an inefficient and fragmented manner. Mental health policies assist to maximize the effectiveness of mental health programmes, to ensure that funds are spent wisely, and to improve coordination among service providers in the community (Funk et al., 2005).

The World Health Organization (WHO) has argued for developing national policies on mental health that are information and evidence based. Though the broad objectives of the policy may remain the same across countries, the starting points are likely to be different across countries (even within the same income category) so much so that background and contextual information become essential for the development of policy and plans.

National mental health policy and plans

A mental health policy provides the overall direction for mental health by defining a vision, objectives, and broad framework for action to achieve the vision. In contrast, the strategic mental health plan is a complementary document that details the specific strategies and activities that will be implemented as well as specifying other crucial elements such as the budget and timeframe, targets, and indicators for activities and strategies. The plan also clarifies the roles of the different stakeholders in implementing the activities of the plan.

The interrelationship between the policy and plan and its elements are schematically represented in Fig. 32.1. An excerpt from a sample mental health plan is presented in Fig. 32.2.

Information required for national mental health policy development and planning

The development of national mental health policies and plans should be guided by scientific evidence, best practice, and human rights standards (WHO, 2009b). This requires, that countries: 1) shift care away from large psychiatric hospitals (deinstitutionalization), 2) develop community mental health services, and 3) integrate mental health care into general health services at primary and secondary health care (WHO, 2001).

Policies need to specifically promote the human rights of people with mental disability in the actions they prescribe. This is an obligation based on the international conventions (International Convention on the Rights of Persons with Disabilities; International Covenant on Civil and Political Rights (1966); International Covenant on Economic, Social and Cultural Rights (1966); WHO, 2009a). In practical terms it means making sure that services are accessible and acceptable to those in need, that they promote the autonomy and liberty of people with mental disability, and that they put an end to the many human rights violations faced by people with mental disability. Policies need to ensure the full and equal enjoyment of all human rights of persons with disabilities (WHO, 2009a).

Conducting a situational analysis is an essential first step for evidence-based decision-making in the development of policy and plans. The situational analysis defines the circumstances prevailing in the country both in terms of the mental health needs and with regard to the existing mental health system, available resources or those that can be mobilized. In many countries, however, situational analyses are informed only by the personal knowledge and beliefs of national experts involved in drafting the new policy which can lead to biased appraisals of need and poor planning decisions.

A combination of quantitative and qualitative research is useful for informing the direction and content of a mental health policy and strategic action plan. Quantitative methods are particularly useful for understanding the epidemiology of mental health problems and service and treatment outcomes, whereas qualitative

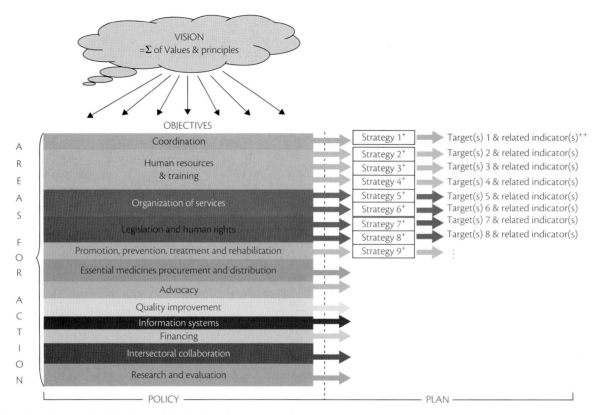

Fig. 32.1 The relation between a health policy and plan (Funk and Freeman, 2010).

Objective: to reduce the number of people in psychiatric institutions
Area for action: service organization
Strategy 1: move people from psychiatric hospitals to the community
Targets: discharge 20% of residents most readily able to move to the community
Indicators: the proportion of people discharged from psychiatric institutions

Activity	Q1	Q2	Q3	Q4	Responsible person	Costs
Identify 20% of patients in hospital who are most readily able to move to the community	X				Mental health team in hospital	Assessment
Discuss with patients and families the reintegration of person in family and community life	X	X			Social worker/nurse from hospital	Visiting, discussing, providing information and support to families
Transfer of medical treatment and care to trained PHC providers in the community		X	X	X	Psychiatrist/mental health team	Initial consultations with PHC medicines in PHC training of PHC staff
Regular supervision and consultation with primary health care staff providing care to the patients		X	X	X	Psychiatrist/mental health team	Regular follow-up and support to PHC staff

Fig. 32.2 Extract from a sample mental health plan.

PHC, primary health care.

research through the use of focus groups and structured interviews is useful for gaining a better understanding of the context in which services are being delivered, including the attitudes and beliefs of service users, families, health workers, and policy makers (WHO, 2004).

Situational analysis

The following are considered to be essential components of a situational analysis (WHO, 2009b):

Country general context: political, demographic, economic, and social factors can all impact on the prevalence of mental disorders and mental health problems in a population, service accessibility, and the perception and treatment of people with mental disorders within the community. For example, in very mountainous countries or countries where travel is difficult for a few months per year due to rainy seasons, it may be difficult to access centralized mental health services reinforcing the need to ensure that mental health service are locally available at the community level. People living in poverty may not be able to afford the costs associated with mental health services and may consequently fail to get the care they require, unless mental health service are covered in health insurance schemes. Demographic data demonstrating a very young population, as is the case in Uganda where almost half of the population (49.3%) is under 15 years of age, may signify the need to make sure that mental health services cater for the needs of young people (WHO, 2009b).

General health context: general information on general health needs, main health challenges, and priorities provides important contextual information to help understand the priority of mental health relative to other health problems in a country as well as some of the mental health issues that may need to be addressed for other high priority health problems. For example, mental health may need to be addressed in the context of countries experiencing high rates of HIV/AIDS given the high comorbidity between mental health problems and HIV/AIDS and links to health outcomes. Similarly, information on the current structure and capacity of the national general health system is required and will guide some of the entry points for strengthening mental health services.

Policy and legislative framework: the drafting of a mental health policy and plan needs to take into account the current policy and legislative environment, and note whether major changes are required. A comprehensive policy and plan in the context of a country implementing an outdated law will not have the desired impact and efforts will need to be made to prioritize the development of a new mental health law in the policy (WHO 2010). Additionally, a mental health policy/plan is more likely to be successful if core elements are integrated into a general health policy and plan and closely aligned with any existing development frameworks at national level (Funk et al., 2010).

Coordination: coordination or stewardship of mental health activities in the country is of central concern for policy development and implementation of the policy/plan. Attempts to implement a policy and a plan will fail if there is there is no coordinating body or if a coordinating body is not sufficiently resourced or supported to carry out its mandate at a high level.

Additionally, the coordinating body should have the inputs and supports from the key stakeholders in the country (WHO, 2004).

Mental health financing: knowing the sources of financing and the budget available for mental health is essential information for realistic planning. Putting in place a policy and plan that relies on a financial commitment far beyond the realities of the country and expected contributions from donors will fail at the implementation phase. Due attention needs to be given to current financial costs incurred by individuals and families in seeking treatment and care in order to understand the degree to which financial factors act as barriers to care and in order to understand how these can be overcome in a new policy framework (WHO, 2003a).

Prevalence of mental health problems and current service utilization: in developing a mental health policy and plan it is crucial to understand the major mental health problems that need to be addressed as well as their prevalence. Not only will this information shape the focus of the policy and plan but it will assist, in a very practical way, the planning of services and the human and financial resources required to drive these services. Information on service utilization can help understand the degree to which some services are being over utilized or underutilized as well as the treatment gap when considered in relation to prevalence rates (WHO, 2003b).

Services for mental health and their organization: analysing information on all aspects of current services for mental health can reveal important gaps and inequities that need to be addressed in a new mental health policy and strategic plan. The situational analysis needs to provide clear and comprehensive information on the location and number of mental health facilities as well as general health facilities and their staffing levels at each health care level (primary, secondary, and tertiary). Where general health facilities also provide mental health services this should be clearly indicated (WHO, 2003c).

Human resources and training: given that human resources are the backbone of all health services, the situational analysis should specify the adequacy of human resources in terms of numbers and types of health and social care workers available (e.g. psychiatrists, psychiatric nurses, general nurses with mental health experience, social workers, and community workers) and describe the skills they have to carry out work in the mental health field. The situational analysis should provide an understanding of the training different health workers receive in mental health and any degree or diploma courses available in the country. It is also important to understand recruitment, retention, and incentive measures in place in a country in order to fully understand the human resource situation for mental health and policies that may be required to maintain a workforce adequate in numbers, skills, and motivation (WHO, 2005a, 2010).

Intersectoral collaboration: collaboration with the non-health sector (e.g. social welfare, education, employment, housing, justice) as well as private providers, non-governmental organizations (NGOs), and faith-based organizations is crucial to provide comprehensive care and support to people with mental disabilities, and to assist in the prevention of mental ill health and the promotion of mental health. It is therefore important to know what resources are available in these different sectors and in the community in order to make optimal use of available resources for the implementation of the policy and plan (WHO, 2004).

The World Health Organization Assessment Instrument for Mental Health Systems (WHO-AIMS)

WHO-AIMS is a tool designed to enable low- and middle-income countries (LAMIC) to assess key components of their mental health systems, and thereby generate essential information that can be used to strengthen mental health policy and service delivery (Saxena et al., 2007; WHO, 2005b). It helps countries to develop information-based mental health policies and plans with clear baseline information and targets. The instrument enables a comprehensive assessment of a country's mental health system, as well as the services and support offered to people with mental disorders that are provided outside the psychiatric services sector (e.g. mental health in primary care, links with other key sectors). Moreover, WHO-AIMS allows countries to monitor progress in implementing policy reforms, the provision of community services, and the involvement of consumers, families, and other stakeholders in mental health promotion, prevention, care, and rehabilitation.

The 10 recommendations of *The World Health Report 2001* (WHO, 2001) served as the foundation for the instrument, as they represent WHO's vision for mental health. In order to operationalize the recommendations (**domains** of interest), a large number of items were generated and grouped together into a number of **facets** (subdomains). Experts and key focal points from resource-poor countries provided input through two consultations to ensure clarity, content validity, and feasibility of the generated items. Based on this feedback, a pilot version of the instrument was released and tested in 12 LAMIC. The instrument was substantially revised and shortened based on data from the pilot study as well as input from international experts. The instrument was then presented at a WHO meeting attended by 14 representatives from LAMIC as well as key resource people from around the world. At this meeting several minor additions and revisions were recommended and were incorporated into a revised version (WHO-AIMS 2.2), which was released for use in country assessments in February 2005.

WHO-AIMS 2.2 consists of six domains:

1 **Policy and legislative framework** This domain covers key components of mental health governance including mental health policies, plans, and legislation. Financing of mental health services and monitoring and training on human rights are also addressed within this domain.

2 **Mental health services** The organizational context of service provision as well as service delivery within mental health facilities are covered within this domain. Equity of access to mental health care is also addressed.

3 **Mental health in primary care** Service delivery within the primary health care system (both physician-based and non-physician-based clinics) is assessed within this domain, as well as interaction with complementary practitioners (e.g. traditional healers).

4 **Human resources** The availability of human resources in mental health as well as training of mental health professionals is assessed

within this domain. The presence and activities of user and family associations and NGOs are also covered within this domain.

5 **Public information and links with other sectors** Public awareness and educational campaigns on mental health as well as collaborative links with key health (e.g. primary health care) and other sectors (social welfare) are addressed in this domain.

6 **Monitoring and research** Mental health information systems and research conducted on mental health are assessed within this domain.

These six domains address the 10 recommendations of *The World Health Report 2001* through 28 facets and 155 items. The instrument consists of input and process indicators, given that in many LAMICs outcome data are extremely difficult to collect.

WHO-AIMS assessments are carried out by a local team. This team is headed by an in-country 'focal point', which in most cases is identified and/or approved by that country's ministry of health. Technical support for the project is provided by WHO staff at the country, regional, and headquarters levels.

To date, WHO-AIMS assessments have been conducted in over 80 LAMIC. An analysis of the first 42 countries to complete an assessment indicated that 62% of the countries used the information gathered through WHO-AIMS to develop or revise a mental health policy or plan or currently have plans to do so, 55% used the assessment for some other planning purpose, 74% of countries presented the results of the assessment in a national workshop attended by key stakeholders, 24% published the results of the assessment in a scientific journal, and 29% of countries used WHO-AIMS to improve their mental health information system (WHO, 2009c). Not only do the data provide baseline information that can be used to develop plans to strengthen or scale up services, but also the process of collecting the data brings together key stakeholders within the countries, placing them in a stronger position to press ahead with the needed reforms.

There is an urgent need for improvement in the provision of mental health care in LAMIC. The saying 'what gets measured gets done' summarizes the importance of monitoring and evaluation for mental health planning. Information gathered through WHO-AIMS enables countries to better gauge the major challenges and obstacles that they face in providing care for their citizens with mental disorders, enabling them to use this information to improve the policy context and strengthen service delivery.

The process of integrating information and evidence into development of policy and plans

The situational analysis is the first basic requirement for establishing a mental health policy and plan. The next steps are to define and agree upon the policy vision, and the underlying policy values and principles which in turn will allow a clearer formulation of specific policy objectives, areas for action, and key strategies. Objectives should broadly aim to improve the health of the population, respond to people's expectations, and provide financial protection against the cost of ill health (WHO, 2001). A number of strategies simultaneously addressing multiple areas for action need to be identified in order to take these objectives forward. These areas which correspond to the main components of the situational analysis include:

financing, legislation and human rights, organization of services, human resources and training, promotion, prevention, treatment and rehabilitation, advocacy, quality improvement, and information systems, research, and evaluation. Once the policy strategies have been determined they must be broken down into specific activities in order to assist implementation. Some of the key planning requirements include the determination of relevant and feasible activities to implement specific strategies, identifying responsible persons for each activity, specifying the duration of each activity, sequencing of activities, specifying outputs and any anticipated obstacles. At this stage specifying targets and indicators for each of the strategies will also help to assess whether or not the plan has been effective following implementation (see Fig. 32.1). Objectives, areas for action, strategies, activities, targets, and indicators can be brought together within a single planning framework. Once brought together, the cost of the whole plan needs to be assessed by calculating the cost of each strategy and the total cost of the plan for each year of implementation. The strategies, activities, time frame, and resources need to be re-planned if large gaps are found between the requirements of the plan and available budget (WHO, 2004, 2010).

Right from the start and throughout the process of establishing a mental health policy and plan it is necessary to have established a policy drafting group with a clear official mandate at the highest level possible in government. Equally important is the need to carry out extensive consultations for its formulation (WHO, 2004, 2010).

The drafting committee should reflect a complement of analytical, technical, and managerial skills that enable the correct interpretation of data from the situational analysis, the strategic use of the data to build the policy and plan, the skilful blending of information and evidence with the viewpoints of the different stakeholders groups (taking into account culture, political issues and processes, and on-the-ground realities) and the skilful writing of the policy and plan using a convincing and well-structured style (Faydi et al., submitted).

The consultative process in formulating the policy and plan is as important as the information and evidence used to build the policy and plan. Policy development is a political process and hence it is essential to conduct wide consultations with all the key stakeholders. Broad consultation with a wide range of stakeholder groups—each with their own specific experience and expertise within the mental health field (e.g. consumer and family groups, general health and mental health workers, government agencies, providers, academic institutions, professional associations, NGOs)—is needed in order to achieve a balanced idea of what is required to improve the mental health situation in a country. It is also required in order to promote ownership of the policy and plan and stakeholder engagement in its implementation. Failure to achieve consensus will lead to a policy and plan that is either ignored or actively sabotaged by different stakeholder groups. The role of the health ministry to listen to the various stakeholders and to make proposals that blend their different views with the evidence derived from national and international experience is crucial in the development of the policy and plan (WHO, 2004, 2010).

Conclusion

A systematic process of collecting, analysing, and using available information is essential to developing and improving mental health policy. Not only does this process lead to a policy that is more appropriate and relevant to the needs of the country but it also facilitates the actual implementation of the policy by involvement of various stakeholders at an early stage.

References

Faydi, E., Funk, M., Kleintjes, S., Ofori-Atta, A., Ssbunnya, J., Mwanza, J., et al. (Submitted for publication). An assessment of mental health policy in Ghana, South Africa, Uganda and Zambia.

Funk, M. and Freeman, M. (2010) Framework and methodology for evaluating mental health policy and plans. *International Journal of Health Planning and Management*, [ePub 2 August 2010].

Funk, M., Saraceno, B., and Drew, N. (2005). Global perspective on mental health policy and service, development issues: the WHO angle. In: Knapp, M., McDaid, D., Mossialos, E., and Thornicroft, G. (eds.) *Mental Health Policy and Practice Across Europe*, pp. 426–40. Milton Keynes: Open University Press.

Funk, M., Drew, N., Freeman, M., and Faydi, E. (2010). *Mental Health and Development: Targeting people with mental health conditions as vulnerable group*. Geneva: World Health Organization.

Saxena, S., Lora, A., van Ommeren, M., Barrett, T., Morris, J., and Saraceno, B. (2007). WHO's Assessment Instrument for Mental Health Systems: Collecting essential information for policy and service delivery. *Psychiatric Services*, **58**, 816–21.

WHO (2001). *The World Health Report 2001. Mental Health: New Understanding, New Hope*. Geneva: World Health Organization.

WHO (2003a). *Mental health financing (WHO mental health policy and service guidance package*. Geneva: World Health Organization. Available at: http://www.who.int/mental_health/policy/essentialpackage1/en/index.html (accessed 11 March 2010).

WHO (2003b). *Planning and budgeting to deliver services for mental health (WHO mental health policy and service guidance package)*. Geneva: World Health Organization. Available at: http://www.who.int/mental_health/policy/essentialpackage1/en/index.html (accessed 11 March 2010).

WHO (2003c). *Organization of services for mental health (WHO mental health policy and service guidance package)*. Geneva: World Health Organization. Available at: http://www.who.int/mental_health/policy/essentialpackage1/en/index.html (accessed 11 March 2010).

WHO (2004). *Mental health policy, plans and programmes (WHO mental health policy and service guidance package)*. Revised edition. Geneva: World Health Organization. Available at: http://www.who.int/mental_health/policy/essentialpackage1/en/index.html (accessed 11 March 2010).

WHO (2005a). *Human resources and training in mental health. WHO mental health policy and service guidance package*. Geneva: World Health Organization. Available at: http://www.who.int/mental_health/policy/essentialpackage1/en/index.html (accessed 11 March 2010).

WHO (2005b). *World Health Organization Assessment Instrument for Mental Health Systems (WHO-AIMS)*. Geneva: World Health Organization. Available at: http://www.who.int/mental_health/evidence/WHO-AIMS/en/index.html (accessed 11 March 2010).

WHO (2009a). *Policy Brief: Developing Effective Mental Health Policies and Plans in Africa: 7 key lessons, Mental Health Policy and Service Development, Department of Mental Health and Substance Abuse*. Geneva: World Health Organization. Available at http://www.who.int/mental_health/policy/development/mhapp/en/index.html (accessed 11 March 2010).

WHO (2009b). *Policy Brief: Key elements of a situational analyses to inform mental health policy. Mental Health Policy and Service Development, Department of Mental Health and Substance Abuse*. Geneva: World Health Organization. Available at http://www.who.int/mental_health/policy/development/mhapp/en/index.html (accessed 11 March 2010).

WHO (2009c). Mental health system in low and middle income countries: a cross national analysis of 42 countries using WHO-AIMS data. Geneva: World Health Organization. Available at: http://www.who.int/mental_health/evidence/who_aims_report_final.pdf (accessed 21 December 2010).

WHO (2010). *Improving health systems and services for mental health*. Geneva: World Health Organization.

CHAPTER 33

Funding of mental health services

Dan Chisholm and Martin Knapp

Introduction

Whether it is a case of setting out to develop, reorientate, or just maintain existing levels of community-based mental health services, policy-makers and planners will run up against the inconvenient but inescapable question of resource constraints. How much money will it take, for example, to build up service coverage and capacity, to introduce effective new intervention strategies, to overhaul prevailing modes of service delivery, or to cater for the changing needs of the population? Decisions made at this strategic level of mental health policy and planning exert a powerful influence over the extent to which those people in need of services will actually be able to access and use them, as well as shape the way in which provision is organized and paid for.

Mental health financing is a far-reaching topic that not only addresses the specific question of what services to purchase and how, but also more normative questions around how much should be allocated to (say) community mental health care (e.g. what can be afforded, given the extent of mental health and broader other health needs in the population?), as well as equity issues (e.g. are funding arrangements fair, in the sense that people in need are not prevented from accessing services on financial grounds?). Indeed, alongside meeting the reasonable expectations of service users and actualizing mental health improvements in the population, fair financing does or should represent a key goal of a mental heath system (WHO, 2006). In this chapter, we endeavour to cover these diverse questions under a number of central financing themes— resource generation and revenue collection, risk pooling and financial protection, plus resource allocation and purchasing—to highlight key funding issues that need to be considered when planning, implementing, or evaluating community mental health services.

Mental health care and market failure

Prior to discussion of these key mental health financing themes, however, we should ask whether individuals should be left to purchase the health services and goods that they need or desire—just like many other commodities such as groceries or transport—or whether there are particular reasons for some kind of collective action or state intervention when it comes to mental health services. In short, is there justification for state intervention in the financing (or provision) of mental health care? There are in fact a number of well-established 'market failures' that commonly arise in the context of health care; that is, reasons why 'regular' market forces cannot be relied upon to achieve socially acceptable outcomes. These include undesired spillover effects (such as the spread of infectious disease within and across populations), and the information imbalance that typically exists between the consumer (patient) and supplier of care (health professional). Such distortions to the 'equilibrium' of the health care market can lead to the undersupply of essential services, excessive prices, or reduced quality of care for consumers, and, of most concern, unmet individual needs. Overarching these problems, there is the inherent uncertainty around a person's future health status, which makes it hard for individuals to predict when they will need to use and pay for health care (this intrinsic uncertainty provides the rationale for insurance against the risk of illness).

Mental health care differs from other health care, with certain market failures less prominent, and others accentuated in comparison to somatic disorders (Beeharry et al., 2002). For example, while the danger of violence to others that can be caused by individuals suffering a psychotic episode or behaving under the influence of illicit drugs would constitute a negative spillover effect that justifies some form of public intervention, for many mental health problems such negative 'externalities' are not a major concern (that is, most of the costs or consequences of illness are internalized). On other grounds, however, mental disorders are especially prone to market failure, perhaps most obviously in terms of information deficits—many people with mental health needs lack insight into their often complicated condition—leading to lower demand than is both personally and socially optimal: individuals may be unaware of their condition and therefore do not seek appropriate treatment. The result will be an undersupply of services that only collective action can redress (and which may even involve treating sick individuals involuntarily). For those with an identified condition, the pervasive stigma attached to mental illness produces a further check on the demand for services. In addition, there is ample international evidence to indicate that mental disorders are disproportionately represented among the poor, either as a result of a drift by those with mental health problems towards more socially disadvantaged circumstances (due to impaired levels of psychological or social functioning), or a greater exposure to adverse life events among the poor (Patel and Kleinman, 2003).

There are also particular problems when it comes to paying for or insuring against mental illness, particularly chronic or lifelong conditions such as schizophrenia or bipolar affective disorder. Uninsured individuals or households face potentially ruinous costs associated with health care expenditures and forgone work opportunities, while those with or seeking private health insurance plans may find themselves excluded or restricted from receiving the services they need. The latter problem of 'adverse selection' occurs because private insurance companies strive to keep premiums competitive by removing or limiting entitlements for high-cost conditions. Conversely, where mental health care is covered, policy holders may actually use more services than they really need because they feel entitled to do so (the problem of 'moral hazard').

In summary, there are sufficiently strong arguments to argue for a collective or public response to mental health problems in the population. As we discuss below, the exact nature of that response or action, e.g. the extent to which governments actually pay for or deliver services, can and does vary considerably, depending on prevailing notions of social choice in a country, as well as existing health system structures and constraints.

Resource generation, revenue collection, and risk pooling

Resource needs for mental health

Providing community-based mental health services involves putting together human, physical capital, and other resource inputs in order to deliver interventions and services capable of improving mental health and related outcomes (WHO, 2003a, 2006). Accordingly, a basic initial requirement of any mental health system is the assessment of what resources are needed in order to deliver services to the target population and meet programme goals. The first logical step in such an exercise is to ascertain what resources are currently available (numbers of mental health professionals, inpatient beds, day care places, etc.), followed by an epidemiologically-driven appraisal of expected service needs and costs at target levels of service coverage (see Fig. 33.1).

The lack of complete or reliable local epidemiological and resource data has thwarted such efforts in many countries, but that is now changing with the generation of national mental heath profiles (see, for example, Jacob et al., 2007). While such profiles may not provide all the detailed information needed by mental health planners to develop community-based services at the national level, they do clearly reveal the paucity of human financial resources relative to the identified need for these resources—and also the absolute shortage of core services inputs in the worst-off countries. Many lower-income countries in fact devote less than 1% of total health funds to mental health, and the poorer the country (measured in terms of average annual income per capita), the more likely they are to allocate less to the mental health sector.

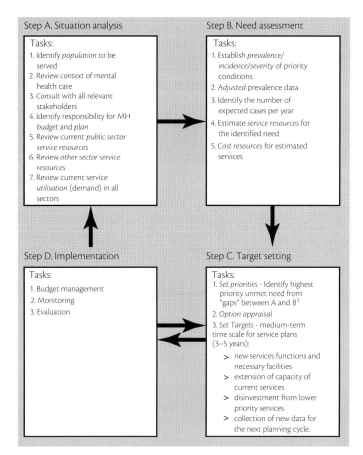

Fig. 33.1 Steps in planning and budgeting for mental health services From WHO, 2003b.

How much a country should be spending on mental health is a question often posed (Lim et al., 2008) but rarely answered, owing to the complex landscape that needs to be mapped out, the multidimensional goals of a mental health system, and prevailing notions of social choice. Nevertheless, analytical tools and methods for financial planning have been developed (e.g. WHO, 2003b) and have been used, for example, to estimate the cost of significantly scaling-up the delivery of a specified package of mental health care in the context of low- and middle-income countries, where services are least well developed yet where the untreated burden of mental disorders is greatest (Chisholm et al., 2007) (Box 33.1).

Funding sources for mental health

Alongside the articulation of programme goals and a viable financial plan for meeting them, consideration needs to be given to how revenues will be sourced in order to pay for salaries, medications, consumables, information systems, and capital infrastructure. Revenue collection is the process by which the health system obtains financial contributions from households, firms, and organizations (plus donors, where applicable). Revenues can be collected in various ways: general taxation; (mandated) social health insurance; (voluntary) private health insurance; out-of-pocket payments; and donations (Knapp et al., 2007). All insurance mechanisms share the goal of spreading the risk of having to pay for services across all members of the pool of contributors. Social health insurance is more specifically organized around mandatory

> **Box 33.1** Financial resources needed to deliver mental health care in low- and middle-income countries (from Chisholm et al., 2007)
>
> A financial analysis was carried out to estimate the expenditures needed to scale-up over a 10-year period the delivery of a specified mental health care package, comprising pharmacological and/or psychosocial treatment for schizophrenia, bipolar disorder, depression, and hazardous alcohol use. Current service levels in 12 selected low- and middle-income countries were established using the WHO-AIMS assessment tool. Target-level resource needs were derived from published need assessments and economic evaluations. The analysis estimated that in order to meet the specified target coverage levels—80% of cases for schizophrenia and bipolar disorder, and 25% to 33% of cases with depression and risky drinking—spending for this package alone would need to be around $2 per capita in low-income countries (compared to $0.10–$0.20 now), and $3–$4 in middle-income countries. So for a middle-income country of 50 million people, total annual expenditure for the package would amount to $150 to $200 million.

contributions by employees and their employers, and is found in many countries of Europe, Asia, and Latin America. In contrast, general taxation applies to all tax payers, not just those in employment: the United Kingdoms's National Health Service, for example, is funded out of general taxation. Private insurance represents the predominant financing mechanism for most citizens in the United States, but there are special (publicly financed) schemes for the indigent and the older people. In many other (mainly poor) countries of the world, but also for uninsured subpopulations of higher income countries, out-of-pocket payments represent the most common means by which health service use is paid for. Table 33.1 provides a summary of some of the distinctive features of these different funding mechanisms, although, as will be made apparent, most countries tend to have in place a combined financing model.

Broadly speaking, the sources of funding for mental health services reflect the pattern for health care in general (Dixon et al., 2006; WHO, 2005). Accordingly, people with mental health service needs living in countries with predominantly tax- or insurance-based systems pay only a small amount or nothing at all at the point of accessing services, while those in countries without

such provisions have to rely on current household income as their primary funding source. Even in mental health systems adequately financed through pre-payment contributions, it is common practice for patients or service users to be charged a small fee (a so-called 'co-payment') at the point of use. This charge—which may be waived for certain services or individuals (such as people with low incomes or congenital health problems)—is levied in order to counter the aforementioned problem of 'moral hazard', whereby fully paid-up members of a risk pool persons have an incentive to use more services than they strictly need. In low-income populations, such fees also have this general intent (as well as shifting some of the financial burden to consumers) but can also have the more negative consequence of putting off potential users in real need of care. Accordingly, there are quite strong equity arguments for abandoning user fees for socioeconomically disadvantaged or other vulnerable groups in the population, including those facing challenging mental health problems.

Fairness in financing mental health

Funding mental health services via mandatory tax-based contributions provides the opportunity to gear payments according to ability to pay; that is, by stipulating contributions as a fixed proportion of income, higher income groups end up 'putting more into the pot' than those with lower incomes. Such a system is described as progressive. By contrast, it is widely acknowledged that out-of-pocket payments represent a regressive form of health financing— they penalize those least able to afford care—and represent an obvious channel through which impoverishment may occur (Dixon et al., 2006; Saxena et al., 2007; WHO, 2003b). Specifically, they lead in many cases to health spending levels that have been labelled 'catastrophic' because they cause households to reallocate their budgets away from other essential needs such as education, food, and housing. The potentially 'catastrophic' impact of private, out-of-pocket payments on the income and savings of households with a mentally ill member was assessed in a recent study in Goa in India: 15% of women with a common mental disorder spent more than 10% of household income on health-related expenditures (Patel et al., 2007). By contrast, a study undertaken in the United States concluded that out-of-pocket spending did not represent a substantial source of financial burden for most service users, since most expenditures were being financed by insurers or managed care organizations (Ringel and Sturm, 2001).

Among pre-payment mechanisms, and as noted already, private insurance markets throw up some particular challenges in the

Table 33.1 Characteristics of different health insurance mechanisms

	National insurance	**Social insurance**	**Private insurance**	**No insurance**
Collection method	General taxation	Employee premiums	Household premiums	Cash (out-of-pocket)
Legal status	Mandatory	Mandatory for workers	Voluntary	None
Pre-paid population	Everyone	Workers only	Those able to pay	None
Fairness/equity	Progressive	Neutral	Regressive	Regressive
Adverse selection	No	No (if working)	Yes	N/A
Moral hazard (users)	Yes	Yes	Yes	N/A
Co-payments	Few	Some	Many	N/A

From Knapp and McDaid, 2007.

context of mental health services, in particular the issue of adverse selection. For example, in Malaysia, health is predominantly financed through private health insurance schemes. However, all of the private insurers exclude mental health services from their plans, leaving mental health services to be financed through general taxation and out-of-pocket payments (Deva, 2004). In the United States, there has been a history of insurers attempting to restrict mental health coverage to avoid enrolling people with higher (expected) mental health service needs, and, more recently, a decision by insurers to carve out mental health care from overall insurance risk and cover enrolees via a separate contract, with mixed results (Frank and Garfield, 2007; Frank and Glied, 2006). That is why the mandatory nature of national insurance schemes is so important, since relaxing this rule provides higher earners with an incentive to opt out and secure for themselves a private health insurance plan that potentially offers more personalized or responsive care arrangements; an obvious knock-on effect of such opting out is that there is then less money to go round for those left in the insured pool, with predictable adverse consequences for service quality and coverage.

Overall, it is safe to say that pre-payment mechanisms such as national or social insurance represent a more equitable mechanism for safeguarding at-risk populations from the adverse financial consequences of mental disorders compared to out-of-pocket expenditures. Furthermore, it can be noted that by mandating universal health insurance, key problems of private or social insurance such as adverse selection can be avoided, and contributions can be geared according to ability to pay.

Despite the desirability of universal coverage, many countries are being hampered from moving towards this goal by a variety of constraining factors, including weak taxation systems and governance structures, inefficient use of existing resources, plus the high transaction costs associated with any fundamental reform. Indeed, in countries with weak (income) tax collection and/or a large informal economy, tax-based financing may not generate sufficient resources for mental health service provision at the population level, which is why many countries have considered social health insurance as a more viable means by which at least one large segment of the population can be covered (often public employees based in urban areas). By so doing, however, such schemes explicitly exclude those working (unpaid) in the household or in the informal sector (which in many countries is very substantial) as well as those unable to work due to long-term or recurrent illness or disability; these gaps in coverage represent a significant shortcoming given the well-known association between low socioeconomic status or poverty and the incidence of mental disorder (Patel and Kleinman, 2003; Saxena et al., 2007).

Mental health care: a mixed economy of financing and provision

Although in certain cases the principal funder may also be the predominant provider, it is more common in the mental health sector to find a 'mixed economy' of financing and provision, in which funding from the various possible sources is expended across an assortment of public, private and also voluntary or non-governmental agencies. Many service delivery models explicitly involve non-governmental actors or sectors, since the specific arguments

in favour of state funding of mental health services (negative spillover effects, information failures) do not apply equally to the state **provision** of mental health services. The precise roles performed by these different providers depend on the prevailing legal, economic, and institutional frameworks of a country, and may also have historical or sociocultural determinants. To illustrate, the role of the non-governmental sector might be quite substantial in a low-income country with a weak state health system—as NGOs or private providers attempt to fill the void left by state provision—but quite limited in the context of strong state control and provision.

Cross-classification of funding and provider types generates a simple matrix representation of the inter-connections characterizing pluralist care systems and their constituent transactions (see Table 33.2). What would go into such a matrix? The simplest task would be to list services (such as inpatient facilities, community nurses, primary care doctors, sheltered work schemes) in the appropriate provider-funding cells of the matrix. More demanding but also more informative would be to record the volumes of provision and/or the total funding or expenditure amounts. Given the multiplicity of service types potentially active in supporting people with mental health problems, it would be preferable if the completed matrix spanned a range of sectors, not being confined to the (narrow) health care system.

Table 33.2 provides some illustrations of the types of link that might be found in a mental health system. In this hypothetical example (for a lower-income country), financing of the mental health system comes mainly from general taxation, but is complemented by contributions from international donors and charitable foundations, as well as via fees or co-payments paid by users of the system to service providers. On the provision side, the state sector is primarily responsible for running government-run hospitals and outpatient services, while non-governmental agencies (whether for-profit or not) carry out a number of activities in their own right, both on the open market and under contract with state sponsors. Mapping the mental health system in this way—even if only descriptively—generates an informative overview of who is doing what now, and can be a useful template against which to consider (for example) the development of or movement towards community-based mental health services.

Paying for mental health care

Following on from questions around how to generate sufficient resources for mental health and to protect the sick against the spectre of financial catastrophe or impoverishment, there remains the central issue of how, where, and to whom should available funds be most appropriately channelled for the purpose of delivering services to the population in need. A number of mechanisms are possible, each with their own underlying incentives, processes, and implications.

Perhaps the most straightforward scenario to consider is one in which both funding and provision of services are controlled by the same agency (most typically a ministry of health). In this case, funds that have been collected (via taxation) can simply be allocated directly to government-run services at the subnational level, most simply on a per capita basis (i.e. budgets are set in proportion to population size alone). Since the budget is fixed, there is strong pressure to keep overall expenditures under this set amount

Table 33.2 Mixed economy of mental health care

Revenue collection (funding)	Mode or sector of provision			
	Public/state sector	**Voluntary/NGO**	**Private (for-profit)**	**Informal sector**
General taxation	(1) State psychiatric hospital (2) Psychiatric outpatient clinics (3) Percentage of primary health care budget used for mental health care (4) Percentage of health promotion budget used for mental health promotion	Pledged state contribution (5%) to an International NGO providing trauma services	Commissioning (contracting out) of specific services, e.g. trauma counsellors in primary care clinics	Grants to identified chronic service users
Social insurance	-	-	-	-
Private insurance	-	-	Voluntary contributions (annual contributions to private Insurance agencies)	-
Charitable	NGO funding of sheltered employment in state-owned facility	(1) NGO providing trauma services (95% of annual budget) (2) Advocacy organization campaigning for rights in psychiatric hospitals	-	Grants to epilepsy sufferers from international epilepsy fund
Foreign governments	Foreign government-subsidies to mental health service providers	-	-	-
Out-of-pocket	Sliding scale service charges for public services	Sliding scale service charges for trauma counselling (NGO)	Fee-for-service payments to private providers and traditional healers	-
No exchange	NA	NA	NA	Family care; neighbourhood support

(i.e. there is very little flexibility for providers to increase their income beyond what has been allocated). However, such a mechanism overlooks the potentially large variations in mental health need at the subnational level, e.g. regions with large cities might be expected to have a larger or more complex case-mix than more rural regions. Accordingly, a number of countries in Europe and elsewhere have constructed allocation formulae in order to better capture these expected variations and better anticipate actual mental health service funding requirements. Budgets can then be based on a fixed fee per person enrolled into the mental health service of a defined catchment area.

The extent to which fixed budgets should be devolved to providers is a commonly recurring financing issue. In principle, devolved budgets and purchasing should increase the likelihood that decision-making is sensitive to user needs and preferences. Through their everyday work, health care professionals should be well placed to recognize individual and (local) community needs and wants, and hopefully to respond to them. Consequently, devolution of financial responsibilities could be seen as one way to help a health system to be more needs-led, although devolved budget-holders would need to have the right information, skills, autonomy, and incentives if they are to budget flexibly, effectively, and efficiently. However, a devolved budget holder may have less information than a central budget holder, fewer technical resources to process what information they have, and less of a financial cushion in the event of a mistaken decision. Holding the budget centrally may leave an organization better placed to pool and spread risks, to wield its purchasing power to achieve better price deals and to use non-price intervention such as subsidies and contracts linked to investment in order to improve quality.

Centralized budgeting might also make it is easier to respond strategically to area-wide needs, whether in terms of purchasing, investment, or shaping of the broader system.

A further concern around allocating public funds **directly** to state providers is that it provides limited incentives for maintaining or improving the quality of services being delivered. This is because providers are essentially free of competition for those funds, and can consequently operate without any real fear of 'losing business' (to use a market-based analogy). There is also the risk that professionals or managers pursue their own rather than nationally mandated objectives. There is therefore increasing interest in, and implementation of, performance-based financing of health services, which links the prospective allocation of resources to the quantity and quality of service provision (via legally-binding contracts). (A better approach still would be to link resource allocation to the actual meeting of needs, i.e. the achievement of better health and quality of life, but this is inherently complex to set up.)

In countries where both financing and provision rest mainly with the state, such as in the United Kingdom, incentive-based funding has been introduced artificially via the imposition of a virtual market in health care, consisting of purchasers or commissioning agencies on the one hand—who are charged with assessing and meeting the needs of a defined population—and (hospital, community or primary care) providers on the other hand, who compete with each other for the available resources. In countries where social or private insurance systems are in place, the contract is between the insurance agency and a range of public as well as private providers.

The main contract types are described in Box 33.2. One central choice in contract specification is the degree of flexibility, particularly with respect to prices. While a pre-determined price

Box 33.2 Types of contract between purchasers and providers

◆ **Block contracts** link service specifications and reimbursement to provider facilities—for instance, buying a defined number of inpatient places—and payment is made regardless of whether the service is actually used. Because block contracts guarantee a level of revenue, small or risk-averse providers may be prepared to accept lower payments in return for predictability. However, purchasers run the risk of having either too few or too many places in the facilities that turn out to be needed. The larger the purchaser (or the purchasing budget) the lower the risk of a mismatch between demand and capacity.

◆ **Spot and call-off contracts** are price-by-case arrangements in that the individual service user is the basis for reimbursement: the provider is only paid if the client uses the service. Purchasers sometimes prefer the flexibility that comes from spot purchasing, but risk paying a premium for this, particularly in markets for highly specialized services. Spot contracts are usually more expensive to operate than block contracts because the latter offer economies of scale in drafting and negotiation. These contracts have a price band set prior to purchase, negotiated by a centralized purchaser, and occasionally with some variation to allow for the needs of individual users. Local decision-makers or care managers or other decentralized agents then call off services from the contract. Spot and call-off contracts shift more of the financial risk onto providers.

◆ **Cost-and-volume contracts** are combinations of block and price-by-case arrangements. A guaranteed level of service is purchased; beyond that level, additional reimbursement is made according to the number of users. There is also the possibility of more easily building in other contingencies.

has the advantage of predictability to the purchaser, the provider may experience cost changes that leave their net revenue (their profits if they are in the commercial sector) uncertain. Moreover, pre-determined prices are not responsive to the individual needs of users. Providers may thus not have the incentive to tailor the services they supply to specific individual circumstances; in particular, they may not offer more intensive treatment and support to those with greater needs. Flexible prices shift some of the risk back to the purchasers, and offer greater incentives to providers to respond to the changing care circumstances.

An alternative mechanism for paying providers is on the basis of 'fee for service', whereby a fixed price is agreed beforehand (e.g. with social insurance or sickness funds) and reimbursed retrospectively following the provision of a service, such as an outpatient consultation or an overnight inpatient stay. In this case, there is a clear incentive for providers to deliver as much care as they can handle, since the more they do the more they receive. Although that does not represent a problem for many essential services, it **can** lead to the over-provision of other, less essential services or even the unnecessary prescription of drugs. Examples in the context of mental heath services might include excessive numbers of psychological sessions for a relatively minor case of depression or anxiety, or the medicalization of—and subsequent drug prescription

for— emotional or behavioural problems in childhood and adolescence. Such an inbuilt incentive to produce or even induce services for which there is strongest demand or highest return—irrespective of the outcomes that they generate—has the potential to undermine other services that are more clinically important or economically efficient. In countries where such a payment model is in place— typically those with social health insurance and mostly private providers, like many countries in central and eastern Europe—there is a consequent need to specify national priorities and develop clinical treatment guidelines that specify normal limits of reimbursable service provision. Accordingly, the main role of government in this context is to formulate national mental health policy and service development strategies, put in place regulatory structures and monitor the overall performance of the mental health system.

Financing the move towards community-based mental health care

Community-based mental health services form one critical component of a comprehensive mental health system (Thornicroft and Tansella, 2004; WHO, 2001), bringing as they do more accessible and responsive care to those in need than hospital-based care (such as outreach and rehabilitation services, for example). In a great many countries, however, the transition to a community-based service model is moving slowly. This is due in no small part to negative social perceptions of mental illness and a lack of political will, but there are also constraints of a financial nature. Over and above the more general health financing objective of moving people with mental health problems away from reliance on out-of-pocket payments towards pre-payment funding schemes, therefore, there is the more specific challenge of how to move funds for mental health away from institutionally-focused services and channel them into the development of community-based care.

At the heart of the funding conundrum for community mental health care is the pre-existing and continuing financial commitment to large-scale hospital institutions for persons with long-term mental health problems. Dating back many generations, governments throughout the world invested in the construction and maintenance of asylums for the mentally ill. With the advent of antipsychotic drugs and the growing emphasis on human rights, together with realization (through research) of the dire standards in many institutions, such a model of care has been increasingly discredited and many countries began a process of deinstitutionalization that is continuing to this day. Nevertheless, in most regions of the world, mental hospitals continue to consume a large proportion of the (government) mental health budget and account for at least three-quarters of total bed capacity (Jacob et al., 2007).

The reasons for this prevailing situation include a lack of strong leadership or political will and the protection of vested interests (in the status quo). In many countries, mental health budgets are simply based on the previous year's allocation and linked to bed occupancy rates, which offers little scope or incentive for change. Over and above these barriers, efforts to change the balance of mental health care have been hindered by a lack of appropriate transitional funding. Transitional or dual funding is clearly required over a period of time in order to build up appropriate community-based services **before** residents of long-term institutions can be relocated. Since such relocation of former inpatients is a gradual movement, it is usually some years before the old institution can be closed (and any proceeds from the sale of land and buildings recouped, as well as staff redeployed to new service configurations). However, governments are typically reluctant to put such dual funding in place because of concerns that they will not be able to recoup much of the additional investment they put into the development and maintenance of community-based services.

Accordingly, where deinstitutionalization has occurred, new funding has generally been patchy and inadequate, resulting in inappropriate care arrangements for a proportion of former inpatients, with the attendant risk that a poorly funded community-based system will fail the people it is intended to support. For mental health policy-makers seeking to move towards community-based mental health care, it is therefore crucial to present an evidence-based case not only on the grounds of equity, human rights, and user satisfaction, but also on the grounds of financial feasibility over a defined transitional period. In addition, it may also be possible to bring arguments of economic efficiency to bear, or at least cost neutrality, although that will depend on the order in which individuals are relocated and the speed with which this happens (Knapp et al., 2006).

A further funding issue relating to the move from hospital-towards community-based mental health care concerns the greater multiplicity of providers and their respective roles, in particular the shifting of responsibilities and associated funding from health to social care and housing systems. Where previously the financial responsibility for long-term institutional care of people with chronic mental health problems clearly rested with the health system, care arrangements in the community typically extend to social or other welfare services (including supported housing and vocational rehabilitation). In the many countries where access or entitlement to these social services is subject to some form of means-testing, individuals whose care would have been paid for by the state under the terms of national or social health insurance may now find themselves having to pay substantially towards that care. It is therefore important that sufficient safeguards are in place—via payment exemption schemes for people meeting a certain threshold level of physical or mental disability, for instance—to protect against such instances of unfair financing for health. One other plausible but so far largely untested mechanism in this regard would be to provide direct payments or individual budgets to service users, who then decide for themselves which services to use. Where pilot schemes have been tried, the results for mental health service users have been broadly encouraging (Glendinning et al., 2008).

Conclusion

While the pursuit of improved health and well-being in the population should unquestionably be the overarching goal of a mental health system, a further objective is to ensure that the financial risks each household in society faces with respect to mental health are distributed fairly, e.g. according to their ability to pay (Dixon et al., 2006; Knapp et al., 2007; WHO, 2003b, 2006). In order to fully meet these objectives, it is necessary to raise and pool enough funds up front so that a comprehensive set of services can be provided to those in need (without regard to income status, ethnicity, age and so on). In addition, it is incumbent on governments to ensure that available resources for mental health service provision—wherever those contributions may come from—are

used to best effect across the range of intervention strategies, service levels, and provider sectors that make up the mixed economy of mental health care.

Earlier in this chapter we reviewed the case for collective action or state intervention concerning the funding of mental health services, and argued that there is solid justification (especially on the grounds of information failure and stigmatized attitudes to mental illness). We might go further and point out that since mental health is an integral part of health, and since health is an integral component of social well-being and happiness, governments would do well to realign their priorities away from those whose primary intent revolves around the creation or retention of wealth towards those that clearly promote societal well-being (and in so doing tackle prominent causes of unhappiness, such as depression and anxiety). Viewed from this broader perspective of what a society should be trying to achieve, it is quite evident that most countries are letting themselves down, often quite badly, when it comes to providing decent and equitable care for their mentally ill populations. It is a sad fact that annual mental health spending in many countries continues to fall far below $1 per capita or just a fraction of 1% of total health expenditure (Jacob et al., 2007). That is equivalent to putting a very low price on human happiness or psychological well-being.

Generating new resources for mental health is therefore of paramount significance in countries with weak or underfunded mental health systems, and a critical step towards building a functional, community-based mental health system. As illustrated in Fig. 33.1, estimation of the additional human, physical, and financial capital needed to develop or scale-up prioritized services or interventions is one task that can usefully be undertaken in order to demonstrate the existing funding gap and to provide a starting point for discussions of how it could be bridged over time. Persuading national governments or international donors to make the large-scale investments needed nevertheless remains a massive challenge. In other, mainly higher-income settings, the shortfall in resources is less stark, and the focus is more likely to be around the reconfiguration of services and associated reallocations of existing resources.

In terms of revenue collection and risk pooling, national insurance was identified as the most likely route to universal coverage, while 'pay-as-you-go' payment mechanisms are clearly the most inequitable. All countries therefore need to try to minimize the contribution of out-of-pocket payments and shift as much as the population to pre-payment mechanisms such as social or national insurance. How collected resources are used to purchase services is a much more flexible and nuanced question, however. The main mechanisms that we reviewed—each subject to its own set of incentives and limitations—included retrospective fee-for-service payments, direct allocation to decentralized providers, and performance-based contracting. Direct (devolved) payments to service users offer a new option in some contexts. Given the ever-increasing concern with cost inflation in the health sector, it seems likely that interest in and implementation of performance-based contracting between providers and insurers of all kinds will only increase over time. Where insurance-based systems are found wanting, not-for-profit non-governmental organizations can go some way to filling the void left by state-sponsored provision. Finally, we sounded some specific words of warning around the economics of deinstitutionalization, where again there may be financial incentives at work which can act **against** the desired goal of comprehensive community-based care that is accessible to all in need.

References

Beeharry, G., Whiteford, H., Chambers, D., and Baingana, F. (2002). *Outlining the scope for public sector involvement in mental health.* HNP Discussion Paper. Washington DC: The World Bank.

Chisholm, D., Lund, C., and Saxena, S. (2007). The cost of scaling up mental health care in low- and middle-income countries. *British Journal of Psychiatry*, **191**, 528–35.

Deva, P. (2004). Malaysia mental health country profile. *International Review of Psychiatry*, **16**, 167–76.

Dixon, A., McDaid, D., Knapp, M., and Curran, C. (2006). Financing mental health services in low- and middle-income countries. *Health Policy and Planning*, **21**, 171–82.

Frank, R.G. and Garfield, R.L. (2007). Managed behavioral health care carve-outs: past performance and future prospects. *Annual Review of Public Health*, **28**, 303–20.

Frank, R.G. and Glied, S.A. (2006). *Better but not well.* Baltimore, MD: The Johns Hopkins University Press.

Glendinning, C., Challis, D., Fernández, J.-L., Jacobs, S., Jones, K., Knapp, M., *et al.* (2008) Evaluation of the Individual Budgets Pilot Programme. York: Social Policy Research Unit, University of York.

Jacob, K., Sharan, P., Mirza, I., Garrido-Cumbrera, M., Seedat, S., Mari, J.J., *et al.* (2007). Mental health systems in countries: where are we now? *Lancet*, **370**, 1061–77.

Knapp, M.R.J. and McDaid, D. (2007). The Mental Health Economics European Network. *Journal of Mental Health*, **16**, 157–65.

Knapp, M., Funk, M., Curran, C., Prince, M., Grigg, M., and McDaid, D. (2006). Economic barriers to better mental health practice and policy. *Health Policy and Planning*, **21**, 157–70.

Knapp, M.R.J., McDaid, D., Ammadeo, F., Constantopoulos, A., Oliveira, M.D., Salvador-Carulla, L., *et al.* (2007). Financing mental health care in Europe. *Journal of Mental Health*, **16**, 167–80.

Lim, K.L., Jacobs, P., and Dewa, C. (2008). *How much should we spend on mental health?* IHE Report. Alberta: Institute of Health Economics.

Available at: http://www.ihe.ca/documents/Spending%20on%20Mental%20Health%20Final.pdf

Patel, V. and Kleinman, A. (2003). Poverty and common mental disorders in developing countries. *Bulletin of the World Health Organization*, **81**, 609–15.

Patel, V., Chisholm, D., Kirkwood, B.R., and Mabey, D. (2007). Prioritizing health problems in women in developing countries: comparing the financial burden of reproductive tract infections, anaemia and depressive disorders in a community survey in India. *Tropical Medicine and International Health*, **12**, 130–9.

Ringel, J.S. and Sturm, R. (2001). Financial burden and out-of-pocket expenditures for mental health across different socioeconomic groups: Results from HealthCare for Communities. *Journal of Mental Health Policy and Economics*, **4**, 141–50.

Saxena, S., Thornicroft, G., Knapp, M., and Whiteford, H. (2007). Resources for mental health: scarcity, inequity, and inefficiency. *Lancet*, **370**, 878–89.

Thornicroft, G. and Tansella, M. (2004). Components of a modern mental health service: a pragmatic balance of community and hospital care: overview of systematic evidence. *British Journal of Psychiatry*, **185**, 283–90.

WHO (2001). *The World Health Report 2001;Mental Health: New Understanding, New Hope.* Geneva: World Health Organization.

WHO (2003a). *Planning and budgeting to deliver service for mental health. Mental health Policy and Service Guidance Package.* Geneva: World Health Organization.

WHO (2003b). *Mental Health Financing. Mental health Policy and Service Guidance Package.* Geneva: World Health Organization.

WHO (2005). *Atlas: Mental health resources in the world 2005.* Geneva: World Health Organization. Available at http://www.who.int/mental_health

WHO (2006). *Dollars, DALYs and Decisions: Economic Aspects of the mental health system.* Geneva: World Health Organization.

SECTION 8

Assessing the evidence for effectiveness

CHAPTER 34

Methods for evaluating community treatments

Peter Tyrer

Introduction

New treatments are constantly being introduced to all forms of psychiatry and for most of these the setting in which the treatment is administered is not of special importance. Thus the introduction of a new and effective drug for a mental disorder will require similar testing in hospital, community, or other settings and does not require special description here. However, all treatments given in the community have a common problem associated with them, compliance, or what is now more appropriately termed 'concordance' or 'adherence' (Mullen, 1997). Because treatment in the community can rarely be supervised satisfactorily, a great deal depends on the motivation of individual patients to continue whatever intervention is being given without the need to be closely monitored. Increasingly, therefore, the evaluation of community treatment is going to involve, 1) some check on whether the treatment is being given appropriately and 2) if not, whether additional treatments are able to be introduced to improve concordance and adherence. New treatments to improve compliance have now been introduced for the major psychoses and shown to be effective (Kemp et al., 1996; 1998; Perry et al., 1999) and these approaches are likely to impinge increasingly on those working in the community and be amongst the areas of competence being evaluated for such workers.

The word 'evaluation' is now being used increasingly to describe any type of description of an intervention, and more and more it is being used inappropriately with regard to community treatments. The word 'evaluate' is a mathematical expression originally used to give a numerical value to something which previously had no such value. It is still used in this sense in related expressions such as 'evaluable', but increasingly it has been broadened in use to describe any form of assessment, whether or not it is quantified accurately.

Three key questions

Before discussing different forms of evaluation of community treatment it is necessary to establish what type of evaluation is proposed

in any one instance, and this is common to evaluations of all treatments in medicine. Up to three main questions are normally being asked in such evaluations and it is important not to blur these because doing so creates confusion. The three questions are:

- Is the treatment (or service) effective? (i.e. does it serve the purpose of the treatment or service?)
- Does the treatment work in conditions of ordinary practice? (i.e. is it efficacious?)
- Is the treatment cost-effective? (i.e. it is worth spending the money required for its implementation?)

Is the treatment effective?

There is no point in any treatment being introduced to clinical practice in medicine unless it is an improvement on no treatment. The first prerequisite of any putative treatment is therefore to develop its efficacy. The way by which such efficacy can be demonstrated has been the subject of considerable dispute over the past few years. Since the pioneering paper by Schwartz and Lellouch in 1967 (see below) a distinction has been made between explanatory and pragmatic trials of treatment effectiveness. Most, if not all, treatments in community psychiatry are determined by pragmatic trials as the circumstances in which treatments are given in ordinary practice may be very different from those which demonstrate the efficacy of a treatment. Such comparisons can be carried out in any setting but may not be necessarily appropriate to ordinary practice. For example, some years ago Soloff and colleagues demonstrated that haloperidol in relatively low dosage (around 7 mg a day) was superior to both antidepressants and placebo tablets in patients with borderline personality disorder treated in a penitentiary. There were no drop-outs from care because all the patients were in a locked environment and, not surprisingly, all patients took their medication as prescribed (Soloff et al., 1986). The prerequisite of efficacy had been established but this is no guarantee that in ordinary clinical usage the treatment would be appropriate for the general population of people with borderline personality disorder. Examination of all the data, as for example in the recent National Institute for Health and Clinical Excellence (NICE) guidelines (National Collaborating Centre for Mental Health, 2009), has shown no good evidence of benefit and the guideline suggests that antipsychotic drugs should be avoided in the treatment of this condition.

Nevertheless, this explanatory phase of investigation is needed to show that the treatment confers benefit; without it there can be no confidence that the treatment is effective. However, in community psychiatry this may have to be carried out by designs that are very different from those in pragmatic trials.

Is the treatment efficacious in practice?

In a pragmatic trial, the circumstances in which the treatment would be used in ordinary clinical practice are being tested and these may be very different from those appertaining in an explanatory trial. Pragmatic trials are more relevant to community mental health services and are also favoured by evidence-based medicine, now accepted as the best way of choosing treatments. A distinction is sometimes made between the words 'effective' and 'efficacious' in this context. If the treatment is superior to a control treatment it can be said to show 'efficacy', but it is only when it has been tested in ordinary circumstances of clinical practice and shown to be superior to other treatments that it can be regarded as 'efficacious'. This might stretch interpretation of the English language too far. 'Effective' refers to the ability of a treatment to bring about a desired effect, and this is virtually the same as 'efficacious', something 'that produces, or is certain to produce, the intended effect (i.e. effective)' (*Shorter Oxford English Dictionary*; Little et al., 1973). The definition of a good service need not therefore be strictly determined by the results of a randomized controlled trial, and although such trials should never be regarded as redundant or unnecessary, evaluation can be greatly reinforced by a range of other sources of information (for review see Thornicroft and Tansella, 1999, pp. 101–5).

Cost-effectiveness

It is no longer satisfactory to merely demonstrate the effectiveness of a treatment. If the cost of this is so much greater than that of existing treatments, and the gain only a small advance, it is difficult to justify its introduction except on a very limited scale. It is fortunate that most treatments in community psychiatry are relatively cheap compared with the high cost of inpatient services. A substantial part of cost-effectiveness of community treatments is the demonstration that inpatient care is reduced as a consequence of introducing the treatment. Even if the reduction in inpatient care is only modest, in most cases it would be more than sufficient to make the cost of treatment less than the alternative (Byford et al, 2010; Knapp and Beecham, 1990).

Stages of evaluation

All evaluations in community psychiatry are complex interventions (ones in which two or more interventions are involved, even if they are not always specified). So it might be thought, for instance, that the assessment of a drug treatment in the community using a placebo comparison was a simple intervention, as the drug/placebo comparison in a randomized trial is now a standard allegedly 'gold standard' comparison. But it is not simple. Whereas in an inpatient sample the administration of the drug can largely be assured in the community there is no certainty that patients will take the medication as prescribed. Many other interventions have up to 10 different components that could all be tested in their own right but in practice are very difficult to tease out from others. In most evaluations in the community the key interventions can be regarded as a set of variables which commonly include: 1) the setting, 2) the personnel involved in the interventions, 3) the specific tested intervention (which may itself have several components), 4) the nature of any relevant comparison treatment and 5) the relationships between the treaters and the treated. This is a little more complicated than is commonly discussed in the evaluation of complex health interventions, but the principles are the same, and follow a graded process occurring in a set of phases (Campbell et al., 2000), somewhat similar to the phases that have now become common parlance in the evaluation of new drugs. I will take the example of one relatively recent community treatment that has now completed all these phases, assertive community treatment, to illustrate each of these.

Phase 0: preclinical or theoretical phase

In the first stage of evaluation it is legitimate to think broadly about an issue and decide whether it is an important subject to examine and research, and then to think about the methods that might be employed. Thus, to take our exemplar, assertive community treatment, there was great concern in the 1960s about the pathological effects of hospital treatment in those with any form of illness that persisted. The nasty eight-syllable word, 'institutionalization' appeared in the literature as a complicating pathology in those who stayed for any time in hospital (Barton, 1966), and so it was natural to look for alternatives in the community. Assertive community treatment grew from this wish; if people could be engaged in treatment outside hospital, preferably in their own homes, the perils of the institution might be avoided. Stein and Test put this notion forward in 1964 and tested it out some years later (Marx et al., 1973). It had a clear theoretical base and was feasible–it was treatment without the institution, probably the core of community psychiatry.

Phase 1: modelling

In this phase the effects of a new intervention or treatment are described and, to some extent, measured before and after its introduction and an idea of its likely effect size obtained. This goes beyond simple description and gives some idea of the impact of the new intervention. However, most open studies exaggerate the degree of change created by the new intervention and invariably further studies show that its impact is considerably less. Nevertheless, these studies serve a valuable purpose in demonstrating: 1) the intervention is feasible in clinical practice, 2) is more likely to have a positive impact than a negative one, and 3) gives some idea of its relative advantages and disadvantages. Other improvements that can be made in such studies include: 1) reduction in numbers of other treatments that are given so confounding is less, 2) formal assessment using rating scales at the beginning and end of the treatment period so that change is measured more precisely, 3) better selection of patients for treatment, 4) formal prepost designs that give some notion of the benefits of the treatment.

In the case of assertive community treatment these initial modelling studies were carried out in the 1970s (Marx et al., 1973; Stein and Santos, 1998) and showed that the risks of treating people with severe mental illness outside hospital were much less than the benefits.

Phase 2 or exploratory trial

In this phase the information gathered in phase 1 is used to develop what appears to be the most optimal form of intervention and to test this in an appropriate study design with a comparison treatment or intervention. This can involve merely testing aspects of the treatment such as acceptability and practicality as these are part of the mix of complex interventions described above. It may also be tested with user groups at this stage in order to develop a strong case for the trial within the community of patients likely to be treated.

Researchers are usually advised to carry out a pilot randomized controlled trial at this stage as this offers many advantages; it informs the development of a definitive trial by helping to decide if a large trial is feasible, the data collected help in deciding the sample size of a larger trial, and problems in recruitment and retention of subjects can be identified and corrected. The pilot trial also has greater scope. Austin Bradford Hill, the inventor of the randomized trial, always pointed out that a good trial answered a 'precisely framed question' but at the stage of the exploratory trial it is often far from certain what that question is. There is sometimes a tendency in the definitive evaluation of complex interventions to either rush to the main research question too early in enquiry or to test out many questions simultaneously; the pilot trial offers the opportunity to be more flexible and choose a different primary research question when the main trial plan is formulated.

There is also a range of interventions that fall short of the requirements of the true randomized controlled trial. These include quasi-randomization in that randomization of the population does not take place but other measures are introduced to make the groups as similar as possible at baseline. The problems of randomization are prominent when community services are being compared (an der Heiden, 1996; Thornicroft et al., 1998)

Phase 3: randomized controlled trials

In the last stage of comparison the new treatment is compared with a standard treatment under the rigorous conditions of a randomized controlled trial. Whilst this has always been the 'gold standard' whereby any new treatment is to be judged, it is important not to be carried away by the scientific arguments for using such trials (which are incontrovertible) without considering alternatives which may be more appropriate **at that particular time in the development of the treatment**. Randomized controlled trials are still relatively new to medicine and particularly to psychiatry and the first major studies, of the treatment of schizophrenia in the United States (Casey et al., 1960) and of depression in the United Kingdom (Clinical Psychiatry Committee, Medical Research Council, 1965), are still within my experience in psychiatry.

Attitudes towards the randomized controlled trial have changed markedly in the last 10 years because of the distinction made between pragmatic and explanatory trials of interventions (Schwartz and Lellouch, 1967). Before this time all was invested in the explanatory trial, a tightly organized and controlled trial of highly selected individuals who were homogeneous for the condition being treated and who were likely to complete the course of treatment. The findings of these studies were then generalized to routine clinical practice. Schwartz and Lellouch pointed out that this approach was not

valid. The explanatory trial was 'aimed at understanding whether a difference existed between two treatments' whereas the pragmatic trial 'aimed at decision by answering the question "which of the two treatments should we prefer?"' (Schwartz and Lellouch, 1967). It is this question that is at the heart of any service evaluation and it is asked at a later stage than the explanatory trial.

Johnson (1998) has recently pointed out that, despite long use of the randomized controlled trial in psychiatry, it continues to be used inefficiently and often wrongly. There are greater problems with psychiatric disorders (and with psychiatric patients) than in other medical conditions and these include: 1) problems of achieving reliable diagnoses, 2) the difficulties of maintaining blind assessments, 3) the common practice of simultaneously giving many treatments, and 4) the difficulties in selecting control groups, particularly for psychosocial treatments. However, these do not excuse the generally laxity of design and poor presentation and interpretation of findings. Johnson recommends that those involved in carrying out clinical trials of treatment interventions in psychiatry should follow seven principles when choosing a suitable design: 1) choose no more than two outcome variables, 2) concentrate on obtaining follow-up information on all randomized patients on a few occasions rather than many, 3) use a multicentre design wherever possible, 4) ensure that the entry criteria are as broad as possible so that the results are likely to be generalizable, 5) forget power calculations and aim to recruit at least 100 patients for analysis in each treatment group, 6) develop the strategy for analysis **before** the trial database is 'unblinded' to reveal treatments, and 7) use recently introduced statistical modelling techniques to enable analysis of all available data rather than restrict this to those with full follow-up information (Everitt, 1995).

Individual randomization may not always be appropriate in mental health service evaluation. For example, if an intervention is directed towards a team intervention, cluster randomization is frequently used and this will affect the numbers needed to show benefit (these are usually larger than when individual randomization is made) (Kerry and Bland, 1998) and may pose important ethical issues (Edward et al., 1999). Randomized incomplete block designs have also been used when full randomized studies are not deemed to be possible.

Because it is rarely possible to blind both patients and investigators in trials of community mental health services there is great potential for bias. Attempts to minimize bias need to be made explicit and one way of ensuring this is to make the investigating (research) team independent of the service providers. The characteristics of those who refuse to participate or who drop out at an early stage of evaluation are likely to differ from those who participate throughout and should be recorded.

The sample size necessary for a trial is dependent on the power calculation which relies on estimating the difference between the effects of two or more interventions and the likely variance of the data. This may be possible if an exploratory trial has been carried out using the same design but in most instances there is a great deal of guesswork in making such estimations. In practice many investigators work backwards. They estimate how many patients they are likely to have available for treatment and then work out the power calculations to fit these figures. This was not the purpose for which power calculations were introduced and the recommendation of Johnson (1998) that investigators should aim for a minimum of 100 patients in each arm of the trial is a better solution.

In the case of assertive community treatment the influential trial that demonstrated its efficacy was published in 1980 and was carried out in the state of Wisconsin in the United States (Stein and Test, 1980; Weisbrod et al., 1980). This indicated both marked clinical efficacy and cost-savings and ACT, as it came to be known, was adopted with varying degrees of enthusiasm across the United States (Stein and Santos, 1998).

Phase 4: dissemination and implementation

This final phase is sometimes neglected by researchers who feel their work has been done when they complete their main trials. The growth of research and development in health service research has achieved greater prominence because of the failure to implement advances quickly enough; this was the main impetus behind the development of the Cochrane Collaboration. Part of this phase is equivalent to post-marketing surveillance after the introduction of a new drug and it is fair to add that health service interventions have been slow to introduce this adequately. However, it has a role in the establishment of audit.

Audit is often undervalued by experienced research workers who are used to working with good resources and no time pressures. However, audit is the best way of ensuring that the benefits of research advance are not only disseminated to clinical practice but are also maintained. In clinical practice good audit ensures quality control so that sound practice is maintained.

Patient preference

Although randomized trials provide the best evidence of efficacy for treatments such as a comparison of new drugs in which patient preference is a very minor factor the situation is different for many psychosocial treatments or those in which drugs and other treatments are being compared. In a consumer society the issue of patient preference in respect of treatment is coming more to the fore. This is particularly true in community settings. One common example is the prescription of antipsychotic drugs in schizophrenia. Although the evidence for the efficacy of these drugs in schizophrenia is overwhelming there is still a large minority of patients who prefer to take other forms of treatment, particularly 'alternative therapies' of unproven and doubtful value. In my personal experience the strong personal belief of such patients that these treatments are the only valid ones does have an influence on response to treatment which goes far beyond the simple placebo effect for the preferred treatment and the nocebo effect (Tyrer, 1991) of the rejected one. The nocebo effect (i.e. the expectation that a treatment will harm) is now as prevalent as the placebo effect in clinical practice. Fifty years ago new treatments were mainly 'wonder drugs' that led to marvel, amazement, and the expectation of improvement. Now we have a more sophisticated and informed population that is likely to look up all the adverse effects on the internet before agreeing to start treatment.

There is also the possibility that there are important interactions between an individual's preferences and the effects of treatment, yet in the standard randomized controlled trial these are not detected. If these are important the results of the randomized controlled trial may be wrongly attributed to the specific content of the intervention alone (McPherson et al., 1997). As a consequence of this there is increasing interest in non-experimental methods in the assessment of efficacy of treatments (Wennberg, 1988) and in

different research designs that take account of patient (or indeed, other people such as clinicians) preferences. Brewin and Bradley (1989) proposed a partially randomized patient-centred design for psychosocial treatments in which patients who had strong preferences for a particular treatment were allocated to it whereas those who had no particular preference were randomly allocated in the usual way. The problem with this approach is that it breaks one of the fundamental principles of the randomized controlled trial, ensuring equivalent populations for all factors apart from the treatments under consideration. If, as has been shown to be the case, patients who have strong preferences differ from others in their level of education and other potentially important factors (Feine et al., 1998) then their results cannot be compared satisfactorily with others.

This does not mean that patient preference trials are inappropriate but it is probably preferable to avoid contaminating the randomized controlled trial by attempting to combine randomization and patient preference in one design. If a patient preference trial is carried out independently of a randomized controlled trial then the results can be compared and policy decisions made after taking account of both sets of findings (Wennberg et al., 1993).

Choice of evaluation for different treatments

Although circumstances vary greatly it is possible to list the most appropriate forms of evaluation for different treatments (Table 34.1). For most drug treatments it is preferable to concentrate on randomized controlled trials as the main method of evaluation as, despite their difficulties in community settings, the ability to make treatments more or less double-blind is a major advantage. However, when multiple drug treatments are being evaluated it is almost impossible to get adequate numbers of patients to test hypotheses adequately and in these circumstances it is better to carry out audit studies and introduce standards to reduce the extent of polypharmacy (Wressell et al., 1990).

For psychosocial interventions the choice is not so straightforward; the difficulties in ensuring blind assessment (or even masked assessment when a small amount of information sometimes is leaked) are often very great. For treatments such as psychotherapy, patient preference should be taken into account more and be linked to single-blind trials, whereas for more clearly defined therapies such as cognitive and behaviour therapy it is appropriate to concentrate on good single-blind trials with tightly defined outcomes.

In the settings of ordinary community practice many treatments are given simultaneously, both pharmacological and non-pharmacological. It has to be admitted that the process of evaluation here is not satisfactory and no sleight of hand in the form of complex assessment procedures and designs can conceal this. At the same time it is quite clear that the solutions to therapeutic questions in these settings are much more important than for most single treatments. It is reasonable to attempt such evaluations only if the investigators are prepared to combine data from several interventions in analysing data. Thus drug and psychological treatments could be combined separately prior to analysis and interactions examined. Ideally studies should be multicentre ones in which sufficient numbers can be generated to test several hypotheses but for many involved in such research the special circumstances of their own community settings seem to make them reluctant

Table 34.1 Common psychiatric treatments and their evaluation in community psychiatry

Treatment	Problems of community evaluation	Most common form of evaluation
Single drug therapy	Adherence	randomised controlled trial
Multiple drug therapy	Adherence	audit
Psychodynamic therapy	Choice of outcomes	preference and randomised controlled single-blind trials
Behaviour therapy	Choice of outcomes	single-blind trials
Cognitive therapy	Treatment fidelity	single-blind trials
Mixed drug and psychological therapies	Choice of control populations	Trials of complex design with insufficient numbers but with opportunities for combining data in meta-analyses
Policy change	Most changes are statutory so little opportunity for adequate controls	(Unsatisfactory) before-after comparisons

to pool resources in this way. As a consequence we have a large number of small-scale studies carried out in different settings with silly differences in methodology which prevent data from being combined or meta-analysis from being carried out successfully. Organizations such as ENMESH (European Network for Mental Health Service Evaluation) could play an important part in fostering a common basis for evaluation that could aid such multicentre studies.

Outcome measures

Although it would be wrong to think that community mental health practice leads to a different set of outcome than other forms of treatment, there is a recurring set of themes involved in community care which has to be borne in mind to process an evaluation. These themes will be discussed in order of importance. This is also relevant in view of the tendency of evaluations of community treatment to attempt to measure large numbers of outcomes on the grounds that all can contribute to the overall effect of a treatment policy.

Cost

Although at various times during the move towards community care emphasis has been placed on improving the quality of life for patients, destigmatizing the mentally ill, and promoting the dignity of self-sufficiency, the major reason why community care has been promoted in psychiatry is that it is considerably cheaper than hospital care. This is illustrated in Fig. 34.1 in which the relative costs of providing care for a population of psychotic patients was recorded over 1 year. The figures shown that, even when community care is specifically focused upon in the practice, its costs are completed dwarfed by the costs of inpatient care. Thus the best-resourced team in the study (Early Intervention Service) (EIS)

shown in Fig. 34.1 still accounted for a much smaller proportion of the total budget than inpatient care despite accounting for a large fraction of the cost of community care in the study. The slogan 'a week in hospital is worth a year in the community' is essentially true even when considerable input is given to the community services.

In all countries of the world we now have to accept that medical services are rationed to some extent and any treatment in the community that is more expensive than other treatments, even if it is more effective, has a hard task in getting preference. In practice, most treatments in community psychiatry do not demonstrate such clear-cut advantages over the best of existing treatments, and the most frequent scenario is that a number of treatments produce equivalent clinical findings but the one that does it most cheaply is the one that is recommended for adoption. In many cases the treatment might appear to be more expensive than the comparison ones but if it saves money by reducing admissions to hospital it would turn out to be cheaper overall. Thus, for example, the atypical neuroleptic drugs are much more expensive than the standard antipsychotic drugs but the case has been made for their adoption in clinical practice because, overall, they save money (Aitcheson and Kerwin, 1997; Guest et al., 1996).

Although cost is an obvious target for outcome measurement it is fraught with difficulties in analysis. Almost invariably costs show a grossly skewed distribution with few outliers costing a very large amount of money and many others costing very little if intervention had been minimal. In terms of analysis, non-parametric statistics are appropriate and yet these data do not deal with real figures. Mean costs constitute real resources whereas median costs are hypothetical even though they are more appropriate for statistical analyses. One of the consequences of this is that most

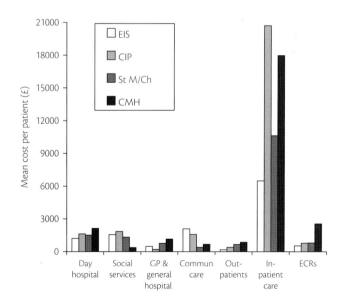

Fig. 34.1 Comparison of costs of randomly allocated community-oriented and hospital-orientated care over one year for 144 patients with recurrent psychotic disorder, illustrating the much greater expense of hospital in-patient care compared with community services. (Derived from Tyrer et al., 1998) Key: EIS - early intervention service (community team); CIP - community intervention project (community team); St M/Ch - St Mary's/St Charles Hospital (hospital team); CMH - Central Middlesex Hospital (hospital team); ECR = Extra-contractual referral (in-patient care away from parent hospital).

analyses of costs tend to be poorly carried out (Barber and Thompson, 1998) and much more rigour is needed in the analysis of data. In our personal work we found the statistical technique called the 'bootstrap method' (Efron and Tibshirani, 1993) to be an appropriate way of dealing with cost data and this allows arithmetic means to be used in analysis despite skewing of the data (Evans et al, 1999).

Generalizability

Good evaluations of treatment lead to findings that can be used widely across a range of settings. In standard research trial methodology this is achieved by broad entry criteria to studies so that the population treated is representative of all those at risk and drop-out rates are kept as low as possible so that the intervention can be analysed within this representative population. Unfortunately it is in this area that many interventions in community psychiatry lead to problems. Community interventions are very dependent on setting. A drug treatment should have its effects shown in all people who take the agent as prescribed, and comparison with a dummy pill under controlled conditions makes it fairly easy to take out the effects of non-specific factors that are independent. Community interventions, including drugs, are different. In the case of drug treatment there is the problem of adherence, particularly with conditions such as schizophrenia, and with different forms of non-drug management, including psychological treatment, there are often great differences between the effectiveness of the personnel concerned and the nature of the 'control' condition in a randomized trial.

The control arm of most community psychiatric interventions is not a placebo; it is another complex intervention. The trouble is that the control group, often called 'treatment as usual', given greater respectability by the initials, TAU, implying it is an independent (Greek) symbol, is anything but a genuine control. The trouble is, it is often assumed to be, and so leads to confusion. Burns (2009) eloquently sounds what he hope will be the death knell of TAU when he restates this position to make sure it cannot be forgotten. Fundamentally, he argues, 'when we conduct (these) community psychiatry studies of complex interventions, we are comparing two interventions and should treat them equally'. An obvious point, but do we listen? No we don't, or at least, not until now. So we have had to go through interminable arguments about why ACT is so much worse in the United Kingdom, with claims that it shows less treatment fidelity that its United States gold standard, even though the real reason has been clear for all to see. I am not the greatest at predicting the future but I wrote 10 years ago that:

> Unlike drug/placebo comparisons, in which the effects of placebo are roughly similar whatever the year, complex psychosocial interventions such as those in a mental health service are changing constantly. I can predict with some confidence that the Cochrane review showing such excellent findings with regard to superiority of ACT in randomized controlled trials will show steadily decreasing benefits of ACT in future revisions. (Tyrer, 2000.)

Yes indeed it has, and simple straightforward community mental health team management does just as well (Malone et al., 2009).

This does not mean that treatment fidelity is unimportant. It can be, particularly in less complex interventions. It is tested most often in studies of psychological treatments that can be formally defined, such as cognitive therapy, but it could equally well be addressed in all forms of treatment, including drug therapy. In respect of drug therapy treatment fidelity is primarily concerned with compliance, adherence or concordance. Although this is true of all forms of treatment it is the essential element in drug treatment since the consumption of the medication constitutes the essential part of treatment fidelity. Pharmacokinetic differences may lead to the drug being less effective in some people compared with others, but these are in no way under the voluntary control of the patient or therapist. In community comparisons of drug treatment it is very difficult to be certain of adherence to treatment, since simple measures such as counting of tablets after each course of treatment does not guarantee that those which have been taken have been consumed by the patient, and the detection of drugs which can be tested in the urine or in other body fluids do not guarantee that the drug concerned has been taken in regular dosage over the total course of treatment.

What seems to be most important in ensuring compliance is education and knowledge. The more a patient knows about the reasons for a treatment and the consequences of not taking it, the more likely they are to comply with a treatment regime. One of the reasons why cognitive and behavioural approaches have been so valuable in recent years is that they essential involve a collaborative approach with the patient which involves an explanation as to why treatment is necessary and which the patient has to adopt if treatment is to proceed successfully (Kemp et al., 1996, 1998; Perry et al., 1999). The best way to achieve adherence is still far from clear and unfortunately compliance or adherence therapy has not proved to be successful in a larger trial (Gray et al., 2006).

For psychological treatments the variance in treatment fidelity may be much greater. If we regard the basic unit of community treatment as the community mental health team, it is clear there is a wide range of experience and knowledge across the range of treatments available and most team members will not be capable of giving psychological treatment competently without training and periodic refresher courses. The standard way of determining treatment fidelity in psychosocial interventions is to tape record interviews and, ideally, have them rated blind by an independent assessor. Although this is a perfectly reasonable procedure to adopt, it is important to realize that it may interfere with the therapeutic session, may not always be representative of all parts of treatment since the therapist and patient know they are being monitored, and it is not usually representative of ordinary practice. It merely tests whether patient and therapist are **capable** of carrying out treatment in a proper manner; it does not confirm that this treatment is being given consistently in this way. Such measures also beg the question, 'what do we do with the results when treatment fidelity is not satisfactory?'. In ordinary practice there is, as yet, no standard way of ensuring that patients are treated by competent therapists (e.g. Kingdon et al., 1996).

Summary

The methodology of evaluation of community treatments is still a young area of science. However, we have moved far from following in the paths of John Conolly at Hanwell and Edward Charlesworth at Lincoln 160 years ago when they removed constraint and encouraged rehabilitation as the first stage of community treatment. These initiatives had face-validity in that they illustrated that patients with mental illness could have a much better quality of life when the right intervention was given. We have become much better informed in the last few years and have moved a long way from the stage of what Thornicroft and Tansella term 'naïve community mental health' in which the chant of the animals in Orwell's *Animal Farm* 'four legs good, two legs bad' could be paraphrased as 'community treatment good, hospital treatment bad'. Thornicroft and Tansella (2004) suggest a more balanced approach:

> In recent years there has been a debate between those who are in favour of the provision of mental health treatment and care in hospitals, and those who prefer to use primarily or even exclusively community settings, in which the two forms of care are often seen as incompatible. This false dichotomy can now be replaced by an approach that balances both community services and modern hospital care.

There is also an urgent need to develop new approaches that are not as time-consuming, expensive, and limited in scope as the randomized controlled trial. It is likely that progress will be made more effectively integrating qualitative and quantitative approaches in this regard. Above all, we need to be aware of the 'saboteur of setting'; the undermining of excellent evidence of a valuable new treatment or form of management by what may first appear as a minor difference in place but which on close examination proves to be a major cruncher.

References

Aitcheson, K.J. and Kerwin, R.W. (1997). Cost-effectiveness of clozapine. *British Journal of Psychiatry*, **171**, 125–30.

An der Heiden, W. (1996). Experimental and quasi-experimental design in evaluative research. In: Knudsen, H.C. and Thornicroft, G. (eds.) *Mental Health Service Evaluation*, pp. 143–55. Cambridge: Cambridge University Press.

Barber, J. and Thompson, S.G. (1998). Analysis and interpretation of cost data in randomised controlled trials: review of published studies *British Medical Journal*, **317**, 1195–200.

Barton, R. (1966). *Institutional neurosis*. London: Butterworth/Heinemann.

Brewin, C.R. and Bradley, C. (1989) Patient preferences and randomised clinical trials. *British Medical Journal*, **299**, 313–15.

Burns, T. (2009). The end of the road for treatment-as-usual studies? *British Journal of Psychiatry*, **195**, 5–6.

Byford, S., Sharac, J., Lloyd-Evans, B., Gilburt, H., Osborn, D.P.J., Leese, M., *et al.* (2010). Alternatives to standard acute in-patient care in England: readmissions, service use and cost after discharge. *British Journal of Psychiatry*, **197**, s20–25.

Campbell, M., Fitzpatrick, R., Haines, A., Sandercock, P. Spiegelhalter, D., and Tyrer, P. (2000). A framework for the design and evaluation of complex interventions to improve health. *British Medical Journal*, **321**, 694–6.

Casey, J.F., Lasky, J.J., Klett, C.J., and Hollister, L.E. (1960). Treatment of schizophrenic reactions with phenothiazine derivatives. *American Journal of Psychiatry*, **117**, 97–105.

Clinical Psychiatry Committee, Medical Research Council (1965). Clinical trial of the treatment of depressive illness. *British Medical Journal*, **i**, 881–6.

Edwards, S., Braunholtz, D., Stevens, A., and Lilford, R. (1999). Ethical issues in the design and conduct of cluster RCTs. *British Medical Journal*, **318**, 1407–9.

Efron, B. and Tibshirani, R. J. (1993). *An introduction to the bootstrap*. London: Chapman and Hall.

Evans, K., Tyrer, P., Catalan, J., Schmidt, U., Davidson, K., Dent, J., *et al.* (1999). Manual–assisted cognitive–behaviour therapy (MACT): a randomised controlled trial of a brief intervention with bibliotherapy in the treatment of recurrent deliberate self–harm *Psychological Medicine*, **29**, 19–25.

Everitt, B.S. (1995). The analysis of repeated measures: a practical review with examples. *The Statistician*, **44**, 113–35.

Feine, J.S., Awad, M.A., and Lund, J.P. (1998) The impact of patient preference on the design and interpretation of clinical trials. *Community Dental and Oral Epidemiology*, **26**, 70–4.

Gray, R., Leese, M., Bindman, J., Becker, T., Burti, L., David, A., *et al.* (2006). Adherence therapy for people with schizophrenia: European multicentre randomised controlled trial. *British Journal of Psychiatry*, **189**, 508–14.

Guest, J.S., Hart, W.N., Cookson, R.S., and Lindstrom, E. (1996). Pharmaco-economic evaluation of long-term treatment with risperidone for patients with chronic schizophrenia. *British Journal of Medical Economics*, **10**, 59–67.

Johnson, T. (1998). Clinical trials in psychiatry: background and statistical perspective. *Statistical Methods in Medical Research*, **7**, 209–34.

Kemp, R., Hayward, P., Applewhaite, G., Everitt, B., and David, A. (1996). Compliance therapy in psychotic patients: randomised controlled trial. *British Medical Journal*, **312**, 345–9.

Kemp, R., Kirov, G., Applewhaite, G., Everitt, B., Hayward, P., and David, A. (1998). *British Journal of Psychiatry*, **172**, 413–19.

Kerry, S.M. and Bland, J.M. (1998). Analysis of a trial randomised in clusters. *British Medical Journal*, **316**, 54.

Kingdon, D., Tyrer, P., Seivewright, N., Ferguson, B., and Murphy, S. (1996). The Nottingham Study of Neurotic Disorder: influence of cognitive therapists on outcome. *British Journal of Psychiatry*, **169**, 93–7.

Knapp, M. and Beecham, J. (1990). Costing mental health services. *Psychological Medicine*, **20**, 893–908.

Little, W., Fowler, H.W., Coulson, J. (Revised and edited by Onions, C.T.) (1973). *Shorter Oxford English Dictionary*. Oxford: Clarendon Press.

McPherson, K., Britton, A.R., and Wennberg, J.E. (1997) Are randomised controlled trials controlled? Patient preferences and unblind trials. *Journal of the Royal Society of Medicine*, **90**, 652–6.

Malone, D., Newton-Howes, G., Simmonds, S., Marriott, S., and Tyrer, P. (2007). Community mental health teams (CMHTs) for people with severe mental illnesses and disordered personality. *Cochrane Database of Systematic Reviews*, **3**, CD000270.

Marx, A.J., Test, M.A., and Stein, L.I. (1973). Extrohospital management of severe mental illness. *Feasibility and effects of social functioning. Archives of General Psychiatry*, **29**, 505–11.

Mullen, P.D. (1997) Compliance becomes concordance. *British Medical Journal*, **314**, 691–2.

National Collaborating Centre for Mental Health (2009). *Borderline Personality Disorder: The NICE GUIDELINE on Treatment and Management. National Clinical Practice Guideline No. 78*. London: British Psychological Society & Royal College of Psychiatrists.

Perry, A., Tarrier, N., Morriss, R., McCarthy, E., and Limb, K. (1999). Randomised controlled trial of efficacy of teaching patients with bipolar disorder to identify early symptoms of relapse and obtain treatment. *British Medical Journal*, **318**, 149–53.

Schwartz, D. and Lellouch, J. (1967). Explanatory and pragmatic attitudes in therapeutic trials. *Journal of Chronic Diseases*, **20**, 637–48.

Soloff, P.H., George, A., Nathan, R.S., Schulz, P.M., Ulrich, R.F., and Perel, J.M. (1986) Progress in pharmacotherapy of personality disorders: a double blind study of amitriptyline, haloperidol and placebo. *Archives of General Psychiatry*, **43**, 691–7.

Stein, L.E. and Santos, A.B. (1998). *Assertive Community Treatment of Persons with Severe Mental Illness*. London: Norton Books.

Stein, L.I. and Test, M.A. (1980). Alternative to mental hospital treatment. I. Conceptual model, treatment program, and clinical evaluation. *Archives of General Psychiatry*, **37**, 392–7.

Thornicroft, G., Strathdee, G., Phelan, M., Holloway, F., Wykes, T., Dunn, G., *et al.* (1998) Rationale and design: the PRiSM Psychosis Study. *British Journal of Psychiatry*, **173**, 363–70.

Thornicroft, G. and Tansella, M. (1999). *The Mental Health Matrix: a manual to improve services*. Cambridge: Cambridge University Press.

Thornicroft, G. and Tansella, M. (2004). Components of a modern mental health service: a pragmatic balance of community and hospital care. Overview of systematic evidence. *British Journal of Psychiatry,* **185**, 283–90.

Tyrer, P. (1991). The nocebo effect – poorly known but getting stronger. In: Dukes, M.N.G and Aronson, J.K. (eds.) *Side effects of drugs annual 15*, pp. 19–25. Amsterdam: Elsevier.

Tyrer, P. (2000). Effectiveness of intensive treatment in severe mental illness. *British Journal of Psychiatry*, **176**, 492–3.

Weisbrod, B.A., Test, M.A., and Stein, L.I. (1980). Alternative to mental hospital treatment. II. Economic benefit–cost analysis. *Archives of General Psychiatry*, **37**, 400–5.

Wennberg, J.E. (1988) Non-experimental methods in the assessment of efficacy. *Medical Decision Making*, **8**, 175–6.

Wennberg, J.E., Barry, M.J., Fowler, F.J., and Mulley, A. (1993) Outcomes research, PORTs, and health care reform. *Annals of the New York Academy of Sciences*, **703**, 52–62.

Wressell, S.E., Tyrer, S.P., and Berney, T.P. (1990). Reduction in antipsychotic drug dosage in mentally handicapped patients: a hospital study. *British Journal of Psychiatry*, **157**, 101–6.

CHAPTER 35

Qualitative research methods in mental health

Rob Whitley

Introduction

In this chapter I set out to introduce the reader to qualitative research in mental health. I describe its main methods of inquiry, and its underpinning foundational and philosophical principles. I give numerous examples of where qualitative research has been fruitfully employed in community psychiatry. I then describe criteria of rigour which can be used to assess the strength and contribution of any qualitative study in mental health. I believe qualitative research continues to offer interesting insights into the prevention, diagnosis, phenomenology, treatment, management, and understanding of psychiatric disorder. It may also assist resolution of current policy imperatives, such as calls for person-centred care, and more thorough evaluations of service effectiveness.

What is qualitative research?

Qualitative research is a broad umbrella term describing a constellation of research methods and paradigms that rely on the collection, analysis, and interpretation of non-numeric data. Qualitative research attempts to access the whole gamut of human experience—investigating knowledge, beliefs, behaviours, attitudes, and emotions. Qualitative research in mental health usually relies on either 1) a series of **in-depth interviews** with individuals from a group of interest, e.g. immigrants with a mental illness who have dropped out of psychiatric treatment (Whitley, et al., 2006a; 2006b; 2007); 2) a series of **focus groups** held with different stakeholders on a topic of psychiatric interest, e.g. with clinicians, patients, and family members to understand stigma associated with mental illness (Schulze and Angermayer, 2003); 3) **participant observation** in a naturalistic setting such as an in-patient ward to understand underlying staff–patient dynamics (Goffman, 1961; Rosenhan, 1973). These three methods can be used in combination. This is known as **triangulation** and is considered a very strong approach as it gives greater perspective and insight into a problem.

The aims of qualitative research

Qualitative approaches share at root an attempt to understand individuals and groups in context. Qualitative research is often used in three specific manners. Firstly, it is used to understand individuals' or groups' generic interaction with core societal institutions such as the education, health, or criminal justice system. Why are men more likely to study certain subjects than women? Why are certain minority groups distrustful of the police? Why do immigrants avoid conventional mental health services? These are the kind of research questions that can be answered by intelligently designed qualitative research that assesses relations between individuals and societal institutions. Secondly, qualitative research can be deployed to understand the lived day-to-day experience of a specific group of people—exploring just how they behave and experience the world around them. What is it like to be an African American with severe mental illness and HIV/AIDS in New York City? How do psychiatrists-in-training change as they progress through their residency? What is it like to be a full-time carer for someone with Alzheimer's disease? These are the kind of questions that can be answered through this type of qualitative research. Thirdly, qualitative research is often used in a very focused manner, in order to evaluate a programme or intervention, or as a needs assessment for a group of people. What are the health needs of elderly people living in inner-city London? How does a fitness intervention influence the social and emotional well-being of people with severe mental illness? What are the barriers and facilitators to implementation of a new psychosocial intervention?

Qualitative research is often concerned with questions of 'why?', 'what?', and 'how?'. Qualitative researchers are particularly interested in reasons given by different stakeholders for actions; these are critically assessed by the researcher who will make appropriate inferences based on his or her knowledge of the data, the context, and the existing literature.

Malinowski (1990) argued that qualitative research aims to understand a phenomenon from a 'native' point of view that above all emphasizes subjective meaning and experience. This involves eliciting as much information as possible about an individual, their worldview, and their sociocultural context. In the famous words of Clifford Geertz (1973), the researcher aims to construct a 'thick description' of the group and phenomena under study. If a study is focused on poor single-mothers with depression, for example, the researcher should design a study that allows for a 'thick description' of poor single-mothers with depression. As such, the researcher should immerse him or herself in the context in which research participants live their lives.

The 'thick description' per se serves a very important function. It brings to life the experience of a group, often a group that is marginalized and misunderstood. It documents challenges and concerns faced by the group in both daily life and in interaction with the health care system. This information can be used by health service planners to create more accessible, appropriate, and culturally competent services. The 'thick description' also serves a second function. It is often used to generate hypothesis or theory that can be tested in new rounds of data collection (Glaser and Strauss, 1967). For example, a recent study explored the experience and meaning of stigma by comparing data from focus groups of patients with schizophrenia, their relatives, and health professionals. The 'thick description' of stigma allowed the authors to theorize that stigma is dimensional and that appropriate interventions should be targeted to these various dimensions (Schulze and Angermayer, 2003). In this manner, stand-alone qualitative studies can build up local 'substantive' theory. As more and more studies are conducted, they can be compared and integrated to generate more general 'formal' theory (Glaser and Strauss, 1967).

The design and execution of qualitative research

The design and execution of qualitative research, if done rigorously, is largely similar to that of quantitative research. The same a priori thought and discussion that goes into the development and design of a quantitative study should also occur in a qualitative study. Like quantitative research, qualitative research is a detailed endeavour, requiring adherence to certain methodological canons. Namely, an innovative research question should be formulated in the light of literature review. A study should be designed that is capable of elucidating the research question. This should take account of the financial, temporal, and human resources available to the investigator. The study should be executed in a timely manner. Incoming data should be interpreted and written up for publication. Stringent training and quality assurance procedures should be in place throughout. All studies should have professional qualitative experts in supervisory or consultancy roles, just as quantitative studies often require advanced statistical expertise (Whitley, 2009).

Though there is much overlap between qualitative and quantitative research, there are also a number of differences, which are summarized in Table 35.1. Those trained mainly in quantitative research will likely be wedded to a positivist model of research that focuses upon large sample sizes, prediction, reliability, and external validity. Those trained mainly in qualitative research will likely be wedded to interpretive-constructivist models of research that emphasize small sample sizes, thick-description, context particularities, and internal validity (Whitley and Crawford, 2005).

It is important to understand some of these broad differences in orientation. Three major differences relate to hypothesis-testing, sample size, and design modification. Qualitative research is rarely hypothesis-driven, but is generally inductive in orientation. Data is explored in light of a research question, rather than tested against a predefined hypothesis or a predefined theory. This is because qualitative research generally aims to broadly understand a phenomenon of interest (e.g. the impact of psychiatric institutionalization), rather than precisely test an extant theory (Whitley, 2007). The second difference relates to sample size. Though a few studies have large numbers of participants (mostly cross-site), generally qualitative studies have a small sample, commonly between 20 and 40 participants. Some studies have fewer than 10 participants—though these are frequently longitudinal in design. The careful and judicious study of lived experience in fewer people is considered optimal in qualitative research as it reaches an intimate depth of knowledge unattainable through other methods (Pope and Mays, 1995). Finally, it should be noted that interim analysis and subsequent modification of design is encouraged in qualitative research. This allows the researcher to hone in on an area of interest that may not have been obvious from the outset.

Another major difference between qualitative and quantitative research is the difference between 'front-end' and 'back-end' work (Miles and Huberman, 1994). Quantitative research can involve

Table 35.1 Broad differences between qualitative and quantitative research[1]

	Qualitative	Quantitative
Epistemology	Inductive	Deductive
Study design	Data-driven	Theory-driven
Departure point	Research question	Hypothesis
Sample size	Smaller	Larger
Analytical units	Words (and behaviours)	Numbers
Analytical process	Repeated iterations during data collection	End-point analysis once all data is gathered
Workload	More back-end work-analysis is lengthy	More front-end, esp. in recruitment and execution

[1] These are somewhat simplified for the purposes of summary. For example, multi-site qualitative studies have large samples, and many epidemiological surveys are not hypothesis driven. This table should be considered a 'rough guide' rather than definitive.

Reprinted with permission from the *American Journal of Psychiatry* (copyright 2009), American Psychiatric Association, first appeared in Whitley, R. (2009). Introducing psychiatrists to qualitative research: a guide for instructors. *Academic Psychiatry*, **33**, 252–5.

an enormous amount of 'front-end' work, e.g. in the setting up and implementation of a randomized control trial. However, once all the data is gathered in, 'back-end' work maybe relatively light, in that statistical packages can be used to help test the hypothesis under observation. In qualitative research, 'front-end' work may be relatively less intense, as researchers recruit a small sample of people and conduct a number of interviews or focus groups to understand a phenomenon. The most challenging part of qualitative research may come at the analysis and interpretation stage, i.e. during the 'back-end' of research, which can be extremely lengthy. Audio-recordings need to be transcribed and should be read (and listened to) many times. Transcripts will need to be coded. Codes need to be related to categories, and theory needs to be produced (Glaser and Strauss, 1967). Computer-assisted qualitative data analysis software may be useful here, however this is an organizational aid and does not conduct the analysis in itself. The researcher still needs to categorize, code, and link data, without losing sight of the overall dataset, and indeed the wider background literature into which it should be ensconced. This is all very lengthy.

Qualitative research in community mental health

Qualitative research has its roots in sociology and anthropology. However there is also a strong tradition of qualitative research within psychiatry and community mental health in particular (Davidson et al., 2008). Qualitative research has been judiciously employed throughout the history of psychiatry, and can trace its lineage back to seminal figures such as Karl Jaspers and Melanie Klein. It continues to be a methodology of choice for those investigating important domains of present day psychiatry such as psychosocial recovery, stigma, cultural competence, and engagement.

Psychiatric deinstitutionalization is one of the developments that was heavily influenced by qualitative research. One of the most influential and well-known studies in psychiatric history was Rosenhan's (1973) 'being sane in insane places'. This is one of the few qualitative papers ever to be published in the prestigious journal *Science*. It was written in 1973 when there were around 200,000 inpatients in psychiatric institutions in the United States. This led to concerns about over-diagnosis and iatrogenesis. Rosenhen explored this matter by employing 'sane' research assistants as 'pseudopatients' to present at psychiatric hospitals, pretending that they heard a voice. This was the only 'psychiatric' complaint given by participants. All were admitted into the hospital. Once admitted, length of hospitalization averaged 19 days. While in the hospitals, pseudopatients engaged in classic participant observation. They experienced and witnessed many 'depersonalizing' events, e.g. being sworn at or ignored by staff. This paper has had a huge impact, being cited over 750 times. It raised questions of the validity of psychiatric diagnostic techniques, as well as the efficacy and humanity of psychiatric hospitalization.

The results of Rosenhen's research were consistent with those of Goffman's, whose best selling book *Asylums* (1963) described and analysed some of the depersonalizing and stultifying effects of psychiatric institutionalization. In this book, Goffman provided a 'thick description' of life in an asylum, and then formulated a grounded concept from his work known as 'the total institution'. This described places where individuals therein were deprived of control and agency, living their lives under strict rules and routines.

Goffman's work was based on 2 years of participant observation at a psychiatric institution where he was ostensibly 'Assistant Athletic Director'. Again Goffman's work strongly influenced the movement for deinstitutionalization, and the transformation towards community care.

When deinstitutionalization finally arrived it demanded a new research question 'what is it like for people with severe mental illness to live in the community?'. This question has been the focus of intense qualitative and quantitative study in the last three decades. Estroff's (1981) monograph *Making it crazy* gives a thick description of life in the community for recently discharged people with severe mental illness, based on 2 years of participant observation with clients receiving outpatient services. Her book richly chronicles the trials and tribulations of living in the community in the context of fragmented services, and patient strategies for surviving and 'making it' in the community. The book cast light on the desperation of many people receiving 'community care' and the nature of fragmented service provision in the post-institutionalization era.

Kirmayer and colleagues have used qualitative methods to understand pathways and barriers to health care among immigrants to Canada (Groleau and Kirmayer, 2004; Kirmayer and Young, 1998; Whitley et al., 2006a,b). This was in response to growing evidence that immigrants tend not to use mental health services, even though they are free at the point of use. This research is thus a pragmatic response to real policy concerns. Young (1995) used qualitative research to investigate post-traumatic stress disorder among returning Vietnam veterans. He found that many veterans were sceptical of the diagnosis and medicalization of their troubles, but 'played along' with the diagnosis and its underpinning technologies for reasons of secondary gain. Antonovsky's (1979) qualitative study of stress and coping among Holocaust survivors raised awareness of medicine's 'pathological emphasis', which tends to ignore the multifarious ways people live meaningful lives in the presence of adversity. This work somewhat presaged the strengths-based focus of the emerging recovery paradigm, now common in community mental health. This paradigm is frequently investigated through qualitative methods, which are ideally placed to elicit and analyse the lived experience of people in recovery from severe mental illness. For example, Deegan (2005) found through qualitative study the importance of activities that give life meaning and purpose in facilitating recovery (e.g. reading, studying, working, parenting)- and that these activities often outweighed clinical services in subjective importance.

Qualitative research has diversified in its investigation of various aspects of life in the community for people with various forms of mental illness. Certain variables have become the frequent focus of attention. These include housing (Padgett, 2007), employment (Becker et al., 2007), religion/spirituality (Russinova and Cash, 2007), culture (Whitley et al., 2006b), stigma (Jenkins and Carpenter-Song, 2008), social support (Davidson, 2003) and community integration (Ware et al., 2007). Though some qualitative studies in psychiatry are published as books (e.g. Davidson, 2003; Luhrmann, 2000; Young, 1995), the vast majority are published as refereed articles in scientific journals. Respected journals which regularly publish qualitative research relevant to community mental health include *The British Journal of Psychiatry*; *Community Mental Health Journal*; *Culture, Medicine and Psychiatry*; *International Journal of Social Psychiatry*; *Psychiatric Services*; *Psychosocial Rehabilitation Journal*; *Social Science and Medicine*;

and *Transcultural Psychiatry*. Any reader interested in perusing a qualitative study in some aspect of community mental health can pick up the current issue of one of the above journals, and they will likely find at least one qualitative study within. If the reader was to conduct such an exercise and find a relevant qualitative study, just how could they differentiate a good qualitative study from a mediocre one? This question is explored next.

Criteria of rigour in qualitative research

When conducting or evaluating a quantitative study, certain criteria of rigour can be deployed to assess the strength and contribution of the study. Two concepts which are central to quantitative research are validity and reliability, both arising out of the positivist framework in which most quantitative research is conducted. Reliability refers to the repeatability of findings—will the same findings be produced in separate repeated studies? An important distinction in reliability is that drawn between inter-rater reliability and test–retest reliability. Inter-rater reliability refers to the extent which two individual raters agree on measurement scores within a study. Test-retest reliability refers to the stability of findings over time–will the same study with the same instruments find similar results with the same participants at different points in time? Validity refers to the strength of the conclusions and presented findings of a study in relation to the study processes. An important distinction is that drawn between internal and external validity. External validity refers to the strength of any generalizations that can be made to contexts beyond that of the study. Internal validity refers to the strength of any inferences and conclusions within the study itself.

Many qualitative researchers have convincingly argued against the application of quantitative criteria of rigour to qualitative research (Barbour and Barbour, 2003; Lincoln and Guba, 1985; Pope and Mays, 1995; Whitley and Crawford, 2005). This is because the social world is constantly in flux, and that it is illogical to expect 'test–retest' reliability in such circumstances. Giddens (1987) well-known 'double hermeneutic' indeed posits that lay people are constantly interpreting the results of social science studies, and adjusting their behaviour accordingly. Likewise an axiom of much social science is that dynamics and processes are locally grounded and it is fallacious to expect to see similar processes elsewhere. Thus an inability to replicate a qualitative study over time and place does not invalidate it in the least; it may simply reflect changing contexts. As such, many qualitative researchers posit that criteria of rigour used to assess quantitative research must be adapted for qualitative research (Strauss and Corbin, 1990).

Lincoln and Guba (1985) posit a four-dimensional framework that can be used to assess what they call the **trustworthiness** (i.e. rigour) of qualitative research. **Credibility** refers to the 'degree of confidence in the "truth" that the findings of a particular inquiry have for the subject with which-and context within which-the inquiry is carried out' (Erlandson et al., 1993). Credibility is thus somewhat similar to internal validity. **Transferability** refers to the extent to which a study's findings can be applied in other contexts or to other people in a similar context. This concept is thus similar to external validity. **Dependability** refers to the extent to which study replication with similar participants and similar contexts would produce similar findings. This concept is somewhat similar to reliability. **Confirmability** refers to the degree to which study

findings are the product of a systematic methodology and analysis, and not of the biases of the researcher. This concept is somewhat similar to objectivity.

Hammersley (1992) posits two criteria of rigour for qualitative research: **validity** and **relevance**. He states that validity can be assessed by identifying the main claims of a study, and assessing the supporting evidence in favour of these claims. This assessment will also include examination of underlying design, methodology, and analytical approach. Relevance refers to an examination of whether the research is addressing issues of societal and/or local concern. If the study is producing knowledge which has no public or local relevance, it is deemed not to be rigorous. Giacomini and Cook (2000) concur with Hammersley, though they also emphasize the importance of clinical relevance in health services qualitative research. In agreement with this position is Malterud (2001), who also emphasizes the importance of validity and relevance. However, she also posits the importance of **reflexivity** as a criterion of rigour. This addresses a critique of qualitative research that it is reliant on the subjective interpretation of data by one or a few researchers. Malterud argues that researchers should thus make a conscious effort to declare their own background and position in disseminated research, ensuring that the effect of the researcher is attended to systematically at every step of the research process. This allows the researcher and the reader to systematically reflect on the investigators role in underlying knowledge production.

It should be stated that some scholars, often known as 'antirealists' have criticized the creation of the above criteria of rigour for qualitative research. Smith and Heshusius (1986) critique the underlying assumption that there are social and cultural realities that exist independent of the researcher. They argue that such criteria betray the critical and interpretative nature of qualitative research. Additionally, the presented criteria of rigour are considered to have only a superficial difference from the traditional positivistic criteria of validity and reliability. As such, these criteria are sometimes rejected as being pseudo-positivistic. At best, researchers can attempt to offer an interpretation of participants' interpretations, which do not reflect a single underlying reality precisely because there is no single underlying reality.

This epistemological position is somewhat extreme and not adhered to by the vast majority of qualitative researchers in psychiatry who may be labelled as 'critical realists'. This describes an approach where scholars assume the existence of reality, with the awareness that such realities are often socially constructed and are by no means inevitable or immutable. Such a foundation allows for the critical conduct of qualitative research in psychiatry. Researchers can attempt to explore, document, and analyse realities through use of participant observation, focus groups, and individual interviews. They can evaluate the rigour of such attempts using concepts of validity, relevance, credibility, transferability, dependability, and confirmability. This position of critical realism is one espoused herein. As such, we believe qualitative research should be conducted with strong efforts to enhance validity, relevance, credibility, transferability, dependability, and confirmability. Fortunately, there are a battery of processes and techniques that are commonly used by qualitative researchers to facilitate such rigour. In the next section, we outline the most common techniques and strategies.

Techniques and strategies to enhance rigour

Techniques and strategies to enhance rigour can be applied at various stages of the research project. In appraising the rigour of qualitative research, readers can assess the level to which such techniques and strategies have been followed. These techniques and strategies can be applied in the design stage, the execution stage, and the analysis/dissemination stage. The list of techniques and strategies blow is distilled from various seminal texts including Lincoln and Guba (1985), Erlandson et al. (1993), Hammersley (1992), and Glaser and Strauss (1967).

A strong method of enhancing validity and credibility is through the **triangulation** of different methods of data collection. A study that uses focus groups, in-depth interviews, and participant observation is stronger than a study that relies on one of those methods. Use of multiple methods obtains different perspectives on a problem under study. This thickens the description of the phenomena under study, giving a wider expanse of data from which inferences can be made. The different perspectives gathered can be compared and contrasted, and any varying findings integrated to deepen the analysis. The degree of confidence in the key findings of the study increases where there is convergence from various data sources (Erlandson, 1993). Triangulation can be built into the design of a study and is a strong signifier of thoughtful planning.

Another factor which plays a strong role in rigour is **sampling**. As previously mentioned, sample sizes in qualitative research vary, but a very small sample should be cause for concern—unless it has been followed up longitudinally using in-depth ethnographic methods. For example a cross-sectional qualitative study that has less than 10 interviews, or less than four focus groups may lack validity, dependability, and transferability. On the other hand, very large samples may also be cause for concern as this could indicate superficiality in the analysis. It may be difficult for researchers to become intimately acquainted with the raw data in a large sample (Miles and Huberman, 1994). A sample of between 20 and 40 participants is an acceptable rule of thumb in qualitative research. Another factor important to bear in mind is the nature and scope of the sample. Homogeneity in qualitative samples is encouraged, as this allows for an in-depth understanding of the group under study, as well as credibility of results. Samples which are socio-demographically or clinically heterogeneous should be treated with caution as they may lack validity, credibility, and dependability. The exception to this rule is when the researcher explicitly attempts to compare and contrast across certain sociodemographic or clinical domains, e.g. examining differences between men and women undergoing a psychosocial rehabilitation intervention.

Another factor related to design, execution and analysis is whether the research was conducted by a **multidisciplinary team**. A multidisciplinary team brings various forms of expertise and perspective to the research project. Sociologists or anthropologists can provide conceptual and methodological expertise, whereas psychiatrists or social workers can provide clinical and other practical expertise. In mixed-methods studies, epidemiologists and statisticians may also join the team to provide expertise in their respective domains. Such collaboration ensures that elementary errors are not made in the research process and that proper methodological procedures have been followed.

In the execution of research, issues of **training** and **supervision** of junior researchers is paramount. Conducting participant observation in a busy clinic is a much more difficult skill than administering a 12-item questionnaire to an individual in a university office. As such, qualitative research papers should show convincing evidence that interviewers, analysts, and project leaders have the sufficient training and experience to conduct the research. This might involve outlining the qualifications of data collectors and analysts, as well as what kind of on-the-job training (and by whom) were received. Another important factor related to training is supervision. How closely were data collectors and analysts supervised? How often did senior researchers shadow research assistants in the field to ensure they were following recommended procedure? Were recordings of interviews and focus groups listened to by senior researchers, and appropriate feedback given to the junior researchers? Affirmative answers to these types of questions suggest rigour, enhancing validity and dependability.

A number of analytical techniques can be used to enhance rigour. A well-known technique is known as **multiple coding**, and involves a number of different individuals coding the same transcripts or pieces of data. Emergent themes can then be compared between different individual coders, and triangulated for consistency, convergence, or discrepancy. The rationale for multiple coding is that the various members of the research team from different disciplinary backgrounds may differentially perceive underlying themes. For example discussion of the influence of religion on recovery will likely be interpreted differently by an anthropologist than by a psychologist. A finding that is agreed upon by four analysts is more credible than a finding derived from a single person.

Another technique commonly employed in the analysis stage is known as **respondent validation** or **member checking**. This refers to a process whereby key themes and findings from a qualitative study are presented to the original research participants, whose opinions on the accuracy of these themes are garnered. For example, researchers might conclude from the raw data of a qualitative study that access to psychiatric care is enhanced when it is integrated with physical health care services. This can be presented to the original participants who can state whether they agree or disagree with this emerging theory. An advantage of this technique is that it can prevent inaccurate portrayals of research participants. It can enhance validity by ensuring conclusions are agreed upon by the people being researched. A disadvantage is that this technique can lead to overly bland or flattering accounts, in that researchers produce a sanitized version of events to avoid offending participants.

Another analytical technique that is often used as a check on rigour is known as **negative (or deviant) case analysis**. This refers to a researcher paying conscious and explicit attention to cases which deviate from the principal findings of the overall study. For example, a needs assessment for carers of people with Alzheimer's disease might find huge gaps in need for most participants, but a minority of participants might not have these gaps. A sensitive research team will interrogate the data to understand why some people have less needs—do they instead rely on family, or friends, or churches, or the like for support? What is it about this subgroup that makes them different? This will then be presented in the results and appropriately discussed.

A final method of evaluating the rigour of a qualitative study is to assess how well the study is ensconced in the existing literature, as well as its use (and contribution to) theory. A good qualitative study should be well ensconced in the existing literature. Other relevant and formative studies should be debated in the introduction and in the discussion. It should be clear how the present study moves this literature forward and advances knowledge on the topic. The findings should also be related to wider social theory. Studies in social and cultural psychiatry often produce findings related to myriad policy or societal factors beyond psychiatry. This may include factors as diverse as immigration policy, multiculturalism in a pluralistic society, fair employment legislation, the role of religion in the public sphere, the advance of modernity, and the use (or credibility) of alternative medicine. An astute qualitative researcher will situate their results in the appropriate social theory, in order to assist thinking and policy-making in this regard. Again teamwork is a factor that can enhance these processes.

Conclusion

Qualitative research has a strong tradition in psychiatry. It continues to make a valuable contribution to the discipline's development. That said, it is worth stating that much qualitative research is of questionable quality. However, this usually reflects lack of judgement, training, experience, or interpretive acuity in the investigators, rather than something inherently defective in the method itself. Where properly applied, qualitative research may be very well suited to answer some of the innovative questions arising out of contemporary community mental health. These include questions related to recovery, service evaluation, and the enhancement of culturally-competent and person-centred medicine.

Further sources

Fortunately, there are many pedagogic resources available for people particularly interested in qualitative research. Numerous 'how to do qualitative research' textbooks exist which can be recommended to students dependent upon their level (e.g. Lincoln and Guba, 1985; Miles and Huberman, 1994; Strauss and Corbin 1990). All these resources give helpful advice on the conduct and evaluation of qualitative research. Many of the journals listed in this book chapter publish qualitative research articles. They can be surveyed regularly by the interested reader. Numerous brief summaries of qualitative research in the health sciences have been published in recent years in key journals. These are useful resources for those planning, conducting, or evaluating qualitative research. Some of these are listed in 'Further reading' below.

Further reading

Buston, K., Parry-Jones, W., Livingston, M., Bogan, A., and Wood, S. (1998). Qualitative research. *British Journal of Psychiatry*, **172**, 197–9.

Davidson, L., Ridgway, P., Kidd, S. Torpor, A., and Borg, M. (2008). Using qualitative research to inform mental health policy. *Canadian Journal of Psychiatry*, **53**, 137–44.

Malterud, K. (2001). Qualitative research: standards, challenges, and guidelines. *Lancet*, **358**, 483–8.

Malterud, K. (2001). The art and science of clinical knowledge: evidence beyond measures and numbers. *Lancet*, **358**, 397–400.

Pope, C. and Mays, N. (1995). Reaching the part other methods cannot reach: an introduction to qualitative methods in health and health services research. *British Medical Journal*, **311**, 42–5.

Whitley, R. and Crawford, M. (2005). Qualitative research in psychiatry. *Canadian Journal of Psychiatry*, **50**, 108–14.

References

Antonovsky, A. (1979). *Health, stress and coping*. San Francisco, CA: Jossey-Bass.

Barbour, R.S and Barbour, M. (2003). Evaluating and synthesizing qualitative research: the need to develop a distinctive approach. *Journal of Evaluation in Clinical Practice*, **9**, 179–86.

Becker, D., Whitley, R., Drake, R. and Bailey, E. (2007). Long-term employment trajectories among supported employment participants with severe mental illness. *Psychiatric Services*, **58**, 922–8.

Davidson, L. (2003). *Living outside mental illness: qualitative studies of recovery in schizophrenia*. New York: NYU Press.

Davidson, L., Ridgway, P., Kidd, S., Torpor, A., and Borg, M. (2008). Using qualitative research to inform mental health policy. *Canadian Journal of Psychiatry*, **53**, 137–44.

Deegan, P.E. (2005). The importance of personal medicine: A qualitative study of resilience in people with psychiatric disabilities. *Scandinavian Journal of Public Health*, **33**, 29–35.

Erlandson, D.A., Harris, E.L., Skipper, B., and Allen, S.D. (1993). *Doing Naturalistic Inquiry: A Guide to Methods*. Newbury Park, CA: Sage Publications.

Estroff, S.E. (1981). *Making it crazy: an ethnography of psychiatric clients in an American community*. Berkeley, CA: University of California Press.

Geertz, C. (1973). *The interpretation of cultures*. New York: Basic Books.

Giacomini, M.K. and Cook, D.J. (2000). Users' guides to the medical literature: XXIII. Qualitative research in health care A. Are the result of the study valid? *Journal of the American Medical Association*, **284**, 357–62.

Giddens, A. (1987). *Social theory and modern sociology*. Cambridge: Polity Press.

Glaser, B. and Strauss, A. (1967). *The discovery of grounded theory*. Chicago, IL: Aldine.

Goffman, E. (1961). *Asylums*. New York. Doubleday.

Groleau, D. and Kirmayer, L.J. (2004). Sociosomatic theory in Vietnamese immigrants' narratives of distress. *Anthropology and Medicine*, **11**, 117–33.

Hammersley, M. (1992). *What's wrong with ethnography?* London: Routledge.

Jenkins, J.H. and Carpenter-Song, E.A. (2008). Stigma despite recovery: strategies for living in the aftermath of psychosis. *Medical Anthropology Quarterly*, **22**, 381–409.

Kirmayer, L.J. and Young, A. (1998). Culture and somatization: clinical, epidemiological and ethnographic perspectives. *Psychosomatic Medicine*, **60**, 420–30.

Lincoln, Y. and Guba, E. (1985). *Naturalistic Inquiry*. Thousand Oaks, CA: Sage.

Luhrmann, T. (2000). *Of two minds*. New York: Alfred A. Knopf.

Malterud, K. (2001). Qualitative research: standards, challenges, and guidelines. *Lancet*, **358**, 483–8.

Malinowski, B. (1990). *A scientific theory of culture and other areas*. Raleigh, NC: University of North Carolina Press.

Miles, M. and Huberman, A. (1994). *Qualitative data analysis*. Thousand Oaks, CA: Sage.

Padgett, D.K. (2007). There's no place like (a) home: ontological security amongst people with serious mental illness. *Social Science and Medicine*, **64**, 1925–36.

Pope, C. and Mays, N. (1995). Reaching the parts other methods cannot reach: an introduction to qualitative methods in health and health services research. *British Medical Journal*, **311**, 42–5.

Rosenhan, D.L. (1973). Being sane in insane places. *Science*, **179**, 250–8.

Russinova, Z. and Cash, D. (2007). Personal perspectives about the meaning of religion and spirituality among persons with serious mental illnesses. *Psychiatric Rehabilitation Journal*, **30**, 271–84.

Schulze, B. and Angermeyer, M.C. (2003). Subjective experience of stigma. A focus group study of schizophrenic patients, their relatives and mental health professionals. *Social Science and Medicine*, **56**, 299–312.

Smith, J.K. and Heshusius, L. (1986). Closing down the conversation: the end of the quantitative-qualitative debate among educational inquirers. *Educational Researcher*, **15**, 4–12.

Strauss, A.L. and Corbin, J. (1990). *Basics of Qualitative Research*. Thousand Oaks, CA: Sage.

Ware, N.C., Hopper, K., Tugenberg, T., Dickey, B., and Fisher, D. (2007). Connectedness and citizenship: redefining social integration. *Psychiatric Services*, **58**, 469–74.

Whitley, R. (2007). Mixed-methods studies. *Journal of Mental Health*, **16**, 697–701.

Whitley, R. (2009). Introducing psychiatrists to qualitative research: a guide for instructors. *Academic Psychiatry*, **33**, 252–5.

Whitley, R., Kirmayer, L.J. and Groleau, D. (2006a). Understanding immigrants' reluctance to use mental health services: A qualitative study from Montreal. *Canadian Journal of Psychiatry*, **51**, 205–9.

Whitley, R., Kirmayer, L.J. and Groleau, D. (2006b). Public pressure, private protest: Illness narratives of West Indian immigrants in Montreal with medically unexplained symptoms. *Anthropology and Medicine*, **13**, 193–205.

Whitley, R. and Crawford, M. (2005). Qualitative research in psychiatry. *Canadian Journal of Psychiatry*, **50**, 108–14.

Young, A. (1995). *A harmony of illusions: inventing PTSD*. Princeton, NJ: Princeton University Press.

CHAPTER 36

Understanding and using systematic literature reviews

Andrea Cipriani and Corrado Barbui

Introduction

Making rapid decisions is a key component of everyday clinical practice. Informed decision-making such as this requires physicians to combine their own clinical expertise and training with high-quality scientific evidence (Guyatt et al., 2000). New scientific knowledge is emerging all the time and all health workers need to update their knowledge continuously. Most busy practising clinicians simply do not have sufficient time to read all the important primary research reports. Over two million articles are published every year in 20,000 biomedical journals (Mulrow, 1994) and even if a clinician restricts his/her reading to high-yield clinical psychiatry journals, he/she would need to read over 5000 articles a year (Geddes et al., 1999). The clinician therefore needs a reliable system of **knowledge management**, that is, systematic reviews and meta-analyses. In this chapter, we will outline the main features and limitations of systematic reviews and will suggest ways in which further syntheses of primary trial data may yield clinically useful information.

Overviews of the scientific literature: systematic reviews and narrative reviews

There are two main approaches to reviewing literature, which differ a lot from each other: **narrative reviews** and **systematic reviews** (see Table 36.1).

Narrative reviews are the traditional approach and usually do not include a section describing the methods used in the review. They are mainly based on the experience and subjectivity of the author, who is often an expert in the area. The absence of a clear and objective method section leads to a number of methodological flaws, which can bias the author's conclusions (Mulrow, 1987). In comparison, systematic reviews (or overviews) are syntheses of primary research studies that use (and describe) specific, explicit, and therefore reproducible methodological strategies to identify, assemble, critically appraise, and synthesize all relevant issues on a specific topic (Carney and Geddes, 2002). There is evidence

that systematic reviews improve the reliability and accuracy of the conclusions; however, the results are rarely unequivocal and require careful appraisal and interpretation (Hopayian, 2001). Clinicians therefore need to integrate the results with clinical expertise and the patient's preferences. There is a further difference between narrative reviews and systematic reviews. New research evidence emerges continuously, and reviews are most useful if they are continuously updated. This tends not to be the case with conventionally published narrative reviews, but the systematic reviews of the *Cochrane Library* are published electronically and can be periodically updated to take into account the emergence of new evidence.

The first stage in conducting a systematic review is the formulation of a clear question. The nature of the clinical question determines the optimal primary study design and hence the a priori inclusion and exclusion criteria. If the question concerns drug efficacy and safety (which treatment is better? Which dose is better tolerated?), the most reliable study design would be a randomized controlled trial (RCT): randomization avoids any systematic tendency to produce an unequal distribution of prognostic factors between the experimental and control treatments, influencing the outcome (Altman and Bland, 1999). However, RCTs are

Table 36.1 Differences between narrative and systematic reviews (modified from Cook et al., 1997)

Item	Narrative review	Systematic review
Question	Often broad in scope	Often a focused clinical question
Sources and search	Not usually specified, potentially biased	Comprehensive sources and explicit search strategy
Selection	Not usually specified, potentially biased	Criterion-based selection, uniformly applied
Appraisal	Variable	Rigorous critical appraisal
Synthesis	Usually a qualitative summary	Quantitative summary

certainly not the most appropriate research design for all questions (Sackett and Wennberg, 1997). For example, for aetiological questions, it would neither be possible or ethical to randomize subjects to many harmful exposures: systematic reviews would therefore need to include cohort and case–control studies. Likewise, a diagnostic question such as 'how well can a screening tool identify patients with psychiatric disorder?' would be best answered by a cross-sectional study of patients at risk of being ill (Mulrow et al., 1995). Systematic reviews of these other study designs have their own methodological problems: guidelines exist for undertaking reviews (and meta-analyses) of diagnostic tests (Irwig et al., 1994) and the observational epidemiological designs used in aetiological research (Stroup et al., 2000).

For all questions, it is crucially important to avoid common and misleading errors that might materially affect and limit the reliability of the results. These errors include both those that occur by chance alone (random errors) and those by systematic bias (Oxman, 1994). As a statistical technique to summarize comparable results from a systematic review, a meta-analysis can estimate the degree of random error by presenting the quantitative results of individual studies and the 'pooled' weighted average result with a confidence interval that provides a good indication of the precision. It shows the extent to which the results are likely to differ from the 'true result' because of chance alone; however, a confidence interval does not provide any indication of the likelihood of bias (Altman and Gardner, 1992). There are several forms of systematic bias that need to be considered in reviews. One of the most important is selection bias, in other words, a systematic bias in the selection of primary research studies that are included in the review. For example, a reviewer may only select those studies that support his prior beliefs. Selection bias, however, may also be due to 'publication bias' (the tendency of investigators, reviewers, and editors to differentially submit or accept manuscripts for publication based on the direction or strength of the study findings) (Gilbody and Song, 2000), 'language of publication bias' (studies finding a treatment effect are more likely to be published in English-language journals, whilst opposing studies may be published in non-English-language journals (Egger and Smith, 1998), and biases introduced by an over-reliance on electronic databases (electronic databases do not offer comprehensive or unbiased coverage of the relevant primary literature—unpublished data (so-called *grey literature*) have to be searched and included).

Systematic reviews seem more likely then narrative reviews to draw attention to the methodological limitations of the primary studies and the possibility of publication bias. In general, they may, therefore, produce more conservative conclusions than narrative reviews. Indeed, the main conclusion of a systematic review may often be that there is little good quality information in literature. Even this conclusion may be useful in that it highlights areas in need of further primary research. When substantial data of adequate quality are available, meta-analyses in the context of a systematic review can make far better use of the available data than can a qualitative narrative review. Not only can meta-analysis formally investigate the reasons for variations in the results of individual studies, but it can also produce sufficient power to allow investigation of clinically important subgroups. Efficient analyses of subgroup effects require individual patient data, but such studies require considerable resource and collaboration between the primary trialists (see below).

The statistical combination of the results: meta-analysis

In order to keep abreast of scientific evidence, physicians need reliable systems for summarizing primary research findings into a form that provides a trustworthy overview of current evidence. Meta-analysis is the statistical combination of the results of several studies into one pooled value and can be a useful way of reducing random error and increasing precision. This is the reason why properly conducted systematic reviews and meta-analyses of RCTs are considered as the best available tool for clinical decision-making and are at the top of the hierarchy of evidence for therapy (see Table 36.2)

Re-analyses of primary data provide overall estimates of treatment effect that have greater power and precision than any of the constituent studies. These overall estimates constitute a summary of evidence that takes into account the results of each individual study included in the re-analysis (usually weighted estimates are calculated, with weights based on each study's sample size). The terms review, systematic review, overview, meta-analysis, and pooled-analysis, although often used interchangeably, refer to different ways of summarizing primary research findings. As shown in Fig. 36.1, re-analyses of data extracted from studies included in systematic reviews are called meta-analyses, while re-analyses of data extracted from studies included in narrative reviews are called pooled-analyses (the term pooled-analysis is also used to describe re-analyses of individual patient data).

It's worth reminding that the term *meta-analysis* was used for the first time in 1977 by Smith and Glass, who carried out a systematic review on the effects of psychotherapy. Generally speaking, statistical re-analyses provide misleading results when applied outside the context of a systematic review. In pooled-analyses the inclusion and re-analyses of a selection of all available studies inevitably leads to biased estimates of treatment effect. The systematic exclusion of unpublished studies (usually studies with negative findings), for example, overemphasizes the effect of new medicines (Whittington et al., 2004). Additionally, it should be considered that the meta-analytical approach is not an essential part of a systematic review. It may be inappropriate to calculate statistical summaries of individual studies when outcomes are, for example, too different.

Table 36.2 Hierarchy of evidence for therapy (modified from Centre for Evidence Based Medicine, University of Oxford: http://www.cebm.net/index.aspx?o=1025)

Ia:	Evidence from systematic review and meta-analysis of randomized controlled trials
Ib:	Evidence from at least one randomized controlled trial
IIa:	Evidence from at least one controlled study without randomization
IIb:	Evidence from at least one other type of quasi-experimental study
III:	Evidence from non-experimental descriptive studies, such as comparative studies, correlation studies and case–control studies
IV:	Evidence from expert committee reports or opinions and/or clinical experience of respected authorities

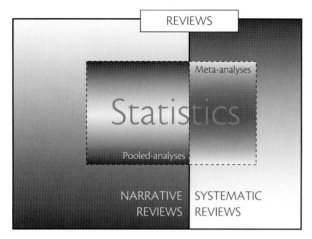

Fig. 36.1 Graphic representation of the concept of narrative and systematic review, meta-analysis, and pooled-analysis.

The inappropriate pooling of data from disparate studies has been exemplified as 'combining oranges and apples', with the likely consequence of reaching meaningless results. However, if studies are not that different, the meta-analytical approach increases the overall sample size and power of the analysis. The quality of studies included in the systematic review is another relevant factor that should always be considered (Moher et al., 1999). Re-analyses of poor quality data provide poor quality results ('garbage in, garbage out'). It has been shown that many qualitative aspects (allocation concealment, randomization, blinding, intention-to-treat analysis) have an effect on the direction of treatment results. Studies of poor methodological quality tend to overestimate the effect of the intervention and real differences may be obscured. When approaching a review article, physicians should initially consider if the review is systematic. If yes, critically appraise the following aspects: 1) authors' affiliation and financial support (reviews supported by drug companies tend to overemphasize the efficacy of the sponsored pharmacological treatments); 2) methods employed to identify and select articles; 3) update of the literature search; 4) quality of primary studies; 5) appropriateness of re-analyses; and 6) statistical significance, clinical significance, and robustness of the results. Ideally, clinicians should integrate the results of systematic reviews with their clinical expertise and with patients' preferences, bearing in mind that high-quality scientific evidence does not take decisions, physicians and patients do (Haynes et al., 2002).

Meta-analysis can be misleading unless it is performed in the context of a systematic review of the literature to avoid systematic biases. Whereas a systematic review can be applied to any form of research question, meta-analysis should not be used indiscriminately, especially when the primary data are inadequate. In psychiatry many trials are small (Johnson, 1983): meta-analysis is a tool that can increase sample size by combining studies, but, even if attractive, it may not always be appropriate. First of all, it is necessary to ensure that the individual studies are really looking at the same question: the criteria used to select including studies and to assess the quality of the studies included should be explicit and consistent with the focus of the review. Results from poor-quality studies can result in misleading conclusions and so inclusion of these studies in a meta-analysis may bias the pooled result

towards an overestimate of the effectiveness of the intervention being evaluated (Detsky et al., 1992). The methodological quality of the included studies is important even if the results or quality of the included studies do not vary: if the evidence is consistent but all the studies are flawed, the conclusions of the review would not be nearly as strong as if consistent results were obtained from a series of high quality studies.

Another important role of meta-analysis is to investigate variations between the results of individual studies (the so called **heterogeneity**). When such variation exists, it is useful to estimate if there is more heterogeneity than can be reasonably explained by the play of chance alone. Attempts should be made to identify the reasons for such heterogeneity, such as variations in trial quality, patient populations, and so on. However, when there is substantial heterogeneity it may then be inappropriate to operate overall pooled estimate (Thompson, 1994). In meta-analyses, the process of combining patient data from different studies increases the precision of the estimates of treatment effects, and consequently the statistical power of the analysis (Lang and Secic, 1997). The typical graph for displaying the results of a meta-analysis is called a **forest plot**. The name forest plot (formerly 'forrest plot'—see Lewis and Clarke, 2001) comes from the idea that this plot appears as a forest of lines. Each line stands for each study included in the meta-analysis. The forest plot allows readers to see the information from the individual studies that are included in the meta-analysis at a glance (Lewis and Clarke, 2001). It also provides a simple visual representation of the amount of variation between the results of the studies, as well as an estimate of the overall result of all the studies together (Sutton et al., 2000) (see Fig. 36.2).

In Fig. 36.2, the names on the first column on the left of the plot are the names of the studies (usually the names of the first author) included in the meta-analysis. Studies can be listed according to subgroups of treatment intervention (i.e. placebo, comparator A, comparator B, and so on) or according to other orders (i.e. alphabetical, by year of publication). Usually, results of these subgroups of studies can be pooled and are shown in the forest plot as subtotals. The overall estimate from the meta-analysis and its confidence intervals (CIs) are reported at the bottom of the forest plot and are represented as a diamond. The centre of the diamond represents the pooled point estimate and its horizontal tips represent the CI. Significance is achieved at the set level if the diamond is clear of the line of no effect (that is below or above 1.0, which corresponds to the vertical line in the graphs). In the 'number of events' column ('lithium' versus 'comparator'), the results of each study are pooled reporting the number of events out of the number of randomized patients (sample) for each treatment group. Accordingly, subtotals and total are also reported. The results of each study are shown as squares centred on the point estimate. The same results are also numerically reported as figures to make the graph clearer and more readable.

The point estimate is the best estimate of what is true for the relevant population from which the sample is taken. In other words, it corresponds to the estimate which has the biggest probability to be the most reliable estimate for that study. The most precise estimates are given the largest plotting symbols. In the graph, the horizontal line which runs through the square shows the CI. The CI is the measure of the uncertainty associated with the point estimate and it is due to the play of chance. Confidence limits are

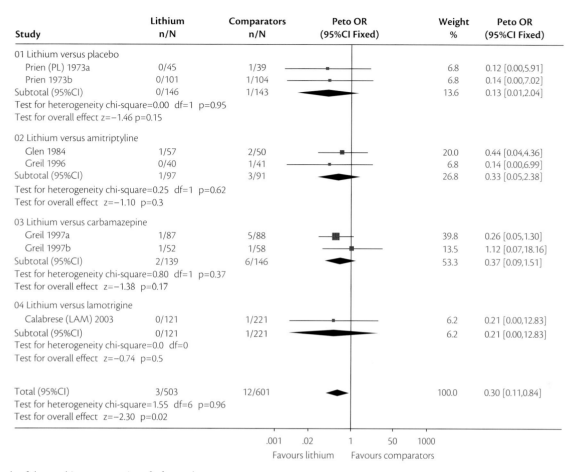

Study	Lithium n/N	Comparators n/N	Peto OR (95%CI Fixed)	Weight %	Peto OR (95%CI Fixed)
01 Lithium versus placebo					
Prien (PL) 1973a	0/45	1/39		6.8	0.12 [0.00,5.91]
Prien 1973b	0/101	1/104		6.8	0.14 [0.00,7.02]
Subtotal (95%CI)	0/146	1/143		13.6	0.13 [0.01,2.04]
Test for heterogeneity chi-square=0.00 df=1 p=0.95					
Test for overall effect z=−1.46 p=0.15					
02 Lithium versus amitriptyline					
Glen 1984	1/57	2/50		20.0	0.44 [0.04,4.36]
Greil 1996	0/40	1/41		6.8	0.14 [0.00,6.99]
Subtotal (95%CI)	1/97	3/91		26.8	0.33 [0.05,2.38]
Test for heterogeneity chi-square=0.25 df=1 p=0.62					
Test for overall effect z=−1.10 p=0.3					
03 Lithium versus carbamazepine					
Greil 1997a	1/87	5/88		39.8	0.26 [0.05,1.30]
Greil 1997b	1/52	1/58		13.5	1.12 [0.07,18.16]
Subtotal (95%CI)	2/139	6/146		53.3	0.37 [0.09,1.51]
Test for heterogeneity chi-square=0.80 df=1 p=0.37					
Test for overall effect z=−1.38 p=0.17					
04 Lithium versus lamotrigine					
Calabrese (LAM) 2003	0/121	1/221		6.2	0.21 [0.00,12.83]
Subtotal (95%CI)	0/121	1/221		6.2	0.21 [0.00,12.83]
Test for heterogeneity chi-square=0.0 df=0					
Test for overall effect z=−0.74 p=0.5					
Total (95%CI)	3/503	12/601		100.0	0.30 [0.11,0.84]
Test for heterogeneity chi-square=1.55 df=6 p=0.96					
Test for overall effect z=−2.30 p=0.02					

.001   .02   1   50   1000

Favours lithium   Favours comparators

Fig. 36.2 Example of the graphic representation of a forest plot.

the lower and upper boundaries/values of a CI, that is, the values which define the range of a CI. The width of the CI gives us some idea about how uncertain we are about the unknown parameter (real estimate). The CI gives an estimated range of values which is likely to include the unknown true estimate and is expressed as percentage. CIs are usually calculated so that this percentage is 95%, but 90%, 99%, 99.9% CIs for the unknown parameter can be produced. It should be remembered that estimates with the widest CIs, which thus have the most visual impact, are the least precise and generally least influential. CIs are more informative than the simple results of hypothesis tests (p value) since they provide a range of plausible values. In the graph the vertical line corresponds to the risk ratio of 1 and means that there is no difference of effect between treatments.

Risk ratio can be expressed either as **relative risk** (RR) or as **odds ratio** (OR). The odds for a group is defined as the number of patients in the group who achieve the stated end point divided by the number of patients who do not. By contrast, **risk** is calculated as the number of patients in the group who achieve the stated end point divided by the total number of patients in the group. As the name implies, OR (or RR) is a ratio of two odds (or two risks). They are simply defined as the ratios of the odds (risks) of the treatment group to the odds (risks) of the control group. An OR or RR greater than 1 indicates increased likelihood of the stated outcome being achieved in the treatment group. If the OR or RR is less than

1, there is a decreased likelihood in the treatment group. A ratio of 1 indicates no difference—that is, the outcome is just as likely to occur in the treatment group as it is in the control group. Statistical significance refers to the likelihood that the results obtained in a study were not due to chance alone. CIs may be used to assess statistical significance. If the CI for relative risk or odds ratio for an estimate includes 1, then we are unable to demonstrate a statistically significant difference between the groups being compared; by contrast, if CI does not include 1, then there is a statistically significant difference.

Clinical significance reflects the value of the results to patients and could be defined as a difference in effect size between groups that is considered to be important in clinical decision-making— regardless of whether the difference is statistically significant or not. The bottom line of the graph is a logarithmic scale. For the purposes of combining results of different studies, it is recommended to work with the natural logarithm of the OR, as this should provide a measure which is approximately normally distributed. The overall treatment effect is calculated as a weighted average of the individual summary statistics. It should be noted that in meta-analysis, data from individual studies are not simply combined as if they were from a single study. Each study estimate is given a weight directly proportional to its precision, that is inversely proportional to its variance and which relates closely to sample size. Greater weights are given to the results of studies that provide more information (number of events, greater sample size), because they are likely to be closer to the 'true effect' we are trying to estimate.

Absolute risk reduction and relative risk reduction

There are many ways of providing estimates for the relationship between two binary ('yes or no') variables. These ways have become increasingly popular in medical reports and nowadays clinicians need to clearly understand the meaning of these values in order to better inform daily clinical practice. The risk (or absolute risk) is the probability that an individual will experience a specified outcome during a specified period. The absolute risk lies in the range from 0 to 1 and can be expressed as a percentage. In scientific literature, the word 'risk' may either refer to adverse events (such as side effects) or desirable events (such as improvement of symptoms). If we have two comparisons, the ratio of the absolute risk for each group is the RR. In other words, the RR is the absolute risk in the intervention group divided by the absolute risk in the control group, that is the number of times more likely (RR greater than 1) or less likely (RR less than 1) an event is to happen in one group compared with another. The closer the RR is to 1, the smaller the difference in effect between the experimental intervention and the control intervention. Conversely, the odds of an event are defined as the probability that an event will occur, expressed as a proportion of the probability that the event will not occur. The difference between absolute risk and odds can be very clear if we use an example to explain the core difference between these two proportions (Bland and Altman, 2000).

Let's imagine we have a dice. All dice have 6 sides and thus there are 6 possible outcomes (namely, number 1, 2, 3, 4, 5, or 6). Let's throw the dice just once and a priori try to quantify the possibility to have one single side (say, number 4). The odds to produce number 4 is 1 (the 'positive' event—that is, number 4) out of 5 (all the remaining 'negative' events—that is, number 1, 2, 3, 5 or 6), that is 1/5. By contrast, the absolute risk of producing number 4 is 1 (the 'positive' event—again, number 4) out of 6 (overall the possibilities, including the desired event), that is 1/6. This example helps clarify that the absolute risk is very close to the odds when events are rare (few events in the numerator and many people in the denominator); however, as event rates increase, the absolute risk and odds can really diverge. The OR is the odds of an event happening in the experimental group expressed as a proportion of the odds of an event happening in the control group. OR has a very convenient interpretation in case–control studies and is used to examine the effects of other variables on a relationship during logistic regression analyses (Bland and Altman, 2000). RR and OR give an idea of the proportional reduction between the two comparison groups.

There are two other ways of reporting results of primary studies. First, the relative risk reduction, which is the proportional reduction in risk between experimental and control participants in a trial. It's worth noting that it could be really misleading to consider only relative indices, without looking at absolute estimates of treatment effect. The absolute risk reduction between the experimental and control groups is calculated by subtracting the absolute risk in the experimental group from the absolute risk in the control group. Clinicians need absolute numbers to make sense of trial results (Streiner, 2005).

Absolute risk reduction can vary a lot according to the hypothetical frequency of the outcome events, even if the relative risk reduction is the same. For instance, absolute risk reduction is dramatically different when comparing the same relative risk reduction in high-risk patients (higher event rate) with low-risk patients (lower event rate) (see Fig. 36.3). Absolute risk reduction and relative risk reduction can be very useful when calculating one measure of treatment effectiveness, the number needed to treat (NNT). NNT is the average number of people who need to be treated with a specific intervention for a given period of time to achieve one additional beneficial outcome (or to prevent one additional adverse outcome). NNT can be calculated as the reciprocal of the absolute risk reduction (see Fig. 36.3). As people cannot be treated as fractions, NNTs are usually rounded up to the largest absolute figure. This provides a conservative estimate of effect. NNTs should only be provided for significant effects because of the difficulty of interpreting the confidence intervals for non-significant results. NNTs are easy to interpret and can help clinicians make decisions about individual patients. However, NNTs can only be applied at a given level of baseline risk and the method of NNT may not apply to periods of time different to that studied in the original trials (Cook and Sackett, 1995).

Individual patient data meta-analysis

The main effect of a trial gives an indication of the average response for an average patient meeting the inclusion criteria, but individual patients in real-life clinical practice deviate from the average to greater or lesser degrees. As we have said before, many trials in psychiatry are small (Thornley and Adams, 1998) and attempting to do a subanalysis of a subgroup of trial participants with a specific characteristic will inevitably reduce the sample size and the statistical power of the results. Estimates of the treatment in subgroups of patients are always more susceptible to random error than the estimate of the average effect for all patients overall effect. Pooling the results from several trials in a meta-analysis can reduce random error and improve precision, but it is often impossible to do subgroup analyses because only the overall results of trials are reported. A potentially useful approach would be to conduct a meta-analysis of the raw data of the trials, to make an 'individual patient data meta-analysis' (Stewart and Clarke, 1995). In an individual patient data analysis it is possible to investigate potentially important baseline characteristics that might affect treatment response or prognosis, e.g. gender, age, race, family history, drug doses, dropping out, age of onset, number of previous episodes. Few individual patient data meta-analyses of the atypical antipsychotics have been attempted.

Dealing with meta-analytical studies, there is a variety of ways to collect data and bring them together in a statistical synthesis (Higgins and Green, 2006). These ways include extraction of data from published reports (the so called, **standard meta-analysis**) or collection of individual patient data that are combined in individual patient data meta-analysis. Individual patient data meta-analyses are sometimes called **pooled analysis** (mostly in the United States). However, as said before, **pooled analysis** may additionally indicate re-analyses of aggregated data extracted from studies included in narrative (not systematic) reviews (Cipriani and Barbui, 2006a). This ambiguity may generate some confusion

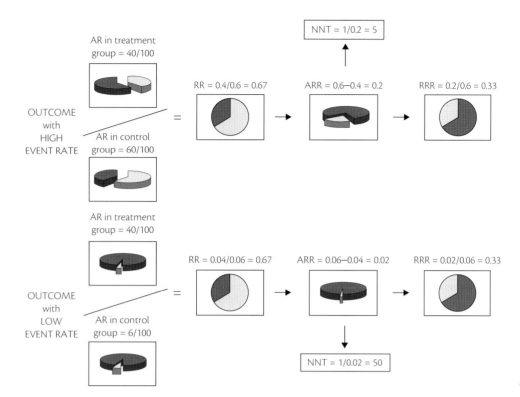

Fig. 36.3 AR, absolute risk; ARR, absolute risk reduction; NNT, number needed to treat; RR, relative risk; RRR, relative risk reduction (see text for details).

and readers of scientific reports should always pay careful attention to what researchers have actually done, irrespective of the terminology employed.

The individual patient data methodology has been used in large-scale collaborative overviews in which data from all randomized trials in a particular disease area were brought together (Rothwell et al., 2004) and also in more restricted reviews in which data from a relatively small number of trials assessing a specific health care intervention were collected and combined (Jeng et al., 1995). Individual patient data meta-analyses usually require more time, resources, and expertise than other forms of review, however the process brings with it a number of advantages (Stewart and Clarke, 1995). The main difference between a standard meta-analysis and an individual patient data meta-analysis is that while the former is based on information that refers to each included **study** (for example, in study No. 1 the mean age of the entire sample is 50 years), the latter is based on information that refers to each included **subject** (for example, in study No. 1 the age of patient No. 1 is 48 years, the age of patient No. 2 is 52 years, and so on). Intriguingly, information that refers to each included **subject** refers to sociodemographic and clinical data but also to outcome data (for example, in study No. 1 patient No. 1 is a responder, patient No. 2 is not a responder, and so on). Individual patient data meta-analyses have advantages over other types of review. For example, individual patient data meta-analyses allow to describe the effects of competitive treatments over time (Jeng et al., 1995). In fact, information that refers to the outcome of each included **subject** is usually collected not only at end point but also at various time intervals after random allocation. Kaplan–Meier analyses of event-free survival on the pooled data are therefore carried out, with stratification by trial where necessary.

The finalized data for each study are then analysed separately to obtain summary statistics, which are combined to give an overall estimate of the effect of treatment. In this way, participants are only directly compared with others in the same study and the entire dataset is not pooled as though it came from a single, homogeneous study. Collecting individual patient data rather than aggregate data brings additional advantages because subgroup analyses testing whether patient-related variables (sex, age, illness severity) are associated with the outcome of interest may be carried out. A practical example may illustrate these concepts. Imagine that we are interested in investigating whether there are clinical characteristics of depressed patients that predict response in trials comparing antidepressants with placebo. Based on clinical reasoning, we may decide to stratify the analysis according to the following patient level variables in a forest plot (Cipriani and Barbui 2006b) (see a hypothetical scenario in Fig. 36.4):

◆ Age at index episode

◆ Gender.

The hypothetical example shows that antidepressants were more effective than placebo, as indicated by the RR reported in the last line of the figure. However, individual patient data meta-analyses allow us to check whether this finding similarly applies to all age groups and to both sexes. In terms of age, Fig. 36.4 reveals that antidepressants were not more effective than placebo in those aged between 18 and 30 years and in those aged between 31 and 40 years. Conversely, the effect of antidepressants is evident in those over 40 years of age. In terms of gender, antidepressants were effective in both sexes, although the RRs were different. Clearly individual patient data meta-analyses are powerful tools that may help take decisions about optimal patient care. However, individual

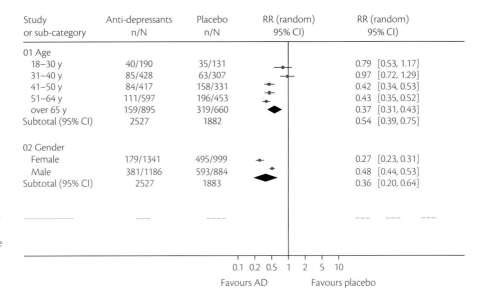

Fig. 36.4 Hypothetical scenario of an individual patient data meta-analysis, with results stratified according to age and gender. AD, antidepressant; CI, confidence interval; RR, relative risk; y, year.

patient data meta-analyses are problematic research exercises because individual patient data remain hardly accessible (Barbui and Cipriani, 2007).

Multiple-treatments meta-analysis

Multiple-treatments meta-analysis is a statistical technique that allows both direct and indirect comparisons to be undertaken, even when two of the treatments have not been directly compared (Higgins et al., 1996; Lumley 2002). In other words, it is a generalization of standard pair-wise meta-analysis for A versus B trials, to data structures that include, for example, A versus B, B versus C, and A versus C trials. Multiple-treatments meta-analysis (also known as **network meta-analysis**) can summarize RCTs of several different treatments providing point estimates (together with 95% CIs) for their association with a given end point, as well as an estimate of incoherence (that is, a measure of how well the entire network fits together, with small values suggesting better internal agreement of the model). Multiple-treatments meta-analysis has already been used successfully in many fields of medicine (Cipriani et al., 2009; Elliott and Meyer, 2007; Psaty et al., 2003) and two fruitful roles for it have been identified (Lu and Ades, 2004):

1 To strengthen inferences concerning the relative efficacy of two treatments, by including both direct and indirect comparisons to increase precision and combine both direct and indirect evidence (Salanti et al., 2008).

2 To facilitate simultaneous inference regarding all treatments in order for example to select the best treatment. Considering how important comparative efficacy could be for clinical practice and policy-making, it is useful to use all the available evidence to estimate potential differences in efficacy among treatments.

Multiple-treatments meta-analyses rely on a strong assumption that studies of different comparisons are similar in all ways other than the interventions being compared. The indirect comparisons involved are not randomized comparisons, and may suffer the biases of observational studies, e.g. due to confounding. In situations when both direct and indirect comparisons are available in a review, any use of multiple-treatments meta-analyses should be to supplement, rather than to replace, the direct comparisons. Expert statistical support, as well as subject expertise, is required for carrying out and interpreting multiple-treatment meta-analyses.

References

Altman, D.G. and Bland, J.M. (1999). Statistics notes. Treatment allocation in controlled trials: why randomise? *British Medical Journal*, **318**, 1209.

Altman, D.G. and Gardner, M.J. (1992). Confidence intervals for research findings. *British Journal of Obstetrics and Gynaecology*, **99**, 90–1.

Bland, J.M. and Altman, D.G. (2000). Statistics notes. The odds ratio. *British Medical Journal*, **320**, 1468.

Carney, S.M. and Geddes, J.R. (2002). *Systematic Reviews and Meta-analyses. Evidence in Mental Health Care.* Hove: Brunner Routledge.

Cipriani, A. and Barbui, C. (2006a). What is a systematic review? *Epidemiologia e Psichiatria Sociale*, **15**, 174–5.

Cipriani, A. and Barbui, C. (2006b). What is a forest plot? *Epidemiologia e Psichiatria Sociale*, **15**, 258–9.

Cipriani, A. and Barbui, C. (2007). What is an indivdual patient data meta-analysis? *Epidemiol Psychiatr Soc*, **16**, 203–4.

Cipriani, A., Furukawa, T.A., Salanti, G., Geddes, J.R., Higgins, J.P., Churchill, R., *et al.* (2009). Comparative efficacy and acceptability of 12 new-generation antidepressants: a multiple-treatments meta-analysis. *Lancet*, **373**, 746–58.

Cook, R.J. and Sackett, D.L. (1995). The number needed to treat: a clinically useful measure of treatment effect. *British Medical Journal*, **310**, 452–4.

Cook, D.J., Mulrow, C.D. and Haynes, R.B. (1997). Systematic reviews: synthesis of best evidence for clinical decisions. *Annals of Internal Medicine*, **126**, 376–80.

Detsky, A.S., Naylor, C.D., O'Rourke, K., McGeer, A.J., and L'Abbe, K.A. (1992). Incorporating variations in the quality of individual randomized trials into meta-analysis. *Journal of Clinical Epidemiology*, **45**, 255–65.

Egger, M. and Smith, G.D. (1998). Bias in location and selection of studies. *British Medical Journal*, **316**, 61–6.

Elliott, W.J. and Meyer, P.M. (2007). Incident diabetes in clinical trials of antihypertensive drugs: a network meta-analysis. *Lancet*, **369**, 201–7.

Geddes, J.R., Wilczynski, N., Reynolds, S., Szatmari, P., and Streiner D.L. (1999). Evidence-based mental health – the first year. *Evidence-Based Mental Health*, **2**, 3–5.

Gilbody, S.M. and Song, F. (2000). Publication bias and the integrity of psychiatry research. *Psychological Medicine*, **30**, 253–8.

Guyatt, G.H., Haynes, R.B., Jaeschke, R.Z., Cook, D.J., Green, L., Naylor, C.D., *et al*. for the Evidence-Based Medicine Working Group. (2000). Users' Guides to the Medical Literature: XXV. Evidence-Based Medicine: Principles for Applying the Users' Guides to Patient Care. *Journal of American Medical Association*, **284**, 1290–6.

Haynes, R.B., Devereaux, P.J., and Guyatt, G.H. (2002). Physicians'and patients'choices in evidence based practice. *British Medical Journal*, **324**, 1350.

Higgins, J.P. and Whitehead, A. (1996). Borrowing strength from external trials in a meta-analysis. *Statistics in Medicine*, **15**, 2733–49.

Higgins, J.P.T. and Green, S. (2006). *Cochrane Handbook for Systematic Reviews of Interventions* 4.2.6. Cochrane Library, Issue 4. Chichester: John Wiley & Sons.

Hopayian, K. (2001). The need for caution in interpreting high quality systematic reviews. *British Medical Journal*, **323**, 681–4.

Irwig, L., Tosteson, A.N., Gatsonis, C., Lau, J., Colditz, G., Chalmers, T.C., *et al*. (1994). Guidelines for meta-analyses evaluating diagnostic tests. *Annals of Internal Medicine*, **120**, 667–76.

Jeng, G.T., Scott, J.R., and Burmeister, L.F. (1995). A comparison of metaanalytic results using literature vs individual patient data: paternal cell immunization for recurrent miscarriage. *Journal of American Medical Association*, **274**, 830–6.

Johnson, A.L. (1983). Clinical trials in psychiatry. *Psychological Medicine*, **13**, 1–8.

Lang, T.A. and Secic, M. (1997). *How to Report Statistics in Medicine*. Philadelphia, PA: American College of Physicians.

Lewis. S. and Clarke, M. (2001). Forest plots: trying to see the wood and the trees. *British Medical Journal*, **322**, 1479–80.

Lu, G. and Ades, A.E. (2004). Combination of direct and indirect evidence in mixed treatment comparisons. *Statistics in Medicine*, **23**, 3105–24.

Lumley, T. (2002). Network meta-analysis for indirect treatment comparisons. *Statistics in Medicine*, **21**, 2313–24.

Moher, D., Cook, D.J., Eastwood, S., Olkin, I., Rennie, D., and Stroup, D.F. (1999). Improving the quality of reports of meta-analyses of randomized controlled trials: the QUOROM statement. Quality of Reporting of Meta-analyses. *Lancet*, **354**, 1896–900.

Mulrow, C.D. (1987). The medical review article: state of the science. *Annals of Internal Medicine*, **106**, 485–8.

Mulrow, C.D. (1994). Rationale for systematic reviews. *British Medical Journal*, **309**, 597–9.

Oxman, A.D. (1994). Systematic reviews: Checklists for review articles. *British Medical Journal*, **309**, 648–51.

Psaty, B.M., Lumley, T., Furberg, C.D., Schellenbaum, G., Pahor, M., Alderman, M.H. *et al*. (2003). Health outcomes associated with various antihypertensive therapies used as first-line agents: a network meta-analysis. *Journal of American Medical Association*, **289**, 2534–44.

Rothwell, P.M., Eliasziw, M., Gutnikov, S.A., Warlow, C.P., and Barnett, H.J. (2004). Carotid Endarterectomy Trialists Collaboration. Endarterectomy for symptomatic carotid stenosis in relation to clinica subgroups and timing of surgery. *Lancet*, **363**, 915–24.

Sackett, D.L. and Wennberg, J.E. (1997). Choosing the best research design for each question. *British Medical Journal*, **315**, 1636.

Salanti, G., Higgins, J.P., Ades, A., and Ioannidis, J.P. (2008). Evaluation of networks of randomized trials. *Statistical Methods in Medical Research*, **17**, 279–301.

Smith, M.L., Glass, G.V. (1977). Meta-analysis of psychotherapy outcome studies. *Am psychol* **32**, 752–60.

Stewart, L. and Clarke, M., for the Cochrane Collaboration Working Group on meta-analyses using individual patient data. (1995). Practical methodology of meta-analyses (overviews) using updated individual patient data. *Statistics in Medicine*, **14**, 2057–79.

Streiner, D.L. (2005). With apologies to Albert: everything is not relative. *Evidence Based Mental Health*, **8**, 93.

Stroup, D.F., Berlin, J.A., Morton, S.C., Olkin, I., Williamson, G.D., Rennie, D., *et al*. (2000). Meta-analysis of observational studies in epidemiology: a proposal for reporting. Meta-analysis of Observational Studies in Epidemiology (MOOSE) group. *Journal of the American Medical Association*, **283**, 2008–12.

Sutton, A.J., Abrams, K.R., Jones, D.R., Sheldon, T.A., and Song P. (2000). *Methods for Meta-Analysis in Medical Research*. Chichester: John Wiley & Sons.

Thompson, S.G. (1994). Why sources of heterogeneity in meta-analysis should be investigated. *British Medical Journal*, **309**, 1351–5.

Thornley, B. and Adams, C. (1998). Content and quality of 2000 controlled trials in schizophrenia over 50 years. *British Medical Journal*, **317**, 1181–4.

Whittington, C.J. Kendall, T., Fonagy, P., Cottrell, D., Cotgrove, A., and Boddington, E. (2004). Selective serotonin reuptake inhibitors in childhood depression: systematic review of published versus unpublished data. *Lancet* **363**, 1341–5.

CHAPTER 37

Developing evidence-based mental health practices

Kim T. Mueser and Robert E. Drake

Effective interventions for individuals with severe mental illnesses such as schizophrenia and bipolar disorder have emerged rapidly over the past 50 years. Numerous pharmacological and psychosocial interventions are now available to ameliorate the symptoms of mental illnesses, to enhance people's functional abilities, and to improve their quality of life (Lehman et al., 2004; Mueser et al., 2003a; Nathan and Gorman, 1998). Further, current clinical research studies frequently evaluate combinations of multiple therapeutic approaches (Jindal and Thase, 2003; Kopelowicz and Liberman, 2003; Lenroot et al., 2003). To a large extent, progress reflects a profound shift in developing, testing, and implementing therapies. Current interventions are designated as **evidence-based** because they have been demonstrated to be effective under scientific conditions (Sackett et al., 1997).

Evidence-based practices (EBPs)

Evidence in health care research denotes factual information that has been developed using rigorous scientific methods. Scientific evidence involves a hierarchy of conditions, some more rigorous than others, but in general differs from opinion or anecdotal information because the information is systematically and deliberately collected under specific conditions designed to control or minimize the effects of bias and other influences. For example, scientific methods include allocation to treatment condition by random assignment, monitored interventions, and standardized assessment procedures. All of these scientific procedures reduce the possibility of false conclusions and maximize the reliability and validity of observations and inferences. In other words, evidence collected under scientific conditions tends to be highly reproducible—to predict what will happen to other clients who receive similar treatments in the future or in other settings.

First consider this simple example. An individual who experienced depression for several months gradually recovered to a normal mood. He might attribute the recovery to a change in diet, to a new relationship, to taking vitamins, to sleeping better, to increased sun exposure, or to a number of other experiences, including treatment,

which temporally coincided with feeling better. This is anecdotal experience. At the same time, his therapist might attribute the recovery to avoiding alcohol for 2 weeks, to dream interpretation, to a new medicine, or to any number of other possible interventions. This, too, is anecdotal observation. These attributions are unlikely to be reproducible in other depressed clients.

Now consider this contrast. The same depressed individual participated in a randomized controlled trial (RCT) in which he was assigned by chance to psychotherapy A rather than to psychotherapy B. He was one of the 80% of clients in psychotherapy A who recovered from depression within 6 weeks, while only 20% in psychotherapy B recovered. His recovery was documented by self-report, by interviews with an assessor who was unaware of which intervention he received, and by objective improvements in his disturbed sleep pattern. In this situation, many personal characteristics and coinciding events during treatment would be controlled by the experimental conditions. We could therefore be more confident in attributing the client's recovery to psychotherapy A because other clients who received this treatment were much more likely to improve than those receiving psychotherapy B, suggesting that the attribution would likely be reproducible in other people with depression. If the results were in fact reproduced by several RCTs, we would consider psychotherapy A to be an **evidence-based treatment**.

The primary problem with relying on personal experience, personal observation, or anecdotal reports is that these types of evidence are highly subject to bias and systematic distortion (Kahnemann et al., 1982). For example, people tend to notice and remember information that supports their pre-existing beliefs rather than to be unbiased scientists. Good science involves the use of rigorous methods to overcome these natural tendencies.

Science does not gainsay the value of personal experiences, individual observations, and anecdotal reports. All provide valuable insights about potentially effective interventions. In fact, all current classes of psychiatric medications were discovered serendipitously by careful observations. Similarly, the growing literature by consumers on the lived experience of recovery (Deegan, 1988; Leete, 1989; Saks, 2007) provides important phenomenological information that may lead to effective interventions. For example, supported employment was largely developed and refined according to reports from clients about their vocational experiences (Becker and Drake, 2003). Science often makes use of accidental discoveries by one person.

EBPs are interventions for which there is a solid scientific basis demonstrating their effectiveness in helping mental health clients to attain valued outcomes. **Best practices**, on the other hand, usually refer to a consensus of individuals in the field as to which interventions are most effective. Best practice recommendations are often made in treatment areas for which there is limited rigorous research to guide more empirically-based judgements as to the optimal intervention. Best practices are sometimes biased by the current beliefs or theories of experts, by the prejudices of guild organizations (e.g. professional groups), or by the marketing of industry. Best practices are often proven incorrect by scientific research. Thus, consistent scientific evidence of effectiveness is required to establish an EBP.

Criteria for EBPs

Numerous groups and organizations have developed standardized criteria for establishing EBPs (Chambless et al., 1998; Hunsley et al., 1999; Sackett et al., 1997). A broad consensus has emerged on the importance of the following criteria: transparency of the review process, standardization of the intervention, controlled research (e.g. RCTs), replication across multiple investigator teams, and impact on meaningful outcomes.

The criteria (e.g. how to find evidence, what qualifies as evidence, how to judge quality of evidence) and the process of review (e.g. who reviews the evidence) should be transparent—open to the field and to the public for observation and discussion. The methods should be described in sufficient detail that independent reviewers can replicate the findings.

An intervention should be standardized so that it can be replicated elsewhere by other clinicians. Standardization typically involves a manual that clearly defines the practice and measures to confirm that the intervention adheres to principles and guidelines. Standardization includes detailed criteria and procedures for assessment, treatment, and outcome measurement. Measures of therapist adherence and treatment fidelity can quantify the accuracy of the implementations to the intended model (Bond et al., 2002; Mueser et al., 2003b; Teague et al., 1998).

The most rigorous methodological design to evaluate an intervention is the RCT, in which clients are randomly assigned (i.e. by chance) to receive one of two or more interventions (which can include 'treatment as usual' or 'wait-list' control groups) and are then followed-up and evaluated after treatment by unbiased assessors to measure important outcomes. Due to random assignment to treatment conditions, significant differences between groups in outcomes can be attributed to the treatment rather than to other factors, such as unobserved or unknown pre-treatment differences between the groups. Several RCTs consistently demonstrating the effectiveness of an intervention constitute very strong evidence.

While RCTs represent the strongest research design for evaluating treatment effectiveness, they are often difficult or impossible to conduct in real-world clinical settings. A less rigorous alternatives to the RCT is the quasi-experimental design, in which clients receiving different treatments are compared to one another, but treatment allocation is not by random assignment (Shadish et al., 2002). For example, clients in one mental health centre receive one treatment and are compared to clients in another centre who receive a different treatment. The most significant limitation of quasi-experimental studies such as this is that the clients in the different treatment groups may differ in important ways that could affect different outcomes. Nevertheless, quasi-experimental designs often provide valuable information regarding the effectiveness of an intervention. Another less rigorous research design alternative to RCTs is the **multiple baseline research design** (Barlow et al., 2008). This approach is usually studied to evaluate the benefit of specific components of treatment in individual clients by first obtaining a stable baseline over several assessments, and then systematically adding treatment components one at a time to evaluate their unique contributions to the overall treatment goals. By varying the length of the no treatment period and number of assessments conducted over baseline between subjects, stronger inferences can be drawn that the treatment components are contributing to any improvements observed in the outcome measures.

Replication means that more then one study finds similar positive effects. Replication is fundamental to research because similar results across multiple studies are unlikely to be due to chance. Reviews also insist that different investigators replicate the findings to minimize the possibility of investigator bias.

Effective interventions should address important goals or improve outcomes that are meaningful to clients, such as symptoms, associated functional impairments, or quality of life. Many outcomes are unequivocally important. People with mental illnesses do not want to be overwhelmed by symptoms or side effects, and nearly all want to live independently, have meaningful work, and have close friends. Other outcomes are more difficult to define. For example, demonstrating that social skills training improves social skills within a treatment group rather than improves relationships in the community is probably insufficient (Heinssen et al., 2000).

Developing an EBP

The process of developing an EBP has received limited attention. For example, Onken, Rounsaville, and colleagues described a three-stage approach: 1) feasibility and pilot testing, 2) RCTs of the intervention, and 3) studies to demonstrate generalizability and implementation (Onken et al., 1997; Rounsaville et al., 2001). Interventions that have passed the first two stages are considered EBPs. Mueser and Drake (2005) previously proposed a four-step process, which we elaborate here: 1) articulating the problem, 2) identifying possible treatments, 3) pilot testing the intervention, and 4) evaluating the intervention in RCTs.

Articulating the problem

All interventions begin with a problem for which an effective treatment is needed. The problem area should be regarded as meaningful (e.g. a distressing symptom that does not respond to standard treatment or a significant functional impairment). The problem should be defined and measured in a reliable and valid way (Nunnally, 1978). Reliable measurement involves reproducibility: inter-rater reliability (i.e. different observers see the same thing), internal reliability (e.g. different items on a scale are related to one-another), and test–retest reliability (i.e. showing stability of the measure over relatively brief periods of time in the absence of intervention). For example, valid measurement corresponds to related measures or behavioural indices and is sensitive to change. Developing an effective intervention requires reliable and valid measures of important outcomes.

Some interventions have broad goals (e.g. reducing hospitalization, incarceration, and homelessness), while others have narrow goals (e.g. independent living skills or competitive employment). Broad outcomes are often difficult to assess (e.g. quality of life), whereas a narrow behavioural target is often assessed more easily and reliably (e.g. employment).

Defining the target population broadly has the advantage of maximizing the number of consumers who may potentially benefit from an intervention, but most interventions are effective only for subgroups. Intervention development includes identifying specifically the individuals who might benefit. Research often starts narrowly and expands to more general populations.

Identifying possible treatments

New interventions are developed by several different approaches: 1) using theories regarding the problem area, 2) using theories of behaviour change, 3) adapting successful interventions used with other populations, 4) adapting successful interventions used for other problems, or 5) discovering interventions serendipitously.

Psychotherapy based on relational frame theory exemplifies the first approach (Hayes et al., 2001). According to this theory, humans' capacity for language and thought enables them to interpret and respond to their thoughts as though they were real-world experiences rather than symbolic representations. Based on this theory, Acceptance and Commitment Therapy (Hayes et al., 1999) teaches clients to accept rather than trying to control unpleasant thoughts and feelings, which are largely beyond their control and have limited basis in reality.

Extending social skills training based on social learning theory (Bandura, 1969) to a wide range of social problems (Liberman et al., 1989), and using motivational interviewing based on the stages of change concept (Prochaska and DiClemente, 1984) to addictive disorders (Miller and Rollnick, 2002) illustrate the second approach. The crux of social learning theory is that people learn from observing others' behaviour, as well as from the consequences of their behaviour. Social skills training involves the systematic teaching of social behaviours through a combination of modelling skills, role-playing, receiving positive and corrective feedback, and practising skills in natural situations. Based on the observation that changes towards healthier behaviour tend to occur through a sequence of distinct stages (pre-contemplation, contemplation, preparation, behaviour change, and maintenance), motivational interviewing helps people articulate their personal goals and explore the steps and barriers to achieving those goals, thereby enhancing the client's own motivation to address substance abuse.

The Individual Placement and Support (IPS) model of supported employment represents the third approach (Becker and Drake, 2003). IPS was adapted from successful supported employment approaches for individuals with developmental disabilities (Wehman and Moon, 1988). Employment specialists work collaboratively with mental health treatment teams to help clients find and succeed in competitive jobs that match their personal preferences.

Adaptations of Assertive Community Treatment (ACT; Stein and Santos, 1998) follow the fourth approach. Originally developed to address the problem of frequent hospitalizations and poor psychosocial functioning, ACT has been used for several other problems, such as homelessness (Lehman et al., 1997), substance abuse (Drake et al., 1998), and involvement in the criminal justice system (Gold Award, 1999).

Finally, serendipity has been the dominant model for developing pharmacological interventions for mental illness. Although this seems less likely to occur for complex psychosocial interventions, many rehabilitation interventions stem from observing techniques that clients have discovered themselves. For example, the teaching of coping skills to manage persistent psychotic symptoms (Tarrier et al., 1993) was initially based on naturalistic studies that demonstrated that clients with schizophrenia often develop their own strategies for coping with distressing symptoms.

Pilot testing the intervention

Pilot testing an intervention establishes feasibility and potential. Secondary goals include standardizing the intervention and developing a measure of fidelity. Pilot testing typically involves providing the intervention to a small number of clients and observing the targeted outcomes. Prior to formal pilot testing, researchers try the intervention with a few clients to examine suitability, mode of delivery, intensity, and need for modifications. Once these aspects are clear, researchers must establish feasibility.

Feasibility includes acceptability and retention. Acceptability refers to willingness to participate in an intervention, while retention involves staying in treatment long enough to achieve benefits. Interventions can only be effective if clients are willing to join and participate. As a general rule, dropout rates of less than 20% are good, in the 20% to 30% range are acceptable, and over 30% are problematic.

Pilot studies also examine whether or not the intervention has potential to improve the targeted outcomes. Researchers disagree about the need for a control group during pilot testing. Those who use a pre-post-follow-up design without a control group must interpret improvements in selected outcomes as meaningful compared to expectations. If functioning in targeted problem areas is relatively stable without treatment, improvements following the intervention can be attributed to the intervention. However, most psychiatric problems fluctuate over time, so improvements could be due to natural history. Controlled research designs that include a comparison group, such as RCTs or quasi-experimental studies, provide stronger evidence, but often lack sufficient statistical power to detect significant differences (Bartels et al., 2004). Researchers should therefore state from the outset that the pilot study aims to show that some clients benefit and to estimate the likely magnitude of the change (called the effect size), not to show statistical significance. However, researchers should also be cautioned that effect size calculations based on relatively small pilot studies are often inaccurate and may lead to the premature rejection of a potentially effective intervention (Kraemer et al., 2006).

Standardizing a manual

The pilot study is usually based on an outline of the intervention programme or a draft of the manual. Because valuable experience delivering the intervention is gained during the pilot study, a formal treatment manual can readily be written based on the pilot. When a draft of a manual exists prior to the pilot study, some modifications are usually made after the study is completed based on the additional clinical experience. The specificity of manuals varies greatly from one program to another, and depends partly on the nature of the intervention. Most treatment manuals include information to orient clinicians to the nature of the problem, as well as some conceptual foundations to the intervention. Specific guidelines are provided regarding the logistics of the intervention, identification of consumers for whom the intervention is designed, curriculum, teaching skills, and guidance for handling common problems. Manuals often provide clinical vignettes to illustrate treatment principles and incorporate specific instruments for assessment and monitoring clinical outcomes. The length of treatment manuals typically ranges from 20 to 200 pages.

During pilot testing, researchers also need to establish methods to verify that an intervention is delivered in a manner consistent with the treatment model. Such verification is crucial to conducting a rigorous assessment of the intervention. Researchers must first establish that the intervention has been implemented as intended before determining its effects. Expert judgements are often used to establish fidelity. In this method, a recognized expert on the intervention obtains information regarding the implementation (e.g. by observing therapy sessions, reviewing case notes, conducting interviews) and provides feedback regarding the degree of adherence to the model. Alternatively, specific behavioural anchor points for rating adherence can be used to train raters and make fidelity ratings. Objective fidelity ratings avoid the expense and potential bias of expert ratings. Fidelity scales have become the standard in the field (Bond et al., 2000). They provide specific information needed to address implementation problems and to explore the relationship between fidelity and outcome.

Evaluating the intervention in RCTs

Rigorous evaluation is the sine qua non of evidence-based interventions. In this section, we briefly address several of the most crucial aspects of RCTs, including the experimental design, the selection of a control group, inclusion/exclusion criteria for the target population, the setting for the trial, and the choice of outcome measures.

The RCT is considered superior to other research designs because it controls for group equivalence. Many important variables are unknown or unobserved, and quasi-experimental designs almost inevitably compare non-equivalent groups. For interventions delivered at the level of the treatment team or mental health agency, a quasi-RCT may, however, be the only option. When treatment teams or mental health centres are randomly assigned to receive the experimental intervention or the control intervention, the true unit of analysis is the mental health treatment team or agency rather than the individual. Statistical techniques exist to deal with the clustering of individuals within groups. In practice, researchers often compare the outcomes of individual clients treated on different teams or in different mental health centres. This design is not considered a pure RCT because each client does not have an independent and equal chance of being in either intervention. Nevertheless, this design has advantages over many other approaches because the agencies or mental health centres are assigned by randomization and are therefore likely to be equivalent.

In selecting the comparison group for an RCT, the common options are an equally intensive intervention, a less intensive intervention, and treatment as usual, placebo treatment, or no treatment (e.g. a waiting list). Each option has advantages and disadvantages. In practice, the selection reflects pragmatic considerations as well as the specific research question.

Pilot work should guide selection of the inclusion and exclusion criteria for the RCT. These criteria inevitably involve a trade-off between efficacy and effectiveness. Efficacy studies use narrowly defined clients to maximize the chance of finding significant differences, whereas effectiveness studies use broad criteria to maximize real-world applicability, or generalizability.

Similar considerations influence site selection because location will affect transferability to other settings. Clinical trials conducted in routine mental health centres rather than in university clinics (i.e. the effectiveness design) maximize potential for applicability to the kinds of settings in which most people receive treatment. By contrast, efficacy studies are conducted in highly controlled settings, with specially trained clinicians, and other constrained conditions for the sake of isolating and controlling the treatment intervention. Traditionally, interventions have been tested first in efficacy trials and then in effectiveness trials. Recently, however, some interventions are developed and tested under effectiveness conditions to insure generalizability from the outset. Needless to say, recruitment, training, high-fidelity implementation, retention, and assessment challenge researchers in multifarious ways.

Measurement should address outcomes, implementation/process, and theory. Outcome measures assess the goals of the intervention (e.g. work, quality of social relationships, symptom severity, relapses, and hospitalization), as identified and measured since the earliest steps of developing an EBP. Primary outcomes reflect the most important targets, while secondary outcomes include areas that may be improved by changes in the primary outcomes. For example, the primary outcome of supported employment is working, measured by percentage of clients who are employed, number of hours they are working, and wages they are earning. Employment may also affect secondary outcomes such as self-esteem, symptoms, and life satisfaction.

Implementation and process measures assess whether the interventions were provided as intended and whether clients received the interventions. These measures can be broadly divided into those that evaluate fidelity to the treatment model and those that record clients' exposure to treatment. Treatment exposure measures include information such as the number, duration, and time of treatment contacts.

RCTs can also provide valuable information regarding how an intervention works, how theoretical constructs interact with functional outcomes, and how different outcomes are related. Theory testing and development can guide the refinement of an intervention to enhance effectiveness.

Summary and conclusions

EBPs are scientifically validated interventions that help people with mental illnesses to achieve improvements in meaningful areas of their lives. Developing and establishing an EBP requires attention to scientific detail, considerable time, and multiple steps. We have described the major steps as: 1) articulation of the problem area, 2) identification of possible treatments, 3) pilot testing the intervention, and 4) controlled evaluation of the intervention.

References

Alverson, M., Becker, D.R., and Drake, R.E. (1995). An ethnographic study of coping strategies used by people with severe mental illness participating in supported employment. *Psychosocial Rehabilitation Journal*, **18**, 115–28.

Bach, P. and Hayes, S.C. (2002). The use of acceptance and commitment therapy to prevent the rehospitalization of psychotic patients: A randomized controlled trial. *Journal of Consulting and Clinical Psychology*, **70**, 1129–39.

Bandura, A. (1969). *Principles of Behavior Modification*. New York: Holt, Rinehart and Winston, Inc.

Barlow, D.H., Nock, M., Hersen, M. (2008). *Single case experimental designs: strategies for studying behavior change (3rd edition)* Boston Addison-Wesley.

Bartels, S.J., Forester, B., Mueser, K.T., Miles, K.M., Dums, A.R., Pratt, S.I., et al. (2004). Supported rehabilitation and health care management of older persons with severe mental illness. *Community Mental Health Journal*, **40**, 75–90.

Becker, D.R. and Drake, R.E. (2003). *A Working Life for People with Severe Mental Illness*. New York: Oxford University Press.

Bellack, A.S., Morrison, R.L., Wixted, J.T., and Mueser, K.T. (1990). An analysis of social competence in schizophrenia. *British Journal of Psychiatry*, **156**, 809–818.

Bellack, A.S., Sayers, M., Mueser, K.T., and Bennett, M. (1994). An evaluation of social problem solving in schizophrenia. *Journal of Abnormal Psychology*, **103**, 371–78.

Bond, G.R., Campbell, K., Evans, L.J., Gervey, R., Pascaris, A., Tice, S., et al. (2002). A scale to measure quality of supported employment for persons with severe mental illness. *Journal of Vocational Rehabilitation*, **17**, 239–50.

Bond, G.R., Evans, L., Salyers, M. P., Williams, J., and Kim, H.-W. (2000). Measurement of fidelity in psychiatric rehabilitation. *Mental Health Services Research*, **2**, 75–87.

Chambless, D.L., Baker, M.J., Baucom, D.H., Beutler, L.E., Calhoun, K.S., Crits-Christoph, P., et al. (1998). Update on empirically validated therapies, II. *The Clinical Psychologist*, **51**, 3–16.

Deegan, P.E. (1988). Recovery: The lived experience of rehabilitation. *Psychosocial Rehabilitation Journal*, **11**, 11–19.

Drake, R.E., McHugo, G.J., Clark, R.E., Teague, G.B., Xie, H., Miles, K., et al. (1998). Assertive community treatment for patients with co-occurring severe mental illness and substance use disorder: A clinical trial. *American Journal of Orthopsychiatry*, **68**, 201–15.

Falloon, I.R.H., and Talbot, R.E. (1981). Persistent auditory hallucinations: Coping mechanisms and implications for management. *Psychological Medicine*, **11**, 329–39.

Gold Award (1999). Prevention of jail and hospital recidivism among persons with severe mental illness. *Psychiatric Services*, **50**, 1477–80.

Green, M.F. (1996). What are the functional consequences of neurocognitive deficits in schizophrenia? *American Journal of Psychiatry*, **153**, 321–30.

Hayes, S.C., Barnes-Holmes, D., and Roche, B. (eds.) (2001). *Relational Frame Theory: A Post-Skinnerian Account of Human Language and Cognition*. New York: Kluwer Academic/Plenum Publishers.

Hayes, S.C., Strosahl, K.D., and Wilson, K.G. (1999). *Acceptance and Commitment Therapy: An Experiential Approach to Behavior Change*. New York: Guilford Publications.

Heinssen, R.K., Liberman, R.P., and Kopelowicz, A. (2000). Psychosocial skills training for schizophrenia: Lessons from the laboratory. *Schizophrenia Bulletin*, **26**, 21–46.

Hunsley, J., Dobson, K.S., Johnson, C., and Mikail, S.F. (1999). Empirically supported treatments in psychology: Implications for Canadian professional psychology. *Canadian Psychologist*, **40**, 289–302.

Jindal, R.K. and Thase, M.E. (2003). Integrating psychotherapy and pharmacotherapy to improve outcomes among patients with mood disorders. *Psychiatric Services*, **54**, 1484–90.

Kahnemann, D., Slovic, P., and Tversky, A. (1982). *Judgment Under Uncertainty: Heuristics and Biases*. New York: Cambridge University Press.

Kopelowicz, A., and Liberman, R.P. (2003). Integrating treatment with rehabilitation for persons with major mental illnesses. *Psychiatric Services*, **54**, 1491–8.

Kraemer, H.C., Mintz, J., Noda, A., Tinklenberg, J., and Yesavage, J.A. (2006). Caution regarding the use of pilot studies to guide power calculations for study proposals. *Archives of General Psychiatry*, **63**, 484–9.

Leete, E. (1989). How I perceive and manage my illness. *Schizophrenia Bulletin*, **15**, 197–200.

Lehman, A.F., Dixon, L.B., Kernan, E., and DeForge, B. (1997). A randomized trial of assertive community treatment for homeless persons with severe mental illness. *Archives of General Psychiatry*, **54**, 1038–43.

Lehman, A.F., Kreyenbuhl, J., Buchanan, R.W., Dickerson, F.B., Dixon, L.B., Goldberg, R.W., et al. (2004). The schizophrenia patient outcomes research team (PORT): Updated treatment recommendations 2003. *Schizophrenia Bulletin* **30**, 193–217.

Lenroot, R., Bustillo, J.R., Lauriello, J., and Keith, S.J. (2003). Integrated treatment of schizophrenia. *Psychiatric Services*, **54**, 1499–507.

Liberman, R.P., DeRisi, W.J., and Mueser, K.T. (1989). *Social Skills Training for Psychiatric Patients*. Needham Heights, MA: Allyn and Bacon.

Miller, W.R. and Rollnick, S. (eds.). (2002). *Motivational Interviewing: Preparing People for Change*, 2nd edn. New York: Guilford Publications.

Mueser, K.T. (2000). Cognitive functioning, social adjustment and long-term outcome in schizophrenia. In: Sharma, T. and Harvey, P. (eds.) *Cognition in Schizophrenia: Impairments, Importance, and Treatment Strategies*, pp. 157–77. Oxford: Oxford University Press.

Mueser, K.T. and Drake, R.E. (2005). How does a practice become evidence-based? In: Drake, R.E., Merrens, M., and Lynde, D.L. (eds.) *Evidence-based Mental Health Practice: A Textbook*, pp. 217–42. New York: John Wiley, 2005.

Mueser, K.T., Torrey, W.C., Lynde, D., Singer, P., and Drake, R.E. (2003a). Implementing evidence-based practices for people with severe mental illness. *Behavior Modification*, **27**, 387–411.

Mueser, K.T., Noordsy, D.L., Drake, R.E., and Fox, L. (2003b). *Integrated Treatment for Dual Disorders: A Guide to Effective Practice*. New York: Guilford Press.

Nathan, P., and Gorman, J. M. (Eds.). (1998). *A Guide to Treatments That Work*. New York: Oxford University Press.

Nunnally, J. (1978). *Psychometric Theory, 2nd Edition*. New York: McGraw Hill.

Onken, L. S., Blaine, J. D., and Battjes, R. (1997). Behavioral therapy research: A conceptualization of a process. In: S. W. Henngler and Amentos, R. (eds.), *Innovative Approaches for Difficult to Treat Populations*, pp. 477–85. Washington, DC: American Psychiatric Press.

Prochaska, J.O., and DiClemente, C.C. (1984). *The Transtheoretical Approach: Crossing the Traditional Boundaries of Therapy*. Homewood, IL: Dow-Jones/Irwin.

Rounsaville, B.J., Carroll, K.M., and Onken, L.S. (2001). A stage model of behavioral therapies research: Getting started and moving on from stage I. *Clinical Psychology: Science and Practice*, **8**, 133–42.

Sackett, D.L., Richardson, W.S., Rosenberg, W., and Haynes, R.B. (1997). *Evidence-based Medicine*. New York: Churchill Livingstone.

Saks, E.R. (2007). *The center cannot hold*. New York: Hyperion.

Shadish, W.R., Cook, T.D., and Campbell, D.T. (2002). *Experimental and Quasi-Experimental Designs for Generalized Causal Inference*. Boston: Houghton Mifflin.

Stein, L.I. and Santos, A.B. (1998). *Assertive Community Treatment of Persons with Severe Mental Illness*. New York: Norton.

Tarrier, N., Sharpe, L., Beckett, R., Harwood, S., Baker, A., and Yusopoff, L. (1993). A trial of two cognitive behavioural methods of treating drug-resistant residual psychotic symptoms in schizophrenia patients: II. Treatment-specific changes in coping and problem-solving skills. *Psychiatry and Psychiatric Epidemiology*, **28**, 5–10.

Teague, G.B., Bond, G.R., and Drake, R.E. (1998). Program fidelity in assertive community treatment: Development and use of a measure. *American Journal of Orthopsychiatry*, **68**, 216–32.

Wehman, P. and Moon, M.S. (1988). *Vocational Rehabilitation and Supported Employment*. Baltimore, MD: Paul Brookes.

CHAPTER 38

Mental health services in low- and middle-income countries

R. Srinivasa Murthy

Introduction

Community psychiatry in low- and middle-income countries (LAMIC) is nearly four decades old (German, 1975; Swift, 1972; WHO, 1975,). The beginnings of organized mental health care in LAMIC can be traced to the important Sixteenth World Health Organization (WHO) Expert Committee meeting held at Addis Ababa, Ethiopia, in 1974 titled 'Organization of mental health care in developing countries' (WHO, 1975). This meeting is important as it not only reviewed the mental health situation in developing countries but outlined a road map for development of services. These guidelines have largely influenced the developments of the last four decades. The important recommendations of this meeting were:

> Basic mental health care should be integrated with general health services and be provided by non-specialized health workers, at all levels;...countries should, in the first instance carry out one or more pilot programmes to test the practicability of including basic mental health care in an already established programme of health care in a defined rural or urban population;...training programmes, including simple manuals of instructions for training of health workers should be devised and evaluated. (WHO, 1975.)

The LAMIC faced the challenge of providing mental health care with very limited psychiatric beds in ancient and custodial care institutions, with limited trained mental health professionals, a general population having very limited knowledge about mental disorders, and persons with mental disorders experiencing stigma and discrimination. Fortunately for the LAMIC, the planning of mental health services occurred around the time of the discovery of antipsychotics and antidepressants and the global recognition of the values of community mental health care. Professionals in LAMIC have addressed the mental health needs of the population using innovative approaches, centred around greater emphasis on use of community resources rather than an emphasis on the highly trained mental health professionals. These innovations have included greater partnership with the families of the persons

with mental disorders, use of general hospital psychiatry units, integration of mental health with general health care, and using non-specialist personnel for focused interventions like suicide prevention, disaster and conflict mental health care, life skills education, and rehabilitation. The result of these initiatives have been, from a situation of nearly no services for the majority of the persons with mental disorders, to today where there is a developing framework for mental health care in the public, private, and voluntary sectors in a large number of LAMIC. In these developments, LAMIC have been influenced by the local situation as well as international developments. For example, in the initial phase, the existing general health care infrastructure was the primary focus of integration of mental health services. Soon, the increased use of family members, volunteers, counsellors, mentally ill persons, survivors of disasters, parents of children with mental disorders, and the education system occurred. In this way the three principles of community psychiatry—meeting population based needs, use of range of resources, and accessibility—were partially addressed (Thornicroft and Szmukler, 2001).

In the last 25 years, the needs of mental health care in developing countries has been addressed by the Harvard group (Desjarlais et al., 1995), the Institute of Medicine (IOM, 2001), the WHO through *The World Health Report 2001* (WHO, 2001), World mental health casebook (Cohen et al., 2002), the World Bank (Baingana et al., 2003), the *Lancet* series on mental health (Horton, 2007), and global review of the developments for integration of mental health into primary care (Gask et al., 2009; WHO-WONCA, 2008). A number of treatment guidelines for specific mental disorders for use in LAMIC have been published (Mari et al., 2009; WHO, 2009) and WHO has developed a package of 13 documents on mental health policy, legislation and mental health care (see Appendix 38.1).

In this chapter, the progress in LAMIC, from the last 40 years of psychiatric services are reviewed towards identification of issues for the future in terms of the priorities, processes, problems, and prospects.

Challenging mental health situation in LAMIC

In contrast to the economically rich countries (Thornicroft and Szmukler, 2001; Thornicroft et al., 2008) the development of community psychiatry in LAMIC has occurred against the background of almost no mental health services. Almost all of the persons with mental disorders were living in the community, most often without any organized services, with the family providing the care in whatever form they were able to do (ranging from isolation to committed care). In a way, community psychiatry has developed in these countries as 'the service' and not as the alternative to institutionalized care.

Barriers to development of mental health care in LAMIC have included 1) custodial institutions (WHO, 2001), 2) limited mental health professionals (Trivedi et al., 2007; WHO, 2005), and 3) stigma of mental disorders (Srinivasa Murthy, 2005; Wig et al., 1980, 1997), resulting in long treatment delays and treatment gaps (Chatterjee et al., 2003; Farooq et al., 2009; Kohn et al., 2004; Srinivasa Murthy et al., 2004; Thara et al., 2008; Thirthahalli et al., 2009, 2010; Wang et al., 2007; World Mental Health Survey, 2004).

Custodial institutions

The mental health infrastructure available in LAMIC were limited to large-size custodial institutions, providing services to a limited population. For example, at the time of India's independence, there were almost no mental health services. For a population of about 300 million, there were only 10,000 psychiatric beds, in contrast to over 150,000 psychiatric beds for about 30 million in the United Kingdom at that time.

In all the LAMIC, the situation of mental hospitals was far from satisfactory as can be seen from the following examples:

> On 15 March 1979, when the 'pavilion' of Ibn Rushd Hospital became the University Psychiatric Centre of Casablanca, there was only one trained psychiatrist and one resident to be in charge of three provinces and four cities namely Casablanca, Mohamedia, El Gidida and Benshimane. The building was in a terrible condition: with almost no electricity, no water supply, no doors (except some metallic ones which did not close), no glass in windows and almost no medication. The ceiling was falling on the heads of the patients and staff, and rats were usual guests of the pavilion. The image of psychiatry was terrible in the community, and the authorities decided to close the ward in the teaching hospital and to transfer the patients to a psychiatric hospital 25 km outside Casablanca. (WHO-EMRO, 2006.)
>
> In southern Yemen, before 1966, patients were kept in the prison, and no formal mental health services were available. The beginnings of organized mental health services were made in Aden in 1966 in an isolated place in Sheikh Othman under the name of Al Salam clinic. (WHO-EMRO, 2006.)
>
> In India, two reviews of the mental hospitals have been undertaken in 1999 and 2008 to identify the needs and the changes that have occurred over a decade (National Human Rights Commission, 1999, 2008). The findings of these evaluations illustrate the challenges these institutions present to mental health care. Over the 10-year period, the improvements were reported in the following: percentage admissions through courts has fallen from about 70% in 1996 to around 20% in 2008; the number of long-stay patients have fallen from 80–90% to about 35%; the custodial care indicators like staff wearing compulsory uniforms (down to 21 from 28), cells use has fallen from 20 institutions; recreation facilities have increased from eight to 29, and rehabilitation facilities from 10 to 23 institutions; budget had doubled in nine institutions, 2–4 times in 13, 4–8 times in four, and more than

eight times in three institutions; the use of electroconvulsive therapy (ECT) had reduced and the modified type increased from nine to 27 institutions. The one area of continuing problem was in the inadequate staff- vacancies continued in spite creation of new positions. Overall, as the Report notes, the changes were more in the last 10 years as compared to the earlier half a century!

Limited mental health professionals

The WHO *Mental Health Atlas* (Trivedi et al., 2007; WHO, 2005) highlights the low numbers of mental health professionals in LAMIC. The figures are worrisome, especially given the pandemic proportions of the figures of the mentally ill. About 52.7% of the countries, covering 69.2% of the world's population, have access to less than one psychiatrist per 100,000 population. All countries in the South-East Asian region and almost 96% of the countries in the African region, accounting for 89% of the population, have less than one psychiatrist per 100,000 population. India counts among them. The figures for psychologists working in mental health care are not too different, and there is also a paucity of social workers and psychiatric nurses too.

Stigma of mental disorders

Stigma is an important barrier to mental health care (Srinivasa Murthy, 2005; Thara, 2007; Thornicroft et al., 2009; Wig, 1997). The most recent of the studies involved 27 participating countries, describing the nature, direction, and severity of anticipated and experienced discrimination reported by people with schizophrenia, by use of face-to-face interviews with 732 participants. Negative discrimination was experienced by 344 (47%) of 729 participants in making or keeping friends, by 315 (43%) of 728 from family members, by 209 (29%) of 724 in finding a job, 215 (29%) of 730 in keeping a job, and by 196 (27%) of 724 in intimate or sexual relationships. Positive experienced discrimination was rare. Anticipated discrimination affected 469 (64%) in applying for work, training, or education and 402 (55%) looking for a close relationship; 526 (72%) felt the need to conceal their diagnosis. Over a third of participants anticipated discrimination for job seeking and close personal relationships when no discrimination was experienced (Thornicroft et al., 2009).

Treatment delay and treatment gap

As a reflection of the limited centralized treatment facilities and limited professionals there are large treatment delays and treatment gaps (Kohn et al., 2004; Phillips et al., 2009; Srinivasa Murthy, 2004; Thirthahalli, 2009; Wang et al., 2007; WHO mental Health Survey, 2004).These studies show that only a few of the ill are receiving care and a large proportion of them came late in the illness for treatment.

International initiatives

The World Health Report 2001 focused on mental health ('New understanding, New hope').The report is significant both as an expression of the importance of mental health at the international level, as well as the commitment of the international organization to the cause of mental health. The report had five chapters, namely, 1) a public health approach to mental health; 2) burden of mental and behavioural disorders; 3) solving the mental health problems; 4) mental health policy and service provision; and 5) the way forward.

The World Health Report 2001, noted

...there have been major advances in the understanding of mental health and its inseparable relationship with physical health. This new understanding makes a public health approach to mental health not only desirable, but feasible. The Report noted mental disorders affect at least a quarter of all people at some time during their lives – and occur in all societies.... The burden on these people, and their families, in terms of human suffering, disability and economic costs, is massive. Effective solutions for mental disorders are available.... Some mental disorders can be prevented, while most can be treated. Enlightened mental health policy and legislation supported by training of professionals and adequate and sustainable financing can help deliver appropriate services to those who need them at all levels of health care. Only a few countries have adequate mental health resources. Some have almost none.... And for the mentally ill, human rights violations are commonplace. There is a clear need for global and national initiatives to address these issues. Countries have the responsibility to give priority to mental health in their health planning and to implement the recommendations given below.

This report made 10 overall recommendations (see Box 38.1)

The World Health Report 2001, further considered the varying needs of countries of the world. With this in mind, the recommendations were presented for the three separate scenarios to guide, LAMIC in particular, towards what is possible within their resource limitations. For each of the scenarios, the most important actions to be undertaken for each of the above 10 recommendations are identified as guide for priority actions (Box 38.1).

Global mental health initiative

On 4 September 2007, *The Lancet* launched a new movement for mental health, through the publication of six key articles. These articles covered the topics of 1) no health without mental health (Prince et al., 2007); 2) resources for mental health: scarcity, inequity and inefficiency (Jacob et al., 2007); 3) treatment and prevention of mental disorders in low-income and middle-income countries (Patel et al., 2007); 4) barriers to improvement of mental health services (Mercier, 2007; Minhas, 2007; Saraceno et al., 2007); and 5) scale-up services for mental disorders: a call for action (Chisholm et al., 2007a). These six papers review the developments in the international literature and present an update on the WHR 2001.

Box 38.1 Recommendations of *The World Health Report, 2001* (WHO, 2001)

1 Provide treatment in primary care

2 Make psychotropic drugs available

3 Give care in the community

4 Educate the public

5 Involve communities, families, and consumers

6 Establish national policies, programmes, and legislation

7 Develop human resources

8 Link with other sectors

9 Monitor community mental health

10 Support more research

Responding to the needs: innovative approaches to care

The mental health professionals in LAMIC have developed a number of approaches to address the mental health needs of the population, within the available resources. A brief account of these is presented below.

Recognition of mental health as of public health importance

In a large number of LAMIC, there is a greater recognition of the importance of mental health as part of public health. This has occurred for a variety of reasons. For example, the conflict situations in a large number of countries in the Middle East and Asia, have brought to attention the vulnerability of the populations to mental distress and disorders and thus the need for organized mental health care to a large proportion of the population. Some examples will illustrate this:

◆ In the Palestine population, even before the start of the mental health programme in 1990, studies had shown a growing number of behavioural disorders, especially among the young people who account for 69% of the wounded.

◆ In Kuwait, following the Gulf War, a special mental health treatment facility called REGAE was started to provide care for persons with post-traumatic stress disorder.

◆ In Lebanon, narcotic production tripled during the years of conflict, and there were an estimated 240,000 young drug addicts. These came under control with specific interventions.

◆ In Sri Lanka, the long internal struggle and conflict has made suicide prevention and trauma care an important part of the country's programme.

Partnership with families

In LAMIC, most people with mental disorders live with their families. The family takes care of them, ensures provision of services, and plans and provides for their future. The role of the family, therefore, becomes crucial when one takes cognizance of the acute shortage of professional care and rehabilitation services. A reflection of this reality is the response of the professionals to form partnerships with families. It is important to recognize that involvement of the families in mental health care started long before the Western countries recognized this possibility. For example, in India, it began in the 1950s (Carstairs, 1974). Indian initiatives relating to families and mental health care have depended on the family support for the mentally ill persons. Since the 1950s, families have been formally included to supplement and support the psychiatric care by professionals. During this period, family members were literally admitted to the hospital along with the mentally ill persons to be part of the care of the patients. This has largely been the pattern in most of the LAMIC. During the 1970s and 1980s, efforts were made to understand the functioning of families with an ill person in the family and their needs ().

During the last 10 years, a more active role for families is emerging in the form of formation of self-help groups and professionals accepting to work with families in partnership (Srinivasan, 2006, 2008). However, reviewing the scene, Shankar and Rao (2005), opine that 'professional inputs have not kept pace' and conclude

> **Box 38.2** Hospital care and home care
>
> An important study of this period was initiated at NIMHANS, Bangalore (Pai and Kapur, 1982, 1983; Pai et al., 1983, 1985) In this study, two similar groups of schizophrenic patients, undergoing two treatment modalities, namely hospital admission and home treatment through a nurse, were compared for the outcome in terms of symptoms, social dysfunction, burden on the family, cost of treatment, and outcome at the end of 6 months. A nurse trained in patient follow-up and counselling visited the home regularly for the purpose of patient assessment and treatment. The results found that the home treatment through a visiting nurse gives a better clinical outcome, better social functioning of the patient, and greatly reduces the burden on the patients' families. Further, the treatment modality is also more economical. A follow-up study observed that the home care group of patients had maintained significantly better clinical status than the controls and this group had been admitted less often. In a subsequent study the focus of family care by visiting nurses was chronic patients with a diagnosis of chronic schizophrenia found that only two of the home care group were admitted to hospital over 2 years in comparison to eight patients in routine care.

that the family movement in India is one of 'unfulfilled promises or great expectations for the future' as follows: 'the vision for the family movement in India would see families from passive carers to informed carers, from receiving services to proactive participation, from suffering stigma to fighting stigma. And it is the responsibility of the mental health system to facilitate this journey of care givers from burden to empowerment' (p. 285).

The value of the availability of family as a resource for professionals in LAMIC can be understood by the challenges faced when families can not be depended on for mental health care as pointed out by Leff (1996):

> Our problem in the West is, that somehow or other we have to make up for the families (emphasis added) who have disappeared and create a supportive structure – not for the patients but for the single relatives who are often desperately trying to cope with schizophrenia. It is, of course, very expensive to create a network of professionals who act as a SURROGATE FAMILY [emphasis added], but we have to provide that form of support, because it is even more expensive to keep hospitalizing patients.

However, many of the leads provided by pilot studies and successes of family care programmes (Box 38.2) have not received the full support of professionals and planners to the extent it could become a routine part of psychiatric care. In the coming years, moving from passive utilization of the families to partnership and true empowerment of the families has the greatest potential in organizing mental health care in LAMIC. The advances in communication technology (mobile phones) and the widening availability of information technology (Internet) should be used creatively to share the caring skills with families, to bridge gap in professional resources. This will be building mental health care from the 'bottom of the pyramid' as it has happened in the other developmental and commercial areas in developing countries (Prahlad, 2006). This area should receive the highest importance in future efforts.

General hospital psychiatry

One important historical change in the field of psychiatry in India and many other LAMIC is the emergence of psychiatric units in general hospitals as the primary centres for mental health care. It has been a slow and silent change but in many ways a major revolution in the whole approach to psychiatric treatment. The general hospital psychiatric units offer numerous advantages over traditional mental hospitals. They are more accessible, easily approachable, are situated right in the community, and above all, less stigmatized. Families can frequently visit and relatives can even stay with disturbed patients. There is no stigma of a mental hospital. There are limited legal restrictions on admission or treatment. Ambulatory treatment on an outpatient basis is available with the use of drugs, ECT, and psychotherapy. Proximity of other medical facilities ensures thorough physical investigations and early detection of physical problems (Behere and Behere, 2000; Wig, 1978).

Formulation of National Programmes of Mental Health (NPMH)

One of the important initiatives of LAMIC is to develop NPMH to address the national level needs. This effort was strongly supported by WHO. One of the first countries to develop NPMH was India in 1982 (GOI, 1982). In the Eastern Mediterranean Region, Pakistan formulated the NPMH in March 1986, followed by other countries (20 of the 22 countries of the Region by 2006) (WHO-EMRO, 2006). There are similar developments in countries of other regions in Africa, South America, and Western Pacific region. The NPMH focus on provision of mental health care for all, integration of mental health care with primary health care, and community participation. Some countries have included care of war victims, prevention, information system, development of mental health infrastructure, and research.

In all of the countries, the national mental health programme has come to be a rallying point for re-examination of the mental health needs and stimulus for innovative approaches to mental health care. One of the professionals, from Middle Eastern countries region, noted the importance as follows: 'The development of a national programme of mental health has provided the much needed sense of direction to the efforts of the mental health professionals in the country.' (WHO-EMRO, 2006).

During the last 10 years, WHO has developed the Assessment Instrument for Mental Health Systems (WHO-AIMS; WHO, 2007a). This has been used to collect information on the mental health systems. The goal of collecting this information is to improve the mental health system and to provide a baseline for monitoring the change. This will enable countries to develop mental health plans with clear baseline information and targets. It will also be useful to monitor progress in implementing reform policies, providing community services, and involving users, families, and other stakeholders in mental health promotion, prevention, care, and rehabilitation. WHO-AIMS reports are available for over 50 countries.

Taking care to the community

In a number of countries efforts have been directed to develop and evaluate the community-based mental health care programmes. Two illustrations from India and China reflect these efforts. During the last few years, important research studies have addressed the situation of persons suffering from schizophrenia living in the community and the effectiveness of community level interventions (Chatterji et al., 2004; Pai and Kapur, 1982, 1983; Pai et al., 1983, 1985; Srinivasa Murthy et al., 2004; Thara et al., 2008; Thirthahalli et al., 2006, 2009, 2010). These studies from India show that about half of the patients with schizophrenia are living in the community without treatment. It is further seen that such patients have significant disability, and cause a lot of emotional and financial burden on the family and caregivers. It is important to note that all of these studies show the benefits of regular treatment in decreasing the disability, the burden on the family, and costs to the families. These studies also emphasize the need for community involvement in the care programmes: 'community-based initiatives in the management of mental disorders however well intentioned will not be sustainable unless the family and the community are involved in the intervention program with support being provided regularly by mental health professionals'. (Thara et al., 2008) If the mindset that chronicity of schizophrenia can be reduced and every person with schizophrenia can improve is coupled with an enthusiastic, aggressive management comprising of both medical and social interventions, then it is possible that many patients can improve or recover and have meaningful, productive lives.

In China, psychiatric care units consist of patients' neighbours, retired persons, and family members, who assist with the care of the mentally ill persons. Today hospital-based services at Shanghai's municipal and district levels are exceptional. Community follow-up occurs at primary care level hospitals and includes outpatient services, medical monitoring, and home visit if required. Rehabilitation is implemented through guardianship networks consisting of groups of trained volunteers (retired workers, family members, community administrators) who supervise individual patients, maintain treatment schedules, and provide family support. One hundred and eighty-four work stations, mainly located in urban areas, also provide rehabilitation services, giving 4628 clients an opportunity to work and receive an income, in addition to obtaining treatment, education, and psychiatric care (Cohen et al., 2002).

Integration of mental health with general health care

This measure is one of the most important initiatives to provide essential mental health care in LAMIC. The chief recommendation of the WHO (2001) was to 'provide treatment in primary care'. The theme of the World Mental Health Day, 2009, was 'Mental health in Primary Health Care: enhancing treatment and promoting mental health' (WFMH, 2009).

The integration of mental health care into general health services, particularly at the primary health care level, has many advantages. These include: less stigmatization of patients and staff, as mental and behavioural disorders are being seen and managed alongside physical health problems; improved screening and treatment, in particular improved detection rates for patients presenting with vague somatic complaints which are related to mental and behavioural disorders; the potential for improved treatment of the physical problems of those suffering from mental illness, and vice versa; and better treatment of mental aspects associated with 'physical' problems. For the administrator, advantages include a shared infrastructure leading to cost-efficiency savings, the potential to provide universal coverage of mental health care, and the

use of community resources which can partly offset the limited availability of mental health personnel.

There is no single best practice model that can be followed in all countries. Rather, successes have been achieved through sensible local application of 10 broad principles (Box 38.3).

WHO supported the movement to provide mental care within general health services in developing countries, and conducted a 7-year feasibility study of integration with primary health care in Brazil, Colombia, Egypt, India, the Philippines, Senegal, and Sudan (Biegel, 1983; Climent et al., 1980; Giel et al., 1981a,b, 1983; Harding et al., 1983a,b; Ladrido-Ignacio et al., 1983; Sartorius and Harding, 1983; Wig et al., 1980). A number of countries have used this approach to organize essential mental health services. For example, India started training primary health care workers in 1975, forming the basis of the National Mental Health Programme formulated in 1982. Currently the government supports over 125 district level programmes in 22 states, covering a population of over 100 million (Agarwal et al., 2004; Chandrasekar et al., 1981; GOI, 1982; ICMR-DST, 1987; Issac and Kapur, 1980; Issac et al., 1982, 1988; Srinivasa Murthy, 2004; Srinivasa Murthy et al., 1988; Thara et al., 2004; Wig and Srinivasa Murthy, 1980; Wig et al., 1981). In Cambodia, the ministry of health trained a core group of personnel in community mental health, who in turn trained selected general medical staff at district hospitals. In the Islamic Republic of Iran, efforts to integrate mental health care started in the late 1980s and the programme has since been extended to the whole country, with services now covering about 20 million people (WHO-EMRO, 2006). Similar approaches have been adopted by countries such as Afghanistan, Brazil (Mateus et al., 2008), Guinea–Bissau (de Jong, 1996), Malaysia, Morocco, Nepal (Cohen et al., 2002), Pakistan (Mubbashar, 1986, 1999) Saudi Arabia, South Africa, the United Republic of Tanzania, Uganda (Ovuga et al., 2007), and Zimbabwe. Some studies have been carried out to evaluate the impact of integration, but more are urgently needed (Cohen, 2002;

Box 38.3 Broad principles of integration of mental health with primary care (WHO-WONCA, 2008)

1 Policy and plans need to incorporate primary care for mental health

2 Advocacy is required to shift attitudes and behaviour

3 Adequate training of primary care workers is required

4 Primary care tasks must be limited and doable

5 Specialist mental health professionals and facilities must be available to support primary care

6 Patients must have access to essential psychotropic medications in primary care

7 Integration is a process, not an event

8 A mental health service coordinator is crucial

9 Collaboration with other government non-health sectors, nongovernmental organizations, village and community health workers, and volunteers is required

10 Financial and human resources are needed

Issac and Guruje, 2009; Kutchner et al., 2005; Srinivasa Murthy, 1998, 2007a; WHO, 2001, 2008).

In a recent review of this area, WHO brought together 12 best practice examples (10 of these are in LAMIC) to show that integrating mental health into primary care is possible across a range of circumstances and conditions, and in difficult economic and political circumstances (WHO-WONCA, 2008). The represented countries have vastly different socioeconomic situations and health care resources. Consequently, their specific models for integrating mental health into primary care vary greatly. While details differ, success has been achieved uniformly through leadership, commitment, and local application of the 10 principles (Box 38.3) Clear policies and plans, combined with adequate resources and close stewardship, training, and ongoing support of primary care workers, availability of psychotropic medicines, and strong linkages to higher levels of care and community resources result in the best outcomes. With the notable exceptions of Belize and the Islamic Republic of Iran, the best practice examples describe mental health integration in provinces, districts, or towns rather than across entire countries. Concentrating on smaller geographical areas facilitated access to detailed information regarding the establishment and maintenance of the programmes, which can help in the planning and implementation of their own services. However, it is also true that integrating mental health into primary care in a small geographical area is far easier than nationwide especially in large countries. There are also issues of making this integration culturally sensitive (Jadhav and Jain, 2009; Kapur, 2004).

Recently, Issac and Guruje (2009: pp. 83–4) have reviewed the field and point out:

> The large unmet need for mental health services in many LAMIC, despite the availability of effective and relatively affordable interventions, calls for an urgent effort to scale up primary care service in those countries. Efforts to scale up services must include a comprehensive review of the training provided for primary care providers in the recognition and treatment of mental health problems and a reorganization of the primary health care system. Assumptions made about the relative autonomy of the primary health care system have led to an unsupported and unmotivated health workforce. A reorganization of primary health care system in the LAMIC must recognize the need for an effective secondary care level., with a sufficient number of specialist mental health workers to provide training and support for primary care providers and back up for difficult cases requiring specialist interventions. Adequate resources are also needed. However, it has been estimated that the investment needed to scale up mental health care is not large in absolute terms, when considered at the population level and in comparison with other health sector investments (Chisholm et al., 2007b). Efforts to integrate mental health efficiently into primary care services are unlikely to work until public funded health systems are better resourced and made more effective.

Utilization of 'non-specialists' for mental health care

Recognizing the need to develop services, against the background of limited trained professionals, professionals in LAMIC have utilized a large variety of community resources for delivery of focused mental health care (Srinivasa Murthy, 2004, 2006; Srinivasa Murthy and Wig, 1983; WHO, 2001). These have included health workers, school teachers, volunteers, and lay workers with specific training to care for specific groups like persons with dementia.

The crucial questions for the involvement of 'non-specialist mental health personnel' are: 1) to what degree should the workers be involved in early identification and diagnosis? 2) To what degree should they be given the responsibility for non-pharmacological methods of treatment? (3) To what degree should the worker be involved in pharmacological and biological interventions? (4) To what degree these workers can work independently or only under the direct and continuous supervision of other professionals? (5) To what degree can they be involved in training of other workers? (6) To what degree should these people be given the responsibility for certification of various types for legal as well as welfare benefits? And (7) to what extent should these workers come under the system of licensing?

In addition, in the involvement of non-specialist personnel, the following safeguards are essential: 1) the scope of the programme should be clearly spelt out to the users and providers of help (**in writing**); 2) all the providers of help should receive **essential** training for the task to be carried out; 3) the providers should be given skills to do what they are expected to do (knowledge alone is not enough); 4) there should be a supportive mechanism to support the providers of care— preferably with some trained professionals once a week and not less than once a month; 5) there, should be clear lines for **referral** to professionals so that inappropriate actions are not taken when more acute need is there (e.g. suicidal risk, violence); 6) there should be clear documentation of the process at all stages, to allow for review both internally and externally; and 7) lastly there should be an **annual audit**, preferably by an outsider to guide the group in its work. In addition, in view of the wide variations in the specialist human resources available in the country, there will be a need to examine in each country the available human resources and identify tasks on the seven areas and allocate responsibilities to the different categories of personnel.

Disaster mental health care and care of persons living in countries in conflict illustrate both the need and feasibility of using community resources for mental health care (Diaz et al., 2006; Srinivasa Murthy, 2007b). The approaches that have been used to address the mental health needs have varied from individual clinical care using both the non-pharmacological and pharmacological interventions, measures to enhance the self-esteem and coping capacity of the general population, measures to improve the life skills of the children through school-based interventions, creation of community support systems, income generating programmes for women, integration of mental health care with general health services, and the rebuilding of the mental health infrastructure of specialist human resources for mental health care. The recently developed Inter Agency Standing Committee (IASC) guidelines (IASC, 2007) have provided support to these initiatives.

Community level rehabilitation

One other important development is the increasing role of the voluntary organizations in developing small-size, locally relevant, community-based psychiatric care facilities like day care centres, vocational training centres, sheltered workshops, half-way homes, and long-stay homes (Patel and Thara, 2003). These facilities have the advantage of limiting long-term institutional care, incorporating the cultural sensitivities of the clientele, and utilization the local resources.

Religion

All major religions give an important place to mental health (Verghen,et al., 2010). Religion has been utilized both at the level of making sense of the illness as well as the involvement of the religious leaders for mental health promotion and mental health care. In a number of religions like Buddhism and Hinduism there are practices like yoga and meditation that have direct value in the treatment of some mental disorders and promotion of mental health.

Traditional practices and traditional healers

In the absence of modern mental health care, a majority of the population has taken the help of traditional healers. The approach of mental health professionals to healers has varied from country to country (Baasher, 1962, 1980; Kapur, 1975; Sebastia, 2009). There are a number of countries, especially in Africa, where there has been active collaboration between healers and professionals. In other countries, like Pakistan (Mubbashar et al., 1999), they have been involved in referral of patients to mental health services.

Public mental health education

Developing programmes to educate the general population about the modern understanding of mental disorders and their treatment has been an important activity of professionals. These efforts have been directed not only to fight stigma and discrimination but to promote mental health, through mental health literacy efforts (Mubbashar, 1999). There is a wide use of the mass media for these efforts in addition to folk measures. With the wider availability of the information technology this area has great potential to bring about changes in the general population. This area also has the potential to stimulate 'self-care' and 'informal care'.

Research

Research forms an important part of the mental health service development (Tomlinson, et al., 2008). Research at national levels has been an important component of activities of the country mental health programmes. Past efforts have been linked to the goals of national mental health programmes. The subject of research has been towards an understanding of mental disorders and the role of biological and psychosocial factors. For example, in India, the Indian Council of Medical Research provided valuable support with a large number of research projects directly and indirectly related to the emerging mental health programme during the 1970s and 1980s (ICMR, 2005). Research on course and outcome of schizophrenia, acute psychoses, old age psychiatric problems, and community psychiatry added the local knowledge to influence the NPMH (Verghese et al., 1989). Lancet Mental Health group (2008) has identified 10 priority research questions (e.g. how effective are early detection and simple, brief treatment methods that are culturally appropriate, implemented by non-specialist health workers in the course of routine primary care, and can be scaled up?) (Tomlinson et al., 2008)

Lessons learnt

Thirty years ago, Professor Allen German, while working in Africa wrote the following:

> The psychiatrist in a developing country, in contrast to one in a more industrialized setting, does not have to face the same degree of frustration resulting from attempts to dismantle an existing inert and cumbersome administrative structure; to determine how to include large numbers of mental hospitals into more efficient and human psychiatric programs; or to deal with large armies of mental health personnel from various disciplines, each of which is preoccupied with and defensive about its own status and intent on holding onto its traditional role. The absence of these barriers provides the psychiatrist in a developing country with a fairly clean canvas on which to develop the themes. (German, 1975.)

Against the this hope at the beginning of the community psychiatry movement, reviewing the progress some lessons can be drawn.

Firstly, during the last four decades there has been a sea change in the importance given to mental health in LAMIC—there is a shift to recognizing the larger mental health needs of the population and including mental health as part of public health programmes.

Secondly, mental health professionals have responded to the challenges of providing mental health care by innovative approaches, relevant to the country situations (community psychiatry in LAMIC is not a 'single model' programme but a wide variety of initiatives involving community resources).

Thirdly, the initiatives have been limited to pockets of population, limited in reach, and have not been adequately supported with funds, by the national governments and international organizations.

Fourthly, extension of the pilot programmes to cover wider population requiring further efforts to develop technical materials (e.g. for non-specialist carers, for families, general public) and at managerial strategies has not occurred.

Fifthly, there are areas of mental health programmes that have not been given adequate attention. The past efforts have laid greater emphasis on care of persons with severe mental disorders, though there have been smaller-scale attempts at promotion of mental health and prevention of mental disorders. The growing recognition of the impact of social changes on the mental health of the population (e.g. increasing suicide rates, domestic violence, violence in children, elderly mental health, migrant populations, displaced populations, etc.) requires that the future mental health programmes should include promotion of mental health, prevention of mental disorders, and care and rehabilitation of persons with mental disorders.

Sixthly, the undergraduate training of basic doctors in psychiatry is extremely limited. The human resource development to meet the total mental health needs have not been fully addressed.

Seventhly, the impact of rapid social change, along with the many changes in the social institutions like the family and community and the ways to help populations experiencing the negative effects of these changes is still not a subject of adequate attention.

Looking to the future

The development of community psychiatry in LAMIC is a developing story. The following are some of the needs to address for the future.

Framework for services

The key issue for the service planners is to determine the optimal mix of services and the level of provision of particular service delivery channels. The absolute need for various services differs greatly between countries but the relative needs for different services, i.e. the proportions of different services as parts of the total mental health service provision, are broadly the same in many countries.

Services should be planned in a holistic fashion so as to create an optimal mix.

Figure 38.1 shows the relationship between the different service components. It is clear that the most numerous services ought to be self-care management, informal community mental health services and community mental health services provided by the primary health care staff, followed by psychiatric services based in general hospitals and formal community mental health services, and lastly specialist mental health services. The emphasis placed on delivering mental health treatment and care through services based in general hospitals or community mental health services should be determined by the strengths of the current mental health or general health system, as well as by cultural and socioeconomic variables.

Areas for interventions

In LAMIC, there is need for interventions at four levels, namely 1) creation of public demand for services; 2) availability of a wide range of services; 3) professional and technical support; and 4) administrative support (Fig. 38.2)

Challenges

The following are the three challenges for community psychiatry in LAMIC, namely, professional level, community level, and policy level (Srinivasa Murthy and Kumar, 2006; Wig, 1989).

Professional challenges

There is a need to simplify mental health care skills and continually review and develop innovative approaches to deliver them, in order to meet the reality of the community needs and expectations. For care to be undertaken by health workers, teachers, volunteers, and family members, there is a need for simple and effective interventions. Professionals have to develop the appropriate information in a simple format and identify the 'level of care' and 'limits of care' to

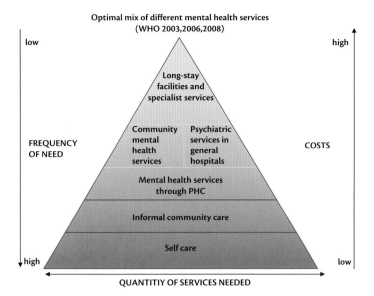

Fig. 38.1 Optimal mix of different mental health services.

be provided by these personnel. These should include choosing priority mental disorders to be addressed in training, limiting the range of drugs to be used by the general practitioners, developing strong referral guidelines and the non-pharmacological interventions to be used by non-physician personnel.

There should be willingness to share the mental health caring responsibilities with non-specialists, overcoming the fear of some professionals of losing their work, identity, and income. The method should be not to convert the non-specialist into a mini-psychiatrist, but to identify what is relevant, feasible, and possible for the specific non-specialist to undertake in his/her work setting.

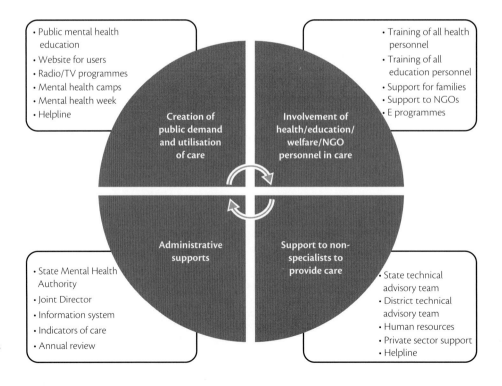

Fig. 38.2 The need for interventions at four levels in LAMIC.

There is a need to decrease the amount of time devoted by specialist mental health professionals to individual clinical care and increase the time for training, support, and supervision of other personnel. This is a big challenge for clinicians who value directly caring for ill people by themselves. This change in role becomes meaningful when it is recognized that training of other personnel has a multiplier effect in providing mental health services to the population.

There is a need to devote significant time to periodic support and supervision of the non-specialists. Reports of mental health care in developing countries have repeatedly shown the importance of support and supervision by psychiatrists to the non-specialist personnel. Fortunately, the easy and inexpensive availability of mobile phones, Internet, and satellite communication for telepsychiatry, allows for distant support to the non-specialists on a continuous and interactive basis.

There is a need for professionals to acquire the skills to work with the community, education sector personnel, welfare sector personnel, voluntary organizations, and policy makers. This includes understanding the planning process, fighting for priority for mental health in health programmes, becoming familiar with legislations and budget procedures, and developing skills to negotiate with different stakeholders.

Community level challenges

In LAMIC, there is a paradoxical situation of limited services and poor utilization of the available services, due to problems of stigma and lack of information in the general population. There is a need for bringing about a major shift in the thinking of the community in terms of understanding of mental health and mental disorders, decreasing the stigma and discrimination of persons and families with mental disorders, and the creation of a wide range of community care facilities and services. There is also a need to develop simple self-care information modules. For those requiring long-term care there is a need to develop measures (e.g. using mobile phones, Internet, community radio) to help in monitoring the progress of mental condition at the home level.

In addressing these needs to cover the total population and in a manner that requires limited travel, there is a need to fully use modern technologies like the world wide web, mobile phones, telemedicine, and community radio to reach and continuously support people with mental disorders and their families. Already some small-scale initiatives have been made and there is a need for both widening these initiatives and a wider application to cover the total population of the country. The use of information technology in spreading agricultural information and consumer goods should give hope for similar success in the mental health area (Prahlad, 2006).

Policy level

There are a number of requirements at this level. The important ones are: 1) greater amount of allocation of funds for mental health programme; 2) recognition of human rights of the persons and families of persons with mental disorders in all development programmes, especially in the areas of education, welfare, housing, and employment; 3) strengthening of the programmes to support the families; 4) legislative support for non-specialists to provide mental health care; and 5) building of a large number of community based care facilities.

Conclusion

In conclusion, development of mental health services all over the world, countries rich and poor alike, have been the product of larger social situations, specifically the importance society gives to the rights of disadvantaged/marginalized groups. Economically rich countries have addressed the movement from institutionalized care to community care, building on the strengths of their social institutions. LAMIC have begun this process in a different way and have made significant progress. There is a need to continue the process by widening the scope of the mental health interventions, increasing the involvement of all available community resources, and rooting the interventions in the historical, social, and cultural roots of countries. This will be a continuing challenge for professionals and people in the coming years.

References

Agarwaal, S.P., Goel, D.S., Ichhpujani, R.L., Salhan, R.N., and Shrivatsava, S. (2004). *Mental Health: An Indian perspective (1946-2003)*. New Delhi: Directorate General of Health Services, Ministry of Health and Family Welfare.

Baasher, T. (1962). Some aspects of the history of the treatment of mental disorders in the Sudan. *Sudan Medical Journal*, **1**, 44–7.

Baasher, T. (1980). Promotion and development of research in traditional medicine: the WHO role in countries of the Eastern Mediterranean Region. *Journal of Ethnopharmacology*, **2**, 75–9.

Behere, P. and Behere, M. (2000). General hospital psychiatry in India. In: Srinivasa Murthy, R. (ed.) *Mental Health in India. Essays in honour of Prof. N.N. Wig*, pp. 169–78. Bangalore: Peoples Action for Mental Health.

Biegel, A. (1983). Community mental health care in developing countries. *American Journal of Psychiatry*, **140**, 1491–2.

Carstairs, G.M. (1974). *Community action for mental health care*. WHO/SEARO/MENT/**22.**

Chandrashekar, C.R., Issac, M.K., Kapur, R.L., and Parthasarathy, R. (1981). Management of priority mental disorders in the community. *Indian Journal of Psychiatry*, **23**, 174–8.

Chatterjee, S., Patel, V., Chatterjee, A., and Weiss, H.A. (2003). Evaluation of a community based rehabilitation model for chronic schizophrenia in India. *British Journal of Psychiatry*, **182**, 57–62.

Chisholm, D., Flisher, A.J., Lund, C., Patel, P., Saxena, S., Thornicroft, G., *et al.* (2007a). Scale up services for mental disorders: a call for action. *Lancet*, **370**, 1241–53.

Chisholm, D., Lund, C., and Saxena, S. (2007b). Cost of scaling up mental health care in low and middle income countries. *British Journal of Psychiatry*, **191**, 528–35.

Climent, C.E., Diop, B.S.M., Harding, T.W., Ibrahim, H.H.A., Ignacio, L.L., Wig, N.N. (1980). Mental health and primary health care. *WHO Chronicle*, **34**, 231–6.

Cohen, A. (2001). *The effectiveness of mental health care in primary health care: the view from the developing world*. Geneva: World Health Organization.

Cohen, A., Kleinmann, A., and Saraceno, B. (2002). *World Mental Health Casebook. Social and Mental Health Programmes in low income countries*. New York: Kluwer Academic/Plenum Publishers.

Desjarlais, R., Eisenberg, L., Good, B., and Kleinman, A. (1995). *World Mental Health: problems and priorities in low-income countries*. New York: Oxford University Press.

Diaz, J.O., Srinivasa Murthy, R., and Lakshminarayana, R. (eds.) (2006). *Advances in disaster mental health and psychosocial support*. New Delhi: American Red Cross.

Farooq, S., Large, M., Nielssen, O., and Waheed, W. (2009). The relationship between the duration of untreated psychosis and outcome in low–middle income countries: a systematic review and meta analysis. *Schizophrenia Research*, **109**, 15–23.

Gask, L., Lester, H., Kendrick, T., and Peveler, R. (eds.) (2009). *Primary care mental health*. London: Royal College of Psychiatrists.

German, A. (1975). Trends in Psychiatry in Black Africa. In: Arieti, S. and Chrzanowski, G (eds.) *New Dimensions in psychiatry – a world view*. New York: Wiley.

Goldberg, D. (1987). Round the world: Pakistan- Revolution in mental health care. *Lancet*, **i**, 736–7.

Government of India (1982). *National Mental Health Programme for India*. New Delhi: Ministry of Health and Family Welfare.

Giel, R., de Arango, M.V., Climent, C.E., Harding, T.W., Ibrahim, H.H., Ladrido-Ignacio, L., *et al.* (1981a). Childhood mental disorders in primary health care: results of observations in four developing countries. A report from the WHO collaborative Study on Strategies for Extending Mental Health Care. *Pediatrics*, **68**, 677–83.

Giel, R., d'Arrigo Busnello, E., Climent, C.E., Elhakim, A.S., Ibrahim, H.H., Ladrido-Ignacio, L., *et al.* (1981b). The classification of psychiatric disorder. A reliability study in the WHO collaborative study on strategies for extending mental health care. *Acta Psychiatrica Scandinavica*, **63**, 61–74.

Giel, R., de Arango, M.V., Hafeiz Babikir, A., Bonifacio, M., Climent, C.E., Harding, T.W., *et al.* (1983). The burden of mental illness on the family. Results of observations in four developing countries. A report from the WHO Collaborative Study on Strategies for Extending Mental Health Care. *Acta Psychiatrica Scandinavica*, **68**, 186–201.

Harding, T.W., Climent, C.E., Diop, M., Giel, R., Ibrahim, H.H.A., Ignacio, L.L., *et al.* (1983a). The WHO Collaborative study on the Strategies for Extending Mental Health Care, II: the development of new research methods. *American Journal of Psychiatry*, **140**, 1474–80.

Harding, T.W., d'Arrigo Busnello, E., Climent, C.E., Diop, M., El-Hakim, A., Giel, R., *et al.* (1983b). The WHO Collaborative study on the Strategies for Extending Mental Health Care, III: Evaluative design and Illustrative results. *American Journal of Psychiatry*, **140**, 1481–5.

Horton, R. (2007). Launching a new movement for mental health. *Lancet*, **370**, 806.

IASC (2007). *Inter Agency Standing Committee Guidelines on Mental Health and Psychosocial Support in Emergency Settings*. Geneva: IASC.

Indian Council of Medical Research – Department of Science and Technology (ICMR-DST) (1987). *A Collaborative Study of Severe Mental Morbidity*. New Delhi: ICMR.

Indian Council of Medical Research (2005). *Mental Health Research in India*. New Delhi: Indian Council of Medical Research.

Institute of Medicine (IOM) (2001). *Neurolological, psychiatric and developmental disorders: Meeting the challenges in the developing world*. Washington, DC: National academy of Sciences.

Issac, M. and Guruje, O. (2009). Low and middle income countries, In: Gask, L., Lester, H., Kendrick, T., Peveler, R. (eds.) *Primary Care Mental Health*, pp. 72–87. London: Royal college of Psychiatrists.

Issac, M.K. and Kapur, R.L. (1980). A cost effectiveness of three different methods of psychiatric case finding in the general population. *British Journal of Psychiatry*, **137**, 540–6.

Issac, M.K, Kapur, R.L., Chandrasekar, C.R., Kapur, M., and Parthasarathy, R. (1982). Mental health delivery in rural primary health care - development and evaluation of a pilot training programme. *Indian Journal of Psychiatry*, **24**, 131–8.

Issac, M.K., Chandrasekar, C.R., and Srinivasa Murthy, R. (1988). *Manual of mental health care for medical officers*. Bangalore: National Institute of Mental Health and Neurosciences.

Jacob, K.S., Sharan, P., Mirza, I., Garrido-Cumbrera, M., Seedat, S., Mari, J.J., *et al.* (2007). Mental health systems in countries: where are we now? *Lancet*, **370**, 1061–77.

Jadhav, S. and Jain, S. (2009). Pills that swallow policy: clinical ethnography of a Community Mental Health Program in northern India. *Transcultural Psychiatry*, **46**, 60–85.

James, S., Chisholm, D., Srinivasa Murthy, R., Kishore Kumar, K., Sekar, K., Saeed, K., *et al.* (2002). Demand for, access to and use of community mental health care: Lessons from a demonstration project in India and Pakistan. *International Journal of Social Psychiatry*, **48**, 163–76.

de Jong, J.T.V.M. (1996). A Comparative public health programme in Guinea-Bissau: a useful model for African, Asian and Latin American countries. *Psychological Medicine*, **26**, 97–108.

Kapur, M. (1997). *Mental Health in Indian Schools*. New Delhi: Sage.

Kapur, R.L. (1975). Mental health care in rural India: a study of existing patterns and their implications for future policy. *British Journal of Psychiatry*, **127**, 286–93.

Kapur, R.L. (2004). The story of community mental health in India, In: Agarwaal, S.P., Goel, D.S., Ichhpujani, R.L., Salhan, R.N., and Shrivastava, S. (eds.) *Mental Health – An Indian perspective (1946–2003)*, pp. 92–100. New Delhi: Directorate General of Health Services, Ministry of Health and Family Welfare.

Kessler, R.C., Angermeyer, M., Anthony, J.C., de Graaf, R., Demyttenaere, K., Gasquet, I., *et al.* for the WHO World Mental Health Survey Consortium (2007). Lifetime prevalence and age of onset distributions of mental disorders in the World Health Organization's World Mental Health Survey Initiative. *World Psychiatry*, **6**, 168–76.

Kohn, R., Saxena, S., Laevav, I., and Saraceno, B. (2004). The treatment gap in mental health care. *Bulletin of World Health Organization*, **82**, 858–66.

Kutchner, S., Chehil, S., Cash, C., and Millar, J. (2005). A competencies based mental health training model for health professionals in low and middle income countries. *World Psychiatry*, **4**, 177–80.

Ladrido-Ignacio L, de Arango, M.V., Baltazar, J., Busnello, E., Climent, C.E, Diop, B.S., *et al.* (1983). Knowledge and attitude of primary health care personnel concerning mental health problems in developing countries. *American Journal of Public Health*, **73**, 1081–4.

Leff, J. (1996). Schizophrenia: aetiology prognosis and course. In: Jenkins R and Field V. (eds.) *The Primary Care of Schizophrenia*, pp. 50–65. London: HMSO.

Mari, J.D.J., Razzouk, D., Thara, R., Eaton, J., and Thornicroft, G (2009). Packages of care for schizophrenia in low- and middle-income countries. *PLoS Medicine*, **6**, e1000165.

Mateus, M.D., Mari, J.J., Delgado, P.G.G, Almeida-Filho, P., Barrett, T., Gerolin J., *et al.* (2008). The mental health system in Brazil: Policies and future challenges. *International Journal of Mental Health Systems*, **2**, 12.

Mercier, C. (2007). *Expert opinion on barriers and facilitating factors for the implementation of existing mental health knowledge in mental health services*, p. 12. Geneva: World Health Organization, Geneva.

Minhas, H. (2007). *Expert opinion on barriers and facilitating factors for the implementation of existing mental health knowledge in mental health services*, p.16. Geneva: World Health Organization.

Mubbashar, M.H. (1999). Mental health services in rural Pakistan. In: Tansella, M. and Thornicroft, G. (eds.) *Common Mental Disorders in Primary care*, pp. 67–80. London: Routledge.

Mubbashar, M.H., Maklik, S.J., Zar, J.R., and Wig, N.N. (1986). Community based mental health care programme: Report of an experiment in Pakistan. *Eastern Mediterranean Region Health Journal*, **1**, 14–20.

National Human Rights Commission (NHRC) (1999). *Quality assurance in mental health*. New Delhi: NHRC.

National Human Rights Commission (NHRC) (2008). *Mental health care and Human Rights* (Nagaraja, D. and Murthy, P., eds.). New Delhi: NHRC-NIMHANS.

Ovuga, E., Boardman, J., and Wasserman, D. (2007). Integrating mental health into primary health care: local initiatives from Uganda. *World Psychiatry*, **6**, 60–1.

Pai, S. and Kapur, R.L. (1982). Impact on treatment intervention on the relationship between the dimensions of clinical psychopathology, social dysfunction and burden on families of schizophrenic patients. *Psychological Medicine*, **12**, 651–8.

Pai, S. and Kapur, R.L. (1983). Evaluation of home care treatment for schizophrenic patients. *Acta Psychiatrica Scandinavica*, **67**, 80–8.

Pai, S. Kapur, R.L, and Roberts E.J. (1983). Follow up study of schizophrenic patients initially treated with home care. *British Journal of Psychiatry*, **143**, 447–50.

Pai, S., Channabasavanna, S.M., and Raghuram, R. (1985). Home care for chronic mental illness in Bangalore: An experiment in the prevention of repeated hospitalisation. *British Journal of Psychiatry*, **147**, 175–79.

Patel, V. and Thara, R. (eds) (2003). *Meeting mental health needs in developing countries: NGO innovations in India*. New Delhi: Sage (India).

Patel, V., Araya, R., Chatterjee, S., Chisholm, D., Cohen, A., De Silva, M., *et al.* (2007). Treatment and prevention of mental disorders in low-income and middle-income countries. *Lancet*, **370**, 991–1005.

Phillips, M.R., Zhang, J., Shi, Q., Song, Z., Ding, Z., Pang, S., *et al.* (2009). Prevalence, treatment, and associated disability of mental disorders in four provinces in China during 2001–05: an epidemiological survey. *Lancet*, **373**, 2041–53.

Prahlad, C. (2006). *The future at the bottom of the Pyramid – eradicating poverty through profits*, Upper Saddle River, NJ: Wharton Publishing House.

Prince, M., Patel, V., Saxena, S., Maj, M., Maselko, J., Phillips, M.R., *et al.* (2007). No health without mental health. *Lancet*, **370**, 859–77.

Ranganathan, S. (1996). *The Empowered Community: a paradigm shift in the treatment of Alcoholism*. Madras: TTR Clinical Research Foundation.

Saraceno, B., van Ommeren, M., Batniji, R., Cohen, A., Gureje, O., Mahoney. J., *et al.* (2007). Barriers to improvement of mental health services in low-income and middle-income countries. *Lancet*, **370**, 1164–74.

Sartorius, N. (1997). Psychiatry in the framework of Primary Health Care: a threat or boost to psychiatry? *American Journal of Psychiatry*, **154**(Suppl. 6), 67–72.

Sartorius, N. and Harding, T. (1983). The WHO collaborative study on strategies for extending mental health care, I: The genesis of the study. *American Journal of Psychiatry*, **140**, 1470–3.

Saxena, S., Thornicroft, G., Knapp, M., and Whiteford, H. (2007). Resources for mental health: scarcity, inequity, and inefficiency. *Lancet*, **370**, 878–89.

Sebastia, B. (2009). *Restoring mental health in India-pluralistic therapies and concepts*. New Delhi: Oxford University Press.

Shankar, R. and Rao, K, (2005). From burden to empowerment: the journey of family caregivers in India, In: Sartorius, N., Leff, J., Lopez-Ibor, J.J., Maj, M., and Okasha, A. (eds) *Families and Mental Disorders*, pp. 259–90. Chichester: Wiley.

Srinivasan, N. (2006). *Together we rise – Kshema family power*. In Srinivasa Murthy, R. (ed) *Mental health by the people*. Peoples Action For Mental Health.

Srinivasan, N. (2008). *We are not alone – family care for persons with mental illness*. Bangalore: Action for Mental Illness (ACMI).

Srinivasa Murthy, R. (1998). Psychiatry in the Third World: managing and rationalising mental health care. *Current Opinion in Psychiatry*, **11**, 197–99.

Srinivasa Murthy, R. (2005). Perspectives on the stigma of mental illness. In: Okasha, A. and Stefanis, C.N. (eds.) *Stigma of mental illness in the third world*, pp. 112–30. Cairo: World Psychiatric Association.

Srinivasa Murthy, R. (2004). The National Mental Health Programme: progress and problems. In: Agarwaal, S.P., Goel, D.S., Ichhpujani, R.L., Salhan, R.N., and Shrivatsava, S. (eds) *Mental Health – An Indian perspective (1946–2003)*, pp. 75–91. New Delhi: Directorate General of Health Services, Ministry of Health and Family Welfare.

Srinivasa Murthy, R (ed) (2006). *Mental health by the people*. Published by Peoples Action For Mental Health, Bangalore.

Srinivasa Murthy, R. (2007). Mental health programme in the 11th five year plan. *Indian Journal of Medical Research*, **125**, 707–12.

Srinivasa Murthy, R. (2007). Mass violence and mental health – recent epidemiological findings. *International Review of Psychiatry*, **19**, 186–192.

Srinivasa Murthy, R. and Kumar, K. (2006). Challenges of building community mental health care in developing countries. *World Psychiatry*, **7**, 101–102.

Srinivasa Murthy, R. and Wig, N.N. (1983). The WHO Collaborative study on strategies for extending mental health care, IV: a training approach to enhancing the availability of mental health manpower in a developing country. *American Journal of Psychiatry*, **140**, 1486–90.

Srinivasa Murthy, R., Issac, M.K., Chandrasekar, C.R. and Bhide, A. (1987). *Manual of Mental Health for Medical Officers-Bhopal Disaster*. New Delhi: Indian Council of Medical Research.

Srinivasa Murthy, R., Chandrasekar, C.R., Nagarajiah, Issac, M.K., Parthasathy, R. and Raghuram, A. (1988). *Manual of mental health care for multi-purpose workers*. Bangalore: National Institute of Mental Health and Neurosciences.

Srinivasa Murthy, R., Kishore Kumar, K.V., Chisholm, D., Thomas, T., Sekar, K., and Chandrasekar, C.R. (2004). Community outreach for untreated schizophrenia in rural India: a follow–up study of symptoms, disability, family burden and costs. *Psychological Medicine*, **34**, 1–11.

Susser, E., Collins, P., Schanzer, B., Varma, V.K., and Gittelman, M. (1996). Topic for our times: Can we learn from the care of persons with mental illness in developing countries? *American Journal of Public Health*, **86**, 926–8.

Swift, C.R. (1972). Mental Health Programme in a developing country: Any reference elsewhere? *American Journal of Orthopsychiatry*, **42**, 517.

Thara, R. (2002). Community mental health in India: a vision beckoning fulfillment? *Canadian Journal of Community Mental Health*, **21**, 131–7.

Thara, R. (2007). We must tackle stigma by offering proven treatments. *PLoS Medicine*, **4**, 965–6.

Thara, R., Padmavathi, R., and Srinivasan, T.N. (2004). Focus on psychiatry in India. *British Journal of Psychiatry*, **184**, 366–73.

Thara, R., Padmavati, R., Aynkran, R.A., and John, S. (2008). Community mental health in India: A rethink. *International Journal of Mental Health Systems*, **2, 11.**

Thirthahalli, J., Venkatesh, B.K., Naveen, M.N., Kishore Kumar, K.V., and Gangadhar, B.N. (2006). Do antipsychotics limit disability in schizophrenia? A naturalistic comparative study in the community. *Indian Journal of Psychological Medicine*, **28**, 14–19.

Thirthahalli, J., Venkatesh, B.K., Kishorekumar, K.V., Arunachala, U., Venkatasubramaniam, G., Subbukrishna, D.K., *et al.* (2009). Prospective comparison of course of disability in antipsychotic treated and untreated schizophrenia patients. *Acta Psychiatrica Scandinavica*, **119**, 209–17.

Thirthahalli, J., Venkatesh, B.K., Naveen, M.N., Venkatasubramaniam, G, Arunachala, U., Kishorekumar, K.A., *et al.* (2010). Do antiopsychotics limit disability in schizophrenia? A naturalistic comparative study in community. *Indian Journal of Psychiatry*, **52**, 37–41.

Thornicroft, G. and Szmukler, G. (2001). *Textbook of Community Psychiatry*. New York: Oxford University Press.

Thornicroft, T., Tansella, M., and Law, A. (2008). Steps, challenges and lessons in developing community mental health care. *World Psychiatry*, **7**, 87–92.

Thornicroft, G., Brohan, E., Rose, D., Sartorius, N., Leese, N., for the INDIGO Study. ((2009). Global pattern of experienced and anticipated discrimination against people with schizophrenia-a cross-sectional study. *Lancet*, **373**, 408–15.

Todd, C., Patel, V., Simunyu, E., Gwanzura, F., Acuda, W., Winston, M., *et al.* (1999). The onset of common mental disorders in primary care attenders in Harare, Zimbabwe. *Psychological Medicine*, **29**, 97–104.

Tomlinson, M., Rudan, I., Saxena, S., Swartz, L., Tsai, A.C., and Patel, V. (2008). Setting priorities for global mental health research. *Bulleting of WHO*, **87**, 438–46.

Trivedi, J.K., Doel, D., Kallivayil, R.A. Issac, M., Shreshta, D.M., and Gambheera, H.C. (2007). Regional cooperation in South Asia in the field of mental health. *World Psychiatry*, **6**, 57–9.

Ustun, T.B. and Sartorius, N. (1995). *Mental illness in general health care: an international study*. Chichester: Wiley.

Verghen, P.J., Van Praag, H.M., Lopez Ibor, J., Cox, J.L., and Moussaoui, D. (2010). *Religion and Psychiatry- beyond boundaries*. Chichester: Wiley-Blackwell.

Verghese, A., John. J.K., Rajkumar, S., Richard, J, Sethi, B.B., Trivedi, K. (1989). Factors associated with the course and outcome of schizophrenia - a multicentric study-results of 2 years multicenter follow up study. *British Journal of Psychiatry*, **154:** 499–503.

Wang, P.S., Angermeyer, M., Borges, G., Bruffarts, R., Chiu, W.T., de Girolomo, G., *et al.* for the WHO World Mental Health Survey Consortium (2007). Delay and failure in treatment seeking after first onset of mental disorders in the World Health Organization's World Mental Health Survey Initiative. *World Psychiatry*, **6**, 177–85.

Wig, N.N. (1978). General hospital psychiatry-right time for evaluation, *Indian Journal of Psychiatry*, **20**, 1–5.

Wig, N.N. (1989). The future of psychiatry in developing countries – The need for national programmes of mental health. *NIMHANS Journal*, **7**, 1–11.

Wig, N.N. (1997). Stigma against mental illness (Editorial). *Indian Journal of Psychiatry* **39**, 187–9.

Wig, N.N. and Srinivasa Murthy, R. (1980). *Manual of mental disorders for peripheral health personnel.* Chandigarh: Department of Psychiatry, PGIMER (2nd printing 1993).

Wig, N.N., Suleiman, M.A., Routledge, R., Murthy, R.S., Ladrido-Ignacio, L., Ibrahim, H.H., *et al.* (1980). Community reactions to mental disorders. A key informant study in three developing countries, *Acta Psychiatrica Scandinavica*, **61**, 111–26.

Wig, N.N., Srinivasa Murthy, R., and Harding T.W. (1981). A model for rural psychiatric services- Raipur Rani experience. *Indian Journal of Psychiatry*, **23**, 275–90.

WHO (1975). *Organization of mental health services in developing countriesTechnical Report Series, 564.* Geneva: World Health Organization.

World Health Organization (2001). *The World Health Report 2001. Mental Health: new understandingnew hope.* Geneva: World Health Organization.

WHO (2005). *Mental Health Atlas.* Geneva: World Health Organization.

WHO (2007a). *Assessment Instrument of Mental health Systems.* Geneva: World Health Organization.

WHO (2007b). *WHO Mental Health Policy and Service Guidance Package.* Geneva: World Health Organization.

WHO-WONCA (2008). *Integrating mental health in primary care-a global perspective.* Geneva: World Health Organization and World Organization of Family Doctors.

WHO (2009). *Pharmacological treatment of mental disorders in primary health care*, World Health Organization.

WHO-EMRO (2006). *Mental health in the Eastern Mediterranean countries: Reached the unreached.* WHO Regional Publications of Eastern Mediterranean, Publication No.29. Cairo: World Health Organization.

WHO World Mental Health Survey Consortium (2004). Prevalence, severity and unmet need for treatment of mental disorders in the World Health Organization World mental health surveys, *Journal of American Medical Association*, **291**, 2581–90.

World Federation of Mental Health (WFMH) (2009). *World Mental Health Day*, 2009. WFMH.

Appendix 38.1 **WHO Mental Health Policy and Service Guidance Package**

1 World Health Organization (2003). *Mental Health Policy and Service Guidance Package: The mental health context.* Geneva: World Health Organization.

2 World Health Organization (2003). *Mental Health Policy and Service Guidance Package: Mental health policy, plans and programmes (updated version).* Geneva: World Health Organization.

3 World Health Organization (2003). *Mental Health Policy and Service Guidance Package: Mental health financing.* Geneva: World Health Organization.

4 World Health Organization (2003). *Mental Health Policy and Service Guidance Package: Advocacy for Mental Health.* Geneva: World Health Organization.

5 World Health Organization (2003). *Mental Health Policy and Service Guidance Package: Organization of Services for Mental Health.* Geneva: World Health Organization.

6 World Health Organization (2003). *Mental Health Policy and Service Guidance Package: Quality improvement for mental health.* Geneva: World Health Organization.

7 World Health Organization (2003). *Mental Health Policy and Service Guidance Package: Planning and budgeting to deliver services for mental health.* Geneva: World Health Organization.

8 World Health Organization (2005). *Mental Health Policy and Service Guidance Package: Improving access and use of psychotropic medications.* Geneva: World Health Organization.

9 World Health Organization (2005). *Mental Health Policy and Service Guidance Package: Child and adolescent mental health policies and plans.* Geneva: World Health Organization.

10 World Health Organization (2005). *Mental Health Policy and Service Guidance Package: Human resources and training in mental health.* Geneva: World Health Organization.

11 World Health Organization (2005). *Mental Health Policy and Service Guidance Package: Mental health information systems.* Geneva: World Health Organization.

12 World Health Organization (2005). *Mental Health Policy and Service Guidance Package: Mental health policies and programmes in the workplace.* Geneva: World Health Organization.

13 World Health Organization (2007). *Mental Health Policy and Service Guidance Package: Monitoring and evaluation of mental health policies and plans.* Geneva. World Health Organization.

All modules can be downloaded at: http://www.who.int/mental_health/policy/essentialpackage1/en/index.html

SECTION 9

Methods for ensuring that effective care is provided

CHAPTER 39

Producing guidelines, protocols, and toolkits

Troy A. Moore, Alexander L. Miller, and Elizabeth Kuipers

Over the past several decades, multiple factors have resulted in the development of guidelines, treatment protocols, and implementation toolkits in all branches of medicine, including psychiatry. First, a number of studies showed that some accepted practices could not be shown to be effective when tested in randomized controlled trials (RCTs: Coffman et al., 1987; Gaebel, 1995; Gaebel et al., 2002; Kinon et al., 1998). The lack of practice effectiveness in randomized studies is often attributed to the interventions not being well defined (Michie et al., 2009).

Second, community surveys showed that many evidence-based practices were either not used, or not used properly (i.e. not used with fidelity to the key details of implementation of the practice) (Buchanan et al., 2002; Cradock et al., 2001; Howard et al., 2009; Young et al., 1998). Fidelity refers to the degree to which a particular programme follows a programme model, which is a well-defined set of interventions and procedures that helps individuals achieve some desired goal (Bond et al., 2000).

Third, studies of incorporation of evidence-based practices into everyday practice showed long delays (Codyre et al., 2008; Rosen et al., 2007; Ruggeri et al., 2008). Meanwhile, evaluation of the impact of continuing medical education programmes demonstrated their ineffectiveness in changing physician practices (Davis et al., 1995). Thus, it became clear that to affect actual medical practices, it would be necessary to put together detailed sets of recommendations, and the means to operationalize them.

Definitions

In this section, we provide definitions of guidelines, protocols, and toolkits because each is different, but they do share some of the same elements. Field and Lohr provided a standard definition of clinical practice guidelines (CPG) in 1990: 'Clinical practice guidelines are systematically developed statements to assist practitioner and patient decisions about appropriate health care for specific clinical circumstances.' (Field and Lohr, 1990). Guidelines cover broad topics or conditions that affect many individuals. The literature often provides multiple ways of treating the clinical situation and the guideline is used to assist practitioners in navigating these different options.

Protocols in science and medicine are a written methodology making explicit the design and implementation of experiments or procedures. They are particularly important when standardization and replication are desired. Protocols in psychiatry are typically developed for an acute clinical situation where there is a high level of certainty in the evidence showing there is a right and wrong way to address the situation. Protocols have a high level of specificity and the intent of following a protocol is to improve outcomes or avoid poor outcomes.

Toolkits are collections of tools and/or strategies. An example of a toolkit in medicine is for the implementation of clinical practice guidelines or evidence-based practices. Toolkits can include worksheets/checklists, template letters, pocket cards, quick reference guides, assessment instruments, and related process and quality measures (National Guideline Clearinghouse, 2009). Toolkits can be thought of an accumulation of multiple protocols addressing a subject with many elements. Figure 39.1 depicts the complex

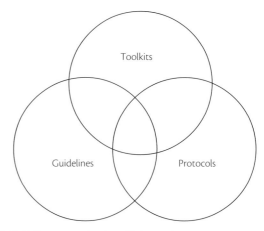

Fig. 39.1 Guideline, protocol, and toolkit interaction.

overlap of elements between guidelines, protocols, and toolkits (GPTs). As we proceed through this chapter, we will compare the goals, risks, benefits, development process, scope, contributors, feasibility, and evidence for the utilization of GPTs. We will primarily focus on pharmacological interventions, but psychological and psychosocial treatments will also be considered.

Goals, risks, and benefits of GPTs

What are the goals of GPTs as commonly used in psychiatry? Ultimately, a well-constructed guideline can be used as a tool for making care more consistent and efficient and for closing the gap between what clinicians do and what scientific evidence supports. Unfortunately, there is literature suggesting practitioners do not necessarily follow guideline recommendations when guideline effect on process of clinical care is examined (Grimshaw and Russell, 1993). Toolkits try to provide a means of support for a practitioner or health care system trying to implement a guideline. Toolkits provide strategies, examples, and monitoring techniques to ensure proper implementation. Guidelines such as the Texas Medication Algorithm Project (TMAP) schizophrenia algorithm (Moore et al., 1997) and the National Institute of Health and Clinical Excellence (NICE) schizophrenia guidelines (National Collaborating Centre for Mental Health, 2009) manuals have many elements of toolkits that can assist in implementing the guideline. Protocols provide a standardization of procedures to ensure similar results are achieved when a different individual performs the same task at a different time and/or place. For instance, administration of an intramuscular antipsychotic can produce very different results in absorption and distribution of the drug if injection technique and injection placement protocols are not followed by the health care provider administering the injection.

The potential risks and benefits of utilizing guidelines and protocols can vary depending on the user's point of view (clinicians, patients, administrators/payers). An example of the risk and benefits of guidelines and protocols utilization on clinical practice is the reinforcement and justification of clinical decisions made by clinicians using guideline or protocol recommendations. At the same time, other clinicians may feel that guidelines and protocols may restrict their clinical practices. Evidence-based guideline recommendations can be used as a tool by health care administrators/payers to determine if clinician prescribing is consistent with the evidence base, such as dosing of antipsychotics. By following evidence-based practice recommendations within guidelines or protocols, administrators and health care systems may restrict certain medications and/or practices that have not been shown to be beneficial, but administrators and health care systems may also make themselves responsible for paying for very costly medications or practices if certain guideline recommendations are followed.

Development of GPTs

Many elements must be considered at the outset of GPT development. First, one must examine what are evidence-based practices. Evidence-based practices are the integration of best research evidence with clinical expertise and patient values (Sackett et al., 2000). Second, data from scientific studies, real-world observations, and clinical experience must be evaluated on their scientific merit to determine their inclusion, and their subsequent weighting when recommendations are made from these data. Should studies with only case–control level data be included? Or is data from one positive RCT enough for inclusion into a guideline? Should data from clinical experience or expert opinion be included? And if expert opinion is included, how should it be weighted versus RCT data? What value do pragmatic design medication trials hold versus typical RCT trials? Will evidence rating systems or quantification be utilized during the evaluation of the literature (such as Agency for Healthcare Research and Quality (AHRQ) evidence ratings)? AHRQ evidence grading reflects the strength of evidence supporting a treatment and the magnitude of net benefit (benefits minus harm), e.g. 'A' equals good evidence supporting the treatment improves outcomes and benefits substantially outweigh the risks (U.S. Preventive Services Task Force, 2010).

It is helpful if the criteria and processes involved in these kinds of decisions are made clear, as those responsible for producing the GPTs must carefully consider these questions. Some decisions are complex, requiring a mixture of scientific merit (whether a paper is included) and expert view (whether the evidence justifies a recommendation).

The pluses and minuses of using the various types of evidence in GPT formation must be evaluated by those producing GPTs. The ultimate issue surrounding evidence inclusion is whether a guideline addresses only those clinical decisions with sufficient RCT evidence or whether it tries to also make recommendations for common clinical decisions where an adequate RCT database is lacking. For instance, the TMAP schizophrenia algorithm tries to only utilize RCTs where appropriate, but includes the best available data under some of the stages of the algorithm. The latter stage of the algorithm examining antipsychotic polypharmacy utilizes case series data and expert opinion because there is a lack of RCTs using two antipsychotics (excluding clozapine augmentation trials) (Moore et al., 2007). The PORT schizophrenia guidelines use strict inclusion criteria for recommendations requiring at least three positive RCTs on a medication management topic before the topic is addressed by the guideline (Kreyenbuhl et al., 2010). NICE guidelines require evidence from at least two well conducted RCTs (National Collaborating Centre for Mental Health, 2009). Consequently, the PORT and NICE guidelines do not address antipsychotic polypharmacy.

Although RCTs are considered the 'gold standard' in formulating GPTs, it is critical to determine if the population that participated in the RCTs is representative of the population that typically receives the intervention, 'the target population'. Some factors that may make study populations differ from 'target populations' include how they were recruited (advertisements vs. clinical settings) or participants joining the study for only altruistic or monetary reasons.

The producers of a guideline that only incorporates RCT data must be prepared not to address some important issues that arise in clinical practice. RCT data provides evidence that one can be confident in the results, but on the other hand RCTs may provide limited external validity. Often clinical trials have very strict inclusion/exclusion criteria that may limit the generalizability of the study results. In practice, the limitations of the available data will need to be acknowledged, and the recommendations that result be duly cautious, pointing out the pitfalls.

What about internal versus external validity? Can results of guideline utilization in Texas, in the National Health Service in the

United Kingdom, or elsewhere be generalized to other populations? Strict inclusion/exclusion study criteria may potentially limit the external validity of the studies used in a GPT. On the other hand, very loose inclusion/exclusion study criteria will limit the internal validity of the studies used to develop the GPT.

An example of a common clinical practice that is difficult to thoroughly evaluate with RCTs is the use of antipsychotic polypharmacy. An RCT examining every possible antipsychotic polypharmacy regimen would be difficult to conduct. It would have to be incredibly large in size to incorporate all the possible antipsychotic polypharmacy regimens and have the power to show differences between regimens. So is it better for a guideline to ignore a treatment with little to no evidence to support its practice (such as non-clozapine antipsychotic polypharmacy) altogether despite a significant segment of the population being treated with antipsychotic polypharmacy because monotherapy treatment has failed in the past, or is it better to provide practitioners with tools (e.g. rating scales) to use in the evaluation of individual patients as a basis for deciding if an intervention that is not supported by RCT evidence is helpful for the individual patient? It is hard to be definitive. If the guideline is trying to provide only firm, concrete evidence from RCTs to its users, then one would not want to include case–control or expert opinion data.

What about industry versus non-industry RCTs? It has become clearer that some industry sponsored studies are not published if there are not positive results. However, rectifying the publication bias can be problematic, as there have been instances of delay and refusal for requests for raw data from unpublished trials during the NICE process.

Do industry sponsored studies hold less weight than non-industry studies? Are the producers of GPTs assuring the RCT study design is not providing an unfair advantage to one of the treatments being studied? Examples of potentially unfair advantage in study design are seen in early studies comparing haloperidol versus second-generation antipsychotics, which used haloperidol doses that are higher than seen in clinical practice today (Davis et al., 2003).

Scope

The scope of any guideline, toolkit, or protocol needs to be clearly delineated. For instance, the TMAP schizophrenia guideline examines antipsychotic medication management in the acute and maintenance treatment phases of adult schizophrenia. Other areas of treatment such as psychosocial interventions are not addressed by the TMAP schizophrenia guideline.

Contributors

Who will be involved in the evaluation process? This may seem like a benign issue, but failure to include necessary topic experts in the development process of GPTs may raise issues about the final results. Is the evaluation group large or diverse enough? Having a small homogeneous GPT development group, might be easy to manage, but could lead to important information or issues being overlooked, minimized, or interject bias into the process. The inclusion of a variety of individuals with differing expertise as contributors to GPTs is an important aspect of the development process. Contributors can greatly influence the direction of the document and in many cases provide first-hand knowledge of the

data being examined. Expert opinion provided in guidelines is commonly presented from researchers, clinicians, academics, administrators, and sometimes consumers, and also covers topics where there may be a lack of literature evidence addressing the topic. Protocol recommendations are usually developed by practitioners highly experienced in dealing with the clinical situation. Any expert opinion utilized in protocol development focuses on issues of implementation, if it is utilized at all.

The TMAP schizophrenia algorithm panel included clinicians, researchers, administrators, and consumers. Clinicians and researchers had expertise in first-episode schizophrenia, chronic schizophrenia, treatment-resistant schizophrenia, or psychopharmacology. An example of the importance of having a diverse group of contributors arose during the most recent TMAP schizophrenia algorithm update. There was debate within the panel over extrapolating results from studies of chronic schizophrenia to first-episode psychosis. Ultimately, the inclusion of a well-rounded group of experts in the field of schizophrenia resulted in a well thought out and thoroughly examined issue that addressed both sides of the debate. If the expert panel had been homogeneous, then some of these important issues about the use of first-generation antipsychotics in first-episode schizophrenia may have been overlooked.

Feasibility

The feasibility of a GPT is an important issue that must be considered. Guidelines do consider the feasibility of implementing their recommendations to some extent, but guidelines are not mandatory and usually do not have funding for implementation. Protocols also heavily rely on their feasibility. A national protocol, such as the acute management of stroke, has to be feasible in terms of personnel, monetarily, time, and equipment for the protocol recommendations to be successfully carried out. Toolkits are also intended to be highly feasible. If toolkit recommendations are not feasible, their recommendations will not be implemented or implemented unsuccessfully. Producers of GPTs can take steps to ensure the inclusion of administrators, practitioners, and consumers in the development process, so they can reveal feasibility issues (such as practicality or cost issues).

The NICE guidelines

In the United Kingdom a government funded body, NICE, is asked to commission reviews of evidence for the treatment of a range of physical and mental health disorders. In 2002 they produced the first mental health review, on schizophrenia, which was also the first one to be updated, in 2009 (National Collaborating Centre for Mental Health, 2009). In the NICE process, it is important to point out that the methodology for looking at evidence is much the same for both medication management and psychological interventions. This means that the quality of the trials included has to meet a threshold of methodologically robust findings for both sorts of interventions, and probably accounts for NICE's insistence on randomized trials for psychotherapy which then share many of the requirements for trials carried out on medication. It is also an important feature as many meta-analyses are criticized for not checking the quality of the trials they include.

The methodological criteria for including studies in the meta-analysis for the recent schizophrenia guideline update

(National Collaborating Centre for Mental Health, 2009) for instance, covered aspects such as a clear description of the trial as randomized, more than 10 patient in each treatment cell, 80% had to have a diagnosis of schizophrenia and adequate information about follow-up data (not more than 50% drop out in any study at follow-up, or not more than 50% of their data unavailable). All studies included also had to be able to get a positive rating on a checklist which looked at whether studies used validated outcome scales, adequate allocation, concealment, and intention to treat analyses. Pharmacological studies had to be within recommended dosages, only trials of licensed medication were included, and not any studies that used rapid titration. For early intervention studies, a priori criteria were a diagnosis of psychosis, not schizophrenia, and participants could be aged 16 and above, instead of 18 and above for all the adult studies. The full check list is available from the NICE website (http://www.nice.org.uk).

The NICE process, as itemized above, required that only RCTs with adequate quality controls were included. These studies were found after a literature and grey literature search of appropriate terms and any queries about the studies were dealt with by discussion with the chair of that topic group. All the meta-analyses were attached to specific clinical, functional, and social outcomes agreed on earlier by the members of the guideline group to be appropriate for that mental health problem. Each meta-analysis was then presented to the group, and an in-depth examination of the results undertaken by the specialist guideline group members selected to be expert in that topic, including service users and carers.

In the most recent update of NICE guidelines for schizophrenia for instance, two main topic groups were convened from members of the main guideline group: medication management and psychological interventions. Individuals chose which topic group they preferred to be in, and each topic group regularly updated the other group about their progress in assessing the evidence. The two service users from the group chose to focus on the medication analyses, and the carer on the psychological interventions. Both groups were, however, in close touch with each other about the results they were finding, and comments could be made and acted upon from any member of the main guideline group. In this particular instance, a third topic group was convened. Members were co-opted into this, to cover access to appropriate treatment by BME (black and minority ethnic) groups. This third topic group was also invited to make comments on any of the results of the meta-analyses as they were produced.

It is also important to stress that the questions the evidence was assembled to answer had been set, a priori, by a scoping exercise carried out by NICE in consultation with relevant stakeholders. It was not therefore possible to answer other questions from the data. This insistence on a transparent, a priori set of questions and assembling of data to answer them, was part of the way that NICE has been able to argue that it is doing methodologically sound analyses, which are not driven by particular pressure groups.

Once evidence has been assembled to answer the questions that have been agreed upon, the guideline group was asked to decide on key recommendations that they would prioritize. These recommendations related to the recommendations from the earlier guideline; these continued to stand unless a substantial amount of new evidence was available to overturn them. This meant that some recommendations remain in place; they were not changed because there was not enough compelling new evidence

to say anything different. If, however, there was a new area with good quality studies that met quality criteria—in this instance, arts therapies—this did form the basis of one new recommendation. The process was thus a mixture of adding in new information to previous analyses, and only making a new recommendation if this new evidence was substantial, or provided substantial evidence of new, robust findings (at least two good quality RCTs).

The methodology for NICE guidelines, how it makes decisions about the questions to be asked, the quality of the evidence that will be used, and all information about the schizophrenia guideline update, is available and can be downloaded from http://www.nice.org.uk/CG82.

The schizophrenia Patient Outcomes Research Team (PORT) guidelines

The schizophrenia PORT guidelines were updated in 2009 (Kreyenbuhl et al., 2010). The PORT guidelines utilize rigorous standards much like the NICE guidelines. The PORT review process entailed using two evidence review groups (ERGs) (one for pharmacological interventions and one for psychosocial interventions). The ERGs selected 41 treatment areas for review. Extensive literature reviews were conducted to identify literature (pre- and post-2002 PORT literature survey) not addressed in the 2003 PORT update for each identified treatment area. The ERGs considered if there was enough evidence (at least three well-designed, positive RCTs by independent investigators) to meet criteria to merit a treatment recommendation. If there was insufficient evidence to warrant a treatment recommendation, a summary statement was written describing the treatment, its indications, evidence summary, and important knowledge gaps that precluded a treatment recommendation.

Toolkits

A further part of the NICE process is to try to encourage implementation of the recommendations contained in the evidence-based guidelines. Currently there is a range of tools available to support local implementation in the United Kingdom. These include web-based implementation resources, and tools aimed at commissioners to help guide the process of commissioning evidence-based services. Information on this process is available at http://www.nice.org.uk/commissioningguides .

Toolkits, such as the Substance Abuse and Mental Health Services Administration (SAMHSA) Assertive Community Treatment (ACT) and Supported Employment (SE) toolkits, address implementing evidence-based practices on a system-level implementation. These toolkits are very detailed resources that cover utilizing evidence-based practices, building an evidence-based programme, training front-line staff, and evaluating a programme after implementation. These toolkits can be found at http://mentalhealth.samhsa.gov/cmhs/CommunitySupport/toolkits/about.asp. The SAMHSA ACT and SE toolkits examine the evidence regarding implementing evidence-based services to help people stay out of the hospital, develop skills for living in the community, and find and keep competitive employment within their communities. Toolkits provide a myriad of suggestions and recommendations for successful implementation of evidence-based guidelines. It is hard to dissect what global elements and recommendations of the complex interventions provided by the toolkits are critical for achieving the desired outcomes of the practice.

Field research on the utilization of the SAMHSA toolkits was conducted in the National Implementing Evidence-Based Practices Project (McHugo et al., 2007). In this project, 53 community mental health centres across eight states in the United States implemented one of five evidence-based practices (EBPs) (SE, ACT, integrated dual disorders treatment, family psychoeducation, or illness management and recovery). Sites were provided with toolkits and human resources to help guide the implementation process. At the end of 2 years, 29 of 53 sites (55%) had high fidelity implementation of the chosen EBP. This study showed most sites implemented EBPs with moderate to high fidelity to the model set forth in the toolkits. Those sites implementing illness management and recovery and integrated dual disorders treatment fared less well overall. Longitudinal fidelity results indicate the use of the toolkit implementation model and similar resources should allow providers to achieve successful implementation of EBPs within 12 months. Subsequent publications revealed the greatest barriers to EBP implementation were leadership, resistance (supervisors, practitioners, and other agencies), utilization of non-EBP services, financing, staffing, and complexity of the intervention (such as with integrated dual disorders treatment) (Bond et al., 2008; Mancini et al., 2009; Rapp et al., 2010).

The Texas Implementation of Medication Algorithms (TIMA) project provides recommendations and implementation strategies learned from a large-scale implementation project within their medication management manuals. The TIMA manuals and the supporting forms are available at http://www.dshs.state.tx.us/mhprograms/TIMA.shtm.

Literature for producing guidelines, protocols, and toolkits

Presently, there is a very small literature base examining how to produce GPTs (Chiles et al., 1999; Frances et al., 1998; Kahn et al., 1997; Woolf, 1992; Woolf et al., 1999). Frances and colleagues (1998) point out that it was surprising how little standardization there was in the development of practice guidelines (Frances et al., 1998). Over a decade later, the same argument can still be made about the lack of guideline standardization. An examination of schizophrenia guidelines shows that each one has different development criteria, with the NICE and PORT guidelines having the most similar development standards (Kreyenbuhl et al., 2010; National Collaborating Centre for Mental Health, 2009). Most of the GPT literature focuses on implementation and utilization outcomes. Those individuals or organizations interested in producing their own psychiatric guidelines mostly have to rely on the examination of the strengths and weaknesses, methods, and design of currently developed GPTs to generate the structure for their own GPT. Figure 39.2 provides a comparison of the elements and qualities of GPTs. A review of articles by Frances et al. and Woolf et al. can provide guideline producers a refresher on the limitations of guidelines and assist in thoughtful development of the methods used to produce the guideline (Frances et al., 1998; Woolf et al., 1999).

A very well-developed list of evidence-based resources has been compiled by SAMHSA. The list includes state, national, and international level evidence-based resources for substance abuse

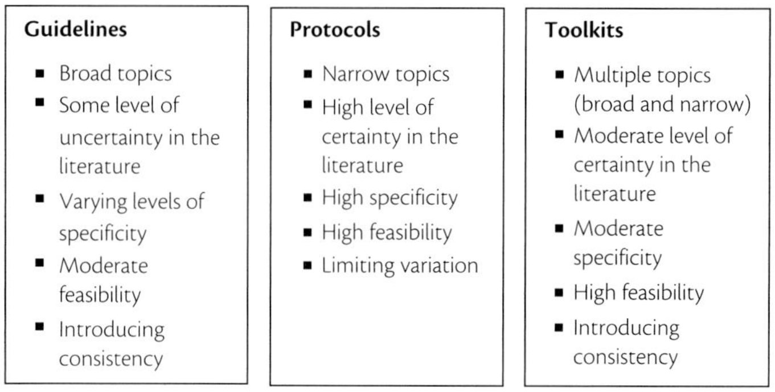

Fig. 39.2 Comparison of guideline, protocol, and toolkit elements and qualities.

prevention, substance abuse treatment, mental health treatment, and the prevention of mental health disorders. The website can be located at http://www.samhsa.gov/ebpwebguide/appendixB.asp. This resource list is a great place to begin an exploration into guideline and protocol development. Within the list is the National Guideline Clearinghouse (NGC), http://www.guideline.gov/, which is the largest database of clinical practice guidelines. It is very comprehensive, but some guidelines may not appear within the NGC if the organization/individuals producing the guideline did not include them into the database. Additionally, if a guideline has not been updated within 5 years it is removed from the active guidelines list and may only be found in the archives.

References

Bond, G.R., Evans, L., Salyers, M.P., Williams, J., and Kim, H.K. (2000). Measurement of fidelity in psychiatric rehabilitation. *Mental Health Services Research*, **2**, 75–87.

Bond, G.R., McHugo, G.J., Becker, D.R., Rapp, C.A., and Whitley, R. (2008). Fidelity of supported employment: lessons learned from the National Evidence-Based Practice Project. *Psychiatric Rehabilitation Journal*, **31**, 300–5.

Buchanan, R.W., Kreyenbuhl, J., Zito, J.M., and Lehman, A. (2002). The schizophrenia PORT pharmacological treatment recommendations: conformance and implications for symptoms and functional outcome. *Schizophrenia Bulletin*, **28**, 63–73.

Chiles, J.A., Miller, A.L., Crismon, M.L., Rush, A.J., Krasnoff, A.S., and Shon, S.S. (1999). The Texas Medication Algorithm Project: Development and implementation of the schizophrenia algorithm. *Psychiatric Services*, **50**, 69–74.

Codyre, D., Wilson, A., Begg, J., and Barton, D. (2008). Dissemination and implementation of the Royal Australian and New Zealand College of Psychiatrists' clinical practice guidelines. *Australasian Psychiatry*, **16**, 336–9.

Coffman, J.A., Nasrallah, H.A., Lyskowski, J., McCalley-Whitters, M., and Dunner, F.J. (1987). Clinical effectiveness of oral and parenteral rapid neuroleptization. *Journal of Clinical Psychiatry*, **48**, 20–4.

Cradock, J., Young, A.S., and Sullivan, G. (2001). The accuracy of medical record documentation in schizophrenia. *Journal of Behavioral Health Services and Research*, **28**, 456–65.

Davis, D.A., Thomson, M.A., Oxman, A.D., and Haynes, R.B. (1995). Changing physician performance. A systematic review of the effect of continuing medical education strategies. *Journal of the American Medical Association*, **274**, 700–5.

Davis, J.M., Chen, N., and Glick, I.D. (2003). A meta-analysis of the efficacy of second-generation antipsychotics. *Archives of General Psychiatry*, **60**, 553–64.

Field, M.J. and Lohr, K.N. (eds.) (1990). *Clinical Practice Guidelines: Directions for a New Program*. Washington, DC: National Academy Press.

Frances, A., Kahn, D.A., Carpenter, D., Frances, C., and Docherty, J. (1998). A new method of developing expert consensus practice guidelines. *American Journal of Managed Care,* 4, 1023–9.

Gaebel, W. (1995). Is intermittent, early intervention medication an alternative for neuroleptic maintenance treatment? *International Clinical Psychopharmacology*, 9(Suppl 5), 11–16.

Gaebel, W., Janner, M., Frommann, N., Pietzcker, A., Kopcke, W., Linden, M., et al. (2002). First vs multiple episode schizophrenia: two-year outcome of intermittent and maintenance medication strategies. *Schizophrenia Research,* 53, 145–59.

Grimshaw, J.M. and Russell, I.T. (1993). Effect of clinical guidelines on medical practice: a systematic review of rigorous evaluations. *Lancet*, **342**, 1317–22.

Howard, P.B., El-Mallakh, P., Miller, A.L., Rayens, M.K., Bond, G.R., Henderson, K., et al. (2009). Prescriber fidelity to a medication management evidence-based practice in the treatment of schizophrenia. *Psychiatric Services*, **60**, 929–35.

Kahn, D.A., Docherty, J.P., Carpenter, D., and Frances, A. (1997). Consensus methods in practice guideline development: A review and description of a new method. *Psychopharmacology Bulletin,* 33, 631–9.

Kinon, B.J. (1998). The routine use of atypical antipsychotic agents: maintenance treatment. *Journal of Clinical Psychiatry*, 59(Suppl 19), 18–22.

Kreyenbuhl, J., Buchanan, R.W., Dickerson, F.B., and Dixon, L.B. (2010). The Schizophrenia Patient Outcomes Research Team (PORT): Updated Treatment Recommendations 2009. *Schizophrenia Bulletin*, 36, 94–103.

Mancini, A.D., Moser, L.L., Whitley, R., McHugo, G.J., Bond, G.R., Finnerty, M.T., et al. (2009). Assertive community treatment: facilitators and barriers to implementation in routine mental health settings. *Psychiatric Services*, **60**, 189–95.

McHugo, G.J., Drake, R.E., Whitley, R., Bond, G.R., Campbell, K., Rapp, C.A., et al. (2007). Fidelity outcomes in the National Implementing Evidence-Based Practices Project. *Psychiatric Services*, **58**, 1279–84.

Michie, S., Fixsen, D., Grimshaw, J.M., and Eccles, M.P. (2009). Specifying and reporting complex behaviour change interventions: the need for a scientific method. *Implementation Science*, 4, 40.

Moore, T.A., Buchanan, R.W., Buckley, P.F., Chiles, J.A., Conley, R.R., Crismon, L.M., et al. (2007). The Texas Medication Algorithm Project Antipsychotic Algorithm for Schizophrenia: 2006 Update. *Journal of Clinical Psychiatry*, **68**, 1751–62.

National Collaborating Centre for Mental Health. (2009). *National Institute for Health and Clinical Excellence Clinical Guideline 82. Schizophrenia: Core interventions in the treatment and management of schizophrenia in adults in primary and secondary care* [serial on the Internet]. Available at: http://www.nice.org.uk/CG82.

National Guideline Clearinghouse (2009). *Glossary*. [Available at: http://www.guideline.gov/resources/glossary.aspx.

Rapp, C.A., Etzel-Wise, D., Marty, D., Coffman, M., Carlson, L., Asher, D., et al. (2010). Barriers to evidence-based practice implementation: results of a qualitative study. *Community Mental Health Journal*, **46**, 112–18.

Rosen, A., Mueser, K.T., and Teesson, M. (2007). Assertive community treatment- Issues from scientific and clinical literature with implications for practice. *Journal of Rehabilitation, Research & Development*, **44**, 813–26.

Ruggeri, M., Lora A., Semisa, D., on behalf of the SIEP-DIRECT'S Group. (2008). The SIEP-DIRECTS Project on the discrepancy between routine practice and evidence. An outline of main findings and practical implications for the future of community based mental health services. *Epidemiologia e Psichiatria Sociale*, **17**, 358–68.

Sackett, D., Strauss, S., Richradson, W., Rosenberg, W., and Haynes, B. (2000). *Evidence Based Medicine*. London: Churchill Livingstone.

U.S. Preventive Services Task Force (USPSTF) (2010). *Grade Definitions. Guide to Clinical Preventive Services, Third Edition: Periodic Updates, 2000-2003* [serial on the Internet]. Available at: http://www.ahrq.gov/clinic/3rduspstf/ratings.htm.

Woolf, S.H. (1992). Practice guidelines, a new reality in medicine, II: Methods of developing guidelines. *Archives of Internal Medicine,* **152**, 946–52.

Woolf, S.H., Grol, R., Hutchinson, A., Eccles, M., and Grimshaw, J. (1999). Potential benefits, limitations, and harms of clinical guidelines. *British Medical Journal*, **318**, 527–30.

Young, A.S., Sullivan, G., Burman, M.A., and Brook, R. (1998). Measuring the quality of outpatient treatment for schizophrenia. *Archives of General Psychiatry*, **55**, 611–7.

CHAPTER 40

Implementing guidelines

Amy Cheung, Paula Whitty, Martin P. Eccles, and Jeremy Grimshaw

Introduction

According to the Institute of Medicine, 'Clinical practice guidelines are systematically developed statements to assist practitioner and patient decisions about appropriate health care for specific clinical circumstances.' (Institute of Medicine, 1990). Guidelines provide a synthesis of what is known about a specific disorder or set of disorders whether it is regarding screening, diagnosis, or management. Compared to systematic reviews, they provide a broad overview of the management of a disorder or of an intervention.

Guidelines may be used as the evidence base for quality improvement activities in health care organizations. Guidelines can also provide the evidence base for other interventions to improve practice (such as part of a computerized decision support tool) (Grimshaw et al., 2005). For example, many North American primary care clinics have adapted the Guidelines for Adolescent Depression in Primary Care (GLAD PC) as the basis for improving depression care for their adolescent patients which has also been incorporated into a web-based decision support tool for paediatricians (CHADIS–http://www.chadis.com) (Cheung et al., 2007; Zuckerbrot et al., 2007). Guidelines are also a good source of information for medical education initiatives. There are many examples of educational activities based on mental health guidelines. One example is the National Collaborating Centre for Mental Health's Schizophrenia guidelines which is the basis of new curricula for training psychiatrists. Finally, guidelines can be used to solve clinical problems that come up as part of patient encounters, e.g. when embedded in online clinical decision support tools such as the Map of Medicine in the United Kingdom (http://www.connectingforhealth.nhs.uk/systemsandservices/mapmed).

The use of guidelines should lead to improved outcomes for service users and their families. However, the quality of guidelines can be variable and mental health professionals and organizations need to identify those that are valid prior to implementation. Furthermore, guidelines are not self-implementing, mental health organizations need to actively disseminate and implement guidelines to ensure their effective uptake.

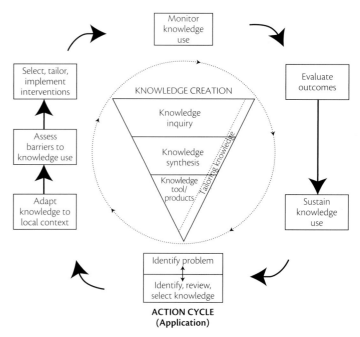

Fig. 40.1 The knowledge to action process framework.

Several frameworks have been developed to address the activities required to implement guidelines effectively, from identifying the need for guidelines in the first place through to monitoring and feedback into future quality improvement activities. One leading framework by Graham and colleagues, which aims to engineer improvements in health care settings, is readily applicable to the whole process of implementing guidelines (Fig. 40.1). Its components are (Graham et al., 2006):

◆ Identification of a problem that needs addressing

◆ Identification, review, and selection of the knowledge or research relevant to the problem (e.g. practice guidelines or research findings)

- Adaption of the identified knowledge or research to the local context
- Assessment of barriers to using the knowledge
- Selection, tailoring, and implementation of interventions to promote the use of knowledge (i.e. implement the change)
- Monitoring knowledge use
- Evaluation of the outcomes of using the knowledge
- Sustaining ongoing knowledge use.

This chapter will describe how mental health professionals and organizations can follow these steps to implement guidelines to improve clinical care. Resources to assist in this process are also listed at the end of the chapter in the appendix.

Identification of a problem that needs addressing

Among mental health professionals, patient encounters in the clinical setting or participation in routine continuing medical education may identify areas of suboptimal care. Among mental health organizations, problems could be identified following a critical incident or routine audit. Health care professionals and organizations may also be prompted to change their practice following the publication of a new guideline or as part of continuous quality improvement strategy.

Identification, review, and selection of the knowledge or research relevant to the problem

Identification of guidelines

Many guidelines are not published in peer-reviewed publications and even among those that are, they can be difficult to identify in bibliographic databases. Fortunately, there are a number of resources available to help mental health professionals and organizations. The appendix lists some common resources for guidelines. Generally, these resources can be divided into three categories:

1 Organizations that produce guidelines (e.g. the National Institute for Health and Clinical Excellence or NICE (http://www.nice. org.uk) in the United Kingdom; the Scottish Intercollegiate Guidelines Network or SIGN (http://www.sign.ac.uk); American Academy of Child and Adolescent Psychiatry or AACAP (http://www.aacap.org)). NICE is one of the largest guideline programmes in the world and produces guidelines that are implemented throughout England and Wales's National Health Service (NHS). This includes a programme of developing guidelines for mental health care, led by mental health clinicians (Kendall and Pilling, 2004). The two most prominent psychiatric associations in North America, the American Psychiatric Association and AACAP, both produce their own guidelines based on research evidence and expert opinion. The AACAP guidelines, also known as practice parameters, are developed through several stages including a literature review, an expert review, and the parameters are also reviewed by AACAP's membership for input and feedback.

2 Organizations that review and recommend, or accredit guidelines. For example, the Ontario Guideline Advisory Committee (http://www.gacguidelines.ca) was developed to assist primary care physicians identify relevant and valid guidelines. The committee reviews guidelines using the AGREE instrument (see next section) and recommends high quality guidelines relevant to the Ontario healthcare system.

3 Organizations that catalogue external guidelines. For example, the Agency for Healthcare Research and Quality's (AHRQ) National Guideline Clearing House (http://www.guideline.gov/) catalogues existing externally-developed guidelines but does not endorse or recommend the use of any specific guidelines. However, guidelines are only included if they are based on systematic literature reviews and were developed under the auspices of relevant health care agencies (e.g. medical specialty associations).

Review and selection of guidelines

Generally, guidelines are more likely to be valid if they are produced by a national or regional guideline multidisciplinary group based upon systematic reviews of relevant evidence. Multidisciplinary groups tend to provide a more balanced perspective than unidisciplinary groups because the diversity of perspectives within the guideline development group allows for: 1) resolution of legitimate conflicts over values (e.g. importance of outcomes such as mortality versus quality of life); 2) interpretation of the available data; and 3) credibility to support implementation of the guidelines after development (Lomas, 1991). In mental health, these multidisciplinary groups should include service user and carer involvement, or have a mechanism of ensuring their input. In general terms, involvement of users and carers is much more advanced in mental health than in other areas of health care. Guidelines are also more likely to be valid if the rationale and strength of evidence underlying recommendations is made explicit. Guidelines should be developed based on a recognized grading system to determine not only the strength of the underlying evidence but also the tradeoffs between the benefits, and the risks, burden, and costs of implementing a specific recommendation in clinical practice. A systematic approach to grading evidence minimizes bias and highlights the uncertainty around the trade-off between risks and benefits by the strength of a recommendation. An example of such a system is GRADE (Grading of Recommendations Assessment, Development and Evaluation). Other common grading systems include the Strength of Recommendation Taxonomy (SORT; Ebell et al., 2004), and systems developed by AHRQ and the Oxford Centre for Evidence Based Medicine (http://www.CEBM.net).

In general, guidelines for psychiatric disorders are developed based on a combination of expert opinion and scientific evidence since these disorders and their management are not generally well studied (even though some psychopharmacological treatments such as antipsychotics have been studied extensively (http://szg.cochrane.org/en/newPage1.html)). Therefore, the explicit link between the strength of the evidence and recommendations is even more important in the field of mental health.

Frequently, there may be several competing guidelines and mental health professionals and organizations have to determine which one is the most appropriate to follow based on considerations of the quality and relevance of the available guidelines.

Fortunately, there are tools available to help with this process. The AGREE instrument (http://www.agreecollaboration.org) is a validated instrument used internationally to appraise the quality of guidelines. The AGREE instrument comprises 23 criteria that map onto six domains and has been translated into several languages (see Table 40.1). Whilst the AGREE instrument is probably the gold standard for appraising guidelines, it may be too unwieldy and time consuming for individual mental health professionals to quickly assess the likely quality of guidelines in day-to-day practice. In this case, there are several simple strategies that professionals and organizations can use to determine whether a set of guidelines is valid. First, we would suggest that professionals and organizations should not use guidelines that do not explicitly discuss its development. Without information on the development methods, it is not possible to determine whether the guidelines are valid. Second, the Users' Guides to Medical Literature series contains two papers on appraising and using clinical guidelines (Hayward et al., 2005; Wilson et al., 2005). These papers describe a series of primary and secondary questions (guides) to help professionals and organizations to appraise guidelines (see Table 40.2). In general, the professionals and/or organization should be convinced that the most important practice options and outcomes have been considered. In mental health, these options and outcomes will look different compared to those for other areas of medicine. In mental health, practice options should include psychological, social, and biological treatments. Outcomes in mental health should focus on improved functioning and quality of life rather than hard outcomes such as mortality. The professionals and/or organizations should also be convinced that a comprehensive literature review has been conducted. Relevant databases for mental health include Medline, CINAHL (Cumulative Index to Nursing and Allied Health Literature), and PsychINFO.

Table 40.1 Guides for appraising guidelines

Primary guide	Secondary guide
Were all important options and outcomes clearly stated?	Was an explicit and sensible process sued to consider the relative value of different outcomes?
Was an explicit and sensible process used to identify, select, and combine evidence?	Is the guideline likely to account for important recent developments?
	Has the guideline been subject to peer review and testing?

Table 40.2 Domains of the AGREE instrument

1. Scope and purpose
2. Stakeholder involvement
3. Rigour of development
4. Clarity and presentation
5. Applicability
6. Editorial independence

Adaptation of the identified knowledge or research to the local context

There are specific issues with the adaptation and implementation of guidelines in mental health including: 1) diagnosis and diagnostic heterogeneity; 2) individual tailoring of psychological treatments and individual expertise of practitioners; 3) course of mental health problems; 4) influence of ethnicity and socioenvironmental characteristics on diagnosis and treatment outcomes; and 5) mental health practitioners' responsibilities to protect the wider public as well as their patients (Kendall and Pilling, 2004).

First, although the diagnoses of mental illness have been operationalized, the validity of the diagnostic criteria has impacted on the evidence base available to guide clinical care. Particularly, some diagnostic groups are too broad and over-inclusive while others are too restrictive and/or do not give consideration to co-occurring illnesses. For example, broader diagnostic groups such as depression and anxiety limit our understanding of the effectiveness of specific treatments due to the heterogeneity of those included in this large group. Conversely, research on very restrictive diagnostic categories such as anorexia nervosa and bulimia has also limited our understanding of a larger service user group who may have eating disorders as well as common comorbid conditions. Second, the application of psychological treatments is dependent on the psychological make-up of an individual, the expertise of an individual practitioner, and the interaction between the two. However, evaluations of such interventions have not accounted for these factors and have instead utilized methodology based on trials evaluating pharmacological treatments. Hence, we have limited understanding of the true impact of such interventions. Third, the natural course of mental illnesses is not predictable, unlike other physical illnesses. This has impacted on our ability to better understand the effectiveness of interventions in altering the progression of mental illnesses. Fourth, patient characteristics such as ethnicity and socioeconomic status can significantly impact on diagnosis and treatment outcomes. For example, symptoms of mental illness may manifest differently in patients from specific ethnic backgrounds which can make accurate diagnosis problematic. Finally, mental health professionals and organizations have the dual responsibility of caring for individuals with mental illness as well as protecting the public such as through involuntary detention. Having a good evidence base for those who are under involuntary detention is particularly important. Each of these specific issues poses further difficulties in the successful implementation of mental health guidelines by professionals and organizations.

Other issues facing mental health professionals and organizations in the adaptation and implementation of guidelines include whether they should use existing guidelines, determine when/how to adapt existing ones to fit a clinical need, and when to develop new ones. Adapting existing guidelines is often the most efficient method when no existing guidelines directly address the needs of a particular clinical setting (Graham et al., 2002). An international collaboration, ADAPTE, was developed to promote the development and use of clinical practice guidelines through the adaptation of existing guidelines (http://www.adapte.org). 'The group's main endeavour is to develop and validate a generic adaptation process that will foster valid and high-quality adapted guidelines as well as the users' sense of ownership of the adapted guideline.' The

ADAPTE collaboration outlines a framework for the adaptation of existing guidelines. In general, recommendations should not be modified if they are supported by very strong evidence (e.g. the use of mood stabilizers in managing symptoms of mania) while recommendations with less evidence may be more appropriate to modify to the local circumstances (e.g. providing education around substance use). The adaptation of guidelines should also be done by a multidisciplinary group of health professionals as this composition ensures the delivery of better health care.

Finally, although professionals and organizations may be tempted to only consider for adaptation those individual recommendations in a set of guidelines that have the strongest evidence base, this process may lead to problems with implementation. For example, organizations could decide to screen for individuals with prodromal symptoms of psychosis due to evidence that early identification will improve prognosis (Phillips et al., 2005). However, if there are no additional resources provided to these families and individuals, the likelihood of them continuing in follow-up will be low given the lack of overt symptoms of psychosis or significant impairment in functioning. Therefore, mental health professionals and organizations must look at the logic chain of implementing a set of guidelines to ensure that the overall change in a clinical setting is successful leading to improved practices or outcomes.

Assessment of barriers to using the knowledge

There are many potential barriers to the uptake of guidelines. These include structural barriers, organization barriers, peer group barriers, professional barriers, and professional–patient barriers. First, structural barriers include those related to the funding model of a healthcare system, accreditation, or regulated roles. For example, although collaborative mental health care in primary care is a recommended practice in many jurisdictions, one of the barriers limiting the uptake of this model is the lack of funding for mental health professionals and organizations to provide indirect consultation to primary care. Second, organizational barriers can also limit the uptake of guidelines. A common example of this type of barrier is the lack of staff training. For example, different psychotherapies are often cited as first-line treatment for mood and anxiety disorders but there is often a lack of staff training for the provision of these treatments in clinical settings. Third, there can be peer-group barriers such as norms for standard of care, and patterns of practice in institutions. An example of this is the use of physical restraints in the inpatient setting. Recent guidelines recommend that physical restraints should only be used when frequent clinical assessments are conducted. However, in many institutions, it is still the norm to order such restraints with no requirements for follow-up clinical assessments (Hellerstein et al., 2007). Fourth, professional barriers such as knowledge and skills can also pose a significant problem. For example, most primary care providers are not trained adequately to handle patients with suicidality who may present in their practices. Therefore, although screening for suicidality is recommended practice for patients with mental illness, the issue of suicidality is often not brought up by primary care providers (Feldman et al., 2004). There may also be professional–patient barriers such as communication issues, and

cognitive issues relating to the limited processing capacity of human beings that can limit the uptake of guidelines. A common example is the inability of mental health professionals to remember a specific protocol for the initiation and follow-up of a prescription medication. A current example in the field of mental health is the use of atypical antipsychotics which are associated with weight gain, diabetes and hyperlipidaemia. However, professionals often forget to monitor for these adverse effects (Mackin et al., 2007).

Potential barriers can be identified using a variety of informal or formal approaches. Commonly, barriers are elicited through informal consultation with key stakeholders. Increasingly though potential barriers are being assessed using more formal theory based approaches usually involving interviews or surveys of mental health professionals and other stakeholders (e.g. practice administrators, patients/families) (Grimshaw et al., in press). For example, in a recent dementia study, the barriers to key behaviours regarding the disclosure of the diagnosis were assessed using a theory-based survey of mental health providers (Foy et al., 2007). The survey was developed based on information from interviews with patients with dementia, their families, and mental health professionals that identified subjective norm, perceived factors in the team environment, and self-efficacy as key influences on practice.

Selection, tailoring, and implementation of interventions to promote the use of knowledge

There is substantial evidence that passive dissemination of guidelines alone is unlikely to optimize clinical care. This has led to the development of a broad range of interventions to promote the use of knowledge in clinical settings. These include professional interventions (e.g. distribution of educational materials, academic detailing, reminders, audit-feedback), organizational interventions (e.g. changing staff roles), financial interventions, regulatory interventions, or a combination of these interventions (e.g. multifaceted) (Gilbody et al., 2003). The choice of dissemination and implementation strategies should be informed by the perceived barriers to knowledge use, identification of potential strategies based upon consideration of their ability to overcome likely barriers and evidence of their effectiveness, and practical considerations (such as available resources and logistical issues). However, commonly there has been little consideration given to these factors; in fact, most interventions have been selected based on 'common sense'. This 'common sense' approach for developing interventions have only shown modest changes in clinician behaviours and, more importantly, in patient outcomes (Gilbody et al., 2003; Grimshaw et al., 2001). However, it is possible for guideline implementers to be more explicit about the design and/or selection of their interventions, e.g. using formal processes such as intervention mapping, and this may improve the effectiveness of selected interventions (Bokhoven et al., 2003). For example, in the study to improve disclosure of the diagnosis of dementia, intervention mapping was used to link the identified factors (subjective norm, self-efficacy) influencing the behaviours with appropriate behaviour change techniques (Bokhoven et al., 2003). The resulting intervention included behaviour change techniques that targeted the specific factors (persuasive communication

Table 40.3 Summary of key findings from overviews of reviews

Intervention (key reference)	Definition of intervention based upon (Bero et al., 2007)	Barriers addressed	Effectiveness	Resource considerations	Practical considerations
Printed educational materials (Farmer et al., 2008)	Distribution of published or printed recommendations for clinical care, including clinical practice guidelines, audio-visual materials and electronic publications	Individual professional knowledge, (attitudes)	6 RCTs General effective Median effect size + 4.6% absolute improvement (range)	Relatively inexpensive	Commonly used in healthcare settings
Educational meetings – didactic (Forsetlund et al., 2009)	Health care providers who have participated in conferences, lectures, workshops or traineeships	Individual professional and peer group knowledge, attitudes and skills	30 RCTs Generally effective Median effect size across 36 comparisons 6% absolute improvement (interquartile range 1.8 to 15.9) Larger effects observed with: higher attendance at educational meetings; with mixed interactive and didactic educational meetings; simpler behaviours; and serious outcomes	Relatively inexpensive (didactic) to modest expense (mixed/interactive - usually higher facilitator to participant ratio than didactic activities)	Commonly used in healthcare settings
Educational outreach (O'Brien et al., 2007)	Use of a trained person who met with providers in their practice settings to give information with the intent of changing the provider's practice	Individual professional knowledge, attitudes using a social marketing approach (Soumerai et al., 1990)	69 RCTs Generally effective *Prescribing behaviours* Median effect size across 17 comparisons 4.8% absolute improvement, (interquartile range 3.0% to 6.5%) *Other behaviours* median effect across 17 comparisons 6.0% absolute improvement, (interquartile range 3.6% to 16.0%)	Relatively expensive due to employment of academic detailers (although can still be efficient) (Mason et al., 2001)	Used in some health care systems. Typically aim to get maximum of 3 messages across in 10-15 minutes (using approach tailored to individual health care provider) and use additional strategies to reinforce approach.(5) Typically focus on relatively simple behaviours in control of individual physician eg choice of drugs to prescribe.
Local opinion leaders (Doumit et al., 2007)	Use of providers nominated by their colleagues as 'educationally influential'. The investigators must have explicitly stated that their colleagues identified the opinion leaders	Individual professional and peer group knowledge, attitudes, (skills)	12 RCTs Generally effective Median effect 10% absolute improvement, (absolute range -6% to +25%)	Moderately expensive due to need to survey target population for each condition.	Rarely used in health care systems. Majority of studies have used the Hiss instrument to identify opinion leaders (who are up-to-date, good communicators, humanistic). Appear to be condition specific. (Doumit, 2006) Coverage across social networks is often uncertain. Temporal stability is uncertain. (Doumit, 2006)
Audit and feedback (Jamtvedt et al., 2006)	Any summary of clinical performance of health care over a specified period of time	Individual professional (and peer group) awareness of current performance	118 RCTs Generally effective Median effect across 88 high quality comparisons +5% (inter-quartile range +3% to 11%) Larger effects seen if baseline compliance is low	Resources required largely relate to costs of data abstraction. May be relatively cheap if data can be abstracted by routine administrative systems.	Feasibility may depend upon availability of high quality administrative data.

(Continued)

Table 40.3 (*Contd.*) Summary of key findings from overviews of reviews

Reminders (Shojania et al., 2009)	Patient or encounter specific information, provided on a computer screen, which is designed or intended to prompt a health professional to recall information	Individual professional cognitive/ memory barriers	28 RCTs Generally effective Median effect across 32 comparisons +4.2% (interquartile range 0.8% to 18.8%)	Resources vary across deliver mechanism. Increasing use of computerised reminders – where inclusion of reminders has relatively modest cost	Insufficient knowledge about how to prioritise and optimise reminders
Multi-faceted interventions (Grimshaw et al., 2004)	An intervention including two or more components	Target multiple barriers of the included intervention components	Grimshaw and colleagues failed to demonstrate a dose response analysis (ie the apparent effects of interventions did not increase with the number of components)	Likely more costly than single interventions	Need to carefully consider how to combine interventions to ensure additive or synergistic effects (eg interventions that include components that target same barriers may not be additive/synergistic)

CDSS, clinical decision support system; RCT, randomized controlled trial.
Used with permission from Grimshaw et al. (in press).

targeting subjective norm and graded tasks—i.e. starting with easy tasks first—targeting self-efficacy) (Eccles et al., 2009).

There is a substantial evidence base about the effects of different behaviour change interventions across all areas of clinical practice. The Cochrane Effective Practice and Organisation of Care group has identified over 6000 primary studies and 200 systematic reviews of interventions to improve health care delivery and health care systems. Table 40.3 summarizes key findings from these systematic reviews across all clinical behaviours—most interventions are effective under some circumstances usually resulting in moderate improvements in clinical care. This reinforces the need to carefully select interventions based upon the factors identified above (Grimshaw et al., in press). There is less specific evidence about the effects of interventions to improve mental health practice. Weinmann and colleagues reviewed 18 implementation studies in mental health care settings and found that few have shown any effective uptake of psychiatric guidelines (Weinmann et al., 2007). Similarly, Gilbody and colleagues conducted a systematic review to examine the impact of educational and organizational interventions to improve depression management in primary care and found that education and passive dissemination strategies were not very effective (Gilbody et al., 2003). However, organizational changes were more effective. Gilbody and colleagues later examined the higher costs associated with these interventions (Gilbody et al., 2006).

At present there is an incomplete knowledge to guide the choice of dissemination and implementation strategies and mental health professionals and organizations need to use considerable judgement when choosing their strategies.

Monitoring knowledge use and evaluation of outcomes

Once a set of guidelines have been implemented, there should initially be a detailed monitoring process to determine uptake and outcomes. For example, this may include a chart audit several months after the implementation of new guidelines to determine whether practice has changed and patient outcomes have improved. Unfortunately, detailed monitoring such as chart audits cannot be sustained over time given the required additional resources.

Therefore, over time, less resource intensive methods for monitoring and evaluation of outcomes will have to be used such as the analyses of data drawn from databases such as electronic medical records or computerized physician order entry systems, once these become more widespread.

Sustaining ongoing knowledge use

After the implementation of guidelines into clinical practice, how does one sustain ongoing knowledge use? First, organizations need to develop processes and policies that promote the sustained use of new knowledge. For example, the responsibility of keeping up to date regarding changes in best practice need to be delegated to someone within the organization, and resources need to be dedicated to the dissemination of these changes. Other resources are also needed to maintain existing incorporation of best practices such as ongoing reminders to professionals. Therefore, professionals and organizations have to be prepared and well-resourced to handle these potential barriers to sustained uptake of knowledge.

Once guidelines have been translated into clinical practice, professionals and organizations also need to monitor the emergence of new knowledge that might make guideline recommendations out of date. Whilst this is often undertaken by guideline development agencies, mental health organizations likely need to share some responsibility for this Furthermore, although there is often concern about guidelines becoming out of date, there is good evidence that guidelines do not generally become out of date quickly. In fact, new evidence that may emerge and shift recommendations are generally related to major clinical trials, therefore allowing for a much less labour intensive process (limited search strategies for new literature) to update older guidelines. Several resources are available to professionals and organizations interested in learning more about this process (Shekelle et al., 2001).

Summary

Although guidelines can be used to improve patient care, successful uptake and change in practice based on new knowledge requires active interventions. There are several steps that mental health professionals and organizations can follow in order to aid in the implementation of guidelines in clinical settings. After identifying an area of clinical practice requiring improvement, professionals and organizations need to find and adapt or, in rare instances, develop guidelines that are appropriate for their setting. The identification of barriers to effective uptake is also a critical step in this process so that professionals and organizations can tailor their implementation strategies to overcome specific barriers. Finally, the ongoing use of knowledge requires changes in processes and policies as well as resources to maintain improvements and to keep up to date with new emerging knowledge.

Although this area of research in mental health is still in its infancy and the evidence for the implementation of mental health guidelines is limited, there is a broader literature that can inform the work of professionals and organizations interested in improving clinical care.

References

Bero, L., Eccles, M., Grilli, R., Grimshaw, J., Gruen, R.L., Mayhew, A., et al. (2007). Cochrane Effective Practice and Organisation of Care Group. About The Cochrane Collaboration (Cochrane Review Groups (CRGs)), Issue 4, Art. No.: EPOC.

Bokhoven, M.A., Kok, G., and van der Weijden, T. (2003). Quality improvement research: Designing a quality improvement intervention: a systematic approach. *Quality and Safety in Health Care*, **12**, 215–20.

Cheung, A., Zuckerbrot, R.A., Jensen, P.S., Ghalib, K., Stein, R.K., Laraque, D., *et al.* (2007). Guidelines for Adolescent Depression in Primary Care–GLAD PC–Part II. Pediatrics. *Pediatrics*, **120**, e1313–26.

Doumit, G. (2006). *Opinion leaders: Effectiveness, Identification, Stability, Specificity, and Mechanism of Action*. Ottawa: University Of Ottawa.

Doumit, G., Gattellari, M., Grimshaw, J., O'Brien, M.A. (2007). Local opinion leaders: effects on professional practice and health care outcomes. *Cochrane Database Syst Rev*, (1), CD000125.

Ebell, M.H., Siwek, J., Weiss, B.D., Woolf, S.H., Susman, J. Ewigman, B., *et al.* (2004). Strength of Recommendation Taxonomy (SORT): A patient-centered approach to grading evidence in the medical literature. *American Family Physician*, **69**, 548–56.

Eccles, M., Francis, J., Foy, R., Johnston, M., Bamford, C., Grimshaw, J.M., *et al.* (2009). Improving professional practice in the disclosure of a diagnosis of dementia: A modeling experiment to evaluate a theory-based intervention. *International Journal of Behavioural Medicine*, **16**, 377–87.

Farmer, A.P., Legare, F., Turcot, L., Grimshaw, J., Harvey, E., McGowan, J.L., et al. (2008). Printed educational materials: effects on professional practice and health care outcomes. *Cochrane Database Syst Rev*, (3), CD004398.

Feldman, M.D., Franks, P., Duberstein, P.R., *Vannoy, S., Epstein, R., and Kravitz, R.L.* (2007). Let's not talk about it: Inquiring suicide in primary care. *Annals of Family Medicine*, **5**, 412–18.

Forsetlund, L., Bjorndal, A., Rashidian, A., Jamtvedt, G., O'Brien, MA., Wolf, F., et al. (2009). Continuing education meetings and workshops: effects on professional practice and health care outcomes. *Cochrane Database of Systematic Reviews*, (2), CD003030.

Foy, R., Francis, J.J., Johnston, M., Eccles, M., Lecouturier, J., Bamford, C., *et al.* (2007). The development of a theory-based intervention to promote the appropriate disclosure of a diagnosis of dementia. *BMC Health Services Research*, **7**, 207.

Gilbody, S., Whitty, P., Grimshaw, J., and Thomas, R. (2003). Educational and organizational interventions to improve the management of depression in primary care: a systematic review. *Journal of the American Medical Association*, **289**, 3145–51.

Gilbody, S., Bower, P., and Whitty, P.M. (2006). The costs and consequences of enhanced primary care for depression: a systematic

review of randomised economic evaluations. *British Journal of Psychiatry*, **189**, 297–308.

Graham, I.D., Harrison, M.B., Brouwers, M., Davies, B.L., and Dunn, S. (2002). Facilitating the use of evidence in practice: evaluating and adapting clinical practice guidelines for local use by health care organizations. *Journal of Obstetric, Gynecologic & Neonatal Nursing*, **31**, 599–611.

Graham, I.D., Logan, J., Harrison, B., Straus, S.E., Tetroe, J., Caswell, W., *et al.* (2006). Lost in knowledge translation: Time for a Map? *Journal of Continuing Education in the Health Professions*, **26**, 13–24.

Grimshaw, J.M., Shirran, L., Thomas, R., Mowatt, G., Fraser, C., Bero, L., *et al.* (2001). Changing provider behavior: an overview of systematic reviews of interventions. *Medical Care*, **39**, II2–45.

Grimshaw, J.M., Thomas, R.E., Maclennan, G., Fraser, C., Ramsay, C.R., Vale, L., et al. (2004). Effectiveness and efficiency of guideline dissemination and implementation strategies. *Health Technol Assess*, **8**(6), iii–72.

Grimshaw, J.M., Thomas, R.E., MacLennan, G. *et al.* (2005). Effectiveness and efficiency of guideline dissemination and implementation strategies. *International Journal of Technology Assessment in Health Care*, **21**, 149.

Grimshaw, J.M., Schunneman, H., Cook, D., *et al.* Integrating and coordinating efforts in chronic obstructive pulmonary disease (COPD) guideline development–guideline dissemination and implementation. In press.

Hayward, R.S.A., Wilson, M.C., Tunis, S.R., Bass, E.B., and Guyatt, G. (1995). Users' Guides to the Medical Literature. VII. How to use clinical practice guidelines. A Are the recommendations valid? *Journal of the American Medical Association*, **274**, 570–4.

Hellerstein, D.J., Staub, A.B., and Lequesne, E. (2007). Decreasing the use of restraint and seclusion among psychiatric inpatients. *Journal of Psychiatric Practice*, **13**, 308–17.

Institute of Medicine (1990). *Clinical Practice Guidelines: Directions for a New Program*, p. 38 (Field M.J. and Lohr K.N. eds.). Washington, DC: National Academy Press.

Jamtvedt, G., Young, J.M., Kristoffersen, D.T., O'Brien, M.A., Oxman, A.D. (2006). Audit and feedback: effects on professional practice and health care outcomes. *Cochrane Database Syst Rev*, (2), CD000259.

Kendall, T. and Pilling, S. (2004). The National Collaborating Centre for Mental Health. In: Whitty, P. and Eccles, M. (eds.) *Clinical Practice Guidelines in Mental Health*, pp. 81–92. Oxford: Radcliffe Publishing.

Lomas, J. (1991). Making clinical policy explicit: legislative policy making and lessons for developing practice guidelines. *International Journal of Technology and Assessment in Health Care*, **13**, 35–9.

Mackin, P., Bishop, D.R., and Helen, M.O. (2007). A prospective study of monitoring practices for metabolic disease in antipsychotic-treated community psychiatric patients. *BMC Psychiatry*, **7**, 28.

Mason, J., Freemantle, N., Nazareth, I., Eccles, M., Haines, A., Drummond, M. (2001). When is it cost-effective to change the behavior of health professionals? *JAMA*, **286**(23), 2988–92.

O'Brien, M.A., Rogers, S., Jamtvedt, G., Oxman, A., Odgaard-Jensen, J., Kristoffersen, D., et al. (2007). Educational outreach visits: effects on professional practice and health care outcomes. *Cochrane Database Syst Rev*, (4), CD000409.

Phillips, L.J., McGorry, P.D., Yung, A.R., McGlashan, T.H., Cornblatt, B., and Klosterkotter, J. (2005). Prepsychotic phase of schizophrenia and related disorders: recent progress and future opportunities. *British Journal of Psychiatry*, **187**, s33–s44.

Shekelle, P., Eccles, M., Grimshaw, J., and Woolf, S. (2001). When should clinical guidelines be updated? *British Medical Journal*, **323**, 255–7.

Shojania, K.G., Jennings, A., Mayhew, A., Ramsay, C.R., Eccles, M.P., Grimshaw, J. (2009). The effects of on-screen, point of care computer reminders on processes and outcomes of care. *Cochrane Database of Systematic Reviews*, (3), CD001096.

Soumerai, S.B., Avorn, J. (1990). Principles of educational outreach ('academic detailing') to improve clinical decision making. *JAMA*, **263**(4), 549–56.

Weinmann, S., Koesters, M., and Becker, T. (2007). Effects of implementation of psychiatric guidelines on provider performance and patient outcome: systematic review. *Acta Psychiatrica Scandinavica*, **115**, 420–33.

Wilson, M.C., Hayward, R.S.A., Tunis, S.R., Bass, E.B., and Guyatt, G. (1995). Users' Guides to the Medical Literature. VII. How to use clinical practice guidelines. B. What are the recommendations and will they help you in caring for your patients? *Journal of the American Medical Association*, **274**, 1630–2.

Zuckerbrot, R.A., Cheung, A., Jensen, P.S., Stein, R.K., Laraque, D., and GLAD PC Steering Group. (2007). Guidelines for adolescent depression in primary care–GLAD PC–Part I. *Pediatrics*, **120**, e1299–312.

Appendix **Electronic Guideline Resources**

Mental Health Specific

CANMAT Canadian Network for Mood and Anxiety Treatments: http://www.canmat.org/

AACAP American Academy of Child and Adolescent Psychiatry practice parameters: http://www.aacap.org/cs/root/publication_store/practice_parameters_and_guidelines

APA American Psychiatric Association: http://psychiatry.org/psych_pract/treatg/pg/prac_guide.cfm

General (includes all medical disorders)

Australia NHMRC National Health and Medical Research Council: http://www.nhmrc.gov.au/guidelines/index.htm

CMA Canadian Medical Association Clinical Practice Guidelines Infobase: www.cma.ca/cpgs/index/html

GAC Guidelines Advisory Committee: http://www.gacguidelines.ca/index.cfm

New Zealand Guidelines Group: http://www.nzgg.org.nz/

NICE National Institute for Clinical Excellence: http://www.nice.org.uk

Scottish Intercollegiate Guidelines Network: http://www.sign.ac.uk/

Overcoming impediments to community mental health in low- and middle-income countries

Benedetto Saraceno, Mark van Ommeren, and Rajaie Batniji

Introduction

As discussed in Chapter 6 by Wang and colleagues, the prevalence of mental disorders across the world—and across low- and middle-income countries (LAMIC)—is high. The median rate across the world of having at least one mental disorder in the last year is 10% (WHO WMHS Consortium, 2004). The impact of these disorders on disability, other aspects of health, and development is substantial. Yet, the vast majority of people with a mental disorder are not in contact with services that offer mental health care (Wang et al., Chapter 6, this volume), Importantly, the association between severe mental disorder and human rights violations is strong (WHO, 2001). Even among people with severe mental disorders, few people receive adequate, humane care (WHO, 2001) and discrimination is pervasive (Thornicroft, 2006). It is clear that there is an urgent need to act.

The World Health Organization (WHO, 2003) developed a mental health policy and planning package to help countries to develop services that provide access to adequate care for people with mental disorder. This package was preceded and followed by evidence-informed and evidence-based advocacy through major publications—such as *World Health Report 2001* on mental health (WHO, 2001), the *World Mental Health Report* (Desjarlais et al., 1995), *Neurological, Psychiatric, and Developmental Disorders* (Institute of Medicine, 2001), *Disease Control Priorities related to Mental Neurological, Developmental and Substance Abuse Disorders* (WHO and Disease Control Priorities Project, 2006), the 2007 *Lancet* Series on Global Mental Health, and the 2008 mental health Gap Action Plan (WHO, 2008). Although most research evidence on interventions comes from specialized care settings in high-income countries, fortunately there are good indications that much of this evidence generalizes to LAMIC (Patel, 2007).

A naïve observer would perhaps expect that with this amount of burden, human rights violations, high-level advocacy, technical guidance, and evidence for interventions, that mental health service development in LAMIC is flourishing. Indeed, it should be. Although it is true that some countries have made major strides, the reality however has been that mental health service development in most LAMIC has been a challenge. This chapter will address some key impediments in developing mental health services in LAMIC and will offer strategies to address these impediments.

Financial resources

As in other areas of health (Laxminarayan et al., 2006), to implement evidence-based policy and practice, financial resources are needed. Resources allocated towards mental health care are insufficient or are ineffectively distributed in (LAMIC) (Saxena et al., 2007). There are many explanations for the low levels of financing for mental health. None of these reasons are independent of one other; rather, they interact and together form a formidable block to the allocation of appropriate funds, whether by foreign donors, ministries of health or ministries of finance. In this section we will describe a variety of reasons for the lack of funding.

In most countries there is a lack of strong, coordinated, and consistent lobbying and political pressure to increase resources for mental health services. Without strong advocacy, mental health will not be high on the public health agenda and political will and funds will remain inadequate

This lack of strong advocacy stems from discrepancies about both the intended purpose of advocacy and the differing targets of advocacy. There appear to be two, implicitly stated disagreements regarding the purpose of global mental health advocacy. First, a disagreement on whom to help—some advocates suggest that the goal is to help the severely mentally ill, while others advocate for support for mild mental health problems. Second, among those who agree on which group to focus their advocacy, there is disagreement on how this should be done—some advocates focus on more a medical model, while others call for a combined medical and social model.

To scale up community mental health services, it is extremely helpful to develop a consensus in advocacy messages among the national mental health community (e.g. service providers, professional associations, senior government leaders in mental health, academics, and national policy-makers), as fragmentation at this level has prevented action in many settings.

Lobbying efforts towards policy and legislation is important but focusing on legislation and policy alone is insufficient. In reality, successful advocacy is also needed to ensure that these are funded, implemented, and translated into services. Coordinated advocacy groups need to continue their work through and beyond the legislative/policy process.

Mental health financing in countries—which is usually extremely low (see Chisholm and Knapp, Chapter 33, this volume)—may be more likely to be increased if there was more advocacy from service users, families, and service providers, including non-governmental organizations (NGOs). People with disorders and their families can be a powerful constituency to press for better mental health care with sufficient funding at local levels. Service-providing NGOs, with close community connections, often serve as advocates and coordinating centres for local advocacy. Such local advocacy will go furthest when in concert with appropriately coordinated national-level advocacy.

Part of the reason for the frequent political (and thus financial) inaction on mental health may unfortunately be attributed to the low level of interest from the public in issues of mental health. Stigma and discrimination pose a challenge to mobilizing the community to be involved in advocacy, perhaps making it especially important that people who receive mental health care are involved in lobbying.

Public advocacy will make investment in mental health more politically palatable, though there is a challenge. In developing coordinated advocacy, the interests of different groups (service users, family members, and mental health specialists) may vary greatly within and between groups. For example, different users have been seen to work towards different objectives, ranging from 1) less or no psychiatric interventions to 2) more, humane community and socially oriented mental health services to 3) better access to new psychotropic medications. (Indeed, some user organizations are funded by industry while others insist on independence from industry.) Similarly, psychiatrists are not a monolithic group. Opposing advocacy from different stakeholders may result in inaction on the part of governments. Thus, it is necessary to develop a clear consensus and plan for action among the national mental health community. Disagreements on goals to be achieved among a community of mental health specialists limits funding and abilities for policy change. Any internal division among mental health experts and decision-makers is an obstacle to coordinated and effective advocacy.

A prominent explanation for the lack of mental health funding concerns the role of donors and the international community as agenda setters. For example, mental health does not appear in the Millennium Development Goals (MDGs; Miranda and Patel, 2005). Unfortunately, in several countries, exclusion of mental health from the MDGs has directly obstructed the financing of mental health services by international donors even in countries where national authorities made mental health a priority (e.g. Afghanistan, Rwanda). When international agencies and donors do not prioritize mental health, there is reduced incentive for national policy-makers to address this issue. Furthermore, ministry of health staff and funds are often directed towards implementing donor-supported programmes.

Communicable disease, especially HIV/AIDS, has been the funding priority for donors and national leaders, and this has been a barrier to securing funds for mental health services in sub-Saharan Africa. This challenge should be converted into opportunity by integrating mental health services into HIV/AIDS programmes (Freeman, 2000). Rather than compete with communicable disease, integrating mental health care into communicable disease health care programmes may be extremely helpful to funding care for the large percentage of people with mostly mild and moderate common mental disorders. Yet, it is unlikely to provide a solution to the problem of organizing care for people with chronic, severe mental disorders.

There seem to be common, but incorrect, beliefs that mental health interventions are ineffective, economically inefficient, and too costly. Perceptions of cost-ineffective services need to be addressed with evidence and political pressure. It should be noted that any discussion of cost-effectiveness depends greatly on the mental disorder being considered (WHO, 2006). The treatment of severe mental disorders may be relatively less cost-effective but they still may provide good value for money (Chisholm et al., 2008).

Critics of the discussion on cost-efficacy point to the human rights of the mentally ill. Because of the prevalence of human rights violations against people with mental disorders (even at times by the professionals who are supposed to care for them), there is a strong moral case for providing effective and humane mental health care (Patel et al., 2006).

Epidemiological data have highlighted the tremendous global burden of mental disease. It is unclear to what extent epidemiological data are helpful in putting mental health on the agenda. In fact, in many cases such data are easily misunderstood or not very informative (e.g. depression prevalence rates typically do not distinguish between mild and severe depression, which are very different public health issues). Moreover, in some circumstances rates of poor quality studies tend to be higher than rates of stronger studies (Steel et al., 2009) and policy makers may be put off by over-advocacy with rates that are not credible. Nonetheless, epidemiological data can have advocacy value if attention to new local evidence prompts health planners to invest in mental health.

Organization of services

The integration of mental health care into general health services occurs mainly in two forms: mental health care delivered by general health workers in primary care settings or through specific programmes addressing physical disease (HIV/AIDS, tuberculosis). Additionally, although not covered here, integration into general health care services could include, for example, liaison psychiatric services in general hospitals.

The term 'dedicated mental health care' is used for mental health care delivered by workers performing full-time mental health work through specific mental health services (e.g. outpatient psychiatry, inpatient care by mental health specialists at general hospitals, mental hospitals). One could also speak of a hybrid model of general care when a worker's time is fully dedicated to providing mental health care in a primary care clinical setting.

How different types of services are organized/configured/mixed within a mental health system tends to have an impact on the effective treatment coverage of people with diverse mental disorders. A mixed model of care, in which mental health care is available at multiple levels of care, is, without doubt, the ideal, but reflection is needed on how services decision-makers should invest their available, limited resources for mental health care (WHO, 2003).

As described earlier in this book (Thornicroft et al., Chapter 12), resources and expertise for mental health care need to be geographically decentralized for people to have access to them, and a system needs to be created that makes treatment for acute and chronic mental illness and the corresponding social and rehabilitation services available at the community level. There is thus a need to move staff and financial resources into the community, and this is an enormous challenge. This requires allocation of funds to different regions and subregions of countries, and the funding should cover general mental health clinics covering a range of disorders, rather than vertical programmes for very specific pathologies.

NGOs often play an irreplaceable role in providing community mental health services. However, in some countries NGOs have difficulties in establishing themselves and, even when established, some NGOs may create their own set of problems. In some locations existing NGOs may be unhelpful by grossly inflating reports on the level and quality of social services that they (the NGOs) provide to the mentally ill. This gives the message that there is no need for government to invest in mental health, as the NGO already has done all the work.

Like in high-income countries, developing community mental health care in LAMIC requires linking mental health more closely with other non-health sector services. Social services are part of, or complementary to, decentralized specialist mental health care, and this should be reflected in the structure of such services. Depending on the setting, linkages that reach beyond the social services sector to traditional and/or religious healers may be appropriate.

Much of the discussion of community involvement in mental health focuses on the crucial role of families and community organizations, especially in rehabilitation, and the need to spread resources and expertise beyond mental health hospitals. There is a need for the 'grassroots' creation and management of mental health programmes, emphasizing collaboration with community members and NGOs. Decentralization and deinstitutionalization—two conceptually distinct but often overlapping processes—open up many opportunities to involve communities and families in mental health care.

Substantial resistance to the decentralization of health resources arises in many countries that have attempted to spread resources to the periphery and to social programmes. Resistance to social services can be substantial, because it involves an understanding of mental disorders outside the medical model.

To assist with these challenges, technical support for LAMIC is needed to develop financing schemes for community-based approaches. It is important to understand the separate sectoral costs (e.g. health care, housing, employment) in attempting to create an integrated, multisectoral mental health programme (WHO, 2003). Problems in mental health financing also arise when mental health policy created at the national level requires financing at the subnational level, where decision-makers may not feel as responsible for implementing national-level policy. This has occurred in South Africa and Pakistan (WHO, 2007).

An important—although often difficult—step in decentralizing mental health resources is downsizing existing mental hospitals

(WHO, 2001). Mental hospitals have poor coverage, tend to put people at elevated risk of human rights violations, and absorb a disproportionate amount of resources (WHO, 2001).

Worryingly, some of the most persistent barriers to the implementation of such community programmes appear to be the vested interests of psychiatrists and other hospital workers. These interests can be an obstacle to funding, deinstitutionalization, and the expansion of a mental health workforce. Concerns about job security have delayed moves to community-based care. The staff and leadership of psychiatric institutions are too often willing and able to exert influence that opposes the political will to reform mental health services. Thus, in pursuit of mental health service reform, psychiatrists should be seen as stakeholders, not just as providers.

Financial incentives and professional self-interest have led too many psychiatrists and mental health staff to resist deinstitutionalization and any restructuring of care to the community level, and to oppose expansion of the workforce and public health models of care. Downsizing hospitals can be an understandable threat to the economic and professional interests of those who work in hospitals. Financial and professional guarantees need to be thus put in place for hospital staff during the period of transformation.

In our experience and in that of a range of experts that we interviewed (Saraceno, 2007, opposition to downsizing hospitals in favour of community-based care most often comes from trade unions and hospital staff of various levels. It is thus important that the reform process incorporates these groups, so that they may be offered roles in the community-based secondary mental health system. It should be recognized that psychiatrists may also resist attempts to expand the mental health workforce to have non-psychiatrists or non-doctors provide management of mental disorders. Such resistance to changing mental health services is often taken up by professional associations, which make it difficult to cultivate the united political will to pursue reforms.

Despite much agreement among international mental health experts regarding deinstitutionalization (Saraceno, 2007), there often exist some controversy and debate in society—especially when it is implemented in a problematic manner. For example, more than 30 years ago, dehospitalization (often confused with the complex process of deinstitutionalization) has led many mentally ill persons living on the streets in North America in places where deinstitutionalization was done without the creation of community-based services. Mental health advocates should be clear that talking about closing a hospital leads to understandable resistance and any talk about closing hospitals should be accompanied with a well-communicated, strong plan about developing care in the community.

Downsizing or closing mental hospitals is likely to result in failure if not accompanied with secondary care and community services. Indeed, the likely reason for Brazil's mental health reform's success is the increase of secondary level care that has co-occurred with the decrease of mental hospital beds. The need to downsize mental hospitals thus coexists with the need to develop community mental health services. Challenges to developing community mental health services may transform into challenges to downsizing mental hospitals. Decision-makers are sometimes unwilling to downsize and/or close mental hospitals—due to the political risk of facing vested interests. Deinstitutionalization is technically complex and cannot occur without adequate community mental health services in place. Thus, any downsizing of mental hospitals should be concurrent with improving community-based inpatient care for the mentally ill. Additional funding will be needed during the transition to community care. Yet, as we discussed earlier, to raise funds unified advocacy is important and this advocacy will be weaker if public health planners and health staff disagree about the need to decentralize. The need for unified, ethical solution is urgent given the inhumane living conditions in many mental hospitals.

Integration of mental health care in primary health care (PHC) is essential to obtain good coverage. However, poorly executed integration of mental health into primary care leads to undertrained, unsupervised primary care workers who are not sufficiently competent in the care (identification and treatment and/or referral) they are supposed to provide. Even if technically competent in clinical management, they may not know how to manage their time in such a way to find time for mental health care during their day. Moreover, without appropriate training and supervision, overburdened primary care staff are at risk of increasing their reliance on pharmaceuticals, leading to narrow biomedical support even for people with subthreshold problems. Integrating mental health in PHC thus requires planning (WHO, 2007). Finally, in many LAMIC essential psychotropic medicines are often not continuously available at the PHC level—a barrier that hinders appropriate care for those people whose disorders can be effectively treated through medication.

Investment in community mental health services and supervision of PHC workers by mental health specialists is critical to the success of the primary care model. This observation is in line with the WHO (1978) Alma-Ata Declaration, which promoted a primary care model 'sustained by integrated, functional and mutually supportive referral systems' as an integral part of a country's health system.

Strengthening the workforce

A commitment to strengthening the mental health workforce by training staff in the community and by expanding the base of providers will require a new role for mental health professionals, one focused on training and supervision, and one that involves the mobilization of families and communities in care and rehabilitation.

Improving the structure of the mental health system in LAMIC depends fundamentally on the availability of an adequate mental health workforce. Mental health training needs to move beyond hospitals and universities and beyond theoretical sessions, to a continual process of supervision and mentorship in the community they serve. This applies to the training of psychiatrists, medical officers, and primary care providers, as well as paraprofessionals in mental health. International collaboration for training can be helpful as countries have much to learn from one other. Training through hands-on supervised clinical work is likely of greatest benefit (WHO, 2007). Training in psychiatric hospitals for undergraduate medical students is particularly unhelpful to teach them how to address mental health in primary care settings. It is suggested that training should take place regularly, in clinical settings in the community and under the dedicated supervision of mental health specialists, rather than through one-off workshops. Therefore, mental health support in the community may depend on a shift in the role of mental health experts from clinical care to one of supervision.

Providers in the general health care system—e.g. community health workers, PHC staff—should be further trained in mental health. Yet, when they are overburdened with other responsibilities, it can be helpful to find, train, and supervise new groups of workers altogether. Training dedicated community mental health workers can be extremely valuable, especially when their roles are recognized and endorsed by governments.

Furthermore, lay individuals in the community can be trained to appropriately refer persons for further care. As for other groups, such training requires adequate post-training supervision from professionals. In particular, it can be valuable to more formally involve families in providing care, and to empower them as advocates. Service users may be involved in care as well, e.g. there can be a role for users as staff in supported housing programmes. To best involve families in care, they need the support of trained personnel, who can provide support and guide the use of medications. Family care may be especially useful in rural areas, providing families are given appropriate support by trained mental health staff.

Involving families makes them stakeholders in mental health. The resulting advocacy can have an impact on policy. In addition to involving families, the involvement of service users in advocacy is likely to lead to increased funding for community mental health services to facilitate responsible deinstitutionalization and greater community integration, as we have discussed above. Thus involving families and users has value both from a human resource and an advocacy perspective.

The involvement of families is complemented by the involvement of the community, and is consistent with using participatory action approaches, which have been common in rural development and which are now also used by some mental health NGOs (Underhill, 2002). Such approaches are also increasingly common in psychosocial programmes in emergencies (IASC, 2007).

As touched upon earlier, making mental health care broadly available necessitates a supervisory role for mental health specialists. Psychiatrists need to focus their efforts on training other health workers. Developing a broader base of mental health care providers in general health services and in community-based mental services, depends on mentorship and community-based training. To restructure care the specialist must be motivated to switch to a training and supervisory role. This may require financial incentives.

Public mental health leadership

Mental health leaders in LAMIC—such as directors of mental health in ministries of health—have responsibility for the complex tasks of increasing funding, making mental health care more broadly available, developing a system for secondary, primary, and community care and reforming hospitals, among other challenges. Such tasks require not only a familiarity with the needs and possible supports for diverse people with mental disorders, but also population-based, public health vision and skills. The skills for such leadership need to be developed, or sought from outside psychiatry, from the academic discipline of public health.

The rarity of public health-minded approaches in mental health care may be due in part to the nature of existing evidence-based interventions which are mostly at the individual level, and also to the training of mental health leaders that tends to have focused on clinical care only. The rarity of adequate public mental health leadership may also be due to a lack of incentives for psychiatrists to take a public health view, and also to a lack of authority for non-psychiatrists attempting to engage such a view.

Training courses for public mental health leaders are needed. Training leaders in public mental health may greatly improve mental health strategies in LAMIC countries. Promisingly, an International Master in Mental Health Policy and Services has commenced in Lisbon, in collaboration with WHO.

International assistance—laterally with other LAMIC or with international agencies—and incentives can play a crucial role in developing public mental health leadership. With concern that any programme should be adapted to local settings, it can be extremely helpful to have lateral, regional, and global cooperation for mentoring and for sharing models of success. International networks— such as Global Forum for Community Mental Health (http://www.gfcmh.com/)—can also play an important role.

Conclusion

Making mental health services available in the community in LAMIC is a must. Community mental health services, compared to institutionalized care, give greater coverage. Also, community care has a lower risk of human rights violations introduced by the care system. Yet, there are impediments to developing community services, as reviewed in this chapter. In particular, the interests of mental health care providers (and often family members as well) favours institutions. Also, there is the challenge that developing mental health care in the community involves start-up costs, which requires a substantial increase in resources, which are most easily raised when key stakeholders agree on how to move to community services.

The formation of national plans for mental health, developed in a participatory manner with service providers and users among other stakeholders, is an excellent vehicle for coordinating advocacy. Such plans are needed not only because good planning helps service development, but also because good plans are a helpful vehicle for fund-raising. By functioning as a coherent proposal for services, a national plan, endorsed by the minister of health, can facilitate sound financing from different levels of government and can be used as a proposal to international donors. Such plans can thus break the vicious cycle between lack of unified advocacy and lack of resources

This chapter also covers other barriers. With respect to human resources, diversifying the mental health workforce is key. Psychiatrists should increasingly move from direct service provision to training/supervising non-psychiatrists (e.g. PHC staff) in mental health care. This change in roles is essential to increase coverage in the community. Incentives—including financial incentives—for such change in roles need to be made available.

This chapter discussed the challenges related to integrating mental health care in PHC, which includes the need for supervision, but also the limited time that PHC providers have for mental health. Greater efforts need to be extended to work with PHC providers on time management for providing mental health care. For example, PHC providers may task-shift some of the work by involving community workers or, alternatively, they may dedicate specific, relatively quiet, times of the week to mental health care, during which they schedule appointments with appropriate amount of time for each patients (Jones et al., 2009). Making dedicated time for mental health care is justifiable given the high prevalence of mental health problems in PHC (Ustun and Sartorius, 1995).

Psychiatrists will continue to play key roles in many countries and, as mentioned earlier, they should lead the clinical supervision of mental health treatment in the health sector. Yet, this chapter provides reasons to doubt whether clinicians are best placed to lead mental health services development in countries unless they have a public health training and perspective to facilitate planning at the population level. There is a need for better access to public mental health leadership training for key decision-makers in LAMIC.

We end this chapter with two observations and a conclusion. The first observation is that integration of mental health into PHC in rural districts works best if secondary care is in place first so that secondary care mental health experts can supervise the integration into PHC. The second observation is that decentralization from tertiary care to community care works best if secondary care is in place first, in order to provide access to care to people who would otherwise go to tertiary care. Accordingly we conclude that countries should consider prioritizing developing mental health in secondary care (e.g. accessible outpatient mental health clinics staffed by multidisciplinary teams, small acute psychiatry wards in general hospital) to be followed by the important work of integrating mental health at the primary care level and decentralizing the tertiary care level.

Acknowledgements

This chapter is based on a written key informant survey with international experts conducted in 2006 to 2007 (WHO, 2007). In this chapter, we represent the entire body of lessons we learned from the study. We thank Jessica Mears for her valuable comments on an earlier draft of this chapter.

References

Chisholm, D., Gureje, O., Saldivia, S., Villalón Calderón, M., Wickremasinghe, R., Mendis, N., *et al.* (2008). Schizophrenia treatment in the developing world: an interregional and multinational cost-effectiveness analysis. *Bulletin of the World Health Organization,* **86**, 542–51.

Desjarlais, R., Eisenberg, L., Good, B., and Kleinman, A. (1995). *World mental health: problems and priorities in low-income countries.* New York: Oxford University Press.

Freeman, M. (2000). Using all opportunities for improving mental health— examples from South Africa. *Bulletin of the World Health Organization,* **78**, 508–10.

IASC (2007). *IASC guidelines of mental health and psychosocial support in emergency settings.* Geneva: Inter-Agency Standing Committee.

Institute of Medicine (2001). *Neurological, psychiatric, and developmental disorders: meeting the challenge in the developing world.* Washington, DC: National Academy Press.

Jones, L., Asare, J.B., El Masri, M., Mohanraj, A., Sherief, H., Van Ommeren, M. (2009). Severe mental disorders in complex emergencies. *Lancet,* **374,** 654–61.

Laxminarayan, R., Mills, A.J., Breman, J.G., Measham, A.R., Alleyne, G., Claeson, M., *et al.* (2006). Advancement of global health: key messages from the Disease Control Priorities Project. *Lancet,* **367**, 1193–208.

Miranda, J.J. and Patel, V. (2005). Achieving the Millennium Development Goals: does mental health play a role? *PLoS Medicine,* **2**, e291.

Patel, V., Saraceno, B., and Kleinman, A. (2006). Beyond evidence: the moral case for international mental health. *American Journal of Psychiatry,* **163**, 1312–5.

Patel, V., Araya, R., Chatterjee, .S, Chisholm, D., Cohen, A., De Silva, M., *et al.* (2007). Treatment and prevention of mental disorders in low-income and middle-income countries. *Lancet,* **370**, 991–1005.

Saraceno, B., van Ommeren, M., Batniji, R., Cohen, A., Gureje, O., Mahoney, J., *et al.* (2007). Barriers to improvement of mental health services in low-income and middle-income countries. *Lancet,* **370**, 1164–74.

Saxena, S., Thornicroft, G., Knapp, M., and Whiteford, H. (2007). Resources for mental health: scarcity, inequity, and inefficiency. *Lancet*, **370**, 878–89.

Steel, Z., Chey, T., Silove, D., Marnane, C., Bryant, R.A., and van Ommeren, M. (2009). Association of torture and other potentially traumatic events with mental health outcomes among populations exposed to mass conflict and displacement: a systematic review and meta-analysis. *Journal of the American Medical Association*, **302**, 537–49.

Thornicroft, G. (2006). *Shunned: Discrimination against People with Mental Illness*. Oxford: Oxford University Press.

Underhill, C. (2002). Mental health and development: from the local to the global. The involvement of mentally ill people in the development process. *Asian Pacific Disability & Rehabilitation Journal*, **2**, 1–15.

Ustun, T.B. and Sartorius, N. (1995). *Mental Illness in General Health Care: an International Study*. Chichester: John Wiley and Sons.

WHO (1978). 'Declaration of Alma-Ata.' International Conference on Primary Health Care, Alma-Ata, USSR, 6–12 September, 1978

WHO (2001). *World Health Report 2001: Mental Health*. Geneva: World Health Organization.

WHO (2003). *Mental Health Policy and Service Guidance Package*. Geneva: World Health Organization.

WHO (2006). *Dollars, DALYs and decisions: economic aspects of the mental health system*. Geneva: World Health Organization.

WHO (2007). *Expert Opinion on Barriers and Facilitating Factors for the Implementation of Existing Mental Health Knowledge in Mental Health Services*. Geneva: World Health Organization.

WHO (2008). *mhGAP Mental Health Gap Action Plan: Scaling up care for mental, neurological, and substance use disorders*. Geneva: World Health Organization.

WHO and Disease Control Priorities Project (2006). *Disease Control Priorities related to Mental Neurological, Developmental and Substance Abuse Disorders*. Geneva: World Health Organization.

WHO World Mental Health Consortium (2004). Prevalence, severity, and unmet need for treatment of mental disorders in the World Health Organization World Mental Health Surveys. *Journal of the American Medical Association*, **291**, 2581–90.

CHAPTER 42

The challenge of integrated care at the programme level

William C. Torrey and Mary F. Brunette

Introduction

Adults with severe mental illnesses need integrated mental health and substance abuse treatment programming. The reasons are compelling: 1) approximately half of adults with severe mental illness also experience a co-occurring substance use disorder (Regier et al., 1990), 2) people with co-occurring disorders tend to have worse clinical outcomes, such as increased symptoms, more hospitalizations, and higher rates of infectious diseases, victimization, and homelessness (Dixon, 1999), and 3) separate or fragmented care is not effective (Ridgely et al., 1987). Despite growing awareness of the importance of these services, integrated programmes are still not widely available for people who need them (Epstein et al., 2004; Presidents' New Freedom Commission on Mental Health, 2003).

Integrated dual disorders treatment (IDDT) is an integrated multidisciplinary team approach to care for adults with co-occurring substance use disorders and severe mental illnesses. The treatment programme grew out of experience with clinical programmes that are effective for this population and has been implemented widely (Mueser et al., 2003). IDDT offers a coordinated package of psychopharmacology, psychosocial interventions, and substance abuse counselling so that those needing the service experience a consistent approach, philosophy, and treatment recommendations. Essential programme elements include a comprehensive, long-term, stage-wise approach to treatment; assertive outreach; motivational interventions; and strategies and supports to help people learn to manage both illnesses and to achieve their functional goals (Table 42.1) (Drake et al., 2001).

This chapter reviews the research on implementing IDDT services and provides practical recommendations for organizational leaders who would like to implement and offer integrated programming for people with co-occurring disorders.

IDDT implementation research

Implementing a new clinical programme in a routine mental health care setting is challenging. A recent review of the research on the general topic of practice implementation in health care concludes that we know what does not work: dissemination of information (research literature and practice guidelines) and training alone are not effective in changing clinical practice, particularly if the practice is complex or multifaceted (Fixxen et al., 2005). The review also concludes that good evidence supports a longer-term, multilevel approach to implementation that not only trains providers, but transforms the system of care in which they work to support the desired practice.

The National Implementing Evidence-Based Practices Project was a multisite examination of practice implementation that used a longer-term, multi-level implementation strategy (Torrey et al., 2005). The project assumed implementations would be more successful if multiple stakeholders (including consumers, family members, mental health authorities, programme leaders, and clinicians) pulled together towards implementing a service, that implementation would take about a year, and would take place with different activities in three phases answering the questions: 1) Why should we do it? (motivating stakeholders); 2) How do we do it? (training and supervising providers, changing practice structures and supports); and 3) How do we maintain and extend the gains? (ongoing clinical supervision, monitoring of outcomes, and attention to ongoing provision of service) (Torrey et al., 2002, 2003). The organizations implementing a new practice were supported by a package of educational materials (films, pamphlets, written material including a workbook), a series of clinician trainings, and expert implementation consultation for a year (Torrey et al., 2005). A separate team studied the implementations using qualitative and qualitative methods. Fifty-three community mental health centres across eight states implemented one of five evidence-based practices: IDDT, supported employment, assertive community treatment, illness management and recovery, and family psychoeducation. Of these, 11 programmes in three states sought to implement IDDT.

Quantitative findings from the project show that high-fidelity implementation of the five studied evidence-based practices took about a year, with fewer gains made after 12 months. More than half

Table 42.1 The essential programme features of integrated services

◆ Integration: mental health and substance use interventions are combined to address the needs of the individual

◆ Staged interventions: treatment offerings are tailored to match the person's readiness to change

◆ Assertive outreach: intensive services actively seek out the individual in a sustained, caring effort to build relationship, engagement, and motivation

◆ Motivational interventions: services help individuals to discover what really matters to them and, through exploration of ambivalence, how they can start to move toward attaining their goals

◆ Counselling: evidence-based individual or group therapy address cognitive or behavioural skills development

◆ Social support: interventions with family and peer groups promote desired behavioural change

◆ Long term: services stay with people over months and years

◆ Comprehensive: treatment offerings address a broad range of needs such as medication management, housing supports, employment support, and links to general medical care

Table 42.2 Functions that facilitate practice implementation

◆ Lining up financing for service

◆ Active use of a consultant-trainer

◆ Senior leadership support

◆ Providing mid-level leadership

◆ Managing staff turnover

◆ Mastering the practice-specific knowledge and skills

of sites were able to implement their chosen practice in a manner that was faithful to the desired model practice. IDDT was harder to implement with high fidelity than supported employment or assertive community treatment. In part, the result may reflect the fact that the fidelity scales have not been carefully calibrated (the IDDT fidelity scale stresses evidence of specific clinical skills such as motivational interviewing whereas the supported employment or assertive community treatment fidelity scales are more focused on clinical structure, like clinician/consumer ratios). But the result may also be a direct reflection of the fact that IDDT present unique administrative challenges: weaving together the clinical skills, cultures, and administrative supports (such as financing) of the mental health and substance use disorder service traditions. Although some programmes implemented IDDT with very high fidelity, others were not able to do so (McHugo et al., 2007).

Qualitative analyses provide a more detailed look at the implementations of IDDT. Brunette and colleagues (2008) used standard qualitative analysis methods to evaluate the research team's ethnographic observations of the 11 implementations, looking for patterns that would shed light on the facilitators and barriers to high-fidelity practice implementation. Programmes that were successful in their implementations had some common features. First, they designated mid-level leaders who actively took on the challenge of implementation. These mid-level leaders did what needed to be done to get the practice running well: hiring and firing staff, changing the structure of clinical supervision, developing new policies, and putting in place new procedures such as substance abuse screening. Second, successful programmes made active use of the consultant-trainers to help them plan the implementations, train key staff in the skills and information they needed to deliver the service, and overcome the inevitable barriers that arise during a change process. Third, the clinical and administrative supervisors really mastered the specific skills and knowledge needed for IDDT so that their clinical and administrative decisions were well informed. Fourth, turnover and job transfer was used by some leaders to move out people who were unable or unwilling to offer the desired model of care and to hire and train capable clinicians

for the new programme. Although chronic, relentless turnover did interfere with implementation where it occurred; some programmes overcame it by redesigning the process of hiring, supervision, and support of new staff. And finally, programmes that successfully implemented IDDT addressed financing so that the programmes were supported over time. Independent qualitative analyses of the IDDT implementations confirmed the opportunity and challenges of staff turnover (Woltman and Whitley, 2007) and reinforced the importance of active, dedicated leadership and of mastering the practice-related skills and knowledge (Moser et al., 2004).

Swain and colleagues (2010) studied the sustainability of the practices that were implemented in National Implementing Evidence-Based Practices Project. Eighty per cent of the implemented practices remained in place 2 years after the original 2-year implementation study was complete. For IDDT programmes, nine out of the 11 (81.2%) programmes were sustained. Factors that helped programmes to sustain were 1) state support for the practice, including direct financing and technical assistance (training and consultation resources); 2) practice proficiency supported by attention to ongoing training and supervision; 3) practice evaluation with regular measurement of fidelity, patient outcome, and practice penetration; and 4) committed agency leadership that believed in the practice and provided space, training, financial support, and a vocal mandate for the practice (Table 42.2). Programmes that did not sustain their practices cited lack of funding and high levels of staff turnover as reasons for discontinuing.

Practical recommendations

Based on our experience and the implementation research reviewed earlier in this chapter, active leadership from multiple administrative levels is vitally important. The mental health authority administrators (regulators and payers), senior organizational leaders, and mid-level programme leaders all have crucial tasks. Their focused efforts, especially when coordinated with one another, can maximize the likelihood of creating and sustaining clinically effective programmes.

Mental health authority tasks

Federal, state, and county level mental health and addiction authority leaders have the opportunity to create an environment where provision of integrated treatment is expected, as well as to create infrastructure to facilitate implementation (Table 42.3) (Moser et al., 2004). In particular, the mental health authority is in a position to bring attention to the need for these services, create a supportive fiscal and legal environment through financing and regulation, and develop training centres that provide knowledgeable

Table 42.3 Facilitating tasks for mental health authority leaders

◆ Bring attention to the need for the service

◆ Facilitate the practice through finance and regulations

◆ Build an implementation-supporting infrastructure that includes implementation consultants and trainers.

consultants and trainers to programmes seeking to implement integrated treatment (Isett et al., 2007, 2008). The implementation research outlined above highlighted three areas of importance. First, financial incentives for integrated care must be in place in order for services to be delivered. Integrated services must be reimbursable at levels that cover the cost of care. Second, state authorities can encourage and fund the development of technical assistance centres that have the capacity to provide consultation, training, and technical assistance for starting and maintaining services (Salyers et al., 2007a). Third, health authorities must ensure that rules and regulations not only allow but encourage the delivery of co-occurring disorders services (Day, 2006). Organizations that provide integrated treatment should plan to interact with state mental health authorities to ensure that the services can be supported. Health authorities will be motivated to focus on service recipients with co-occurring disorders because the cost of their care is higher when the illnesses are unstable (Dickey and Azeni, 1996). The State Health Authority Yardstick (SHAY) (Finnerty et al., 2009) is a structured measure of whether a behavioural health authority is involved in all of the activities shown to improve the implementation of a particular practice region- or statewide. Health authorities can systematically evaluate themselves with this tool and use it as a guide to make changes necessary to support practice implementation by organizations over which they have authority.

Senior organizational leaders' tasks

The mental health authority can create a facilitative environment for implementation, but with or without the help, senior organizational leaders and mid-level programme leaders must do the hard work of redesigning care to meet the needs of the people with co-occurring disorders (Rapp et al., 2008).

Define the programme scope and mission

Organizations look to senior leaders to set the tone and establish priorities. Since implementing requires a substantial amount of work, it will only occur if senior leaders believe and communicate through words and action that establishing an effective co-occurring disorders programme is essential to the overall organizational mission. Senior leader communication can take the form of public meetings, written documents, and private conversations. This communication is most likely to resonate with staff if the proposed change addresses an urgent need that is felt by many, flows out of the overall accepted mission of the organization, and is consistent with the values that motivate mid-level programme clinical leaders and direct care staff. The message will be more effective if senior leaders passionately address the question: 'Why do this?,' remembering that this question will likely be on the minds of staff members long after the senior leaders have answered it for themselves.

Senior leaders decide on the parameters and details of the co-occurring disorders programme. The organization's goals and resources will guide this planning process. The parameters of a co-occurring disorders initiative can be as narrow as establishing a team of trained clinicians to serve a small, well-defined subgroup of patients or as large as screening all patients for co-occurring illness, creating multiple specialized teams, establishing several layers of care, and training all clinicians to recognize and treat people with co-occurring illnesses. Integration is at the heart of effective service. Integration can occur by creating new co-occurring disorders teams, incorporating substance abuse treatment in mental health programmes, building mental health services into substance abuse programmes, or creating joint programmes that report to two agencies or agency divisions. Laying out an overall vision and a detailed plan for the programme and implementation process should be done early so that everyone can work toward the same goal rather than pulling in different directions.

Line up financing

Establishing how financing will be obtained is an essential role for senior administrators. Financing rules can either support or hinder the clinical goals of the programme. Rather than allowing services to be forced apart by reimbursement rules, administrators should ensure that the financing of integrated treatment services allows behavioural health and substance abuse treatment to occur together in an integrated fashion. Since mental health and substance abuse services are typically purchased by separate departments within health authorities or administered by different departments within insurance agencies, planning and negotiation may be required to ensure that the funding will be completely integrated at the programme level. Senior leaders need to establish with funders that co-occurring disorder treatment can be provided and that the services will be adequately reimbursed prior to implementing a co-occurring disorders programme. Reliable financing allows a programme to function over time.

To work out financing that truly supports the clinical aims of the programme, senior administrators must become well-versed in both the intricacies of the financing systems and core clinical issues of co-occurring disorders services. Financing affects clinical care since it has an impact on how mid-level programme leaders and clinicians are managed and behave. For example, people with co-occurring disorders use more services than those who do not have both disorders. In a purely capitated payment system this well-established characteristic of the population creates a disincentive to serve people with co-occurring disorders. Administrators who function in a capitated financing system are therefore wise to negotiate for added incentives to engage and treat this population. Without that added financial reinforcement, financial pressures over time will lead the programme to exclude the people who are more ill and in the greatest need of this specialized service. Cutting through the complexity of the financing systems requires perseverance and a consistent commitment to placing the patients' health interests first.

Assign mid-level programme leadership responsibility

A critical task for senior leadership is to designate and support a competent programme director for the co-occurring disorders programme. This director will be responsible for redesigning care and must own the implementation process. The programme director's role is to oversee the development, operations, and improvement of all co-occurring disorders services. The implementation research underlines the importance of this hand-on leader in successful implementation.

The ideal candidate for this role knows the organization well and has the trust of senior leadership as well as the direct care clinicians and staff. Additionally, experience with developing and improving programmes is very helpful. Some programmes have successfully implemented using a pair of mid-level leaders who work together well with one leader being an operations leader and the other being a respected clinician. Together they champion and enact change with combined administrative and clinical authority.

Monitor progress

Once a programme director is assigned, senior leaders can help him or her to succeed by demonstrating a sustained interest in the integrated treatment programme. Senior leaders can help programme leaders to establish a regular reporting process and measures of programme success. When elements of the programme are going well, senior leaders can reinforce the programme leader and staff by acknowledging and celebrating aspects of the programme that are succeeding. When components of the programme are not progressing, questions from senior leaders help to focus attention and resources to those areas that need to be improved. See Table 42.4.

Mid-level programme leadership tasks

Improving the health of any defined population over time requires effective clinical interventions, operations that support their efficient delivery, and funding to pay for the services. The programme leader's job is to put those elements together to help real clinicians treat real people in need of the service. The work is active, practical, problem-solving, and creative.

Learn the practice

In order for the programme leader to succeed, he or she must have a practical understanding of the co-occurring disorders treatment. During implementation, the programme leader makes many practical decisions (hiring, arranging training, measuring outcomes) and these decisions will only be as good as the knowledge of the practice on which they are based. Of particular importance is the understanding of the stages of change theory and the need for different types of services to be available for patients who are in different stages of change (Brunette and Mueser, 2006). The studies of implementation show that some programmes fail because leaders have not ensured that the providers absorbed the core knowledge of the practice.

Programme leaders can learn about integrated treatment from materials such as workbooks, videos, and detailed practice guidelines, such as the IDDT fidelity scale (Brunette et al., 2002). They can attend trainings and read the many books and articles on the subject. Visiting an organization that has a well-established integrated programme and learning from the programme leader there can be very beneficial. Of course, working with an experienced implementation consultant/trainer is optimal, when such a person is available.

Table 42.4 Facilitating tasks for senior organizational leaders

◆ Define the programme scope and mission
◆ Line-up financing
◆ Assign mid-level leadership responsibility
◆ Monitor progress—stay actively interested and celebrate success

As the programme leader becomes familiar with the desired practice he or she can then assess the services that are currently delivered by their organization. Since co-occurring disorders are so common, all aspects of clinical service are affected. The programme leader can learn about the current situation by sitting in on clinical team meetings and speaking to leaders of services including emergency, residential, medical, vocational, family education, and clinical case management services. Informally rating current fidelity using the fidelity scale can help to identify obvious gaps.

Hire, train, and supervise staff

Effective integrated care, like all of behavioural healthcare, is a very human process that requires skilled, trained clinical providers. The aim is to have providers who have mastered the knowledge and skills required to deliver the service, work together as a team, and consistently seek ways to improve the service. When a programme leader embraces the mission, he or she can often build and maintain a team's enthusiasm and pride at being experts in challenging work that not everyone can do—an important professional and human accomplishment.

In creating a new programme, momentum is important. Gaining support from existing respected clinicians by getting them involved early can be very helpful. A small number of respected and knowledgeable providers can bring other providers along and attract new staff with their contagious enthusiasm.

Staff turnover rates are often high in human service organizations and present a challenge to evidence-based practice implementation (Brunette et al., 2008; Woltmann et al., 2008). Programme leaders can make good use of staff turnover when they are able to replace providers who are impeding change with new staff who contribute to the desired programme. But chronic, high-level turnover is a difficult barrier to overcome; higher rates of turnover are related to lower rates of faithful programme implementation (Woltmann et al., 2008). Chronic high-level turnover puts a large training burden on the programme and leaves the remaining staff with caseloads that may be too large to manage clinically, especially when they are simultaneously trying to learn new clinical skills. Providing adequate support and supervision during a new programme implementation can prevent high turnover.

Programme leaders need to build an ongoing programme of training and supervision for new and experienced clinicians. New clinicians need initial training as part of their orientation. Providing a standardized set of required group trainings, readings, and videos gives all staff members a common educational base. But initial training is not enough. Training alone has been shown to increase knowledge (Salyers et al., 2007b), but not practice skills and patient outcomes (Forsetlund et al., 2009). Programme leaders should develop a weekly clinical supervision that focuses on the clinical skills required in providing co-occurring disorders treatment. Group supervision is preferred over individual supervision because it efficiently provides more learning opportunities as well as peer support for clinicians providing the service (Rapp, 1998). The supervisor's aim is to teach and reinforce the principles of care through their application to specific clinical challenges that come up on a week-to-week basis. The supervision process entails starting with the specific current clinical challenge, identifying what clinical principle applies to that challenge, expanding on that general principle to teach it well, then going back to apply that principle to the specific clinical situation at hand. This supervision process helps the presenting provider with his or her immediate challenge. It also provides all of the clinicians in the supervision group with an opportunity to go through the clinical thought process that they can apply to similar challenges in their own work. Training content is easy to forget, but group supervision by a knowledgeable supervisor regularly reinforces treatment principles until they are built into the fabric of day-to-day care.

Implementation also entails scanning for and removing disincentives and barriers to the desired clinician practice. For example, in many systems of care face-to-face service is incentivized because of reimbursement. While staying fiscally sound is essential for the long-term health of the programme, leaders need to find a way to get staff to training and supervision or they will not learn the required skills.

Redesign the practice for effective integrated care

Clinical care takes place within an operational context that can either support or hinder the programme's effectiveness. A programme leader's job is to creatively redesign the flow of care so that the people being served will reliably encounter the clinical services they need to do well. This means thinking through what the patients need (from a welcoming atmosphere to effective screening, education, and treatment services) and making it easy and natural for the programme staff and clinicians to offer what is needed.

In his chronic care model, Wagner (2005) has summarized the components of treatment that improve the health of people with long-term difficulties. Caring for populations of people with persistent vulnerabilities involves creating a system of care that: 1) identifies the population the programme aims to serve, 2) educates them about their condition and treatment options, 3) engages them in a process of taking an active role in caring for themselves, 4) offers them services that have been demonstrated to work, 5) functions as a team on their behalf, 6) measures clinical process and outcome variables, and 7) feeds back reports on these variables so that the care system can 'see' itself and continually improve (Dietrich et al., 2004). Service agencies caring for individuals with co-occurring disorders are often missing some or all of these elements. The programme leader must assess which elements are missing and then develop them.

Identification of people who have co-occurring disorders is the first element of a population-focused care programme. The programme leader can build in systematic screening at intake and periodically thereafter. A variety of brief screening instruments for substance use disorders have been shown to be valid for persons with serious mental illness (Maisto et al., 2000; Rosenberg et al., 1998). In addition, urinalysis can often be useful for detecting substance use that clients may fail to report using on self-report measures or during interviews.

Creating educational opportunities for the people being served is very important. Studies have shown that people with persistent health difficulties do better over time when offered interventions that help them develop the skills, knowledge, and confidence to actively participate in managing their illnesses (Wagner et al., 2001). Creating organizational resources that provide the opportunity for service recipients to easily access information allows them to more meaningfully participate in the treatment decisions that deeply affect their lives (Torrey and Drake, 2010). Decision support systems for service recipients and providers are

currently being developed and tested and, as more providers have access to electronic medical records, will increasingly support care (Deegan et al., 2008; Mueser and Drake, in press). Regardless of the current level of technical support, programme leaders can establish educational opportunities in the care process.

Building process and outcome measurement into care processes improves services and allows clinicians and leaders to assess how they are doing in meeting their goals. 'Audit and feedback' is one of the strategies to changing clinical practice that has been shown to change clinician behaviour (Jamtvedt et al., 2006). Data collection must be built into routine record keeping if it is to reliably occur. Modern electronic record systems can collect relevant outcome data during routine documentation while paper records require an added data entry step. Reports can enhance direct clinical care (i.e. showing the patient a graph of hospital use over time to celebrate success), inform provider supervision (i.e. comparing patient group participation rates across clinicians), and allow programme evaluation (i.e. assessing programme fidelity score against national norms).

Data and reports based on data provide a catwalk from which care processes and outcomes can be observed and evaluated, allowing both individual provider treatment and entire service programmes to improve over time (Batalden and Stoltz, 1993). Conversely, programmes are blind to their own effectiveness if they do not have data and meaningful reports on quality measures. In an integrated treatment programme, reports that show that the percentage of new referrals with co-occurring disorders is lower than expected can alert the programme leader to investigate the screening process to see if it is working as designed. Or, if reports show that a substantial number of service recipients are not progressing in their recovery despite good programming, the information can support the programme leader's advocacy for resources to expand a particular clinical service, such as residential programming.

In co-occurring disorders programmes, important elements of programme quality that can be measured include programme fidelity to the model, programme delivery processes, and programme outcome measures. The fidelity scale for IDDT provides a detailed operational definition of the elements of an effective integrated programme. Periodic measurement using this scale can provide information that will guide implementation and focus improvement efforts. Process reports are also important. Relevant process information includes the number of patients who are screened for substance use disorders and the percentage service recipients that are attending co-occurring treatment groups. Finally, patient outcomes are important as improving lives is the aim of clinical care. Leaders can monitor outcomes through reports of clinician-measured patient progression through stages of treatment, including tracking rates of stable remission from substance use disorders. Other outcomes, such as rates of homelessness, hospitalization and employment, track important elements of function.

Establish treatment groups and (if possible) residential care

Co-occurring substance use disorders and mental illnesses affect many aspects of life including symptoms, housing, work, family and community relations, and legal status. For this reason, people with co-occurring disorders benefit from services that have been shown to support recovery in these domains of life. They need comprehensive services, including services that target symptoms, such as psychopharmacologic treatment and training in illness management, and services that directly address function, such as supported employment, case management, family psychoeducation, and social skills training. Research suggests that group treatment and specialized residential care directly affect substance use outcomes in this population (Drake et al., 2008).

Setting up group treatment is a priority for implementation leaders, since studies consistently show positive benefit for substance use outcomes and other non-symptom outcomes (Drake et al., 2008). The group format allows participants to learn skills to manage both the mental illness and the substance use disorder (Weiss et al., 2007), as well as to identify with each other and support each other's recovery through sharing experiences and coping strategies. Substance use often takes place in a social context (Dixon et al., 1991) and the group can become a powerful social force for recovery. In addition, groups have the advantage of being an economical way to offer treatment as they require less clinician time than individual treatment.

Different kinds of groups have been shown to be helpful, including educational groups, stage-wise treatment groups (persuasion, active treatment, relapse prevention groups), and social skills groups. Larger programmes may be able to offer many different groups whereas smaller programmes will want to focus their fewer numbers of groups to match the people they are serving—an engaging educational group for people willing to consider learning more about co-occurring illnesses and an active treatment/relapse prevention group for those more committed to achieving and maintaining abstinence. Establishing ties to community self-help groups, such as Alcoholics Anonymous, can make it easier for people with co-occurring disorders to engage in these beneficial community supports (Mueser et al., 2003).

For individuals who do not respond to interventions of lower intensity or who are homeless, residential treatment with integrated services stabilizes individuals and improves their ability to recover (Brunette et al., 2004). Establishing a residential treatment programme is more complex than developing groups, but is a much needed intensive level of care. These programmes are most effective if they provide flexible, low intensity, long-term monitored care with built-in supportive treatment interventions (Drake et al., 2008). Patients who participate in the longer-term programmes experience improvements in substance use and other many functional outcomes (Brunette et al., 2004). See Table 42.5.

Conclusion

Many people with severe mental illness and co-occurring substance use disorders have not had access to the services that have been demonstrated to facilitate functional and symptomatic recovery, such as co-occurring disorders groups. Implementing and leading a programme of integrated care is a creative process that can lead to satisfying results. The aim is to offer services that you would want for yourself or a loved family member should you need such a service. The work is important and achievable.

References

Batalden, P.B. and Stoltz, P.K. (1993). A framework for the continual improvement of health care: Building and applying professional and improvement knowledge to test changes in daily work. *The Joint Commission Journal on Quality Improvement*, **19**, 424–45.

Brunette, M.F. and Mueser, K.T. (2006). Psychosocial interventions for the long-term management of patients with severe mental illness and co-occurring substance use disorder. *Journal of Clinical Psychiatry*, **67**, 10–17.

Brunette, M.F., Drake, R.E., Lynde, D., and IDDT Group (2002). *Toolkit for Integrated Dual Disorders Treatment*. Rockville, MD: Substance Abuse and Mental Health Services Administration.

Brunette, M.F., Mueser, K.T., and Drake, R.E. (2004). A review of residential programs for people with severe mental illness and co-occurring substance use disorders. *Drug and Alcohol Review*, **23**, 471–8.

Brunette, M.F., Asher, D., Whitley, R., Lutz, W.J., Wieder, B.L., Jones, A.M., et al. (2008). Implementation of integrated dual disorders treatment: a qualitative analysis of facilitators and barriers. *Psychiatric Services*, **59**, 989–95.

Day, S.L. (2006). Issues in Medicaid policy and system transformation: Recommendations from the President's Commission. *Psychiatric Services*, **57**, 1713–18.

Deegan, P.E., Rapp, C., Holter, M., and Riefer, M. (2008). A program to support shared decision making in an outpatient psychiatric medication clinic. *Psychiatric Services*, **59**, 603–5.

Dickey, B. and Azeni, H. (1996). Persons with dual diagnoses of substance abuse and major mental illness: their excess costs of psychiatric care. *American Journal of Public Health*, **86**, 973–77.

Dietrich, A.J., Oxman, T.E., Williams, J.W.J., Schulberg, H.C., Bruce, M.L., Lee, P.W., et al. (2004). Re-engineering systems for the primary care treatment of depression: A cluster randomized controlled trial. *British Medical Journal*, **329**, 602–5.

Dixon, L. (1999). Dual diagnosis of substance abuse in schizophrenia: *prevalence and impact on outcomes: Schizophrenia Research*, **35**, S93–S100.

Dixon, L., Haas, G., Weiden, P.J., Sweeney, J., and Frances, A.J. (1991). Drug abuse in schizophrenia patients: Clinical correlates and reasons for use. *American Journal of Psychiatry*, **148**, 224–30.

Drake, R.E., Essock, S.M., Shaner, A., Carey, K.B., Minkoff, K., Kola, L., et al. (2001). Implementing dual diagnosis services for clients with severe mental illness. *Psychiatric Service*, **52**, 469–72.

Drake, R.E., O'Neal, E.L., and Wallach, M.A. (2008). A systematic review of psychosocial research on psychosocial interventions for people with co-occurring severe mental and substance use disorders *Journal of Substance Abuse Treatment*, **34**, 123–38.

Epstein, J., Barker, P., Vorburger, M., and Murtha, C. (2004). *Serious mental illness and its co-occurrence with substance use, 2002*. Rockville MD: Substance Abuse and Mental Health Services Administration, Office of Applied Studies.

Finnerty, M.T., Rapp, C.A., Bond, G.R., Lynde, D.W., Ganju, V., and Goldman, H.H. (2009). The State Health Authority Yardstick (SHAY). *Community Mental Health Journal*, **45**, 228–36.

Fixxen, D.L., Naoon, S.F., Blasé, K.A., Friedman, R.M., and Wallace, F. (2005). *Implementation Research: A synthesis of the Literature*. (FMHI pub no. 231.) Tampa, FL: University of South Florida, Louis de la Parte Florida Mental Health Institute, National Implementation Research Network.

Forsetlund, L., Bjorndal, A., Rashidian, A., Jamtvedt, G., O'Brien, M.A., Wolf, F., et al. (2009). Continuing education meetings and workshops: effects on professional practice and health care outcomes. *Cochrane Database of Systematic Reviews*, **2**, CD003030.

Table 42.5 Facilitating tasks for mid-level programme leaders

- ◆ Learn the knowledge and skills of the practice
- ◆ Hire, train, and supervise staff
- ◆ Redesign the practice for effective integrated care
- ◆ Establish co-occurring treatment groups and (if possible) residential services

Isett, K.R., Burnam, M.A., Coleman-Beattie, B., Hyde, P.S., Morressey, J.P., Magnabosco, J., et al. (2007). The state policy context of implementation issues for evidence-based practices in mental health. *Psychiatric Services*, **58**, 914–21.

Isett, K.R., Burnam, M.A., Coleman-Beattie, B., Hyde, P.S., Morressey, J.P., Magnabosco, J., et al. (2008). The role of state mental health authorities in managing change for the implementation of evidence-based practices. *Community Mental Health Journal*, **44**, 195–211.

Jamtvedt, G., Young, J.M., Kristoffersen, D.T., O'Brien, M.A., and Oxman, A.D. (2006). Audit and feedback: Effects on professional practice and health care outcomes. *Cochrane Database of Systematic Reviews*, **2**, CD000259.

Maisto, S.A., Carey, M.P., Carey, K.B., Gordon, C.M., and Gleason, J.R. (2002). Use of the AUDIT and the DAST-10 to identify alcohol and drug use disorders among adults with a severe and persistent mental illness. *Psychological Assessment*, **12**, 186–92.

McHugo, G.J., Drake, R.E., Brunette, M.F., Xie, H., Essock, S.M., and Green, A.I. (2006). Methodological issues in research o interventions for co-occurring disorders. *Schizophrenia Bulletin*, **32**, 655–65.

McHugo, G.J., Drake, R.E., Whitley, R., Bond, G.R., Campbell, K., Rapp, C.A., et al. (2007). Fidelity outcomes in the National Implementing Evidence-Based Practices Project. *Psychiatric Services*, **58**, 1279–84.

Moser, L.L., DeLuca, N.L., Bond, G.R., and Rollins, A.L. (2004). Implementing evidence-based psychosocial practices: lessons learned from statewide implementation of two practices. *CNS Spectrums*, **9**, 926–36, 942.

Mueser, K.T. and Drake, R.E. (in press). Treatment of co-occurring substance use disorders using shared decision making and electronic decision support systems. In: Rudnick, A. and Roe, D. (eds.) *Serious Mental Illness: Person Centered Approaches*. Abington: Radcliffe Press.

Mueser, K.T., Noordsy, D., Drake, R.E., and Fox, L. (2003). *Integrated Treatment for Dual Disorders: A Guide to Effective Practice*. New York, Guilford.

Presidents' New Freedom Commission on Mental Health. (2003). *Achieving the Promise: Transforming Mental Health Care in America*. (Pub no SMA-03-3832.) Rockville, MD: Department of Health and Human Services.

Rapp, C.A. (1998). *The Strengths Model: Case Management with People Suffering from Severe and Persistent Mental Illness*. New York: Oxford University Press.

Rapp, C.A., Etzel-Wise, D., Marty, D., Coffman, M., Carlson, L., Asher, D., et al. (2008). Barriers to evidence-based practice implementation: results of a qualitative study. *Community Mental Health Journal*, **44**, 213–24.

Regier, D.A., Farmer, M.E., Rae, D.S., Locke, B.Z., Keith, S.J., Judd, L.L., et al. (1990). Comorbidity of mental disorders with alcohol and other drug abuse: results from the Epidemiologic Catchment Area (ECA) Study. *Journal of the American Medical Association*, **264**, 2511–18.

Ridgely, M.S., Osher, F.C., Goldman, H.H., and Talbott, J.A. (1987). *Executive Summary: Chronic Mentally Ill Young Adults with Substance Abuse Problems: A Review of Research, Treatment, and Training Issues*. Baltimore, MA: University of Maryland School of Medicine. Mental Health Services Research Center.

Rosenberg, S.D., Drake, R.E., Wolford, G.L., Mueser, K.T., Oxman, T.E., Vidaver, R.M., et al. (1998). The Dartmouth Assessment of Lifestyle Instrument (DALI): A substance use disorder screen for people with severe mental illness. *American Journal of Psychiatry*, **155**, 232–8.

Salyers, M.P., McKasson, M., Bond, G.R., McGrew, J.H., Rollins, A.L., and Boyle, C. (2007a). The role of technical assistance centers in implementing evidence-based practices: Lessons learned. *American Journal of Psychiatric Rehabilitation*, **10**, 85–101.

Salyers, M.P., Rollins, A.L., Bond, G.R., Tsai, J., Moser, L., and Brunette, M.F. (2007b). Development of a scale to assess practitioner competence in providing integrated dual disorders treatment. *Administration & Policy in Mental Health*, **34**, 570–81.

Swain, K., Whitley, R., McHugo, G.J., and Drake, R.E. (2010). The sustainability of evidence-based practices in routine mental health agencies. *Community Mental Health Journal*, **46**, 119–29.

Torrey, W.C. and Drake, R.E. (2010). Practicing shared decision making in the outpatient psychiatric care of adults with severe mental illnesses: Redesigning care for the future. *Community Mental Health Journal*, 46, 433–40.

Torrey, W.C., Drake, R.E., Cohen, M., Fox, L.B., Gorman, P., and Wyzik, P. (2002). The challenge of implementing and sustaining integrated dual disorders treatment programs. *Community Mental Health Journal*, **38**, 507–21.

Torrey, W.C., Finnerty, M., Evans, A., and Wyzik, P. (2003). Strategies for leading the implementation of evidence-based practices, *Psychiatric Clinics of North America*, **26**, 883–97.

Torrey, W.C., Lynde, D., and Gorman, P. (2005). Promoting the implementation of practices that are supported by research: The National Implementing Evidence-Based Practice Project, *Child and Adolescent Psychiatric Clinics of North America*, **14**, 297–306.

Wagner, E.H., Austin, B.T., Davis, C., Hindmarsh, M., Schaefer, J., and Bonomi, A. (2001). Improving chronic illness care: translating evidence into action. *Health Aff* (Millwood), **20**, 64–78.

Wagner, E.H., Bennett, S.M., Austin, B.T., Greene, S.M., Schaefer, J.K., and Von Korff, M. (2005). Finding common ground: Patient centeredness and evidence-based chronic illness care. *Journal of Alternative and Complementary Medicine*, **11**, S7–S15.

Weiss, R.D., Griffin, M.L., and Kolodziej, M.E., Greenfield, S.F., Najavits, L.M., Daley, D.C., et al. (2007). A randomized trial of integrated group therapy versus group drug counseling for patients with bipolar disorder and substance dependence. *American Journal of Psychiatry*, **164**, 100–7.

Woltman, E. and Whitley, R. (2007). The role of staffing stability in the implementation of integrated dual disorders treatment: An exploratory study. *Journal of Mental Health*, **16**, 757–79.

Woltman, E.M., Whitley, R., McHugo, G.J., Brunette, M., Torrey, W.C., Coots, L, et al. (2008). The role of staff turnover in the implementation of evidence-based practices in mental health care. *Psychiatric Services*, **59**, 732–7.

SECTION 10

Looking to the future

CHAPTER 43

Summing up: community mental health in the future

Graham Thornicroft, Robert E. Drake, Kim T. Mueser, and George Szmukler

Introduction

Several fundamental tenets inform our view of community mental health care. First is an understanding of a community's needs for mental health services. Policy makers must appreciate epidemiological needs to implement services from a public health perspective. Second, mental health care must balance several opposing forces: population needs and local resources, hospital-based and community-based services, and human rights versus public safety concerns. Third, mental health services must align with basic human rights and health care values. Fourth, effective mental health care must incorporate evidence-based approaches. Fifth, putting intended services in place with high fidelity and cultural sensitivity must involve the complicated and poorly understood science of implementation. This step includes planning, organization, financing, workforce training, and quality assurance. Sixth, community mental health must address the community as well as mental health services. Addressing public attitudes, stigma, and community resources, as well as developing a consensus for good mental health care, are all critical. Finally, these systems of care must be flexible enough to evolve as our knowledge of needs, values, evidence-based practices, and implementation science changes over time. This final chapter addresses each of these tenets.

The balanced care model

Countries vary widely in how they define, interpret, and implement community-orientated care (World Health Organization 2001, 2008a,b). Nevertheless, they all must balance competing priorities. Mental health care must align epidemiological needs with community resources. From the point of view of the balanced care model (see Chapter 14), most mental health services should be provided in community settings close to the populations served, with hospital stays and incarcerations reduced as far as possible, and with inpatient services usually located in acute wards in general hospitals (Thornicroft and Tansella, 2009).

Differing priorities apply to low-, medium-, and high-resource settings:

- In low-resource settings the focus is on establishing and improving the capacity of practitioners in primary health care facilities to deliver mental health care, with limited specialist back-up. Most mental health assessment and treatment occurs, if at all, in primary health care settings or in relation to traditional/religious healers. For example, in Ethiopia, most care is provided within the family or in the close community of neighbours and relatives: only 33% of people with persistent major depressive disorder reach either primary health care or traditional healers (Fekadu et al. 2008; Hanlon et al. 2008).

- In medium-resource settings, in addition to primary care mental health services, an extra layer of general adult mental health services can be developed as resources allow, in five categories: 1) outpatient/ambulatory clinics; 2) community mental health teams; 3) acute in-patient services; 4) community-based residential care; and 5) work, occupation, and rehabilitation services.

- In high-resource countries, as well as the services described above, more specialized services dedicated to specific patient groups and goals may be affordable in the same five categories. These may include, for instance, specialized outpatient and ambulatory clinics, assertive community treatment teams, intensive case management, early intervention teams, crisis resolution teams, crisis housing, community residential care, acute day hospitals, day hospitals, non-medical day centres, and recovery/employment/rehabilitation services.

We have assumed the balanced care model approach throughout this book in considering community-orientated care. In low-resource settings community-orientated care will be characterized by:

- A focus on population and public health needs
- Case finding and detection in the community

◆ Locally accessible services (i.e. accessible in less than half a day)

◆ Community participation and decision-making in the planning and provision of mental health care systems

◆ Self-help and service-user empowerment for individuals and families

◆ Mutual assistance and/or peer support of service users

◆ Initial treatment by primary care and/or community staff

◆ Stepped care options for referral to specialist staff and/or hospital beds if necessary

◆ Back-up supervision and support from specialist mental health services

◆ Interfaces with non-governmental organizations (e.g. in relation to rehabilitation)

◆ Networks at each level, including between different services, the community, and traditional and/or religious healers.

Community-orientated care therefore draws on a wide range of practitioners, providers, care, and support systems (both professional and non-professional), though particular components may play a larger or lesser role in different settings depending on the local context and the available resources, especially trained staff.

In preparing this summarizing chapter we have drawn upon a series of resources including:

◆ Material from the relevant literature included in the preceding chapters

◆ The recent World Psychiatric Association Task Force on the lessons learned and the mistakes to avoid in the implementation of community mental health care (Thornicroft et al., 2010). For the work of this group electronic searches were supplemented by searches of the reference lists of all selected articles, and key references (Benegal et al., 2009; Mbuba and Newton 2009; Patel et al. 2009; Thornicroft and Tansella, 2009; Thornicroft et al., 2008)

◆ The special edition of *The Lancet* on Global Mental Health (Chisholm et al., 2007; Jacob et al. 2007; Moran et al. 2010; Patel et al. 2007; Prince et al. 2007; Saraceno et al., 2007; Saxena et al., 2007)

◆ The *PLoS Medicine* series of papers on treatment guidelines relevant to community mental health care in low- and medium-resource settings (Benegal et al., 2009; Patel et al., 2009; Patel and Thornicroft, 2009)

◆ Relevant World Health Organization (WHO) publications which provide information regarding community mental health services worldwide were also sourced (World Health Organization, 2005a, 2008b,c, 2009).

Human rights and basic health care values

Underpinning the successful implementation of community-orientated mental health care is a set of principles that relate on the one hand to the value of community and on the other to the importance of self-determination and the rights of people with mental illness as persons and citizens (Bartlett et al., 2006; Thornicroft and Tansella 1999). We expect that in the future, community mental health services will increasingly emphasize the importance of treating and enabling people to live in the community in a way that maintains their connection with their families, friends, work, and community. This process acknowledges and supports the person's goals and strengths to further their recovery in their own community (Slade, 2009).

A fundamental principle supporting these values is the notion of people having equitable access to services in their own locality in the 'least restrictive environment'. While recognizing the fact that some people are significantly impaired by their illness, a community mental health service seeks to foster the service user's rights to self-determination and participation in processes involving decisions related to their treatment. These values need to be upheld, often in the face of public pressures to prioritize safety concerns and to re-institutionalize people with mental disorders in hospitals, nursing homes, jails, and prisons. Given the importance of families in providing support and key relationships, their participation (with the permission of the service user) in the processes of assessment, treatment planning, and follow-up are also key values in a community model of service delivery.

Various conventions identify and aim to protect the rights of service users as persons and citizens, including the recently ratified United Nations Convention on the Rights of Persons with Disability (UNCRPD) and more specific charters such as the UN Principles for the Protection of Persons with Mental Illness and for the Improvement of Mental Care adopted in 1991 (United Nations 1992, 2006). International, regional, and national documents specify the rights of the person to be treated without discrimination and on the same basis as other persons; the presumption of legal capacity unless incapacity can be clearly proven; and the involvement of persons with disabilities in policy and service development and in relation to decision-making which directly affects them (United Nations, 2006). We strongly endorse the principles of the UNCRPD and associated treaties and conventions.

Evidence-based approaches to mental health interventions and decisions

Evidence-based mental health care comprises three fundamental approaches: evidence-based practices, evidence-based decision-making, and quality assurance (Drake et al., 2003). Chapters 11 to 14 discuss many of the techniques that are used to develop and validate evidence-based practices. These techniques target specific interventions that are efficacious and effective for specific populations. For example, the evidence indicates that a client with serious mental illness who wants to work should receive supported employment and that a client who experiences serious mental illness and chronic homelessness should receive assertive community treatment (Dixon et al., 2010).

But evidence-based practices have limits, and many treatment decisions are much more complex than deciding who should receive a basic intervention such as supported employment or assertive community treatment. Typical mental health clients often have multiple comorbidities, lack basic psychosocial supports, live in communities with limited mental health resources, or have histories of failing numerous trials of evidence-based interventions. Further, for most treatment decisions, a single, clear best practice does not exist. Instead, several interventions with variable effectiveness and side effects are available. These decisions require a shared approach to making complex decisions. The mental health practitioner and the client discuss the best current scientific information; the practitioner provides expertise on diagnoses, the course of illnesses, and available treatments; and the client offers expertise on personal goals and preferences. Together they negotiate treatment plans that balance these three inputs in a process of shared decision-making (Drake et al., 2009a,b, 2010a).

At the team, programme, agency, or system level, evidence-based care requires systematic attention to outcomes. Quality is often addressed by training and supervision. But outcomes must be measured to be certain of quality. Data are systematically gathered on clients, services, and outcomes to assess whether the clients are remaining in services, are receiving services that are appropriate to their needs, and are improving in relation to expected outcomes based on established benchmarks. The process of monitoring data in this fashion to detect problems in the flow of assessment and treatment to improve services is a necessary step for high-quality mental health care.

Implementation

Implementation differs substantially from intervention. One challenge common to many countries worldwide is the difficulty in putting effective community mental health interventions into faithful implementations.

Policies, plans, and programmes

We further distinguish here between:

◆ National policy (or provincial or state policy in countries where health policy is set at that level): an overall statement of strategic intent (e.g. over a 5–10-year period) that gives direction to the whole system of mental health care.

◆ Implementation plan: an operational document setting out the specific steps needed to implement the national policy (e.g. what tasks are to be completed, by whom, by when, with which resources, and identifying the reporting lines, and the incentives and sanctions if tasks are completed or not completed).

◆ Mental health programmes: specific plans either for a local area (e.g. a region or a district) or for a particular sector (e.g. primary care) that specify how one component of the overall care system should be developed.

According to the WHO's *Mental Health Atlas* (World Health Organization, 2005a) 62.1% of countries worldwide had a mental health policy, and 69.6% had a mental health programme in place in 2005 (with 68.3% and 90.9% of the global population covered respectively). Many of the countries without such policies were low- and middle-income countries (LAMIC). Even where comprehensive evidence-based mental health policies are in place, problems in implementing these policies are common (Knapp et al., 2007; World Health Organization, 2008c). Some of the reasons may include health staff not complying with policies due to difficulties in accepting and implementing changing roles (World Health Organization, 2008c), the lack of accessible evidence-based information or guidelines for health staff, inadequate funding mechanisms, inadequate training of health care personnel, the lack of mechanisms for training and coaching health staff, poor supervision and support, and an overall lack of human resources (Knapp et al., 2007). Detailed and highly practical implementation plans (taking into account available resources) must include guidelines, training, supervision, fidelity assessment, and alignment of financing and organizational regulations (Bond et al., 2009; Greenhalgh et al., 2004; McHugo et al., 2007; Proctor et al., 2009).

Scaling up services for whole populations

A further challenge that needs addressing worldwide is the massive gap between population needs for mental health care (true prevalence of mental illness) and what is actually provided in mental health care (treated prevalence) (World Health Organization, 2008b), highlighting the importance of scaling up services for whole populations. The substantial burden of mental disorders has not been translated into investments in mental health care (Jacob et al., 2007). The treatment gap is particularly pronounced in LAMIC, where commonly over 75% of people with mental disorders receive no treatment or care at all, and less than 2% of the health budget is spent on mental health (World Health Organization, 2008b). Whilst the high-income countries of the world have an average of 10.50 psychiatrists and 32.95 psychiatric nurses per 100,000 population (median figures), in low-income countries there are only 0.05 and 0.16 respectively (World Health Organization, 2008b). Furthermore, even within countries the quality and level of services often vary greatly according to, for instance, patient group, location (with service provision usually being higher in urban areas), or socioeconomic factors (World Health Organization, 2001).

Similarly, only 10% of global mental health research is directed to the health needs of the 90% of populations living in LAMIC, and only a fraction of this research activity is concerned with implementing and evaluating interventions and services (Saxena et al., 2006). Methods to estimate resource needs are necessary in scaling up services, as well as a rethinking of professional roles, for instance in terms of task-shifting. A systematic methodology for setting priorities in child health research has been developed taking into consideration that interventions should be effective, sustainable, and affordable to reduce the burden of disease (Rudan et al., 2008). A similar methodology was applied by the *Lancet* Global Mental Health Group which focused on four groups of disorders whilst setting priorities for global mental health research: depressive, anxiety, and other common mental disorders; alcohol- and other substance-abuse disorders; child and adolescent mental disorders; and schizophrenia and other psychotic disorders (*Lancet* Global Mental Health Group, 2007). In conclusion, it was recommended that interventions should be delivered by non-mental health professionals within existing routine care settings, and specialists should play a role in capacity building and supervision (Patel, 2009). A comprehensive review of packages of care for six leading neuropsychiatric disorders (alcohol abuse, attention deficit hyperactivity disorder, dementia, depression, epilepsy, and schizophrenia) have also recently been proposed as means to extend treatment in LAMIC (Benegal et al., 2009; de Jesus Mari et al., 2009; Mbuba and Newton, 2009; Patel and Thornicroft, 2009; Patel et al., 2009). An extensive set of treatment guidelines, also suitable for LAMIC, will be published by the WHO in 2010 as a part of their mental health Gap Action Programme (mhGAP).

The community as context for mental health care

Community awareness

Further common barriers that need to be decisively tackled in the future are mental health-related stigma and discrimination. These pervasive and pernicious problems have many ramifications. On one extreme, public misperceptions and fears can result in excessive criminalization and incarceration of people with mental illnesses (Choe et al., 2008). On the other hand, effective awareness-raising campaigns can result in increased presentation of persons with mental illness to primary health care (Eaton and Agomoh, 2008).

Three main strategies have been used to reduce public stigma and discrimination: protest, education, and social contact (Corrigan and Penn, 1999). Protest, by stigmatized individuals or members of the public who support them, is often applied against stigmatizing public statements, such as media reports and advertisements. Many protest interventions, e.g. against stigmatizing advertisements or soap operas, have successfully suppressed negative public statements and for this purpose they are clearly very useful (Wahl, 1995). However, it has been argued (Corrigan and Penn, 1999) that protest is not effective for improving attitudes toward people with mental illness.

Education interventions aim to diminish stigma by replacing myths and negative stereotypes with facts, and have reduced stigmatizing attitudes among members of the public. However, research on educational campaigns suggests that behaviour changes are often not evaluated. The third strategy is personal social contact with persons with mental illness (Thornicroft, 2006). In a number of interventions in, e.g. secondary schools, or with the police, education and personal social contact have been combined (Pinfold et al., 2003). Social contact appears to be the more efficacious part of the intervention. Factors that create an advantageous environment for interpersonal contact and stigma reduction may include equal status among participants, a cooperative interaction, and institutional support for the contact initiative (Pinfold et al., 2005).

For both education and contact, the content of programmes against stigma and discrimination matters. Biogenetic models of mental illness, although not scientifically accurate in light of knowledge regarding social and environmental factors, are often highlighted because viewing mental illness as a biological, mainly inherited problem may reduce shame and blame associated with it. Evidence supports this optimistic expectation (i.e. that a biogenetic causal model of mental illness will reduce stigma) in terms of reduced blame. However, focusing on biogenetic factors may increase the perception that people with mental illness are fundamentally different, and thus biogenetic interpretations have been associated with increased social distance (Phelan et al., 2006). Therefore, a message of mental illness as being 'genetic' or 'neurological' may be overly simplistic and unhelpful for reducing stigma, indeed in many LAMIC conveying a message emphasizing the heritable nature of mental illness fuels stigma, e.g. making marriage more difficult.

Anti-stigma initiatives can take place nationally as well as locally. National campaigns often adopt a social marketing approach, whereas local initiatives usually focus on target groups. An example of a large multifaceted national campaign is *Time To Change* in England (Henderson and Thornicroft, 2009). It combines mass-media advertising and local initiatives. The latter try to facilitate social contact between members of the general public and mental health service users as well as target specific groups such as medical students and teachers. The programme is evaluated by public surveys assessing knowledge, attitudes, and behaviour, and by measuring the amount of experienced discrimination reported by people with mental illness. Similar initiatives in other countries, such as *See Me* in Scotland (Dunion and Gordon, 2005), *Like*

Minds, Like Mine in New Zealand (Vaughan and Hansen, 2004), or the World Psychiatric Association anti-stigma initiative (Sartorius and Schulze, 2005) along with similar programmes in other countries, including Japan, Brazil, Egypt, and Nigeria, have reported positive outcomes (Eaton and Agomoh, 2008).

In sum, overall there is evidence for the effectiveness of measures against stigma and against discrimination (Thornicroft et al., 2009). On a more cautious note, individual discrimination, structural discrimination, and self-stigma lead to innumerable mechanisms of stigmatization. If one mechanism of discrimination is blocked or diminished through successful initiatives, other ways to discriminate may emerge (Link and Phelan, 2001). Therefore, to substantially reduce discrimination, stigmatizing attitudes and behaviours of influential stakeholders need to change fundamentally.

Developing a consensus for change

In most countries transforming mental health services to focus on community-orientated care has proven a major task. Perhaps the most important factor is the range of people involved in providing services and the recognition that service users and their families should be involved in care planning and service development. In all this has meant that there is a complex mix of people who have an investment in the development and delivery of mental health services, the majority of whom have to be brought on board when significant change is contemplated. Large and smaller scale ventures such as those in the United Kingdom, New Zealand, and Australia have proven that the collaborative engagement of a wide variety of supportive stakeholders is critical to successful implementation of community orientated mental health care.

Change requires the support of politicians, board members and health managers whose primary focus may not be on mental health, clinicians, key members of the community including non-governmental organizations providers, service users and their families, and traditional and religious healers. To involve them in the imperative for change will require different strategies and a change management team that includes people with a variety of expertise and different networks to undertake them. Overall, having clear reasons and objectives for the shift to community orientated care is essential. Messages should be concise, backed by evidence and consistent.

Developing consensus for change requires a lot of work meeting and communicating with people. The main means of communication need to include written material and opportunities to meet with stakeholder groups. Politicians and administrators will require a compelling business case. However, others will need summaries of plans, slide presentations, and the opportunity to meet and work through proposals and concerns. Emails and website information and surveys are now valuable supplements to the process. In all communications the emphasis must be on a willingness to communicate in good faith and to do so openly and honestly to convince people of the benefits of the change process and determination to see it through.

This said, it is important to bear in mind that in some cases prejudice and self-interest will have to be confronted. It is helpful, at the beginning of the process, to identify both those who are likely to support change, and those who are likely to oppose it. A willingness to listen to concerns and to find ways of incorporating these if possible into the planning and implementation process is essential because when such an attitude is communicated there is an opportunity for people to feel included in the process. That done, boldness and firmness will communicate to remaining detractors the seriousness of the intent to implement change; it will also encourage supporters to believe that their aspirations for better mental health care will be realized, and thus embolden them in turn.

Engaging stakeholders requires both formal and informal opportunities to meet, receive advice, and work through issues. The establishment of reference groups early on in the change process is a key formal mechanism to achieving this. These should include all the key stakeholders, in particular service users, families, clinicians, and service providers, with service providers being essential to facilitate integrated systems of care further on in the process. While it is important to structure the overall process with formal meetings and communications it is also important to be willing to convene informal meetings upon request to 'trouble-shoot' situations of concern. For practical purposes the consultation process takes place at a number of levels and should result in an amalgam of 'bottom-up' and 'top-down' contributions to the change process. In this reports on progress are an essential way of maintaining trust and building excitement to the process of successful implementation.

It is also important to bear in mind that good mental health services have established processes for ensuring the voices of service users, their families, and community providers are heard on an ongoing basis. It is then not simply a matter of achieving discontinuous change but ongoing quality improvement in which consumers of mental health services know they have a major stake. Without such effective and united consortia, policy makers may find it easy to disregard the different demands of a fragmented mental health sector, and instead respond positively to health domains (e.g. HIV/AIDS) which demonstrate the self-discipline of united approach with a small number of fully agreed priorities.

Lessons learned

Several key mistakes are commonly made in the process of attempting to implement community mental health care. First, a carefully considered sequence of events must link hospital bed closure to community service development. It is important to avoid closing hospital-based services without having successor services already in place to support discharged patients and new referrals, and also to avoid trying to build up community services while leaving hospital care (and budgets) intact. In particular, there needs to be at each stage of a reform process a workable balance between enough (mainly acute beds) and the provision of other parts of the wider system of care that can support people in crisis.

A second common mistake is to attempt system reform without including *all* the relevant stakeholders. Such initiatives especially need to include psychiatrists, who may otherwise feel subject to 'top-down' decision-making and react, either in the interests of patients or in their own interests, by attempting to delay or block any such changes. Other vital stakeholders to be directly included in the process will often include: policy makers and politicians, health service planners, service users and carers, service providers including those in state and private practice, national and international non-governmental organizations, and those working in alternative, complementary, indigenous, and religious healing traditions, and relevant national and professional associations.

Typically those groups not fully involved in a reform process will make their views known by seeking to undermine the process!

A further common mistake is linking inappropriately the reform of mental health care with narrow ideological or party political interests. This tends to lead to instability as a change of government may reverse the policies of their predecessors. Such fault lines of division or fragmentation may also occur, e.g. between service reforms proposed by psychologists and psychiatrists, or between socially and biologically orientated psychiatrists, or between clinicians and service user/consumer groups. Whatever the particular points of schism, such conflicts weaken the chance that service reforms will be comprehensive, systemic, and sustainable, and they also run the risk that policy makers will refuse to adopt proposals that are not fully endorsed by the whole mental health sector.

Payment systems

A fundamental component in the successful implementation of mental health service provision is that of funding (Saxena et al., 2007). As indicated earlier, funding for mental health services in LAMIC tends to be very low. This may be due in part to a stigmatizing attitude toward mental illness, and to an absence of the recognition of the economic benefits that can accrue from improved mental health care. Ideally, the share of its health funding that a country devotes to mental health care will be informed by careful consideration of the comparative health benefits of spending on alternative forms of care. The data needed to carry out such an analysis are, however, typically not available in LAMIC.

Furthermore, what funding there is also tends to be concentrated on inpatient services—as this entire article implicitly presupposes. Correcting this is, initially, a matter of budgetary reallocation: using funds that could have been used for other purposes to increase funding for community-orientated care.

The issue then arises of how to pay public providers (hospitals, stand-alone programmes—institutional or voluntary sector, and possibly independent individual providers such as psychiatrists) for the services that they render. The simplest forms of payment are global budgets for facilities and programmes, which may be carried over from year to year with minor adjustments for inflation, and salaries for individual providers. These simple payment mechanisms have the advantage of administrative simplicity. At the same time, they have at least two important drawbacks. First, they provide no incentive for increasing either the quantity or the quality of service provision. Second, population shifts are likely to cause the demand for the services of different providers to evolve, and without taking changes in local demand into account inequities in payment across providers are likely to emerge and grow over time. This in turn will compromise access to overburdened providers, while possibly resulting in overprovision (e.g. excessive lengths of stay) by other providers. Accordingly, countries with the technical and administrative capacity to introduce more complex payment systems should consider doing so.

For hospitals, a fairly simple alternative which is applicable where care is sectorized is to modulate budgets on the basis of the population of the facility's catchment area. Countries with the technical capacity to do so may wish to adjust the payment level per person on the basis of socio-demographic variables known to be related to the need for inpatient mental health care (e.g. poverty).

For hospitals that have overlapping catchment areas, a combination of prospective payment (payment on the basis of number of admissions) and retrospective payment (payment on the basis of bed-days actually provided) may be preferable to exclusive reliance on one or the other. Pure retrospective payment encourages over-provision of services; pure prospective payment, given the difficulty of assessing reliably the degree of need for care of a person admitted for a psychiatric condition, may encourage under-provision.

For stand-alone programmes or individual providers, the two main options beyond a fixed budget or a salary are fee-for-service and capitation. Fee-for-service payment encourages a higher volume of services without regard to outcomes. If certain services (e.g. prescription of medications) are paid at a higher rate per unit time than others (e.g. psychotherapy), then fee-for-service payment will also influence the mix of services provided. In addition, fee-for-service payment tends to maximize contacts with patients who are less ill, more compliant, and easier to treat. Difficult or more severely ill patients receive less care unless payments are adjusted by severity—so-called case-mix adjustments. Efficient uses of clinical time such as telephone or computer contacts are ignored because they are not reimbursed.

Capitation payment encourages increasing the number of people served. It may lead to greater accountability for the care of specific patients. In and of itself, however, unless there is competition for patients across providers, it provides no incentive for quality. Furthermore, programmes often fill up to capacity and have difficulty shifting patients to less intensive services.

Countries with the technical and administrative capacity (and political leeway) to do so should consider introducing incentives for increasing quality, either for hospitals, programmes, or individual providers. Following Donabedian's seminal work, quality is commonly conceptualized as related to structure, process, and outcomes (Best and Neuhauser, 2004). Adjusting payments to hospitals, programmes, or individual providers on the basis of structure or process indicators (e.g. formal qualifications of staff, achievement of a certain score on a model fidelity scale) assumes that these indicators actually predict quality. To the extent that they do, then providing incentives for achieving a high score on those indicators is likely to be beneficial, with a neutral effect on which types of patients the provider will seek to serve. Adjusting payments based on outcomes (e.g. physiological indicators of metabolic syndrome, rehospitalization rates, employment rates) has the advantage of being directly related to a system's ostensible goals. It encourages, however, selection of less ill patients. More research is needed on how to design effective systems for encouraging quality of community-oriented mental health care that are practicable in countries with more or less developed technical and administrative capabilities. In sum, payment systems influence patient selection, quality and amount of treatments, and outcomes, in more or less favourable ways, and different ones require varying degrees of technical and administrative capacity to be implemented successfully. Determining the optimal system or combination of systems for a particular health care system or locale probably depends heavily on history, infrastructure, financial resources, human resources, and other factors.

Human resources

Human resources are the most critical asset in mental health service provision. The gradual transformation to community-based care has resulted in changes in the ways human resources have been utilized (World Health Organization, 2005b). The essential changes have been a reallocation of staff from hospital to community-based service settings, the need for a new set of competencies which include recovery and rehabilitation, training of a wider range of workers, including informal community care workers, within the context of the practical needs of a country (Deva, 1981). Further, in many LAMIC trained psychiatrists work under conditions of heavy and relentless clinical activities, and may not have dedicated time during the week for any service development duties.

Another perspective to human resource development has been the increasing emphasis on integration of mental health into a primary care setting, thereby increasing access to the vast majority of the underserved. This has necessitated the training of general health staff in basic skills in mental health care, such as detection of mental disorders, provision of basic care, and referral of complex problems to specialist care. In most developing countries, need has been for a well-rounded generalist who is capable of coping with most psychiatric problems with little access to any mental health practitioner. Further important issues are: lack of insurance, out of pocket expenses, and the economic burden falling on families.

The broadening scope and the shift to community-based mental health services introduce greater levels of complexity, affecting the role of psychiatrists, broadening it to areas such as promotion and social inclusion. Psychiatrists need to work in more settings, with more staff groups. Planning and management will take a more central place. Psychiatrists are seen to possess a unique expertise, and occupy leading positions in most countries, functioning as advisers to governments and chairing drafting groups that are responsible for the production of policies and action plans. There are countries where such groups comprise only psychiatrists. They have therefore a unique opportunity to shape the process of reform in the best interest of patients, families and carers, the public, and staff.

While psychosocial rehabilitation is an important part of the overall process of successful management of chronic mental illnesses, its practice is still rare compared to the use of medicines to 'cure' illnesses (Deva, 2006). In many developing countries, training is scarce for occupational therapists, psychologists, or social workers. In countries with few psychiatrists, numerous medical, administrative, and leadership duties leave psychiatrists little time to work with rehabilitation units. Even so, in many LAMIC other resources are available, e.g. strong family and community networks, faith groups, informal employment opportunities, which might be mobilized to support the rehabilitation of people with longer-term mental illnesses.

Organizational development, quality assurance, and service evaluation

Starting the reform process is a challenge worldwide, which may also in part be due to difficulties in imagining how a new system works. Thus, initiation of community mental health care services generally requires strong leadership among stakeholders based on community-orientated care concepts. Focusing on the structures and processes, organizational development is necessary to increase the potential for an organization to accomplish its goals. It enhances the organization's awareness, knowledge, and techniques required for the changes. It is practical to learn from successful models by using basic tools including timetables, assessment forms, job descriptions, and operational policies (Thornicroft and Tansella, 2009).

As part of the process of establishing a new system, and of maintaining it subsequently, coaching and maintenance activities are needed to make services robust and sustainable; manualization of operational procedures, reference materials, and ongoing supervision are essential. The manual is designed to assist organizations achieve continuous improvement in their community services. As community-orientated care becomes established in several regions, service components are gradually standardized, and manualized standard care becomes available.

Quality assurance is feasible even in settings with limited resources. Quality monitoring can be incorporated into routine activities by selecting target services, collecting data, and using the results for system problem-solving and future direction. External evaluation takes place at different levels. Local government checks whether service providers meet the requirement of laws or acts, while payers focus on examining the necessity of services provided. Professional peers and consumers also participate in independent evaluation.

Since the primary purpose of mental health services is to improve outcomes for individuals with mental illness, it is crucial to assess outcomes of treatments and services. Also, the results can be used to justify the use of resources. More research is therefore needed to provide the best possible services that would directly link to better outcomes for those in need of care.

Information technology

The incorporation of information technology into mental health service provision is emerging as a valuable tool (Institute of Medicine, 2010). Information technology can be used to expand access, capacity, quality, and efficiency across countries worldwide. The following concepts are reviewed in greater detail elsewhere (Drake et al., 2010b).

The Internet and other electronic resources can be primary sources of case identification. They provide information regarding psychiatric symptoms, illnesses, treatments, and services. In many countries people use the world wide web to explore their symptoms before they seek professional or non-professional help. Computerized information can help people to define their problems and access services, even in remote areas, by providing personal information on needs and local information on service alternatives.

As computer literacy increases, people with mental illnesses in many settings have demonstrated willingness and ability to enter personal information on demographics, medical histories, and current symptoms that facilitate diagnosis. To address the problem of illiteracy, software can be easily adapted for aural and touch-screen use. Diagnoses can be confirmed or refined by professionals, but self-entry of data obviously increases the efficiency of assessment and reduces costs. Paradoxically, research shows that people are often willing to disclose more information to a computer than to a trained interviewer!

The three fundamental pillars of evidence-based medicine are research evidence, clinical expertise, and patient preferences. Patient decision aids, which are often computerized to add personal testimonies and explanations of treatment alternatives and risks, enable patients to better express their preferences, based on accurate understanding of the choices and clarification of their own values. Computerized decision tools can also modify treatments and summarize current treatment evidence for practitioners, thereby enhancing clinical expertise and the use of research evidence. For example, information systems are commonly used to check for medical errors, such as incorrect medication dosages, and adverse medication interactions.

When patients live at a great distance or when they fail to attend appointments, electronic communications can easily stimulate outreach efforts to ensure that they receive the education, services, and monitoring that they need, e.g. the use of telemedicine to support access in remote sites (Griffiths et al., 2006). Personal computers, phones, and other electronic devices can be used to provide reminders for using coping skills and taking medications.

Another form of electronic service provision involves guided self-treatment, e.g. computerized cognitive behavioural treatment for anxiety, depression, or addiction. Early studies show outcomes that are equivalent to professionally delivered interventions.

As people come to professional attention, an electronic case registry can track amount and quality of treatment. Services received should be consistent with treatment plans and also with evidence-based practices; these quality assurance indicators can be monitored and summarized daily through electronic records. Even in remote areas people can be served and monitored according to evidence-based guidelines through telemedicine and other electronic communications.

Few mental health programmes monitor outcomes in real time in order to assess the effectiveness of services in relation to established benchmarks. Patient data entry via web-based systems can serve this purpose.

When patients do not respond to treatment or when they reach other decision points, they should be considered for alternative interventions according to best available evidence, personal preferences, and clinical judgement. Guidelines for making such decisions, called treatment algorithms, can be made available electronically at the point of decision-making.

For many reasons, including concerns regarding privacy, people want to own and control their own personal health records, including current diagnoses, treatments, and allergies. Electronic records facilitate this capacity. People can easily carry their medical information and treatment preferences on a small computer memory device.

Despite the promise of information technology, its impact may be limited for now in low-income settings. In Ethiopia, for example, illiteracy rates among rural women are 73%, health centres struggle even to have phone contact with district or regional services, and there are major problems arising from unreliable electricity supplies, low-quality hardware, and inadequate protection from computer viruses.

Conclusions

We have described here a series of commonly occurring challenges and obstacles to implementing a community-orientated system of mental health care. At the same time we have identified related steps and solutions which may work in responding positively and effectively to these barriers (Saraceno et al., 2007; Thornicroft et al., 2008), as set out in Table 43.1. We therefore recommend that people

Table 43.1 Obstacles, challenges, lessons learned, and solutions in implementing community-orientated mental health care

Obstacles and challenges		Lessons learned and solutions
Society	1. Disregard for, or violation of, human rights of people with mental illness	Oversight by: civil society and service user groups, government inspectorates, international NGOs, professional associations. Increase population awareness of mental illness and of the rights of people with mental illness and available treatments.
	2. Stigma and discrimination, reflected in negative attitudes of health staff	Encourage consumer and family and carer involvement in policy making, medical training, service provision (ex. board member, consumer provider), service evaluation (consumer satisfaction survey)
	3. Need to address different models of abnormal behaviour	Traditional and faith-based paradigms need to be amalgamated, blended, or aligned as much as possible with medical paradigms.
Government	4. Low priority given by government to mental health	Government task force on mental illness outlines mission as a public health agenda. Mission can encompass values, goals, structure, development, education, training, and quality assurance for community-oriented mental health system from a public health perspective Establish cross-party political support for the national policy and implementation plan Effective advocacy on mental health gap, global burden of disease, impact of mental health conditions, cost effectiveness of interventions, reduce life expectancy, use of WHO and other international agencies for advocacy, linking with priority health conditions and funds, positive response of untoward events Identifying champions within government who have administrative and financial authority.
	5. Absence or inappropriate mental health policy	Advocate for and formulate policy based upon widespread consultation with the full range of stakeholder groups, incorporating a rationalized public health perspective based on population needs, integration of service components Consumer involvement in policy making
	6. Absent, old or inappropriate mental health legislation	Create powerful lobby and rationale for mental health law. Modernize mental health law formulated and implemented relevant to community orientated care Watchdog or inspectorate to oversee proper implementation of mental health law.
	7. Inadequate financial resources in relation to population level needs	Help policy makers to be aware of the gap between burden of mental illness and allocated resources, and that effective treatments are available, and affordable Advocate for improved mental health expenditure using relevant information, arguments and targets, e.g. Global Burden of Disease (GBD), mhGAP unmet needs Recruit key political and governance champions to advocate for adequate funding of initiatives
	8. Lack of alignment between payment methods and expected services and outcomes	Design a system that directly relates required service components and financially reimbursable categories of care, e.g. for evidence based practices Provide small financial incentives for valued outcomes Create categories of reimbursement consistent with system strategy Develop and use key performance indicators Reserve transitional cost to reallocate hospital staff to move to community
	9. Need to address infrastructure	Government to plan and finance efficient use of, e.g. buildings, essential supplies, and electronic information systems and other to direct, monitor, and improve the system and outcomes
	10. Need to address structure of community-oriented service system	Design the mental health system from local primary care to regional care to central specialty care and fill in gaps with new resources as funding grows
	11. Inadequate human resources for delivery of mental health care in relation to the level of need in the population	Assessment of population level needs for primary care and specialist mental health care services Build capacity of health workers engaged in providing general health care and mental health care in community Training current health and mental health professionals in community orientated mental health care
	12. Brain drain, failure to retain talent, staff retention, and weak career ladders	UN agencies/International NGOs assure sustainability of their projects/programmes Exchange programmes between countries Set period of time medical students/registrars have to serve in their countries or rural area Task shifting/function differentiating of the psychiatrist to use their ability in their area of speciality Create financial incentives and reputation systems for psychiatrists who engage in community mental health Train other (less 'brain drainable') health professionals to deliver mental health care Payment for education may be attached to the allocation and preservation of resources to address equitable distribution and to prevent emigration without appropriate reimbursement

(Continued)

Table 43.1 (*Contd.*) Obstacles, challenges, lessons learned, and solutions in implementing community-orientated mental health care

Obstacles and challenges		Lessons learned and solutions
	13. Non-sustainable, parallel programme by international NGO	Close relations with ministries and other stakeholders and international NGO Mental health plan in place so NGOs can help achieve these goals sustainably Government to be proactive in collaborating with NGOs and private- public partnership
Organization of the local mental health system	14. Need to design, monitor, and adjust organization of mental health system	This includes plan for local, regional, and central mental health services based on public health need, full integration with primary care, rational allocation of multidisciplinary workforce, development of information technology, funding, and use of existing facilities. All stakeholder groups can be involved in developing, monitoring, and adjusting plan Set implementation plan with clear coordination between services Development of policy/implementation plan with number of service needed per population (e.g. New Zealand service 'Blueprint') Role differentiation of the hospital, community, and primary care services, and private and public services, using catchment area/capitation system with flexible funding system Prioritization of target groups, especially people with severe and persistent mental illness
	15. Lack of a feasible mental health programme or non-implementation of mental health programme	Make programme highly practical by identifying resources available, tasks to be completed, allocation of responsibilities, timescales, reporting and accountability arrangements, progress monitoring/evaluation systems
	16. Need to specify developmental phases	Planners and professional leaders to design 5- and 10-year plans.
	17. Poor utilization of existing mental health facilities	Improve awareness of benefits of facilities and services Specify pathways to care Inbuilt monitoring quality of care, especially process and outcome phases
	18. Need to include non-medical services	Include families, faith-based social services, NGOs, housing services, vocational services, peer-support services, and self-help services: All stakeholders involved in designing system Task shifting, i.e. moving key tasks such as initial assessment and prescribing using a limited and affordable formulary to specially trained staff who are available at the appropriate local level Identify leaders to champion and drive the process More involvement in planning, policy making, and leadership and management Include in psychiatrist training programmes
	19. Lack of multisectoral collaboration, e.g. including traditional healers, housing, criminal justice, or education sectors	Development of clear policy/implementation plan by all stakeholders Collaborate with other local service to identify and help people with mental illness Provision of information/training to all practitioners Establish multisectoral advisory and governance groups Familiarization sessions between practitioners in the Western and in the local traditions.
	20. Poor availability or erratic supplies of psychotropic medication	Educate policy makers and funders about the cost/benefits of specific medications Provide infrastructure for clozapine monitoring Monitoring prescribing patterns of psychotropic medication Drug Revolving Funds, public-private partnerships
Professionals and practitioners	21. Need for leadership	Psychiatrists and other professionals need to be involved as experts in planning, education, research, and overcoming inertia and resistance in the current environment.
	22. Difficulty sustaining in-service training/adequate supervision	Training of the trainers by staff from other regions or countries Task shifting of the psychiatric functions, e.g. prescribing to trained and available practitioners Lobby hard to ensure this is a priority and integral to the mental health plan
	23. High staff turnover and burnout, or low staff morale	Introduction of recovery oriented services Collect case examples of recovery Build trust by involving staff leaders in oversight and decision-making committees Sponsor social events to enable staff to team build in non-work situations Emphasize career-long continuing training programmes Training of supervisors Provide opportunities for attending out of area professional meetings Equip with sufficient skills and support
	24. Poor quality of care/concern about staff skills	Ongoing training and supervision Create and disseminate guidelines for professionals Third-party evaluation Encourage and reward quality by awards and similar processes

(Continued)

Table 43.1 *(Contd.)* Obstacles, challenges, lessons learned, and solutions in implementing community-orientated mental health care

Obstacles and challenges		Lessons learned and solutions
	25. Professional resistance, e.g. to community orientated care and service-user involvement	Government and professional societies promote the importance of community oriented care and service user involvement Task shifting/function differentiating of psychiatrists to use their abilities more broadly in their area of speciality and work with a range of stakeholders including consumers and carers/families Develop training in recovery-orientated psychosocial rehabilitation as part of training of new psychiatrists, including at medical schools in LAMIC Collect case examples of recovery and successfully implemented community mental health initiatives
	26. Dearth of relevant research to inform cost-effective services and lack of data on mental health service evaluation	More funding on research, for both qualitative and quantitative evidence of successfully implemented examples of community orientated care
	27. Failure to address disparities (e.g. by ethnic, economic groups)	All key stakeholders involved; advocacy for underrepresented group to develop policies and implementation plans
Users, families, and other advocates	28. Need for advocacy	Users and other advocates may be involved in all aspects of social change, planning, lobbying the government, monitoring the development and functioning of the service system, and improving the service system
	29. Need for self-help and peer support services	Users to lead these movements
	30. Need for person-centred care	Users and other advocates must demand at all levels that the system shift to value the goals of users and families, that shared decision-making become the norm, and that person-centeredness becomes a central value in assessing services and outcomes Continuing professional education on human rights and staff attitudes emphasizing paying attention to preferences of consumers and carers Consumer involvement at all levels, national level, local level, and patient care level

NGOs, non-governmental organizations.

interested in planning and implementing systems of mental health care which balance community-based and hospital-based service components, give careful consideration to anticipating the challenges identified here, and to learning the lessons from those who have grappled with these issues so far (Thornicroft et al., 2010).

References

Bartlett, P., Lewis, O., and Thorold, O. (2006). *Mental Disability and the European Convention on Human Rights*. Leiden: Martinus Nijhoff.

Benegal, V., Chand, P.K., and Obot, I.S. (2009). Packages of care for alcohol use disorders in low- and middle-income countries. *PLoS Medicine*, **6**, e1000170.

Best, M. and Neuhauser, D. (2004). Avedis Donabedian: father of quality assurance and poet. *Quality and Safety in Health Care*, **13**, 472–3.

Bond, G.R., Drake, R.E., McHugo, G.J., Rapp, C.A., Whitley, R., and the National Evidence-Based Practices Project Research Group. (2009). Strategies for improving fidelity in the National Evidence-Based Practices Project. *Research on Social Work Practice*, **19**, 569–81.

Chisholm, D., Flisher, A.J., Lund, C., Patel, V., Saxena, S., Thornicroft, G., and Tomlinson, M. (2007). Scale up services for mental disorders: a call for action. *Lancet*, **370**, 1241–52.

Choe, J.Y., Teplin, L.A., and Abram, K.M. (2008). Perpetration of violence, violent victimization, and severe mental illness: balancing public health concerns. *Psychiatric Services*, **59**, 153–64.

Corrigan, P.W. and Penn, D.L. (1999). Lessons from social psychology on discrediting psychiatric stigma. *American Psychologist*, **54**, 765–76.

de Jesus Mari, J., Razzouk, D., Thara, R., Eaton, J., and Thornicroft, G. (2009). Packages of care for schizophrenia in low- and middle-income countries. *PLoS Medicine*, **6**, e1000165.

Deva, P. (2006). Psychiatric rehabilitation and its present role in developing countries. *World Psychiatry*, **5**, 164–5.

Deva, P.M. (1981). Training of psychiatrists for developing countries. *Australian and New Zealand Journal of Psychiatry*, **15**, 343–7.

Dixon, L.B., Dickerson, F., Bellack, A.S., Bennett, M., Dickinson, D., Goldberg, R.W., *et al.* (2010). The 2009 schizophrenia PORT psychosocial treatment recommendations and summary statements. *Schizophrenia Bulletin*, **36**, 48–70.

Drake, R.E., Cimpean, D., and Torrey, W.C. (2009a). Shared decision making in mental health: Prospects for personalized medicine. *Dialogues in Clinical Neuroscience*, **11**, 319–32.

Drake, R.E., Wilkniss, S.M., Frounfelker, R.L., Whitley, R., Zipple, A.M., McHugo, G J., *et al.* (2009b). The Thresholds-Dartmouth partnership and research on shared decision making. *Psychiatric Services*, **60**, 142–4.

Drake, R. E., Deegan, P., Woltman, E., Haslett, W., Drake, T., and Rapp, C. (2010a). Comprehensive electronic decision support systems. *Psychiatric Services*, **61**, 714–17.

Drake, R.E., Deegan, P.E., and Rapp, C.A. (2010b). The promise of shared decision making in mental health. *Psychiatric Rehabilitation Journal*, **34**, 7–13.

Drake, R.E., Rosenberg, S.D., Teague, G.B., Bartels, S.J., and Torrey, W.C. (2003). Fundamental principles of evidence-based medicine applied to mental health care. *Psychiatric Clinics of North America*, **26**, 811–20.

Dunion, L. and Gordon, L. (2005). Tackling the attitude problem. The achievements to date of Scotland's "See Me" anti-stigma campaign. *Mental Health Today*, **5**, 22–5.

Eaton, J. and Agomoh, A.O. (2008). Developing mental health services in Nigeria: the impact of a community-based mental health awareness programme. *Social Psychiatry and Psychiatric Epidemiology*, **43**, 552–8.

Fekadu, A., O'Donovan, M.C., Alem, A., Kebede, D., Church, S., Johns, L., *et al.* (2008). Validity of the concept of minor depression in a developing country setting. *Journal of Nervous and Mental Disease*, **196**, 22–8.

Greenhalgh, T., Robert, G., MacFarlane, F., Bate, P., and Kyriakidou, O. (2004). Diffusion of innovations in service organizations: Systematic review and recommendations. *Milbank Quarterly*, **82**, 581–629.

Griffiths, L., Blignault, I., and Yellowlees, P. (2006). Telemedicine as a means of delivering cognitive-behavioural therapy to rural and remote mental health clients. *Journal of Telemedicine and Telecare*, **12**, 136–40.

Hanlon, C., Medhin, G., Alem, A., Araya, M., Abdulahi, A., Tesfaye, M., *et al.* (2008). Measuring common mental disorders in women in Ethiopia: reliability and construct validity of the comprehensive psychopathological rating scale. *Social Psychiatry and Psychiatric Epidemiology*, **43**, 653–9.

Henderson, C. and Thornicroft, G. (2009). Stigma and discrimination in mental illness: Time to Change. *Lancet*, **373**, 1930–2.

Institute of Medicine (2010). *Key Capabilities of an Electronic Health Record System Institute of Medicine*. Washington DC: Institute of Medicine.

Jacob, K.S., Sharan, P., Mirza, I., Garrido-Cumbrera, M., Seedat, S., Mari, J.J., *et al.* (2007). Mental health systems in countries: where are we now?. *Lancet*, **370**, 1061–77.

Knapp, M., McDaid, D., Mossialos, E., and Thornicroft, G. (2007). Mental health policy and practice across Europe: An Overview. In: Knapp, M., McDaid, D., Mossialos, E., and Thornicroft, G. (eds.) *Mental Health Policy and Practice Across Europe*, pp. 1–14. Maidenhead: Open University Press.

Lancet Global Mental Health Group (2007). Scale up services for mental disorders: a call for action. *Lancet*, **370**, 1241–52.

Link, B.G. and Phelan, J.C. (2001). Conceptualizing stigma. *Annual Review of Sociology*, **27**, 363–85.

Mbuba, C.K. and Newton, C.R. (2009). Packages of care for epilepsy in low- and middle-income countries. *PLoS Medicine*, **6**, e1000162.

McHugo, G.M., Drake, R.E., Whitley, R., Bond, G.R., Campbell, K., Rapp, C.A., *et al.* (2007). Fidelity outcomes in the national Implementing Evidence-based Practices project. *Psychiatric Services*, **58**, 1279–84.

Moran, P., Borschmann, R., Flach, C., Barrett, B., Byford, S., Hogg, J., *et al.* (2010). The effectiveness of joint crisis plans for people with borderline personality disorder: protocol for an exploratory randomised controlled trial. *Trials*, **11**, 18.

Patel, V. (2009). The future of psychiatry in low- and middle-income countries. *Psychological Medicine*, **39**, 1759–62.

Patel, V., Araya, R., Chatterjee, S., Chisholm, D., Cohen, A., De Silva, M., *et al.* (2007). Treatment and prevention of mental disorders in low-income and middle-income countries. *Lancet*, **370**, 991–1005.

Patel, V. and Thornicroft, G. (2009). Packages of care for mental, neurological, and substance use disorders in low- and middle-income countries: PLoS Medicine Series. *PLoS Medicine*, **6**, e1000160.

Patel, V., Simon, G., Chowdhary, N., Kaaya, S., and Araya, R. (2009). Packages of care for depression in low- and middle-income countries. *PLoS Medicine*, **6**, e1000159.

Phelan, J.C., Yang, L.H., and Cruz-Rojas, R. (2006). Effects of attributing serious mental illnesses to genetic causes on orientations to treatment. *Psychiatric Services*, **57**, 382–7.

Pinfold, V., Huxley, P., Thornicroft, G., Farmer, P., Toulmin, H., and Graham, T. (2003). Reducing psychiatric stigma and discrimination— evaluating an educational intervention with the police force in England. *Social Psychiatry and Psychiatric Epidemiology*, **38**, 337–44.

Pinfold, V., Thornicroft, G., Huxley, P., and Farmer, P. (2005). Active ingredients in anti-stigma programmes in mental health. *International Review of Psychiatry*, **17**, 123–31.

Prince, M., Patel, V., Saxena, S., Maj, M., Maselko, J., Phillips, M.R., *et al.* (2007). No health without mental health. *Lancet*, **370**, 859–77.

Proctor, E.K., Landsverk, J., Aarons, G., Chambers, D., Glisson, C., and Mittman, B. (2009). Implementation research in mental health services: an emerging science with conceptual, methodological, and training challenges. *Administration and Policy in Mental Health and Mental Health Services Research*, **36**, 24–34.

Rudan, I., Chopra, M., Kapiriri, L., Gibson, J., Ann, L. M., Carneiro, I., *et al.* (2008). Setting priorities in global child health research investments:

universal challenges and conceptual framework. *Croatian Medical Journal*, **49**, 307–17.

Saraceno, B., Van Ommeren, M., Batniji, R., Cohen, A., Gureje, O., Mahoney, J., *et al.* (2007). Barriers to improvement of mental health services in low-income and middle-income countries. *Lancet*, **370**, 1164–74.

Sartorius, N. and Schulze, H. (2005). *Reducing the Stigma of Mental Illness: A Report from a Global Association*. Cambridge: Cambridge University Press.

Saxena, S., Paraje, G., Sharan, P., Karam, G., and Sadana, R. (2006). The 10/90 divide in mental health research: trends over a 10-year period. *British Journal of Psychiatry*, **188**, 81–2.

Saxena, S., Thornicroft, G., Knapp, M., and Whiteford, H. (2007). Resources for mental health: scarcity, inequity, and inefficiency. *Lancet*, **370**, 878–89.

Slade, M. (2009). *Personal recovery and mental illness. A guide for mental health professionals*. Cambridge: Cambridge University Press.

Thornicroft G (2006). *Shunned: Discrimination against People with Mental Illness*. Oxford: Oxford University Press.

Thornicroft, G. and Tansella, M. (1999). Translating ethical principles into outcome measures for mental health service research. *Psychological Medicine*, **29**, 761–7.

Thornicroft G and Tansella, M. (2009). *Better Mental Health Care*. Cambridge: Cambridge University Press.

Thornicroft, G., Tansella, M., and Law, A. (2008). Steps, challenges and lessons in developing community mental health care. *World Psychiatry*, **7**, 87–92.

Thornicroft, G., Brohan, E., Rose, D., Sartorius, N., and Leese, M. (2009). Global pattern of experienced and anticipated discrimination against people with schizophrenia: a cross-sectional survey. *Lancet*, **373**, 408–15.

Thornicroft, G., Alem, A., Atunes dos Santos, R., Barley, E., Drake, R., Gregorio, F., et al. (2010). WPA guidance on steps, obstacles and mistakes to avoid in the implementation of community mental health care. World Psychiatry, (in press).

United Nations (2006). *Convention on the Rights of Persons with Disabilities*. New York: United Nations.

United Nations (1992). *UN Principles for the Protection of Persons with Mental Illness and for the Improvement of Mental Health Care. Adopted by UN General Assembly Resolution 46/119 of 18 February 1992*. New York: United Nations.

Vaughan, G. and Hansen, C. (2004). "Like Minds, Like Mine": a New Zealand project to counter the stigma and discrimination associated with mental illness. *Australasian Psychiatry*, **12**, 113–17.

Wahl, O.F. (1995). *Media madness: Public images of mental illness*. New Brunswick, NJ: Rutgers University Press.

World Health Organization. (2001). *The World Health Report 2001 – Mental Health: New Understanding, New Hope*. Geneva: World Health Organization.

World Health Organization (2005a). *Mental Health Atlas – Revised Edition*. Geneva: World Health Organization.

World Health Organization (2005b). *Human Resources and Training in Mental Health*. Geneva: World Health Organization.

World Health Organization (2008a). *The Global Burden of Disease: 2004 Update*. Geneva: World Health Organization.

World Health Organization (2008b). *Mental Health Gap Action Programme - Scaling Up Care for Mental, Neurological, and Substance Use Disorders*. Geneva: World Health Organization.

World Health Organization (2008c). *Policies and Practices for Mental Health in Europe - Meeting the Challenges*. Geneva: World Health Organization.

World Health Organization (2009). *Mental Health Systems in Selected Low- and Middle-Income Countries: A WHO-AIMS Cross-National Analysis*. Geneva: World Health Organization.

Index